Mast Cells United:

A Holistic Approach to Mast Cell Activation Syndrome

Amber Walker

Published in the United States by Kindle Direct Publishing

ISBN: 978-1-7337117-0-8 (paperback)

ISBN: 978-1-7337117-1-5 (digital)

Editor: Jennifer Leopoldt Roop

Cover Designer: Ryan Biore

@mastcellsunited

www.facebook.com/MastCellsUnited/

www.mastcellsunited.com

email: mastcellsunited@gmail.com

To my love, EGH—thank you for being an unparalleled and unwavering beacon of hope, joy and laughter.

Contents

Content Outline: Roadmap

Chapter 1: My MCAS Story

Chapter 2: The Mast Cell

- Mast Cell Overview
- Mast Cell Mediators
- Chemical Mediator Specifics
- The Role of the Mast Cell in Immunity
- Mast Cell Triggers

Chapter 3: Mast Cell Activation Disease

- The Lingo
- The Experts
- Symptoms of MCAD
- Classification of MCAD
- Mastocytosis
- Mast Cell Activation Syndrome (MCAS)

Chapter 4: Special Topics in MCAD

- What causes MCAS?
- The Tryptase Conundrum
- Histamine Intolerance vs. MCAS
- MCAS and Hymenoptera venom
- Current Considerations for MCAS

Chapter 5: Many Systems, One Diagnosis

- The Many Faces of MCAS
- Cardiovascular and Circulatory System
- Dental Health
- Diabetes Spotlight
- Ears, Eyes and Nose

Chapter 8: Common Root Issues

- Canaries in a Coal Mine
- Toxic Overload
- Bacterial Infections: Spotlight on Lyme Disease/Vector-Borne Illness
- Viral Infections: Spotlight on Epstein-Barr Virus

Chapter 9: Conventional Treatment Approaches

- MCAS Treatment Strategy
- Initial Considerations Following MCAS Diagnosis
- Mainstream Medications for MCAS Treatment
- Preventive Medications to Address Bone Mineral Density Issues
- Pain Management and Hospital Medication Considerations for MCAS
- Medications to be Avoided
- Management of Other Symptoms/Comorbidities

Chapter 10: Natural Treatment Options

- A Team Approach
- Alternatives and/or Supplements to Medication Regimen
- Nonpharmacological Pain Management
- MCAS and Vaccination Decisions
- Venom Immunotherapy
- Considerations for Conception and Pregnancy
- A Note on Pediatrics

Chapter 11: Dietary Considerations for MCAS

- Overall Dietary Considerations
- Elimination Diets
- Histamine Considerations with MCAS
- What is Optimal for Healing?
- Fruits, Vegetables, and Other Foods That *May Be* Helpful for the MCAS Patient
- Plants, Herbs, and Other Sources That *May Be* Helpful for the MCAS Patient
- The Importance of a Well-Trained Nutritionist

Chapter 12: Holistic Healing

- What is Holistic Care?
- Expectations for Life with MCAS
- Widespread Trigger Elimination
- Detoxification
- Exercise and MCAS
- Neuropsychological Treatment Approaches
- Strategies for Emotional Healing
- Additional At-Home Practices for Healing
- Spirituality
- Financial and Accessibility Considerations
- Community-Based Resources
- Conclusions

Preface

My grandmother on my mom's side, my Italian *Noni*, was the humblest and kindest person that I've ever met. Throughout her life, she always had a huge smile on her face and an affinity for quality time (and food!) with loved ones. When I was 25, she died after a valiant fight with multiple myeloma, a cancer of the bone marrow. As she battled this particularly brutal form of cancer, I never once heard her complain. She handled her illness with a poise and grace unlike anything I've ever witnessed. It wasn't until after her death that I learned that she had struggled for much of her adult life with invisible symptoms that were system-wide and didn't add up. Invisible symptoms just like mine.

We are currently facing epidemic proportions of patients who are coming out of the woodwork with similar stories: a generation-to-generation worsening of chronic, unexplained, invisible illness. Nearly two years ago, I made the decision to dig deeper into this problem; I wanted to discover how my recent diagnosis of mast cell activation syndrome (MCAS) related to everything else I was experiencing, and I realized that many of my peers had the exact same questions. More than that, I wanted to figure out how to alleviate the root cause of invisible suffering, empower fellow patients with holistic tools and halt this worsening epidemic in its tracks. I dove full-time into working on this book and never looked back.

I have my doctorate in physical therapy, but I am not a classic "medical doctor," nor do I intend to imply that by writing this book. I am also a patient who has been through countless trials and tribulations in the system. When I was diagnosed with MCAS, I pored over every study and bit of literature I could find. Unfortunately, there are not many books out there on the subject yet.

I enjoyed the case studies and very valuable clinical insight from Dr. Lawrence Afrin in his book "Never Bet Against Occam: Mast Cell Activation Disease and the Modern Epidemics of Chronic Illness and Medical Complexity." Dr. Afrin is one of the leading experts on the diagnosis and treatment of this disease. His book is an incredibly valuable resource for medical practitioners and patients alike.

I also enjoyed Pamela Hodge's patient perspective in "My Crazy Life: A Humorous Guide to Understanding Mast Cell Disorders." My heart goes out to her and others who react to everything in their environment. I can relate to so much of what she has gone through.

Dr. Xiu-Min Li and Henry Ehrlich have a chapter about mast cell activation syndrome in their book "Traditional Chinese Medicine, Western Science, and the Fight Against Allergic Disease." A number of reputable Internet resources also exist for this relatively new diagnostic subgroup of patients.

However, despite these wonderful resources, I still felt that as a newly diagnosed patient, I lacked a book-based resource with clear-cut organization of the diagnosis and long-term management of MCAS for patients, families and medical professionals. I felt frustrated in my dependence on medications to function at even 50 percent in my daily life and wanted greater knowledge about more natural treatment approaches and ideas for how to combine diet, natural supplements and lifestyle management with pharmacology in order to find more healing and stability of symptoms. I decided that if I was going to devote a great deal of time to in-depth research and experimentation, I might as well share my findings with others who likely have the same questions.

Above all, I want patients to have tools and answers to end their vicious cycle of hopelessness and despair. One factor that prompted me to write this book in the first place was news of a string of patient suicides and anaphylaxis deaths in Facebook support groups. I want patients to feel less alone and more informed. I want patients to have a physical, hard copy overview to hand to their doctors, and I want doctors to have something to spark their interest as a starting point for learning about MCAS.

My aim in writing this book is to provide a blend of both approaches: the clinical and patient worlds. I'll include concrete scientific research results, content from interviews with some of the world's leading MCAS experts, and will also comment on patient trends and anecdotes, which will be clearly delineated. My hope is that this book will become a useful beginner's guide for medical professionals, patients and families that encompasses the whole picture—little snippets of the patient perspective, a review of common facets to clinical presentation organized by system, the latest research regarding diagnosis and treatment, natural approaches and other resources—in one organized package. I'm Type A by nature (or maybe just when flared!) so I will attempt to leave no stone unturned!

I will re-emphasize that I do NOT have my MD degree and this book is NOT intended to diagnose or treat anyone, nor should it be a substitute for medical advice. I

encourage readers to reach out to qualified professionals if they suspect that they may have mast cell activation disease.

I began writing this book with a bit of a naïve optimism, like a budding first-time trail marathon runner lining up at the gates with a little water and some of those energy gels, thinking, "It can't be that bad!" (…Only to realize later that I would run out of fuel, forge a quarter mile of glacial rivers, get lost a few times, impale my thigh with a tree branch, vomit uncontrollably for 10 miles, sprain both ankles, and narrowly dodge bears and bees along the painful path…. Yup, that was my first trail marathon experience!)

As I've pushed forward it's become more and more clear that my topic of choice for my first book is one that is exponentially difficult to present. Mast cells are present virtually in every tissue, and their mediators act on essentially every single body system. On top of that, each patient may have a different predominance of chemical mediators impacting their symptoms, and their symptoms may look surprisingly different despite having the same cell origin. And each patient presents with a unique background of what triggers his or her mast cells into overdrive.

When compared to discussing something like rheumatoid arthritis, a disease with more clear-cut diagnostic criteria and decades of peer-reviewed research, I felt like I was faced with the colossal challenge of summarizing something that is a black hole of possibilities with very few concrete, research-based facts. One day I suddenly came to the realization of why nobody else has written a book quite like this yet—they are all much smarter than me!

Humor and daily headaches from being buried in detailed scientific literature for two years aside, I actually quite enjoyed the process in spite of its many challenges. I hope that you will keep one fact in mind as you read my literature interpretations: *MCAS research is very much in its infancy.* There is a LOT that we don't know and a lot that will change in what we know about this disease moving forward. I hope to be a small part of the catalyst for increased awareness and holistic management of MCAS, and I recognize that this book will probably need to be revised in a few short years as more evidence emerges.

I have conducted research myself as both a doctoral student and post-graduate practitioner and feel that I am qualified to help readers interpret study results. I feel compelled to present and summarize the findings as best as possible in one place. However, I acknowledge that as best as I try to include "all" of the high-quality evidence, I will inevitably miss things. And I also acknowledge that some (if not most) of the studies out there have methodological limitations and small sample sizes. I have done my best with what we currently have available to us, given the scarcity of MCAS research available.

Of course, the challenge of summing up this condition is nothing compared to actually living with it. Above all, I hope that I can do this condition justice for my fellow MCAS patient community, their families/friends/caregivers and the future practitioners who will help guide patients to a better understanding of their mystery symptoms. I hope that readers will be able to extract useful information and tools from this book in order to keep putting one foot in front of the other with hope. And I hope that we, as a society, will evolve from superficially treating symptoms to deeply targeting root issues in the chronic illness patient population.

Noni, this one's for you!

Chapter One

My MCAS Story

Note: This first chapter discusses my own experience with chronic illness as a first-person account. Chapters 2-12 are designed to be more of a medical text format investigating various angles of expert opinion, and they do not include personal commentary. Feel free to jump ahead to the chapter or topic that interests you, keeping in mind that some topics will reference information from earlier chapters.

As I strolled around the eclectic yogi community of Ubud, Indonesia, I was still on a high from my past 24 hours that began with a sunrise volcano summit and ended with delicious Balinese cuisine and a coffee plantation tour. Maybe it was the famous luwak-infused brew (made from the defecated coffee cherries of the sloth-like civet), but I felt especially alive and invincible as I took in the late afternoon scene at the Wanara Wana Nature Reserve Temple Complex.

It was 2014 and I was nearing the tail end of a several-month solo international backpacking trip, affectionately termed "30-tirement." I've always been passionate about travel and made great effort to experience new cultures while I was between jobs. The year I turned 30, while exploring Colombia with a group of friends, I had the epiphany that I needed to see more of the world NOW.

I had an open house style garage sale to get rid of most of my belongings, something that had become a habit every few years for me, strapped on a backpack and took off with a one-way ticket to Australia. At the time, I was training for the Boston Marathon and ended up having a several-month *running* tour of Australia, New Zealand, Indonesia and Thailand—a great way to see the sights!

I ran portions of Australia's Great Ocean Road trail with a 45-pound pack, dodging snakes, racing the tides to make beach crossings and sharing serene moments with unsuspecting wallabies in my path. I ran the city of Sydney, Australia, until I knew it like the back of my hand, and then took the ferry over to Manly Beach, where I surfed until I couldn't lift my limbs anymore. In New Zealand, a friend showed me the beauties of small agricultural town life on the north island, where I ran through farm country and over volcano cirques and then learned how to drive on the "wrong" side of the road to check out surfing hot spots. I ran laps and did speed workouts at Bangkok universities so I wouldn't have to deal with Thailand's city traffic and stoplights.

However, the highlight was definitely Indonesia. The culture was fascinating and vibrant, and the surfing was an out-of-body experience. I stayed with a local family on a small island near Bali. I took to the hilly dirt paths of the quiet Indonesian island in the beating sun between surfing sessions. The island had no motorized vehicles and I got around the hills on a mountain bike or on foot, exploring secluded beach coves, snorkeling with manta rays, and embracing Indonesian holidays and culture. It was truly the experience of a lifetime.

Following my stay on the small island, I headed over to Ubud for a quick self-guided tour inland before my flight home. On my last evening, I entered the gates to the Wanara Wana Nature Reserve Temple. The site was thriving with macaque monkeys, which I regarded as a common and unremarkable sight in Indonesia. At the gates to the attraction, I quickly side-stepped the vendors selling bananas as I had no intent to interact with the monkeys and simply wanted to photograph the famous temples.

In the sweltering heat and humidity, I stopped to sit in the shade and talk to a few fellow tourists. Mid-conversation, a tiny baby monkey leapt from behind me onto my left shoulder! It startled me and I jumped to my feet in surprise. A split second later, the (apparent) mother monkey was on me like a great white shark on a gentle baby dolphin!

She tore into my right deltoid with her incisors and clawed at my face with her hands. At that point I had two monkeys on me; the adorable baby was still innocently perched on my left shoulder, seemingly oblivious to the angry mother whose teeth pierced deep into my right arm. I was screaming and doing a little circular dance in efforts to carefully put the baby back on the ground and simultaneously detach the mother from my other side, as sharp pain seared down my right arm.

With blood flying and monkey spectators squawking, a crowd of humans also began to gather to witness the spectacle. Eventually a nice man helped me remove the monkeys, but the damage was already done. I headed to an emergency medical clinic with a migraine headache and blood dripping down my arm. A few hours later, I was cleaned and bandaged and freshly vaccinated. Even though I was told that "these monkeys all line up for their shots each year," I wasn't about to take any chances.

I remained skittish of any small moving animal (bird, squirrel, cat, etc.) for many months and ended up needing a series of follow-up rabies vaccines once home. Within a day of my first vaccine in Indonesia, I developed severe flu-like symptoms, flushing, severe mood swings and a strange headache. The side effects lasted about five days.

When I returned to the United States, I was due for my second rabies vaccine. This time, my post-shot reaction was greatly intensified. In addition to the previous symptoms, I developed intense all-body muscle pain, extreme thirst, mental confusion, extreme fatigue and a very real impending sense of doom.

Three days and two flights later, I toed the line for the Boston Marathon. I'd qualified with a time of 3:20 in Utah the previous summer, and Boston would be my third marathon. To be honest, I felt terrible on race morning. I was still experiencing the vaccine side effects, but I tried to ignore them. After all, I'd just flown across the world to be there.

When the race gun went off, I tried to stay positive. I started at my goal pace and maintained it for the first 10 miles fairly easily. About halfway through the race, I developed intense muscle sensations (not quite cramping pain, but strange rigidness all over my body) and gastrointestinal distress, with eventual difficulty breathing and feeling like I was going to faint. I somehow pushed through to the finish line, though I did have to walk sections. After the race I was doubled over in pain and could not speak well or coordinate my movement. I suffered acute vomiting and diarrhea for several hours. My blood pressure was concerningly low. It took me nearly three hours to walk the mile from the finish line to where I had checked my pre-race gear bag because I was doubled over on the sidewalk or else in a porta potty.

I'd never experienced symptoms quite like that with exercise. This was long before I was aware of my mast cells going awry, and I blamed the incident entirely on the vaccine side effects and poor hydration. I now suspect it was a mast cell mediator "storm" triggered by the recent vaccine and intensity of exercise.

The remaining series of rabies shots came and went with equally miserable side effects, always with severe symptoms for days after the vaccine. The doctor in the clinic didn't seem too concerned about them, and from what I gathered, the rabies vaccine can do that to you. (Better than having rabies, obviously!)

Unfortunately, my symptoms never returned to their prior baseline after the international travel, subsequent vaccines, and marathon—three triggers that became a tipping point for my system. Up to that point, most people who knew me would probably consider me an athletic and thriving physical therapist. But beneath the surface, I had been harboring a number of chronic undiagnosed ailments since I was a teenager and often felt like I was in "survival mode" in terms of health.

It's hard to imagine that a person capable of running marathons could truly be in that much trouble. As symptoms became more and more in my face, I continued to force myself to run and exercise regularly because it was such an important aspect of my stress relief and mental health. Because I had seen so many doctors without gaining much information about what was going on, I kept that side of my life somewhat hidden from others out of embarrassment for not having a true medical diagnosis to explain my struggles.

But when I look back at my entire life, I recall things from prior to my teenage years that were also problematic. The truth is, my MCAS story started decades before I began traveling the world as a young adult.

An Alaskan Youth

I was born in Anchorage, Alaska, to two loving and wonderful parents, and at age 2, I was elated when my sister Brittany was born. I had a fairly happy and carefree childhood growing up in Alaska. I grew up with a deep appreciation for the great outdoors and sports and art, with very little time engrossed in pop culture or television. I spent my first 18 years embracing the unparalleled beauty of my home state before leaving for college, graduate school and career opportunities.

I never considered myself one of those kids who was "allergic to everything," though I did have some issues. When I was an infant, I had a severe allergic reaction to sulfa drugs. I was also very colicky and had lactose intolerance symptoms from a young age. For as long as I can remember, I've had digestive issues and abdominal pain. I accepted it as normal to be chronically constipated, and one of my earliest memories as a toddler is my dad sitting on the bathtub with my favorite toys and a cup of orange juice, consoling me and distracting me while I was perched on the toilet trying to have a bowel movement.

I had hives and/or a rash on my skin nearly daily from elementary school and on, which was attributed to the chlorine in the swimming pool where I practiced on a team five times per week. Small dark spots developed on my skin, especially prominent on my extremities. When my parents took me to see an allergist, I was told I had chronic urticaria and was instructed to take an antihistamine such as Claritin or Zyrtec twice daily. My skin issues were somewhat controlled in my youth as long as I stuck to daily antihistamines. My skin was also very sensitive and reactive to touch and clothing, and light scratches displayed what I now know to be dermatographism. I experienced skin issues like ringworm and had multiple mole removal procedures done.

In my youth, I was diagnosed with asthma and was put on a variety of medications that didn't seem to help much. I had instant allergic reactions to dogs, horses, hamsters, rabbits and cats and remember many miserable birthday parties, visits to friends' houses and trips to the petting zoo. I had one season with a spontaneous habitual neurological tic in my eyes that caused abnormal blinking and eventually went away on its own.

I began having repeated sinus infections and ear infections. I took countless antibiotics for these. (I cringe even trying to ballpark the number…) As a competitive swimmer it seemed I was always sick. I would finish my antibiotics for a sinus infection and a few weeks later would have a relapse infection. Sinus infections became a way of life for the entire 16 years of my competitive swimming career.

In my early years I developed food allergies, the most mentally detrimental being my allergy to chocolate, which I luckily outgrew as a teenager. I reacted to pine nuts and eventually all tree nuts. In high school I also started having anaphylactic reactions to shellfish, some of which required emergency room visits.

For as long as I can remember, Raynaud's disease has always been a normal part of my everyday life. Raynaud's is a condition that affects the blood vessel circulation in the skin. The small vessels vasospasm, creating a painful and visible loss of circulation, typically affecting the fingers and toes. For my entire life, I've had it fairly severely in my hands, feet and nipples. It's triggered by getting out of bed in the morning, reaching into the fridge, touching a cold or metallic object, preparing food and changing out of my pajamas. It's even triggered by a slight breeze while sitting in a hot tub in the heat of summer. Fans and air conditioning are automatic triggers, even when it's above 90 degrees. It had a chronically annoying presence in my life as I was growing up in Alaska.

I always liked school and got good grades, but secretly had a very difficult time focusing and concentrating, particularly when there was background noise. I felt I had to study longer than my peers to get the same grades. I was sensitive to excess sensory stimulus but tried to hide it as best as I could, especially as I became more aware of social norms. I also struggled with either being hyper-focused or unable to focus at all. In high school, I began to feel more and more like I was "out of it" or in a near constant brain fog and usually had trouble getting school tasks done unless I was isolated in a very quiet environment. I often felt sensitive and inexplicably irritable and emotional a lot of the time.

As I entered my teenage years, I thought it was normal to have a bowel movement every few days, and eventually it became every week or two. That was all I'd really known. I also thought it was normal to get "hangry" all the time, to feel ill when I hadn't eaten in a while, but to also feel ill after I ate. I tried all the food-related trends, hoping to ease my abdominal symptoms, with no results.

My freshman year of high school, I sustained a soccer ball hit to the face which resulted in a broken nose. Over the years that followed, I developed stress fractures in the metatarsals of both feet nearly 10 different times as a track and cross-country runner, to the point where I had several pairs of shoes to match the height of my walking air cast boot. I originally attributed the fractures to having been a swimmer for so many years. When I suddenly started running in high school, I assumed that my bones just weren't used to the impact, as explained by one doctor, and I didn't think much more about it.

Eventually I grew accustomed to the warning signs and forced myself to back off the activity whenever I felt a stress fracture coming on in my foot or shin from running, or in my spine while backpacking around South America with a heavy pack. I could never convince a doctor to look at my bone mineral density because I was a "healthy-looking young woman" and they all assumed I was over-training.

When I was 17, I developed fairly noticeable fatigue and irritability and was diagnosed with iron-deficiency anemia. Then at age 19, my swollen neck and groin lymph nodes, abdominal pain and fatigue all seemed to increase around the same time, shortly after a car accident. My lymph nodes were noticeably enlarged, but every doctor I saw in the years to come saw me as a healthy, athletic teenager and very few would even palpate the nodes or listen to my concerns.

For me, that was one of the first pivotal moments when I realized that something was off. The lymph nodes certainly give us clues regarding toxic load, infectious burden and other factors that the body is responding to. I suspect that the car accident triggered a certain level of stress that contributed to an increase in symptomatic baseline at that time in my life. I also suspect that this was when hidden factors like Epstein-Barr virus and/or Lyme disease infection could have been creating symptoms, though I was unaware of it at the time.

College Years

I'd always seemed to attract mosquitos and had noted extreme reactions to insect bites since I was a toddler. Having grown up spending lots of time in the Alaskan wilderness, I'm pretty surprised (and lucky!) that my first *stinging* insect encounter occurred in the middle of the city at age 19. I was home from college for the summer and was helping a friend with some yard work when a yellowjacket stung me on the leg. I didn't think much of it and kept working, but I quickly developed a swollen face and hives all over my body and rushed to the emergency room, where it took a few doses of epinephrine to stop the reaction. The welt on my leg was red and swollen for about a year after that incident, and I was grateful that I was only stung one time.

I was advised to get venom testing at my local allergy clinic and eventually learned that I was severely allergic to all seven types of Hymenoptera venom, including wasps, bees, yellow jackets, and hornets. Once I could afford to do so and was on solid insurance, I began getting venom immunotherapy shots, but this wasn't possible until over 10 years later.

In my early 20s I experienced chest pain and heart palpitations along with what seemed to be the occasional arrhythmia, symptoms that have come and gone ever since. At the onset of these symptoms, I had a normal EKG test and doctors claimed it was anxiety. My blood pressure became perpetually low, typically 80-100/40-60. I began to experience issues with adrenaline rushes occurring when they shouldn't, difficulty sleeping, lightheadedness and frequent near fainting.

I began to notice a right-sided pain under my ribs and a bizarre referral-type pain underneath my right shoulder blade. It came and went but seemed especially bad every time I had a flare in other allergy and inflammatory type symptoms. Based on my knowledge, it seemed to be my gallbladder, although it wasn't behaving like typical gallstones or chronic gallbladder inflammation. An eventual HIDA scan showed no abnormalities.

I began having other strange symptoms in college. I had frequent signs of urinary tract infections, both with and without positive tests. My cholesterol and glucose levels would be extremely high or low for no good reason, despite my high fitness level and decent diet. I felt lightheaded and dizzy a lot, but I assumed it was the altitude while I was living and training in Utah on the collegiate swim team. I had severe cold intolerance and occasional heat intolerance. I began to experience strange reactions to taking medications and more anaphylaxis to dietary triggers.

At age 20, I sustained a low back injury while diving into the pool at the start of a race that caused me to miss part of a season of collegiate athletics. I underwent countless steroid injections and was told I was a surgical candidate due to the radiculopathy (nerve symptoms and weakness) in my right leg. It was then I discovered that I was reactive to most pain medications and contrast injections for imaging and also did poorly with medical procedures. Luckily, I managed to rehabilitate the injury with physical therapy and avoided surgery, which eventually inspired me to pursue a career as a physical therapist.

It seemed that as a collegiate competitive swimmer, I was in a near-constant state of sinusitis, ear infections and eye irritation. None of my teammates seemed to experience the same issues, or at least not nearly as often. I learned to push through these symptoms and did my best to ignore them. However, in the height of my senior year of competitive division one collegiate swimming at the University of Utah, I had an especially bad sinus infection and bilateral ear infections while in Florida for a winter training camp. On the flight back to Utah, my right eardrum ruptured, sending blood and pus all over the place. (It also sent the 10-year-old girl next to me to a new seating arrangement!)

Once it ruptured, I felt so much better, though both ears were still infected. Doctors in Utah confirmed the right-sided rupture and, sure enough, I was required to be at practice the next day and in a competition that Friday, so I attempted to use some wax to prevent water from entering the inner ear. It didn't really work and I spent many moments vomiting into the pool gutters and gripping the edge of the pool in vertigo until it healed. I'm not exaggerating (though I realize I'm painting an honest but fairly merciless picture of swimming coaches!). Luckily for me, I eventually regained hearing in that right ear, though I still have some issues sometimes.

Within a month of the eardrum rupture, my housemate arrived home one day to find me lying in bed shivering under a down comforter, decked out from head to toe in snowboarding clothing with the heat cranked up as high as possible. I was dizzy and confused, spiking a high fever and unable to take a deep breath without having a coughing fit. I was propped up with pillows because I felt like I was drowning in my own lung fluid when I tried to lie flat. My heart rate was about 160 at rest.

This time, my symptoms had started out as what seemed like the stomach flu for a week and then moved to my lungs. My coach had the motto of "if you're not in the emergency room, you'd better be at practice," so I had continued to show up for twice-daily workouts despite feeling worse and worse.

By the time we left for our out-of-state competitions, I was in pretty bad shape. I was ridiculously cold and weak and dizzy; I huddled in a hot shower between my races. I found myself gasping for air even during a basic slow warm-up and had a constant productive cough. I honestly don't remember how poorly I must have raced that weekend; I was just glad to have it behind me.

I finally checked myself into the urgent care clinic once back in Utah and their chest X-ray showed pneumonia. I was put on antibiotics and ended up having a few relapses over the next few months but eventually was able to recover enough to complete the end of that season and my swimming career. However, my lungs were never really the same. From that point forward, any time I picked up even the slightest cold or sore throat, an upper respiratory infection and lung rattling and wheezing would return and persist for weeks or months.

At the end of college, I began to have increased dental and periodontal issues. Despite a regular routine of gentle oral hygiene, I had severe gum recession to the point where some of my front teeth were loose. My grandmother had a history of gum recession and surgeries for gum grafting, so maybe it was a genetic thing? Either way, I ended up needing a gum grafting procedure at age 22.

The procedure itself was fairly uncomfortable as I was reactive to the numbing agent and could not tolerate it, so I had to experience it with intact sensation as they removed strips of gum from the roof of my mouth and transplanted them across my upper and lower teeth. The recovery was fairly annoying, too, since I could not tolerate the narcotic pain medication I was prescribed and also did poorly with nonsteroidal anti-inflammatory medications. It was a long healing process, longer than normal, but at the time I didn't think much of it.

The Abdominal Attacks

When I was in my late teens, I experienced my first abdominal "attack." This was distinct from my normal, perpetual gastrointestinal annoyances. These episodes consisted of intense abdominal pain that usually doubled me over, with extreme distention (to the point of looking pregnant or like I had ascites) and the inability to eat or drink anything (not even water sometimes) for anywhere from two to seven days.

Doctors said I had irritable bowel syndrome, but nothing dietary seemed to trigger the symptoms or alleviate them. I would simply wake up in the morning and they would be there. They were occasionally triggered by lack of sleep, but as a general pattern they occurred with no rhyme or reason. Countless years of food diaries and different, often extreme, elimination diets and eating plans showed no apparent dietary trend in my severe abdominal pain and swelling episodes.

The pain was not the cramping associated with diarrhea, but rather an intense inflammatory-type pain that often expanded around my entire lower abdomen and radiated to my back when I was especially swollen. I felt like glass was cutting into my insides. It was not a classic "intestinal" pain, nor was it bloating, despite the fact that I looked bloated and distended. It seemed like something was getting enlarged or inflamed, which was causing ischemia or blockage to the rest of my intestines, but yet at the same time it did not feel like a pain originating from inside my intestines. Occasionally it was accompanied by vomiting and it was sometimes followed by diarrhea. The episodes were almost always accompanied by mental confusion and anxiety, delirium and dehydration (especially the attacks that lasted several days). I could never seem to adequately explain it to doctors.

I have vivid memories of certain episodes that were so painful that I became semi-conscious and vomited uncontrollably in public places. While most of my attacks would start in the middle of the night or first thing in the morning, my first severe episode began while I was driving home from the pool after teaching swimming lessons. I remember thinking afterward, as only a dramatic teenage can claim, "If I have to experience that pain again, I will die."

At first, my years as an athlete training for two to four hours a day instilled in me a stubborn work ethic that helped me through the episodes. Thus, I trained through the symptoms and forced myself to put on a happy face and pretend everything was normal. I still got out there and tried to do what made me feel alive, to the best of my abilities, without complaining. And from an outsider's view, I've been told that I looked like a normal, energetic athlete. However, as the episodes got more severe and more frequent, I found myself less and less able to hide them.

For the first five years after my abdominal episodes began as a teenager, I only had a handful of episodes per year. I assumed they were connected to food poisoning or some kind of bacterial infection. In my mid-20s, the attacks became monthly and bi-monthly, and by the time I was in my 30s, there were times when they were almost daily. I would lose weight and become dehydrated and mentally confused from the episodes and then have a few days of "normalcy" before falling into another episode. During episodes, I began to notice other symptoms such as a low blood pressure and fast heart rate. It wasn't until I was in my 30s that I began to associate throat and sometimes facial, brain or extremity swelling with them.

I have countless memories of abdominal attacks derailing my plans—having to leave college classes to lie in bed and wait out the pain, lying down on running trails because the symptoms got so intense, vomiting while hiking in Grand Teton National Park, being stuck in the fetal position in a tent while my friends partied by the campfire a few feet away, and being doubled over in emergency room–level pain traveling on public transit in foreign countries. It would take me nearly 17 years of suffering before I finally had a diagnosis for these painful attacks.

Because I had no acceptable diagnosis responsible for these attacks for so long, I became accustomed to going into survival mode in daily life, a little bit through my college years and then regularly as a graduate student in physical therapy school. The pain grew to be so severe that I was barely able to stand or talk during episodes. I isolated myself from everyone when these occurred and began to live alone without roommates in my mid- to late-20s. I was ashamed that I was in so much pain from "irritable bowel syndrome," even though I knew that deep down I had a much more serious issue going on. I jumped from doctor to doctor in desperation. I prayed that I wouldn't get an abdominal episode on a test day, during travel or on a race day. On attack days, I took refuge in the fetal position in my bed and was unable to eat or drink until the intensity of the symptoms subsided, which usually took several days; this got to be problematic in graduate school, as well as once I entered the working world.

Graduate School

After completing five years of undergraduate studies in Utah, I decided to pursue physical therapy education in Denver, Colorado. During this time frame of my mid-20's, my neurological symptoms grew especially worrisome. I began having numbness and tingling in my extremities and episodes of weakness and vision difficulties. The numbness and tingling came and went all day long and was especially bad when I was showering in hot water, something that can trigger increased symptoms in demyelinated nerves, and something that I later learned is also a trigger of mast cell activation. My balance was worsening and some of my upper motor neuron tests were positive when performed by physical therapy classmates. I saw several neurologists and eventually had a brain MRI to rule out multiple sclerosis (MS). Fortunately, it was not MS, and they never found the cause of the symptoms, most of which spontaneously resolved within a year.

I experienced other novel symptoms as a graduate student. I began having episodes of vertigo and nausea, which was later determined to be BPPV (benign paroxysmal positional vertigo). I began to notice brittle nails, lines on my nails, scalloping and a white coating on my tongue, and hair loss that varied from mild to clumps. I saw countless doctors who ruled out everything from hypothyroidism to mono to cancer. I began to notice more and more flushing and low-grade fevers for no reason. I had eye blurriness and irritation and my optometrist told me that I had suddenly, out of the blue, developed an allergy to saline solution for contact lenses, so I switched to the daily type of contacts.

I developed intermittent insomnia and night sweats that would completely soak the bed. I had always considered myself a positive person, but I began to feel more and more anxious and depressed, with occasional manic-like windows of time. The mental struggles seemed to have a "chemical" feeling and they came and went without reason. I began to wonder if I was bipolar.

In addition to slow bone healing with stress fractures and increasing bone loss on dental exams, I also noticed that wounds and skin issues took an extremely long time to heal. Sometimes a small wound the size of a paper cut would take one to three months to close up.

At the end of my first year of grad school, I was exposed to carbon monoxide and other gases at the same time for several hours in the house I lived in, and was acutely ill for several days. I didn't put two and two together at the time, but a lot of my chronic symptoms worsened in the weeks and months following the gas exposure.

Orthopedic Blues

I always joked that I went to physical therapy (PT) school to learn how to fix myself, but there may be some truth to that. In addition to the low back pain with lumbar radiculopathy that began in college, I also experienced several years of jaw pain and TMJ dysfunction and began to have frequent joint subluxations, ankle and wrist sprains, joint swelling, IT band pain, knee meniscus problems, plantar fasciitis and inflammation in my patellar/Achilles/elbow tendons. I was a passenger in a car accident and began to have more severe neck instability and pain issues. As a physical therapist, I suspected that I had something bigger or more systemic going on, and I was often too busy or plagued by abdominal attacks to devote time to properly addressing my orthopedic issues, which would often spontaneously subside with the passage of time.

While living in Denver, I had some urinary incontinence issues and one ER visit for symptoms of cauda equina, a compression of the nerve roots of the spine that can lead to paralysis. After several days this spontaneously resolved. The tests continued to be normal and I began to think I was going crazy with such an abundance of strange and spontaneous symptoms.

In all fairness, some of my mishaps were definitely fueled by poor choices. I'll never forget the floating bluegrass festival on the Colorado River in 2008. I was part of a large group of inner tubers going down the river as large rafts came by with live music. We decided to stop at some warm springs located at a popular spot for cliff jumping.

I made the mistake of hiking up to the cliff to check out the view. Once up there, I was peer pressured to make the jump, with people who stopped at the bottom chanting my name. I made the 60-foot jump without hitting the rocks below, and the free-fall was a wild, never-ending slow-motion rush of absolute adrenaline.

12

When I hit the water, I immediately had an intense searing pain at the base of my spine and could not move my legs. The river was fairly fast-moving, but I was able to get to shore using my arms alone. After a few minutes, I was able to walk but my legs were numb and we eventually determined that I had fractured my tailbone.

It was odd that the impact of the water could cause such a fracture, especially considering how many of my friends made the exact same jump in the same way. The recovery seemed unusually slow and with large amounts of swelling (though the tailbone is certainly a difficult bone to immobilize). Fortunately, I regained feeling in my legs, but the other concerns took a while to heal. I sat on an inflatable donut for most of a year and it took a few years to be able to sit through a movie without tailbone pain. After the fracture healed, I continued having nerve pains in my groin, hip and legs that also persisted for a few years despite attempts to rehabilitate the injury with the help of my physical therapy mentors.

One Month in Ethiopia

During my last month in PT school, I was part of a group that traveled to Ethiopia for a month-long clinical rotation. The trip sparked in me a deep passion for global health and resulted in a wonderful cross-cultural learning experience as we worked with several Ethiopian physical therapists. We experienced an acute care setting unlike any I'd ever seen, where there was such a shortage of surgical hardware that patients had to return to the operating room after they'd healed so that someone else could use the screws, plates and bolts for another surgery. There were some horrors that still haunt me, like the conditions of the hospital, or the burn unit that was not able to provide pain medication during wound debridement. There were more joyous moments; one of my highlights was working with a visually-impaired young woman so that she could hold her daughter and walk for the first time since she experienced a stroke. We also spent time at a hospital and an orphanage in a remote village.

I had a wonderful time in Ethiopia, despite multiple episodes of intense vomiting and missing work because of my other symptoms while traveling. I was having anaphylaxis as a response to my anti-malarial medication, so I stopped taking it. A few months after my return, I began to develop unexplained moderate to high fevers accompanied by sweats and fatigue. They seemed to come and go, and I was tested for malaria (which was negative).

There were several strategies I tried over the years for coping with the chronic symptoms; my most effective tactics for cultivating inner peace were travel and focusing on others. Once I finished graduate school at Regis University, I felt a strong calling to begin my career as a physical therapist abroad.

One Year in Peru

As a brand-new physical therapist, I volunteered for a year in northern Peru in 2010-2011 with a nonprofit called Catholic Medical Mission Board (CMMB). It was the experience of a lifetime. I lived with a host family who became true family to me in every sense and who put up with my *gringa* Spanish. I was afforded the opportunity to explore different parts of the country and South America.

My main worksite was an outpatient clinic run by a lively bunch of Catholic nuns. I also spent several mornings a week working at a school for children with disabilities, had a brief stint doing home health and enjoyed several months of eye-opening work at an inpatient acute care setting. In addition, I worked on a research study assessing the quality of life for patients with disabilities and their caregivers in an impoverished area and later relayed the findings to the Peru Ministry of Health in Lima. Based on the findings, I created a community-based rehabilitation program for children in the area where I lived, which was implemented by a team of local community members.

I also lectured at local hospitals and colleges monthly and facilitated several annual continuing education conferences in northern Peru for physical therapists, speech therapists, nurses and occupational therapists over the years to come. Regis University began to send students down for several weeks a year to work with the local team in home visits with the children, and eventually the program model expanded to other communities around the country. It was an incredibly beautiful experience, and Peru has now become a second home to me.

While in Peru, I experienced a big flare of the symptoms, which I attributed to the unclean water and food I was inadvertently ingesting while living with a host family and making home visits. It was difficult because when I would be working in patient's homes, I would inevitably be offered food or a beverage, and it was rude to say no. I essentially accepted that after one year, no matter what I did I would probably have some sort of parasitic infection. I developed several new food intolerances. I began to have more insomnia, skin issues, irritability, brain fog/memory loss, more regular fevers and chills, severe constipation and diarrhea, abdominal discomfort, anal fissures and crippling fatigue.

The abdominal attacks I'd been experiencing since teenage years caused me to miss more days at work as a volunteer physical therapist and public health leader. While in Peru I also experienced acute episodes of food-borne illness which didn't help matters.

One particularly memorable episode of chills, flushing, cramps, vomiting and diarrhea occurred on an overnight bus from Lima to Trujillo in the heat of summer. My boss and I were shocked when, in the middle of the night, the large bus window pane shattered on top of us! Apparently, *los bandidos* on the highway had thrown something to break the window in order to get the bus to stop, a common strategy for highway robbery. The window pane was huge and the glass flew everywhere. The row of seats in front of us had the worst of it, but luckily everyone was okay. Afterward, the window curtains flapped wildly in the new breeze, and I sat back and soaked it in, too sick to mind the shards of glass everywhere. Finally, some air-conditioning! The bus barreled ahead and eventually we arrived at our destination unscathed.

Parasite Party Pooper

On one of my Lima work trips, I spent my last evening surfing near Miraflores. As I exited the ocean and was walking on rocks with my surfboard, I cut my left foot near the big toe. I continued to walk barefoot across rocks, mud and grass before I was able to find a place to rinse my foot. The wound was not especially large but it certainly grew inflamed. The following day I noticed a red squiggly line snaking up my foot toward my ankle. I quickly assumed I had an infection and began tracking the line with a marker. It inched its way up to my upper calf, and I really began to freak out.

At that point, I was back in the northern Peru community I lived in, which—in all honesty—had some sketchy hospital options (…speaking from experience, since I had worked in some of them!). I decided to go into my medical clinic as a patient, but the following morning, the red line had completely vanished. I cheerfully thought, "Great, I dodged that bullet!" and went about rather naively with my daily routine. Within a few months, I developed a strange sensation that things were crawling under my skin, intense sugar cravings, night sweats, fevers, fatigue, skin rashes, insomnia, brain fog, a heightened level of gut symptoms with intense ear, eye and rectal itching.

Now, these symptoms (aside from the crawling sensation and sugar cravings) were not completely new to me, so it took me awhile to suspect parasites. One characteristic that helped clue me in was the fact that the symptoms seemed to be cyclical and related to the moon cycle. Each month I would get a strange patch of a bumpy welt-like red rash, almost in a line, in a completely new area of my body. These patches would hang out in one area for a week or two before disappearing and then reappearing in a new area.

After several months of this, I experienced the same type of rash on my abdomen around my belly-button. It was itchy but also fairly painful and distinct looking from the usual urticaria I was accustomed to. One of these red welts was near my belly-button, right at the spot where I had a hole from a prior body piercing. As I pushed on it, a half-inch long worm emerged from the hole. It was dead, but there was no mistaking what I was looking at.

At this point, I had been living in Peru for over 10 months and had a completely new perspective on things like parasites, which had already been determined to have a 68% prevalence in my neighborhood, based on a recent study by Paz and colleagues.[1] I was living in an area of extreme poverty, and I'd become mentally hardened to much of the reality of my community's daily life at that point. I decided to think of my new parasite as a neighborhood "rite of passage" of sorts.

I photographed the worm and threw it in a Ziploc baggie. I sent photos to my nurse friend and my sister (who happened to be in physician assistant school at Stanford at the time, taking a class with a prominent infectious disease specialist, as luck would have it) to see if they had any ideas. The next morning, I marched triumphantly to the medical clinic where I worked, certain that my friend Dr. Julio could tell me what it was. Dr. Julio was no expert in infectious disease, and he stared at me as if I were crazy! He ordered parasitic testing and we determined that I had a case of *Strongyloides stercoralis* as well as *Blastocystis hominis*. (He also prescribed me azithromycin for bronchitis, even though my airways were apparently irritated by worm migration. I never understood the logic there.)

At that point, I was having trouble breathing and was also coughing up things that looked like eggs and pulling worms out of my nose. I had poor lighting in the bathroom I was using, but once I was able to use a different toilet I realized that I was also pooping out an alarming number of eggs and worms. I was grateful that I was able to access the medications I needed to calm down the acute spreading of the parasite, and more grateful I didn't react too terribly to it. After several doses (to target both adult and larvae), I did feel better. And my parents were kind enough to mail down a care package of herbal remedies for extra peace of mind.

Now looking back, I realize that the contraction of the parasite(s) was a pivotal moment for me in which my baseline of health took another plunge, as my mast cells were in full attack mode and created a great deal of havoc on my already-ailing gastrointestinal system and other areas.

Additional Stressors in Peru

I wish I could say that parasites were my only worries while I was living in Peru. Unfortunately, I also had encounters with several types of bugs that also seemed to cause mast cell flares. The churches in Peru are open-air buildings, and in my neighborhood (and most of the country) packs of wild dogs roamed around freely. While I was attending the baptism of a friends' daughter, a wild dog ran across the altar and then decided to sit down right next to me. Out of the corner of my eye, I saw some nearly-microscopic movement coming from the surface of the dog's hair. By the time I realized it was fleas, the ceremony had already started. The fleas began biting me and I was wiggling and squirming around in my seat, trying to move farther away. Unfortunately, the church was packed and I was unable to get away before it was too late. I was covered in flea bites, which were annoyingly painful to experience and equally frustrating in terms of trying to quarantine clothing to make sure I didn't infest the whole house! The welts from the bites swelled up quickly and I looked like I had the chicken pox on my arms, legs and low back for a good four months.

Later in Lima, I was victim to a hostel bed bug infestation, which was also a pretty gross experience. I mention these experiences because fleas and bed bugs are vectors that can carry different bacterial diseases and viruses, which could explain why I became so flared and experienced a new baseline after they happened. But, more on this theory later…

Peru was certainly not a stress-free time for me, and not only because of my health issues and demanding work schedule seven days a week. While I loved the culture and many aspects of daily life there, I lived in a neighborhood with high crime rates and could never fully let my guard down. In my first month, a coworker arrived to the clinic covered in blood by the man in the taxi next to her who had been shot in the head for his cell phone. Shortly thereafter, my boss went missing for several days, and narrowly escaped with her life by fleeing on foot when the captor's vehicle got a flat tire. The nuns I worked with were forced to remove money at an ATM at gunpoint. My host sister and a friend were kidnapped in a taxi and escaped by leaping out of the moving vehicle.

I was attacked by wild dogs and guard dogs on several occasions over the course of one year. On one occasion we had to take cover because a building one street over was bombed by extortionists. Once I began public speaking and teaching at physical therapy events, I had some concerning phone calls from the sister of a male attendee who claimed that her brother was stalking me and was dangerous. Near the end of my time in Peru, a (different) man wielding a knife kidnapped me and locked me in his home, demanding that I become his wife and take him to America. Fortunately, I narrowly escaped on foot later that same day.

17

It saddens me that while I was able to remove myself from those kinds of daily stressors after one year, such violence (and much worse) continues to be a regular reality for so many people around this world. Peruvian culture is incredibly beautiful and I hope that my honesty in regards to this part of my story does not deter people from visiting the country. I was living in an impoverished area of one of the most dangerous cities in South America, and many other (touristy) areas of Peru are considered safe to visit.

The Peruvians that I know are people with a family-first, "God's got this" mentality. When I lived there, I was completely mesmerized by the slowness of life, the presence in the moment, and the love for God that was shared outwardly by young people my age. Many of the families that I worked with were living in extreme poverty but were the most joyful people I'd ever met. To this day I often still struggle with the contrasting culture in the U.S.

Looking back, I am in complete awe that I was able to put aside so many of my physical symptoms in order to complete the work in Peru. I know that my ability to do so only came from the hand of God guiding me through each moment, one step at a time. Each day was a struggle, because I was highly symptomatic and simultaneously working in a physically taxing environment that required constant mental clarity in order to communicate effectively in Spanish. I was completely passionate about the work, which made it easier to put in long hours, but I also grew sicker and increasingly fatigued as the year went on. When I returned to Alaska at the end of my volunteer commitment, I vaguely remember sleeping for what seemed like a month straight.

Post-Peru Problems

When I returned to the states, I underwent additional testing and parasitic treatment. Again, malaria tests were negative. But I still felt terrible. I relocated back to Utah and continued to push through the symptoms as best I could for several years while working as a physical therapist. Every time I went to the doctor, the routine blood work and tests were normal.

Finally, at age 29 I had an endoscopy/colonoscopy that looked normal. The doctor also performed a small bowel follow-through that was normal. However, my celiac blood test was on the low range of positive, so I commenced a gluten-free diet. Unfortunately, the dietary changes did not improve symptoms dramatically. I was continually handed samples of laxatives (which did nothing for me) and told that my pain was caused by irritable bowel syndrome.

I began to miss larger chunks of work for the abdominal attacks and began wearing baggier clothes to hide the swelling and take the pressure off my midsection. While working on my feet all day, it took all the strength I had to be attentive to my patients while I was having

18

episodes of abdominal pain. Often, I could barely carry on a conversation due to pain. After my time in Peru, I felt as if I was in survival mode on a daily basis. I felt completely helpless and in deep despair at not knowing how to prevent the severe abdominal episodes, nor how to reduce the plethora of constant chronic symptoms I was experiencing on the side.

The year I turned 30, I decided that I could no longer push through all of the symptoms with my career as a physical therapist. I had decreased my hours to part time, but it didn't seem to help. When I found out I had a nephew on the way, I decided to leave Utah and move back to Alaska after some traveling and the Boston Marathon (hence, my "30-tirement" adventure). Then I did a road trip up through Canada to Anchorage, where, feeling refreshed and also desperate for income, I changed my mind and decided to give my career in healthcare another go.

Back in Alaska

The fevers, fatigue, brain fog, abdominal pain and night sweats reached a new high in my early 30s. I developed more and more intense migraines and difficulty concentrating. I began to notice a strange body odor, a "stale and sour" smell. I was having strange facial nerve pain. My Raynaud's symptoms began happening over 10 times per day in the winter, often for 20-60 minutes at a time (or often for half a day while on a trail run!), to the point where I was having damage to the nerve endings in my hands. The numbness began interfering with my ability to perform some of my tasks as a physical therapist, particularly tasks that involved needles and manual therapy.

Once I had new health insurance, I underwent numerous trials of allergy testing, and interestingly my IgE-positive foods were almost always different. For example, one summer I tested positive to skin prick testing to 32 allergens including green beans, rice, oats, potatoes, carrots, tree nuts and shellfish. The experience made me question whether IgE-mediated allergy testing (outside of true anaphylaxis) can be faulty and prohibitive in terms of promoting a healing diet, and I struggled to eliminate all 32 foods, plus the other ones that historically tended to cause me GI distress, plus the elimination of gluten/grains and dairy and sugar and… you get the point.

Subsequent food testing was negative with the exception of tree nuts and shellfish (which I've always had a true allergy to). Patch testing showed a very mild response to garlic and carrots, but those foods seemed to have no actual relation to my episodes. I also tested positive for nearly every environmental allergen and went to great lengths to use HEPA air filters and hypoallergenic bedding. Certain pets/animals were a small trigger, and I definitely had seasonal allergies to pollens, trees, etc. Despite my efforts, elimination of known triggers had no effect on the majority of my chronic symptoms.

Mental Weariness and Despair

I began to feel like a shell of the person I once was, though on the outside I still attempted to put my best foot forward. My social life fluctuated as I would try to "power through" the symptoms for several months and then crash physically and mentally and become more of a homebody for a period as I tried to take better care of myself.

Around this time the anxiety and depression were out of control, so I finally sought help. I was diagnosed with attention deficit hyperactivity disorder (ADHD) as an adult and was put on a number of medications for that and anxiety/depression, none of which seemed to work. I was not a big fan of taking medications and did not trial the drugs for very long. And deep down I knew that something else was at the root of all of my issues.

I began to notice more symptoms associated with autism, like difficulty in social environments, obsession with rules and routine, the need to perform repetitive movements to soothe myself, and poor tolerance to loud noises, bright lights and additional excess sensory stimulus. These symptoms increased dramatically when I was experiencing a flare-up in other mast cell-type symptoms.

I tried therapy sessions, which I enjoyed, but I only seemed to be getting worse physically. I went through countless ups and downs of finding a new doctor or specialist who seemed genuinely interested in helping me, the process of them theorizing about a cause, testing for it with extremely high hopes, and facing the inevitable crashing realization that the tests were negative (or false positive). I began to have serious hopes for an answer—even if it was really bad news—that could explain what I was going through.

I experienced countless doctors who told me it was in my head. I had numerous doctors say it was all stress. This cycle of physician-deemed psychosomatics was extremely frustrating and left me feeling pathetic and hopeless as I left with real symptoms and no answers. But I never doubted the validity of what I was experiencing, and I knew it was a matter of time (and money) before I got to the bottom of it. Still, I remained a bit fake with family and friends because I was so ashamed that I was going to great lengths to figure this out and was not getting any "real" or socially accepted answers. I put up a lot of walls and tried to put a smile on my face in public but found myself in extreme lows when I was alone.

Most of all, I just wanted to know what "it" was so that I would know what to focus on to attempt to prevent/alleviate the daily suffering instead of feeling so helpless. It seemed I had three distinct things going on: the severe abdominal attacks, separately-occurring frequent mild-to-severe anaphylactic episodes and a bunch of other chronic systemwide symptoms. I hated how self-centered I felt while searching desperately for health answers all the time. The times that I let my guard down to confide in others about the struggles often left them saying, "But you look normal!"

I suppose that was OK, because my big aim amidst all of this was to appear normal. I used social media as a way to prevent me from falling into the depths of despair. I aimed to post a fun, upbeat or positive photo as much as I could. I knew that my likelihood of staying positive was higher if I took it one day at a time and found something fun to get me active and out of the house each day. I knew that if I relinquished my efforts to stay active, I would only sink into more problems. I knew that if I didn't "use it," I would most certainly "lose it" in terms of my physical activity and exercise habits. Yet looking back, I know that I pushed myself too much and was way too hard on myself, as opposed to letting my body have the rest and healing that it needed.

Running and other physical exercise had been a staple for so much of my life, and for a long time, I refused to give them up. Even though I knew that the high-intensity exercise often made all my symptoms worse, it also helped me manage stress and enjoy the beauty of nature. Mountain trails became the only place where I felt less anxious and more at peace. I refused to fall down the slippery slope of stopping the one thing I had left to escape from my reality of health issues. I began to embrace running-related pain because it gave me a sense of control and distracted me from the other symptoms. (Of course, on weeks I was having an abdominal attack, physical activity was out of the question.)

I often ran alone because my systemic symptoms and athletic performance were so variable on a day-to-day basis, and I didn't want to make plans and then have to break them if I had a sudden episode come on. As I became more depressed, I began running alone in more daunting and dangerous conditions in Alaska, half willing mother nature to somehow end my suffering. Yet I carried an extensive first aid pack including at least four Epi-Pens at all times. I didn't truly want my life to end, but I was hitting rock bottom and couldn't get out of the crushing reality of daily, chronic, debilitating symptoms. I could (barely) put on a happy face all week to family, friends and patients; I needed my mountain escape whenever possible to be truly real with my depression and frustration with feeling so ill and yet not having a diagnosis that made sense.

Rheumatology Possibilities

At age 31, one week after a flu shot and a period of high stress, I began having intense joint pain with some swelling, in addition to the other symptoms, most notably constant fever/chills, abdominal issues, night sweats and fatigue. I was unable to exercise, struggled with work and on some days even had difficulty standing long enough to cook an egg. Exercise became out of the question. I was also having severe blood pressure and heart rate fluctuations, and the near-fainting episodes seemed to get worse and worse to the point where I was concerned for the safety of some of my own patients working with me.

Blood work was positive for rheumatoid arthritis, so I was started on prednisone. As I was waiting to see a rheumatologist, I tapered off the prednisone and had a bizarre episode of severe neck pain with dural tension, headaches and fevers that put me in the emergency room. Inflammatory markers were sky high and they suspected meningitis. They never figured out what it was, but I was out of commission for a few weeks and my C reactive protein (CRP) was through the roof.

Four months later when I got in to see the specialist, my joint inflammation had calmed down and the imaging and second round of blood work for rheumatoid arthritis was suddenly negative. They decided I had some sort of "mixed connective tissue disorder." I was more puzzled than ever. Around that time, they also found an ovarian cyst that originally looked to be a large mass but later was proven to be benign.

Light in the Darkness

There was a bright light amid my struggles that particular season. At a mutual friend's engagement party, I reconnected with a friend from high school, Graham, and we ended up dating shortly after that. Graham is by nature extremely outgoing, positive and compassionate, has a great sense of humor and is very open-minded. He's the optimal blend of career drive and laid-back Type B personality (that I hope will eventually rub off on me). He doesn't sweat the small stuff at all. He's a family guy and would do anything for his friends and loved ones. And, of course, he's exceptionally handsome. He made our long-distance relationship fun and exciting and we began writing each other letters, sending care packages, talking for hours at a time on Skype and planning weekend trips together.

One unique beauty of our relationship was that we'd known each other for half of our lives. While he was a high school crush of mine and may have been mentioned a *few* times in my teenage diary, we never ended up dating back then. Our long-standing friendship made long-distance dating easier since we already knew and trusted each other and were comfortable around each other's families. In addition to being all-around awesome, Graham was also incredibly understanding and supportive in terms of the health issues that were unfolding in his new girlfriend.

Back to the Drawing Board

That spring, I began to have near-constant severe abdominal episodes. I revisited my diet and tried a candida cleanse, a Paleo approach, the low FODMAP diet and eventually just straight-up meat and a select few vegetables/fruits and nothing else. Despite my desperate attempts to control the gastrointestinal symptoms, they were only getting worse and had returned to being present daily to the point of my missing more and more work. I saw a nutritionist who gave me handouts on my allergies and celiac disease but basically left me with no more answers on what I could do for myself dietarily.

I went back to the drawing board and saw a new GI specialist. He did another endoscopy (normal) and looked for some "zebras," too—my celiac artery originally looked 90% blocked, but the follow-up CT showed it was normal. Liver and gallbladder imaging were normal despite tenderness and what seemed like enlargement and classic referral pain patterns.

For several decades I'd struggled off and on with throat hoarseness, difficulty raising my voice and frequent clearing of my throat. Sometimes my throat also felt swollen. This reached a new level while I was in my 30s. I was constantly teased by my swimmers when I was a high school coach because I could barely raise my voice above the noise of the pool deck. Despite all sorts of exercises and consultation from a speech therapist, these symptoms seemed to come and go as they pleased with no discernible trend, apart from a generalized "sterile inflammatory" type pattern that tended to correspond to my system-wide flares.

My immune system seemed to fluctuate (over the course of several months or years at a time) between being hyperactive and underactive. It seemed I would go 2 years without catching a single cold or other illness (which I found unusual, considering I was around ill patients all day, plus my niece and nephew when they were sick). In other windows of time, it seemed I was immunosuppressed and constantly sick, unable to get healthy for more than a week at a time before I would have another bout of the flu, a sinus infection, cold or respiratory infection.

Exploratory Surgery

As I continued to suffer through the workday with unexplained symptoms, in the spring of 2016 my lower abdominal pain episodes began to involve severe bladder spasms and pain. I found myself running to the bathroom between almost every patient. I returned to the OB/GYN at the suggestion of my GI specialist, and they thought I might have endometriosis and interstitial cystitis. So, I underwent a laparoscopy with cystoscopy which looked completely normal. However, my surgeon noted an abnormal amount of colon distention during the procedure and suggested I repeat the colonoscopy.

I was ashamed as I watched my scars heal slowly. I was absolutely mortified that I had just undergone surgery for something that wasn't even there! They call Lyme disease "the great mimic," but I personally think that expression would suffice for MCAS as well. In financial desperation, I went against doctors' advice and skipped the colonoscopy (which I'd had a few years prior) since I was switching health insurance and had a new deductible to meet.

I began to cut my hours down at work, going down to four days a week, and then three, and eventually two days in the physical therapy clinic with patients. I had done the exact same thing a few years prior when I was working in Utah. I seemed to have this pattern of a year or two where I could push through symptoms, followed by a breaking point where I would "reset" everything and then slowly crawl out of the deep hole that I assumed was career burnout.

However, the reduced working hours in Alaska seemed to have no effect on my symptoms. I was feeling more and more despair and helplessness with the abdominal attacks that were causing me to either miss work or be present but mentally struggle to provide quality care to patients. It was very difficult because the episodes were so unpredictable and I was still unable to identify consistent triggers. The added burden of a bunch of system-wide symptoms like extreme fatigue and brain fog was making work especially difficult. I normally was on my feet all day and practiced quite a bit of manual therapy and dry needling with patients, in addition to therapeutic exercise, but when I began to contemplate changing patient's plans of care in order to accommodate my physical ability limitations for the day, I knew that something had to change.

I revisited my gastrointestinal specialist who essentially told me that there was nothing medically wrong with me. He said that "gas" could cause abdominal discomfort and that extra stretching and pressure can be quite painful. (This really pissed me off. I definitely know the difference between flatulence and the pain I was experiencing.) He told me that my symptoms were caused by stress and suggested that I change my career. I tried to explain that the symptoms were what was causing me stress because they prevented me from performing my best at work, but he convinced me that it was the other way around.

As I approached the summer of 2016, I knew deep down what I had to do. I met with my boss and gave him my two weeks' notice. I imagine he wasn't too surprised at that point. I had been in a manual therapy residency program the prior year and had dropped out halfway through due to health issues, marking the first time I'd ever "quit" something without finishing it. He was the instructor of the program and was very kind about it. In fact, the company I'd been working for was nothing but completely supportive and empathetic to me the entire time I was there, despite my missed work and what I imagine looked to outsider eyes like a big flailing hypochondriac. They were, in many senses, family to me, and leaving their work environment was one of the hardest things I've ever had to do. It was also hard to leave patient care, as getting to know patients was one of the highlights of the profession for me. But I had, yet again, hit my breaking point and could no longer push through the physical symptoms in that environment. I also decided to leave my swim coaching position.

In the previous summer, a friend and I had started work on a small paddleboarding business that was set to open on June 1, 2016. In hindsight, starting a small business was definitely not the stress-free work environment I was seeking to help my health, but it was a wonderful ride! One of the best parts was that I could work from home a lot and set my own schedule, building it around my symptoms. Nonetheless, throughout summer 2016 I felt like I was still in survival mode as I was working overtime to get the new small business up and running.

Venom Immunotherapy

That summer, I returned to the allergist. He didn't have any solutions for my system-wide issues, but was insistent that I was a high-risk Hymenoptera venom allergy patient who needed regular injections. I began venom immunotherapy (VIT) because I was told that there was a good chance I would die if re-stung again without undergoing the allergy shot treatment protocol. My allergist attempted to help my system tolerate the ramping up of venom dosage by taking steroids and antihistamines. However, every time I had a venom test or venom injection, I seemed to be more and more reactive. While the allergist was attempting to ramp up my dosage to the maintenance level, I went into anaphylactic shock in the office and needed a few shots of epinephrine to stabilize.

What was scarier was the fact that instead of presenting with hives and swelling and a gradual reaction like my first sting episode, my anaphylaxis to venom grew into an immediate throat closure accompanied by a drop in blood pressure and high heart rate, burning on the insides of my eyes, mental confusion/sense of impending doom and abdominal cramps. It happened quickly (in a matter of seconds) and was terrifying. Around that same time, many of my other triggers (foods and environmental) began to mirror that quick anaphylaxis that went straight to my throat without hives or other signs.

From my personal experience, VIT was horrible. It induced miserable systemic symptoms that often lasted until my next injection, in addition to my arm swelling up to the point where it would not fit into clothing for several weeks at a time. I experienced a surge in flushing, headaches, nausea, vomiting, abdominal cramping, fevers, difficulty breathing and swallowing, dizziness, low blood pressure, fatigue, extreme emotional fluctuations and severe brain fog. System-wide side effects lasted one to two weeks after the shot, with extreme mood fluctuations and anxiety. I began to experience heightened reactions to all sorts of environmental factors in the months that I started VIT, things that I had never previously reacted to—perfumes, cleaning supplies, secondhand cigarette smoke, even being in a house that was near a farm!

VIT ended up triggering anaphylaxis for me on many occasions, and I spent numerous days stuck in the clinic where I had to be monitored. It never triggered facial swelling or hives, so I had a hard time getting some clinic staff to take my concerns seriously. However, despite my systemic side effects, I knew that with my outdoor lifestyle, it was important to minimize the risk of death by stinging insect, and I forced myself to continue with VIT for another nine months of misery. At that point, I was still oblivious to the fact that I had an underlying issue that caused my mast cells to go awry.

Could It Be Crohn's?

The abdominal episodes reached an all-time high at the end of summer 2016. Running a small seasonal business had been more stressful than anticipated (even though my "office" was on a paddleboard on most days). Similar to the need to push through symptoms in the physical therapy clinic, I often experienced abdominal episodes while working with paddleboarding clients and it took everything I had to put on a happy face and get through the day. However, I had already lost one career and was stubbornly determined to maintain what I had left—my small business dream—at all costs.

Finally, in the fall of 2016 I returned to the GI specialist. He did a colonoscopy and saw signs of Crohn's disease. The lesion biopsies showed acute ileitis in the terminal ileum but no granulomas. Nonetheless, maybe because he was sick of seeing me, he told me that the findings were significant and that given my history I did have Crohn's. He put me on a steroid treatment (budesonide) and sent me on my way. I didn't feel like it all added up, but I was so happy to finally have some sort of diagnostic explanation. While my primary issue of constipation didn't make sense with the typical diarrhea presentation of Crohn's, I still celebrated having a name for my symptoms—and something that made more sense than irritable bowel syndrome.

Interestingly, I had a terrific first month response to the Crohn's medication without a single abdominal attack like those that had been plaguing me. This was the first time in years that I was not suffering with some degree of that abdominal pain. Unfortunately, after one month on the budesonide, I had a relapse and symptoms came back with a vengeance.

The financial stress amid all of this certainly did not help matters. I spent nearly my entire savings as a physical therapist as I had countless medical tests and procedures while also having to switch health insurance plans three times in the state of Alaska, where medical care is quite expensive. In the fall of 2016, I decided to relocate to Washington for the winter to live closer to Graham. I still was co-owner of the Alaska-based paddleboarding company and decided to try being a "snowbird" in Seattle.

Symptom-Filled in Seattle

Once I was in Seattle, I found a new GI specialist. She took one look at me and said, "I don't think you have Crohn's. This just isn't adding up." Plus, I was not responding to the Crohn's medications. She ordered more expensive GI imaging (all negative) and then handed me probiotics and laxatives. I was on my own again.

I was getting worse and worse and in even more despair at being answer-less and kicked to the curb by the medical system. I attempted to continue the venom immunotherapy in Washington despite the sides effects and increasing anaphylaxis. The doctors and nurses in Washington didn't seem to take my concerns seriously and would insist on increasing my dosage since I wasn't up to the traditional "maintenance dosage" standards when I left Alaska. I continued to note that the more I went, the more sensitive I was to my environment and the more likely I was to have anaphylaxis to the tiniest triggers. Finally, I just stopped going.

As my sensitivity to my environment and anaphylactic episodes increased, my low blood pressure become more and more of a concern. At the peak of one flare, I was experiencing 20 to 30 near-fainting episodes per day, virtually any time I exerted myself or changed positions. Many days I would have to stop in the middle of the workday or after walking up a flight of stairs and lie flat with my feet elevated. Sometimes "safe" foods would trigger blood pressure drops. A change in body position was a sure way to experience severe episodes of dizziness and blurred vision. I finally purchased a blood pressure (BP) monitor for home use and realized that my BP was dropping to below 80/40 in these episodes and was otherwise hovering around 95/60.

My adrenaline baseline seemed to be at a strangely high level as I began to have more and more issues with anaphylaxis. I would have adrenaline rushes from the slightest daily activities; noises (like a door shutting) or visual stimuli (like someone walking by my desk at work) would startle me into an adrenaline rush that would previously have been expected in association with near car accidents or pre–cliff-jumping moments. The adrenaline rushes would happen all day long and I could not seem to get my system to relax. Nighttime was the worst, as I would start to nod off and then suddenly have a huge rush of adrenaline and a racing heart for several minutes that would startle me; sometimes this would happen all night long, and my insomnia grew to be severe. The insomnia was often accompanied by an intense burning in my calves and pain in my feet and hands while in bed. It made my sleep quality especially poor for months at a time, and the lack of sleep would trigger a vicious cycle of abdominal attacks and severe drowsiness during the day. Eventually I was told that I had adrenal fatigue but was not offered any remedies.

I also began to experience postural orthostatic tachycardia syndrome (POTS) more severely when I was living in Washington. When I would stand up, I would experience a very intensely racing heartbeat. It began to interfere with my ability to exercise, perform normal daily activities around the house and maintain a standing position for very long. Turning over in bed woke me up all night long as my heart rate raced to 130-150 beats per minute every time I moved. Between the sudden adrenaline rushes at rest and the heart rate fluctuations with positional changes, my sleep quality was terrible and I had constant circles under my eyes.

Mast Cells and Mold

I was growing sicker and sicker in Washington and lucked out with a temporary public health job that eventually let me do some work from home. At that point I was nearly homebound all the time and was very reactive to the slightest odors and triggers. I moved several times over the course of six months in efforts to escape homes that had obvious signs of black mold as well as buildings that seemed newer and safer but still triggered reactions.

This wasn't my first experience with mold. When I was in college, I took two separate trips to New Orleans with my church for post-Hurricane Katrina relief efforts. We donned cheap safety masks and went about with sledgehammers and crowbars knocking down walls, removing mold-covered belongings, and chasing cockroaches and rodents out of the fridges that had been untouched for six months to two years. As a young 20-something, I remember thoroughly enjoying the physical labor of gutting homes. Looking back, I also remember that after both trips, I had several visits to doctors for various mysterious ailments, without attributing the mold spore and endotoxin exposure as a potential cause. After those trips, it seemed that I had more and more reactions to certain buildings. I recall several musty places that I lived in graduate school and beyond where I began to experience migraines and other unexplained symptoms.

Between secondhand exposure to cigarette smoke from passersby on the streets and around my apartment, bus vibrations and perfumes on public transit, and water-damaged buildings, I was a complete wreck on a daily basis after a few months in Seattle. I was reacting to my boyfriend's car, the neighbor's dryer sheets, the same apple I had eaten yesterday; reactions went from predictable clearly "toxic" substances to random and idiopathic triggers. I was experimenting with at-home efforts to help my body "detox" like supplements, enemas, and lymphatic drainage with little results.

At that point I had to increase the dose of my antihistamines to control my chronic urticaria and other symptoms and became more concerned about my antihistamine "cocktail" taken three times a day. But every time I tried to taper off my antihistamines, the hives got worse. They were already spreading to my face, neck, throat, chest, and more and more on my extremities. I still would get episodic hives around my face when I ate something that I was reactive to, but the extremity hives seemed to be a low-level constant in my daily life.

Outside of the hives, I also experienced an increasing amount of skin flushing, eye floaters, restless legs, facial nerve issues, hypoglycemia, ringing in the ears, severe grogginess bordering on narcolepsy, heartburn, hair loss, acne and eczema. The longer I was in Seattle, the more that I felt achy, chilled and feverish like I constantly had the flu. And, much to my dismay, the flu-like symptoms persisted pretty much daily for close to one year after they began, which was miserable in itself.

I also began to note an interesting correlation between my anxiety level and my antihistamine dose. If I forgot a dose, I would most certainly be plagued by an intense "chemical-like" anxiety episode. Within 30 minutes of swallowing an H1 or H2 blocker, the anxiety would be replaced with a deep sense of peace.

Answers in Seattle

In early 2017, I qualified for a new insurance plan and got connected with a functional medicine doctor (who I'll call Dr. C) who would forever change my life. Dr. C took an extremely thorough history and also provided me with compassionate care. I had been listening to podcasts on Crohn's disease and the Specific Carbohydrate Diet, which led me to a podcast on small intestinal bacterial overgrowth (SIBO). I asked Dr. C if she would order the test for SIBO. She agreed but said that she thought that the root of all my problems was actually a histamine intolerance issue.

I admit, I was a bit of a skeptic. I'd never even considered that histamine could be connected to my abdominal pain, and I'd never tried a low-histamine diet. I was so convinced that I had SIBO; nonetheless, I agreed to try her suggestions.

The temporary low-histamine diet proved mildly helpful and my symptoms did match a lot of what are seen with histamine intolerance, but I still wasn't completely sold. So, I did what any stubborn patient would do—I decided to try a *high*-histamine diet so I would "truly know" if histamine was my issue. I spent a day eating bacon and leftovers topped off with a glass of wine. Within half a day I was extremely flared with an intense migraine, joint pain, eczema, fatigue, constipation, a POTS flare-up, heart palpitations, low blood pressure, ringing in the ears, etc. I thought to myself, "OK, now we're definitely on to something!"

The week that followed my high-histamine experimentation was a blur as my symptoms worsened and I ended up having three episodes of idiopathic anaphylactic shock. I could not stabilize unless I was on a high dose of round-the-clock antihistamines such as Benadryl. As I started to come out of it, I had a strange episode of mental confusion and difficulty with my brain's executive function, hoarseness, severe POTS problems, blurred vision, extreme thirst, and liver and gallbladder-area pain. Plus, my resting blood pressure was bumping back and forth between 175/100 to 80/40, with my pulse fluctuating from 40 to 155 at rest for no reason. The doctors weren't sure what to do with me. I was given the advice to just keep taking Benadryl around the clock.

I began to investigate histamine more and stumbled upon information about mast cell activation disorders. I read Dr. Afrin's book[2] about mast cell activation syndrome (MCAS) in nearly one day. Immediately light bulbs began going off, but I pulled myself back in from getting my hopes up about being diagnosed with yet another "false positive" condition. Nonetheless, the next time I saw Dr. C, I came prepared with a list of tests useful in identifying MCAS. She was unfamiliar with the condition but agreed to order the lab work for tryptase and a 24-hour urine sample looking at histamine and prostaglandins.

Dr. C also had me get a Spectracell nutrient panel done, which showed that I was severely deficient in many vitamins and minerals. She speculated that the choline/inositol deficiency could be related to some of my fatigue, anxiety, brain fog and memory issues.

The test for SIBO involves drinking a lactulose beverage and then submitting breath samples into a tube at intervals for three hours. This measures the gas levels emitted and can predict where in the GI tract abnormal bacteria may be present. It took a while for the test to come back, but when it did it was positive for methane-dominant SIBO. I was overjoyed—finally, something could explain the abdominal issues! Dr. C was surprised and we discussed the treatment options, which included herbal/antibiotic options and dietary plans similar to what I was already doing. While I was happy to have a diagnosis that was more abdomen-specific, it still didn't seem like SIBO explained the severe 2-7 days attacks that I had been prone to getting for so many years.

Less than a week after this new diagnosis of SIBO, I received the MCAS lab results back and learned that my liver enzymes were elevated and also that my prostaglandin D2 test value was 1345! (Normal is 100-280.) When I got my prostaglandin test results I sobbed uncontrollably. It was an incredibly powerful feeling to know that we had finally uncovered concrete signs of a condition that could explain the decades of strange symptoms. 1345 was not the "slightly positive but not off the charts" level that my last decade of testing had shown for just about everything else. There was no denying that the test was positive. (Finally, I had proof that I wasn't crazy! There was something chemically off, and it was confirmed!) I knew that I still had to have further testing to confirm the clinical diagnosis, but I felt certain that MCAS was the missing piece of the puzzle for me.

I followed up with an allergist who wanted to have an additional positive test to confirm that it was MCAS. He had some of my old intestinal biopsies sent to a new lab for mast cell specific staining to give us more information. There was some concern for mastocytosis, since I had a history of severe Hymenoptera venom issues, near-fainting with blood pressure drops during anaphylaxis, as well as a propensity for bone fractures and liver enzyme abnormalities. He also suggested a standing tryptase lab order, since my tryptase the previous month had been normal but had never been tested during an episode.

The biopsy results seemed to take forever to come back. Based on gastrointestinal tissue samples from nearly two years prior, the *KIT* mutation was negative, but the other tests confirmed that I did have positive (abnormal) results with CD25 staining for mast cells and a higher than average number of mast cell aggregates consistent with monoclonal MCAS. I was never able to get the tryptase level drawn during the right window of time within an episode, and because my baseline tryptase was normal, my doctor did not think a bone marrow biopsy was urgently necessary. He worked with me to trial more medications for monoclonal MCAS and suggested I focus on getting to a more stable baseline before resuming venom immunotherapy.

As an experiment, I attempted to psychologically will myself to be better. In the past I had used this strategy to try and ignore symptoms, but this time I mentally thanked my mast cells for their attention to detail all day long but also reassured them that my everyday triggers were not threats to the system (and often were good for my healing). But no matter what kind of a mental approach I had, there was no denying or ignoring the physiological reactions that kept occurring.

I began the search to find the right combination of pharmacological management and natural treatment approaches, in addition to the right lifestyle changes and healthcare team, to aid me in the process of addressing MCAS. I trialed a number of mast cell-specific medications, including cromolyn sodium, which was not particularly helpful in my case. I was able to stabilize better once I upped my dosage of twice-daily H1 and H2 blockers and leukotriene antagonist medication. The addition of compounded ketotifen and low dose naltrexone to my antihistamine and anti-leukotriene medications were some of the bigger game-changers in helping my initial symptoms stabilize.

I hated to be taking that many medications, but it was huge for my quality of life and anaphylaxis prevention. I told myself that the increase in drugs was only for a season, until I could better address the underlying triggers that plagued my system.

The severe abdominal attacks were deemed to be associated with anaphylaxis and my chronic gastrointestinal symptoms were attributed to chronic mast cell mediator release. However, antihistamines and epinephrine never seemed to influence the abdominal attacks that would last for days, so I remained puzzled about that aspect of my symptoms.

During that time frame, I was also diagnosed with Ehlers-Danlos syndrome (hypermobile type) which I had already suspected given my history of joint/connective tissue issues and POTS problems. But nothing made more sense in terms of my system-wide symptoms than the new diagnosis of MCAS. As a whole, it was extremely validating to finally have an explanation that made sense for a lifetime of confusing issues. I went from feeling joyful—elated!—at having answers to the stark realization that I was up against a LOT of challenges to recover my health and vitality. When you have multiple underlying mechanisms occurring, which do you address first? Where was I to even begin? Little did I know, I still had more information to uncover on this journey before I would begin to heal.

Functional Medicine Gold Mine

My diagnosis with monoclonal MCAS in early 2017 marked the start of a more novel and focused functional medicine approach. Indeed, the diagnostic process was not over, as that spring I also was tested for parasites and yeast overgrowth because my SIBO was not clearing up despite adhering to a strict treatment plan. The fatigue was also unrelenting. Given my severe intolerance to moldy buildings, I was also tested for chronic inflammation secondary to mold toxins. I continued to test repeatedly positive for chronically elevated liver markers and experienced a new type of right-sided trunk pain. Intermittent flare-ups of neck pain appeared to coincide with systemic flare-ups more so than traditional musculoskeletal factors.

Eventually I discovered that I now had four types of parasites and multiple bacterial infections in my bloodstream and gastrointestinal tract. Klebsiella and mycoplasma pneumonia bacteria were elevated and my naturopath was working with me to resolve some dysfunction in the ileocecal valve that connects the small intestine to the large intestine. I focused hard on gut health and attempted to address the infections in a variety of ways, but remained frustrated that my gastrointestinal symptoms weren't improving.

My mold-related testing came back (unsurprisingly) with a resounding positive result and I did a trial of cholestyramine, a compounding pharmacy toxin binding agent. After a few weeks of taking it, I felt back to a more stable baseline and was then able to more effectively address my mast cell activation symptoms with a more holistic and natural approach. The mold toxin binding treatment was especially helpful for eliminating my POTS symptoms, shortness of breath, and heart palpitations. If I had missed the step of addressing mold in my journey, I have no doubt that I would be much worse off today and still stuck in the frustrating battle of many antihistamine medications and "putting a Band-Aid" on my symptoms.

While treating mold illness was an important piece of the puzzle, it did not remove all of my symptoms by any means. Still, it enabled me to feel cleansed of some of the junk clogging my system so that I could more efficiently focus on addressing other areas. After a few weeks on cholestyramine, I ended up discontinuing it because it triggered anaphylaxis, but those two weeks were enough for me to notice a significant change in my baseline of overall symptoms.

The Pursuit of a Stable Baseline

I returned to Alaska in the summer of 2017 for the small business, and my symptoms initially improved once I left (moldy) Seattle. However, they were still surprisingly disabling, and I struggled to maintain an active lifestyle after I returned to my home state. At that point, I was working on this book about MCAS, working full-time on small business administrative tasks, and meeting clients for paddleboarding lessons and day trips. I was planning a race event and doing some freelance writing for a running website.

I found it a big struggle to get out of the house each day or to maintain the physical exercise routine I aimed for. Even at home, unanticipated secondhand exposure to wet paint, cleaning supplies, perfumes and other chemicals seemed to interrupt my life on a regular basis, and it seemed like I was engaged in an uphill battle to stay away from anaphylactic reactions. I felt "hungover" each day despite the fact that I didn't drink. The fatigue, migraines, abdominal issues, blurred vision, hair loss, and food reactions persisted daily. As my abdominal attacks and chemical sensitivities were still uncontrolled, I found myself leaving the house less and less, and making fewer plans because I didn't want to commit to something and then let people down or force myself to go when I needed to take care of myself at home.

I was still experiencing more spontaneous reactions to foods that I could previously tolerate. I completed a strict elimination diet as part of a trial of the specific carbohydrate diet (SCD) recommended for SIBO, with a low-histamine approach, and then found that I had a difficult time adding "safe" foods back in. Several months of eating like this made me feel even worse than before, and I was frustrated because I got down to only a handful of safe foods.

Eliminating the highest culprits on the histamine list (like bacon/cured meats, alcohol, and aged cheese) was definitely helpful, but I realized that there were a lot of problems with trying to follow the histamine number charts. Truly following the low-histamine diet left me feeling even worse, and it cut out healthy options that I loved like avocado and other fruits and vegetables. Plus, the logic did not make sense to me. Histamine was just one of the many chemical mediators that tends to be high with MCAS, and food-ingested histamine was not nearly as consistently potent as simply hugging someone with perfume on or other types of triggers on my reactivity scale.

I also toyed with the idea of removing salicylates, oxalates, night shades, and dietary sources containing the carbohydrate alpha-gal, but ultimately decided (with the help of a few short trials) that I needed to gain diversity in my diet, not cut it off. Fortunately, none of those categories of foods seemed to make a difference either way in my personal symptoms.

My food reactions were all over the map, and I began to realize that if I decreased my overall load of inflammation and triggers from other lifestyle factors (such as exposure to chemicals and mold), my diet could become more diverse again. I also realized that I needed to commit to 100% organic food choices and the complete elimination of all preservatives and processed foods for optimal success. I became better at reading labels and eventually had no need to read them as my grocery store choices turned to fruits, vegetables, and the occasional grass-fed meat or fresh-caught filet of salmon.

I began to fill my days with precautions that seemed a little ridiculous but necessary, such as only drinking filtered water, avoiding plastic at all costs, and using very basic and expensive allergen-free beauty products and hand soap. I avoided leaving the house within an hour of eating or taking medications (to try to avoid reactions in public). I got used to driving the long way around a farm or house that had horses and hay, since those triggered anaphylactic episodes even when I was in the car.

I was constantly on the lookout for other drivers who smoked, as their secondhand smoke drifting out the window would trigger anaphylaxis as it entered my car vents. I changed the air settings back and forth as I drove and scanned other drivers. I had to leave business meetings and social gatherings due to anaphylactic responses triggered by different perfumes. I crossed the road if I saw a cigarette smoker. I had to switch churches multiple times because of the incense and/or the proximity to people who wore perfume. The slightest whiff of an air freshener, secondhand perfume on my clothing from a hug, cleaning supply or charred cooking fume would leave me flared for days.

The smallest things were immensely fatiguing. I could muster up the mental energy to agree to meet friends for dinner, but then by the time I had showered I felt like I could barely lift my arms to dry my hair. I prioritized my small business activities and church, but by the summer of 2017, the rest of the time I was mostly homebound.

The fatigue definitely took a toll on relationships. Family members assumed I was too busy to call or visit, but in truth I was too tired to muster the strength to talk on the phone or leave the house. I struggled to stay upbeat and put my best foot forward in my long-distance relationship.

One of the things that I hated the most was the stoicism that chronic illness breeds. I often felt alone and like I was trying to survive each day on my own, even with people around me, so in order to do that I had to muster up every ounce of strength I had to "get through it." I felt like it turned me into a serious, non-smiling, non-laughing monster. Gritting my teeth through the pain became the norm, and it was very hard to pay attention to anything outside of that when I was in physical survival mode.

In some ways, the physical slowing down that became a necessity helped me to heal internally. I used to think that my worth was dependent on what I accomplished or did as opposed to who I was. Somewhere in my subconscious I still believed that I had to earn my salvation. And I felt truly unloveable and struggled with feeling like a failure. When you stay busy, you can kind of ignore this internal backdrop of damaging self-talk. But when you're forced to slow down, these types of mindsets become front and center.

Slowly I began to turn these around. I listened to audiobooks, gobbled up podcasts, changed my prayer life, and dove into self-help books. I'd read that if I just told myself the opposite long enough, I would eventually start to believe it. "I am enough" became a new mantra. Despite my best efforts to change my mindset, I still had many low points that were usually triggered when my symptoms were flared, when I was in the ER, or where I was in bed with a five-day episode of abdominal angioedema. It was extremely difficult to be positive and selfless when experiencing certain levels of pain. I did my best to cultivate joy despite whatever circumstances came my way, but it was extremely challenging. I began to open up more about my struggles to people in my life. I had previously suffered through emergency room visits in secret, without notifying loved ones, but I began to be more honest with everyone.

Toward the end of summer 2017, my functional medicine doctor recommended some additional testing and I was also diagnosed with Lyme disease (and eventually with coinfections including bartonella and babesia). I began to realize that there are many misconceptions about the condition. Conflicting information exists regarding how Lyme disease can be spread, how many of us are likely exposed to it, and how the body often expresses symptoms once the immune system is run down. While I had a history of two separate red rashes followed by classic symptoms of Lyme disease after trips to Montana and Panama, my naturopathic doctor was under the impression that I may have been exposed in utero. Either way, a mere six months after my monoclonal MCAS diagnosis, I was glad to have another diagnostic label that helped explain my mast cells going awry. It was tempting to blame everything on Lyme disease and the coinfections, but I knew that my situation was much more complex than that.

Another Move

As the summer came to a close, I was attempting to sell my small business because my health continued to deteriorate and also because it was financially straining and difficult to find short-term work while trying to live in two states. (It was hard on my relationship, too.)

As I parted ways with Alaska for good this time, my soul felt heavy. I was letting go of the successful small business I'd built with a friend and opportunities to be involved in the swimming, paddleboarding, triathlete and physical therapy communities that I loved. It was extremely hard to say goodbye to my sister, brother-in-law, niece, and nephew knowing that I would be missing so many milestones with them. I put freelance writing and photography passions on hold and also accepted that I was no longer well enough for my affiliate faculty role leading groups of PT students down to rural Peru for alternative clinical experiences and public health work. I basically wiped my slate clean to focus on healing, and though painful, it was also a sigh of relief after trying to juggle so much while being chronically unwell.

The drive down the Alcan highway that fall was memorable—and not in a good way. Road trips always seemed to trigger attacks, and similar to the previous year, on day two of the trip I began to have an abdominal angioedema episode that left me feverish, delirious, and severely dehydrated. I swelled quickly and as the pain intensified, I realized that I needed emergency room care, but we were in the middle of nowhere part-way down the Cassiar Highway in Canada. All I could do was pray and curl up in the fetal position as my boyfriend drove.

This time, the episode would last six days and would be one of the worst attacks I'd ever experienced. I wasn't sure if it was the stress of moving and being in the middle of nowhere in an emergency medical scenario or the vibrations of the car, but it was miserable. Luckily, Graham is an incredible partner who took good care of me and was willing to do most of the driving, and I got through the episode just in time to make the journey to Minnesota.

An MCAS Community

I'd been working on this book about MCAS for five months when I learned of a great opportunity in St. Cloud. A healthcare organization was hosting a continuing education event that covered MCAS, Ehlers-Danlos syndrome (EDS), and complex regional pain syndrome (CRPS) all in one day! I knew immediately that I had to go—not only as a physical therapist and as a patient, but as an author attempting to clarify MCAS as accurately as possible.

It was an incredible opportunity to meet the experts in the field, and I reached out to the presenters to arrange interviews with them. Fortunately, they obliged to my requests and even invited me to a post-event dinner. Dr. Afrin patiently answered all of my questions for hours. Other specialists in MCAS opened my eyes to new facets of the disease. I was able to listen to heroes of mine like Dr. Pradeep Chopra connect the dots between CRPS and MCAS. I became re-inspired to get back into the clinic and help patients who were suffering with chronic pain and began to dream about opening a PT clinic that was specific to patients with the MCAS-EDS-POTS trifecta.

However, one of the biggest highlights was the opportunity to meet fellow patients with MCAS. While I'd communicated with many on social media, it was extremely empowering to have a face-to-face conversation with others who just "got it."

I returned to Washington briefly in which time I was attempting to live in a tent and in hotels due to my level of mold reactions. Even with a mask on, I was going to the emergency room with anaphylaxis and abdominal episodes after spending minutes to hours in my Seattle apartment. I felt like a failure for deciding to leave Washington, when more than anything I just wanted to be there to support my boyfriend's career. But I knew that no matter how much I mentally willed myself to get through living in a place that constantly triggered my mast cells into distress, it was not enough, and I wasn't sure how much longer I could handle that type of survival mode. My parents graciously invited me to stay with them in Arizona in order to pursue more naturopathic care and get back on my feet.

Abdominal Angioedema

Prior to my move to Arizona, I began to peruse patient forums about abdominal angioedema as I assumed that this aspect of my struggles was connected to MCAS somehow. This led me to stumble upon a description of hereditary angioedema (HAE), a condition that I'd never heard of. To make a long story short, I pursued the testing for it, and the tests came back affirmative for HAE, so I began another process of specialist visits and medication trials.

If I was happy when I learned about MCAS, I was absolutely ecstatic to learn that I had HAE. Finally, I had answers for the brutal abdominal attacks that had been plaguing me since my teenage years, and the other bizarre swelling I'd noted for much of my life! Who knew that it was all connected?! I had a name for the enemy that had gradually reduced my ability to work, have an active lifestyle, and even eat and drink water for days on end. If only I'd put two and two together sooner! (It turns out that the average length from onset to diagnosis of hereditary angioedema is 8.3 years,[3] but I had gone double that.)

This new diagnosis was a HUGE deal for me. It gave me hope that I would be able to return to a normal work environment in the future. It also reinforced my "gut feeling" (pun intended) that my episodes were not solely gastrointestinal in nature. The fluid caused by the blood vessels inappropriately leaking caused ascites-like pressure in my abdominal cavity, which explained the type of pain and swelling they caused.

My first question amid all of this was, "Does this mean that I don't have MCAS?" After all, HAE is on the differential diagnosis list when doctors are evaluating a patient for the potential to have MCAS. However, it was clear that I had two separate types of attacks occurring. My allergist happened to be one of the leading doctors in the field of HAE (a rare disease) and he told me that 1) I had the clinical diagnosis of both diseases, and in my case, was probably unlucky/suffering from a perfect storm of environment and genetics. Because I had monoclonal MCAS, my MCAS was *not* likely secondary to anything else, though it was probably flared by other factors and 2) In his experience, there was a pattern of several patients presenting with both conditions at once, though the common mechanism was not entirely understood.

Bradykinin is a chemical mediator released by mast cells that triggers the movement of fluids to other tissues during HAE attacks. Patients with HAE lack the enzyme needed to break down/remove bradykinin, so logically the two conditions could feed off each other. We also discussed how most patients with both conditions have a certain subset of classic MCAS symptoms that respond well to epinephrine and antihistamines, but that their HAE seems largely unaffected by mast cell medications and tends to present in distinct, longer-lasting episodes.

Interestingly, there appears to be a higher prevalence (nearly five times the rate!) of systemic mastocytosis in patients with HAE.[4] I learned that as many as one-third of patients undiagnosed or undertreated for HAE actually die due to laryngeal swelling that leads to asphyxiation, and about half of patients with HAE experience a laryngeal attack in their lifetime, so emergency meds were not something to take lightly.[5,6] Ironically, the (previously) outrageous cost of an EpiPen now looked enticing when compared to my new rare disease medication options; the cost for the new HAE rescue med alone was over $100,000 per month at the dose I was prescribed.

For the first time in my life, I had a treatment option that I could use during abdominal attacks, and it worked to prevent symptoms from worsening! The bad news was, I generally needed more than one dose of the medication per attack, and I was having attacks at least 75% of the calendar month at that time. Insurance only approved 3 per month initially, so I was still pretty disabled in terms of attack length and severity. It was bad timing, as one of the few prophylactic meds for HAE was in a shortage, so I was put on a waiting list for access to something more preventative.

Naturopathic Care

I was beginning to feel like I was carrying around a longer and longer chronic illness cover letter, so I prepared a single-page summary of my most pertinent health conditions and medications/supplements, as well as a spreadsheet of my labs. Then, for each individual visit, I would summarize a few bullets of my goals and questions for the particular specialist or practitioner I was seeing. These summary pages were extremely instrumental as I saw new doctors, and also ensured that I focused on the main issues at hand in my short time with each visit. They helped me stay organized, and I was told that they helped my providers put the pieces together as well.

Despite a season of incredible answers, I was yet to realize that things would still get worse before they got better. Shortly after my HAE diagnosis, my naturopathic doctor performed more baseline testing which revealed that I had both acute and chronic Epstein-Barr virus, multiple heavy metal toxicities, hormonal abnormalities. adrenal issues, excess inflammatory markers, and Hashimoto's thyroiditis. He also performed additional testing (beyond the Western Blot) that reconfirmed Lyme disease. When combined with the previously diagnosed issues like parasites, mold illness, SIBO, and detoxification organs that were on overdrive, it was clear that there were over a dozen underlying issues that were likely influencing my mast cell activation symptoms and abdominal distress.

I opted for the most natural approach for thyroid treatment and began some new supplements, with the help of my doctor, to boost my detoxification and toxin-binding capabilities. Over the course of several months, I also trialed quercetin, luteolin, bromelain, mangosteen, CBD oil, alpha-lipoic acid, L-glutamine, selenomethionine, new probiotics, different types of magnesium, estrogen-reducing supplements, B vitamins, lypo-spheric vitamin C, zinc, melatonin, biotin, ashwagandha, milk thistle extract, spirulina, digestive bitters, Parasym plus, homeopathic drops, and other mast cell and immune-targeting supplements, in a meticulous one-at-a-time process.

A friend recommended I read the book "Medical Medium" and I committed to adhering to the majority of the dietary recommendations strictly for about a year. While the book is controversial since the author does not have a medical background, I believe that the big picture approach, focusing on an abundance of life-giving organic fresh produce (both vegetables and fruit) and avoidance of toxins, is so important for healing.

I began to treat healing like a full-time job, incorporating twice-daily juicing and a fruit, vegetable, and herb-heavy diet that continued to avoid additives, processed foods, dairy, caffeine, gluten/most other grains, and sugar. I ate blueberries with honey or some dates when I had a craving for something sweet. I began to reincorporate vegetables and fruits that I had previously avoided and slowly found that I was able to tolerate things like raw apples and Brussels sprouts again. The high-FODmap foods were occasionally irritating but I began to phase them in slowly.

Herbal tea, coconut water, and lemon water became my beverages of choice. I enjoyed teas containing red clover, nettle, lemon balm, peppermint, and dandelion root. I focused on quality sleep and dramatic lifestyle changes, with very light physical activity at first. Yoga, prayer, meditation, and reading were front-and-center priorities. I addressed sources of psychological trauma from the past head-on. I began shift my mindset more consistently in the right direction.

As fall turned to winter and I settled in Arizona, I commenced regular IV treatments at a naturopathic office that included ozone sessions and natural substances that help the body to remove toxins, viruses and bacteria. My new clinic offered pure, preservative-free IV infusions and was very attentive to preventing MCAS reactions and flare-ups. My doctor believed that if we could clear my blood of the junk clogging my system, my MCAS would resolve or at least be minimal. I half-expected to have a reaction to every IV I had, but amazingly, I did well (in terms of avoiding anaphylaxis) with a slow and gradual approach.

My first few months of IVs were rough in some ways, and chronic symptoms were definitely flared up as my body struggled to detoxify a presumably massive load of issues. But after a few weeks of the IV treatment combined with my prior dietary and supplement changes, I was able to halve my mast cell medications from what I had needed to take in Washington. (I do attribute *some* of this to moving away from a moldy environment.) I was still very symptomatic but no longer having spontaneous reactions to any foods. I still had to wear a mask around perfumes, passing cigarette smokers, cleaning supplies, etc., but I felt that I was making progress in other ways.

After a month of IV treatment, my neurological symptoms began resolving, and my anxiety lessened. My skin looked less yellow, my eyes looked whiter, and I noticed that I was losing less hair and even had some new hairline area growth for the first time in five years! The asymmetry in my face had improved and my face was less swollen. The best progress of all, however, was that my sluggish gastrointestinal system started moving a little more consistently. I was so grateful for this time devoted to healing and for the gracious generosity of my parents.

Around this time, a care package of items that had been in my boyfriend's apartment and car in Washington sent me into a big reaction. I decided to take drastic steps to ensure that I was not re-contaminating myself with mold toxins. I got rid of all permeable items and essentially started over with clothing and all other personal belongings. I was already sort of used to a "less is more" mentality from all the moving I'd done throughout my adult life. I kept a few things that had sentimental value quarantined in a box in the garage, but as a whole, it wasn't too hard to get rid of everything. And at that point I was pretty desperate. Shortly after the dramatic mold-exposed belonging purge, my headaches nearly vanished, I had fewer neurological symptoms, and my insomnia was less severe.

I began to find a balance in my mindset—one of fighting hard, but also of letting God handle it. This was difficult, because I wanted so badly to be in control of any and every trigger for mast cell reactions and HAE attacks. I was so desperate to get back to work and was getting more financially stressed by the day. But I did my best to foster healing while also embracing the chance to surrender.

I began to listen to my body more and avoided overcommitting to social engagements or groups or even hikes I wanted to do, instead forcing myself to set boundaries without feeling guilt about it, because I needed to prioritize healing. I feel extremely blessed that I was able to do this at a time in my life where I did not have many responsibilities and did not yet have children to care for. At the same time, I felt the maternal clock ticking and was hopeful that I would get to a place where having children would be an option someday soon.

I began to try new approaches to detoxification and more regularly appreciated colonic enema therapy. I added in techniques to improve lymphatic drainage and jumped on board (ha ha) with rebounder training every day to stimulate lymphatic flow. I incorporated massage and dry needling treatments when able and practiced yoga, breathing exercises and meditation. I listened to binaural beats and had sessions with a sound healer. I attended psychotherapy sessions and tried a type of therapy called Tension and Trauma Releasing Exercises. I joined a church group and worked on new aspects of spirituality. I began to reintegrate creative outlets like photography and painting. I incorporated parasympathetic nervous system techniques into my daily routine. Quiet time spent in prayer and spiritual healing sessions were other keys that have helped to facilitate emotional healing.

However, in spite of many lifestyle changes and additions, the HAE episodes were very much alive with a vengeance; that winter, I endured severe levels of pain and swelling for 2-5 days at a time, followed by a day or so of relief, and then another attack. They got so bad that for a 6 month stretch I was having near-daily abdominal attacks and periodic throat swelling that resulted in weight loss and deconditioning. My outings outside of the house were limited mainly to doctor appointments and the grocery store for several months, and I tried to fit in a gentle bike ride or walk between attacks.

I was also experiencing issues with head pressure and had a period of time where I had symptoms of Chiari malformation and intracranial pressure issues. Throughout my adult life, those types of headaches and head pressure symptoms would come and go for months at a time, with seemingly no rhyme or reason. But in the winter of 2017, I was having especially severe and excruciating headaches, neck pain and stiffness, difficulty swallowing, blurred vision, head pressure, and brain fog that all seemed to go hand in hand. A clear fluid was leaking (sometimes gushing!) out of my nose when I would change positions, which was later connected to a suspected extracellular fluid leak. I began to investigate the role of the vagus nerve and started taking supplements that would boost neurotransmitters and vagal tone, which helped temporarily with anxiety and digestion but had a questionable effect on my headache pain.

It wasn't until I used my HAE emergency meds during a headache that it became more obvious that the intracranial pressure issues were likely connected to swelling around the brain from HAE, as all symptoms completely disappeared with medication administration. I also began to make more retrospective observations about HAE triggers; for example, my venom immunotherapy in 2016-2017 preceded a significant increase in the frequency of HAE attacks. I noticed that my left arm (where I'd originally had all my injections) continued to swell for years after stopping the venom injections, especially when my HAE was flared up. To this day, the venom injection sites continue to swell up several times a week and anytime I exercise with my left arm.

Despite these new considerations and feeling grateful to finally have big picture answers about my abdominal attacks, I was growing in despair that the attacks were becoming so frequent. I was at a general loss to figure them out. I was eating clean and going to great lengths to eliminate toxins and promote a well-rounded, healing lifestyle. The attacks persisted even after I finished the IV treatments, eliminated medications, added probiotics, and further addressed parasite and SIBO issues. I could not connect any particular foods as triggers to attacks, but began to notice that previously benign factors like caffeine or exposure to a chlorinated swimming pool were consistent HAE attack triggers. However, most of the time, I would simply wake up in the morning and they would be there.

I tried to stay positive and focused on my "passion projects." I began making a website of resources for patients with MCAS. I continued to work on this book. I brainstormed ideas for

MCAS advocacy and ways for patients to connect to each other on a more personal, one-on-one basis.

In the spring of 2018, I had a large ovarian cyst rupture and went from having near-daily attacks to HAE symptoms less than 50% of the time. It was a huge turning point for me and reinforced the theory that estrogen was strongly connected to my HAE issues. I finished the IV treatments and continued addressing concerns like SIBO, mold and parasites with my naturopath. But I was largely improved to the point where, on "good" days I could walk by a smoker or hike up a mountain without major issues (preferably, not in that order)!

At Home in Colorado

In the fall of 2018, I moved to Colorado where, after nearly three years of a long-distance relationship, Graham and I finally lived in the same place. I was thrilled! In spite of several dental-related HAE attacks, health-related housing snafus and one water leak 5 days after we moved into our 3rd housing option, my entire system seemed to do better in Colorado. I still had occasional MCAS reactions, like when my boyfriend tried a new deodorant, or when he returned from a work trip to Houston with mold spores permeating his pores. (All I can say is, what a trooper! His patience has been such an incredible blessing.)

I had switched to a new magnesium supplement around the time of the move, which seemed to significantly help with my gastrointestinal motility issues. I had also continued to work with my naturopathic care team on determining which supplements were most effective, and was now stable on a once-daily dose of ketotifen, plus magnesium, soil-based probiotics, estrogen-reducing supplements, selenomethionine, CBD oil, and a supplement containing antioxidants, adaptogens from mushrooms, and vitamins/minerals. I continued to take GI Detox Plus, a toxin binder, a few times a week as able. I used Firazyr as rescue medication for HAE throat and abdominal swells as needed, and was still waiting to get a prophylactic HAE medication option approved by insurance.

But at the end of the day, I knew that my improvements were not related to one particular supplement, medication or diterary approach, but rather, the cumulative effort of diagnosing and treating the root issues that contributed to my perfect storm of chronic illness factors. While the dietary changes and herbal supplements were important, I never felt like those factors alone were enough to counteract the overload of systemic issues I had going on, at least initially. (Though I do like to think that my healing was accelerated by those factors.) It was not until I addressed viral and bacterial infections that I began to notice significant progress. And my recent success also required a period of over one year (during, as well as post-IV treatments) as I attempted to persevere through the times when the progress seemed glacially slow, or even reversed, as I attempted to unclutter my system from so many different toxic burdens.

As my own health journey evolved, I became more and more engrossed in research for this book. It was overwhelming yet invigorating in so many ways. I was fortunate to have the chance to interview a number of experts in the field and attempted to communicate with a wide range of medical professionals in order to present a thorough summary of MCAS in this book.

My book research led me to investigate a type of testing and treatment called CranioBiotic Technique (CBT). Devised by Dr. Tony Smith in Idaho, CBT evaluates the system for underlying root issues such as viruses, bacterial infections and gastrointestinal problems utilizing energetic muscle testing. If abnormalities are present, a treatment is conducted that alerts the brain to 1) what infection or health stressor is likely present, and 2) where it appears to be present, so that the immune system can effectively target and remove the problem naturally. The technique also includes a simple form of allergy testing and treatment.

While I was trained medically in a classic mainstream environment, I found myself fascinated by CBT and other holistic healing methods. As I stabilized more and more under a quality naturopathic care program, I began to dream of resuming patient care again—but this time, with a more integrative approach. I attended a training conference for CBT in the fall of 2018 and was astounded by the results. Subsequent evaluation(s) indicated that my immune system was still struggling to resolve health stressors including clostridium difficile, strep, staph, toxoplasmosis, Epstein-Barr virus, parasites, SIBO, Lyme disease and its coinfections, mycoplasma pneumonia, aspergillus, candida, protozoal infections, borrelia, and other viruses.

The treatment received as I practiced the technique with colleagues dramatically improved my own health, and I gained further confidence as I noted improvements in chronically unwell colleagues, friends and family members who I went on to treat with CBT. The first person I treated was able to reverse the thyroid disease that had plagued her for years—her blood work came back normal within a few months! More and more affirmations of the effectiveness of the approach began to reveal themselves, and I decided to embrace CBT as an important tool in my box of options for patients with chronic pain and fatigue, not as a physical therapist but as a holistic medicine provider.

Unfortunately, CBT (as a tool for both diagnosis and treatment) does not yet have any randomized controlled trials to support its benefits. It was the first time that I pursued professional continuing education for a technique that was not "evidence based" and yet it seemed to be the most effective resource I'd come across. I went back and forth through the mental tug of war of wanting to promote this incredible tool and also knowing that colleagues could be skeptical of it.

At the end of the day, I believe that if the technique is approached the right way (without making outlandish diagnostic claims) and used in conjunction with other tools, it's unethical to *not* consider using it when I know it could benefit a patient. The technique itself is natural in the sense that it involves gentle finger/hand pressure on points on the body and the skull, posing no risk to patients. When compared to the antibiotics and other medications that are often first-line options with these patients, CBT offers a way for the body to potentially restore health naturally by moving the immune system in the right direction to eliminate health stressors on its own. Patients with chronic illness are likely influenced by a set of unique and specific factors, and I believe that treating the symptoms without aiding the immune system in addressing underlying systemic issues (such as gastrointestinal inflammation/dysbiosis, viral and bacterial infections) remains a suboptimal Band-Aid approach treatment for this patient population.

Addressing the complete picture of mind, body and spiritual wellness was essential for my own progress in healing from chronic illness, and it was something that I was excited to share with patients. I was also profoundly and pleasantly surprised to note that my chronic orthopedic inflammatory issues (such as neck and back pain) essentially spontaneously resolved once I properly addressed the bacterial, viral, and detoxification issues my body was fighting for so long. It became clear that a similar approach could be of great benefit for patients with chronic musculoskeletal pain, chronic fatigue and fibromyalgia, instead of simply focusing on the particular location(s) of pain in isolation.

Over time, I devised a dream model for patient "functional PT" care that incorporates an assortment of focuses including restoring parasympathetic nervous system activation, addressing trauma and PTSD, targeting underlying health stressors including viruses, bacterial infections, and gastrointestinal dysfunction, starting programs for special populations (such as patients with Ehlers-Danlos syndrome and POTS), integrating nutritional and detoxification resources, and incorporating visceral manipulation and craniosacral techniques, all in combination with my traditional physical therapy tools like manual therapy, dry needling, and patient-specific exercise—perhaps the topic of my next book!

A Full-Circle Journey

Over time, I regained enough stability to resume certain passions of mine and increased physical activity on most days of the week. I was certainly not feeling 100% but was so grateful that I could consider returning to some type of modified work. And in late 2018, I found myself able to consider international travel again—one of my biggest passions!

As I headed over to South Africa in November of 2018 for a wedding celebration with Graham and a group of old friends, I marveled at how far I'd come from a place of rock bottom over the past 3 years. Aspects of travel were still difficult—the inevitable exposure to other passengers perfumes or cleaning supplies for long periods, restaurant cigarette smoke, food choice difficulties, walking by those ridiculous duty free stores in airports, insecticide sprayed inside the airplane in Africa while onboard(!), lack of filtered water, laundry challenges, lack of sleep, immune system issues—but it was still so empowering to resume that aspect of my life that I'd assumed I'd have to give up or modify greatly as a result of medical conditions. And each time I encountered an environmental challenge, I attempted to reframe it mentally and to flood my soul with gratitude for the fact that I was there in the first place, as opposed to a need to control my situation.

Today, I still struggle with wanting to be in control of my health, but I feel like I've made significant progress in terms of my MCAS symptoms, and I am able to manage things with mostly a natural supplement-based approach combined with diet and lifestyle modifications that promote a focus on fruits and vegetables that supply the body with antioxidants and complexes that are natural mast cell stabilizers. Anaphylaxis and epinephrine injections are becoming a distant memory. Chronic symptoms fluctuate but are greatly improved. HAE attack triggers remain a problematic enigma, but have decreased in intensity and frequency. I keep putting one foot in front of the other in the hopes that I will see further healing in this area soon as well.

I continue to be amazed that Graham remains by my side, and that he never doubted me or questioned the validity of what I was experiencing. My saint of a boyfriend has been with me from the "drowning in invisible symptoms stage" to multiple misdiagnoses, the diagnostic clarity of MCAS and HAE, the pursuance of further resources in terms of root causes, and the fusion of mainstream and naturopathic journeys to healing. Fortunately, he also knew "the old me" when we were teenagers and has the interesting perspective of knowing innate aspects of my personality but also having awareness of the MCAS-associated chemical mediator-induced frenzy that became especially apparent in adulthood.

I'm blessed with a wonderful additional support system including my loving parents and sister and brother-in-law, my boyfriend's amazing parents, a fantastic bunch of extended family, and one-of-a-kind friends all over the map. My nieces and nephew bring me daily joy and remind me to not sweat the small stuff. My parents have been unwavering in their love and support and words will never sufficiently express the gratitude I have for them opening their home to me in my biggest time of need.

Faith for the Journey

Throughout this journey, the process of psychological healing, for me, was greatly enriched when I was able to fully grasp the depths of God's love for me and the powers of grace and mercy in my life. It meant active efforts to break down the patterns of struggles with feelings of "not enough" or needing to earn my salvation and stay busy in order to be worthy. And, at the end of the day, it meant that I had to place my trust completely in God and lift my fears and the desire to be in control upward while simultaneously shifting my focus outward. I certainly cannot say that I mastered these concepts in practice, but I did my best.

Over the past several years, I've had numerous experiences with the repeated theme of the Bible story from the book of Mark, chapter 5. In 2016, two women randomly approached me at a public park in Utah and discussed this particular Bible story and then prayed with me to have faith in God's healing power, even when circumstances seemed so chronically debilitating and hopeless. These two women appeared radiant, almost angelic, and it was as if they already knew me and the struggles that were on my heart that day.

A month later, at a healing mass/prayer service in Arizona, as some ministers were praying with me, one of them suddenly stopped and said "God wants you to revisit Mark 5. Don't be afraid to reach for Jesus like the sick woman." Again, I was completely floored.

Even as I've been writing this book, that particular passage has continued to resurface in moments I needed it most. In the past year, I've had half a dozen people discuss this Bible story with me, often out of the blue, and always in moments when I felt I was in complete (silent, unspoken) despair from the challenges of chronic illness.

Mark 5:24-34 (NIV)[7]

So Jesus went with him. A large crowd followed and pressed around him. And a woman was there who had been subject to bleeding for twelve years. She had suffered a great deal under the care of many doctors and had spent all she had, yet instead of getting better she grew worse. When she heard about Jesus, she came up behind him in the crowd and touched

48

his cloak, because she thought, "If I just touch his clothes, I will be healed." Immediately her bleeding stopped and she felt in her body that she was freed from her suffering.

At once Jesus realized that power had gone out from him. He turned around in the crowd and asked, "Who touched my clothes?"

"You see the people crowding against you," his disciples answered, "and yet you can ask, 'Who touched me?'"

But Jesus kept looking around to see who had done it. Then the woman, knowing what had happened to her, came and fell at his feet and, trembling with fear, told him the whole truth. He said to her, "Daughter, your faith has healed you. Go in peace and be freed from your suffering."

There are a few messages I take away from this repeated theme of Mark 5 in my life. The first is that God sees our suffering and does not wish it upon us. *It is not punishment.* God truly wants us to be well. He wants us to live in peace and be freed from our suffering.

The second is that faith can move mountains. Despite being shuffled from doctor to doctor, and despite carrying a heavy burden of hopelessness, this woman had the courage to reach out, and, *in an instant*, she received miraculous healing. Her faith healed her, despite what she had been through, in spite of the odds, and in spite of a long journey exhausting all potential medical answers and cures.

Contextually, in those times, this woman's disease ostracized her from her own community and deemed her "unclean." Nonetheless, she boldly reached out and received a compassionate and loving response. Jesus wants us to reach for Him and to follow Him, and to *persist in following Him.*

The backstory to the woman with a bleeding disorder was about a man whose daughter was gravely ill. In fact, Jesus was on His way to the man's house when He was slowed by the crowd and the woman who touched him. When the man learned that his daughter had passed away before they'd had time to make it to her, Jesus instructed the man, "Don't be afraid; just believe."[7] He then went on to miraculously revive the man's daughter.

Fear and anxiety often seem overbearing, but focusing on the fact that "God's got this" and "this, too, shall pass" has helped me tremendously. I've lost count of how many times those words have lifted me up as I've struggled with weariness and despair along this path. Fear can be blinding and paralyzing all at once. But faith, even when blind, has carried me through the depths of survival mode as my healing journey has continued to unfold.

Putting It Together

For so long, I could not see how my health experiences could possibly be used for some greater good. Now, however, with deep gratitude, my story has come full circle in some ways, and I look forward to resuming patient care this year with a new approach. I plan to specialize in working with patients who have MCAS, EDS, dysautonomia, and many of the other conditions discussed in this book and am teaming up with other holistic practitioners in northern Colorado to offer patients a diverse toolbox of customizable treatment options. I also hope to get involved with university and continuing education resources in efforts to bridge more of a functional medicine approach into physical therapy practice.

As I look back at my entire patient experience, a number of patterns emerge. For one, my body did not do well with vaccines. Physical trauma in the form of car accidents, insect venom and animal attacks likely contributed to elevations in my symptomatic baseline. Chronic environmental factors like four hours a day of chlorine exposure and living situations that involved water-damaged buildings were likely sources of inflammation, alongside short-term acute toxin exposure like carbon monoxide. Repeated antibiotic use coupled with the standard American diet (until my mid-20's) certainly did not help matters. My body was pushed to the limits in terms of physical activity, workplace stress, and lack of sleep. Emotional trauma from abusive swimming coaches and Peru experiences got pushed under the rug.

For me, while the diagnosis of MCAS brought significant clarity, the profound healing occurred once I stopped focusing on MCAS as a diagnosis and instead began to methodically address *underlying root issues* with the help of several practitioners with a naturopathic type approach.

The following areas were key in my case:

- Addressing chronic inflammation as the result of exposure to mold toxins
- Working on global detoxification system struggles, particularly in the liver, gut and lymphatic system
- Reducing continual exposure to hidden environmental toxins in cleaning supplies, living spaces, beauty products, etc.
- Eliminating exposure to vaccinations and venom immunotherapy
- Reducing any form of food-based contamination, such as pesticides, processed foods, artificial sugar, coffee, gluten, other grains, additives and preservatives, dairy, etc.
- Addressing intestinal dysbiosis, candida and SIBO

- Addressing viral infections like Epstein-Barr virus

- Addressing bacterial infections like Lyme disease and its coinfections

- Factoring in ovarian cysts, hormonal fluctuations and their relationship to symptoms

- Pursuing natural approaches to promoting thyroid and adrenal health

- Addressing parasitic and protozoal infections

- Factoring in neurotransmitter deficiencies

- Reducing sympathetic (fight or flight) nervous system activation and fostering parasympathetic (rest and digest) nervous system activation

- Addressing heavy metal toxicity

- Maintaining some degree of physical activity while avoiding strenuous exercise

- Attending to emotional trauma and focusing on spirituality

I never took a direct approach to some of my diagnoses like POTS or EDS, and found that their symptoms, like my mast cell activation issues, resolved substantially when I addressed the above issues in a naturopathic manner.

While monoclonal MCAS and HAE clearly have genetic influences, I refuse to accept a genetic stance of learned helplessness. I think that the complex interactions of epigenetic factors and the above factors have all contributed to the perfect storm of MCAS and HAE in my life. *A perfect storm that, via extensive trial and error, became apparently more and more reversible with the proper approach.*

When I first started this journey as a newly diagnosed MCAS patient, I was instructed by a doctor to eliminate all dietary sources of histamine, with no instruction on a time frame and with no attention to my individualized reactions. Eliminating most histamine-containing foods caused me to feel slightly better for a number of days or weeks, but then I got sicker and down to very few "safe" foods and had very few healthy options left. When I instead focused on eliminating viruses, mold exposure, chemical toxins, heavy metals, and other everyday triggers to my mast cells, I was able to reintroduce virtually all foods (except my few true anaphylactic allergies I've had my whole life) and was able to reduce my mast cell medications dramatically. In other words, while elimination of high histamine dietary items may have felt helpful for a short while initially, it was nowhere near as powerful as eliminating other triggers for my long-term health. And for me, the resulting nutrient-devoid, low-histamine diet was far from ideal for healing from other issues.

When all was said and done, I estimated that I'd seen over 100 specialists over nearly 18 years, including gastroenterologists, ENTs, neurologists, rheumatologists, nutritionists, speech therapists, physical therapists, internal medicine doctors, urologists, cardiologists, emergency medicine practitioners, gynecologists, orthopedic doctors and surgeons, pulmonologists, dermatologists, ophthalmologists, asthma specialists, psychiatrists, psychologists, allergy/immunology specialists, family medicine doctors, naturopaths, functional medicine doctors, infectious disease/parasite specialists, and one unidentified and questionable specialist who performed a rectal exam in Peru (ha!).

It goes without saying that no two patients with MCAS are alike, and my personal example is certainly not a "classic" case of MCAS, as there's no such thing. Likewise, the things that I tried for treatment should not serve as a blueprint for patients struggling with the disease. *It's imperative that patient care is guided by the help of a holistic team of practitioners at all times.*

Over the course of the past year and a half, I've heard the stories of hundreds—if not thousands—of patients who have MCAS and a whole host of other medical problems and diagnoses, just like me. Why are so many patients testing positive for MCAS plus *x, y and z*? If we zoom out and take a giant step backward from MCAS, it begs the questions: Am I really so unlucky that I have these 10 to 20 diagnoses? Can it be that MCAS is causing all of them, or is it actually that my immune system and detoxification capabilities are weakened to the point where I'm like that sticky fly trap paper, collecting new bugs left and right, which are contributing to my mast cell activation issues?

Thus, I believe that we can't point a finger of blame at "just Lyme disease" or "just MCAS." Holistic healing involves stepping away from labels and diagnoses. We need a huge overhaul of our belief system about where these problems come from; we need to shift away from stopping once we have labels for these symptoms and focusing our intervention on a passive (medication only) approach. We need to ditch learned-helplessness sentiments and empower ourselves to make important lifestyle changes that may be difficult but will later reap rewards. We need to focus on a more proactive lifestyle change that addresses all potential triggers that could account for this immune system tornado of viral, bacterial, and toxin debris that together leave a very destructive path. We need to address our immune system as a whole and we need to provide the right environment to facilitate healing.

I recognize that my story will resonate with some MCAD sufferers, while others won't find many commonalities. The variety of chemical mediators, genetic variability, and environmental factors lend to a consistently unique constellation of symptoms among sufferers despite sharing the exact same disease. My understanding is also that many people with MCAS have comorbidities that make their situation even more unique. The presence of Epstein-Barr virus and Lyme disease are two examples that commonly coexist and overlap with MCAS and manifest in different ways, nonetheless making the differentiation of symptom origin tricky at best. And I now know that my description of abdominal attacks is more hereditary angioedema–driven than caused by MCAS, though I suspect that MCAS plays a role in the attacks and that the two conditions feed off each other.

My resume is a colorful example of my many efforts to make changes and start over in the hopes that my career or a certain stressful job was triggering symptoms. I've blamed so many things over the years and experienced false hope that "if I just try harder, or if I just change this one aspect of my life, I'll feel better." It took me a long time, but I now realize that this mindset only strives to gain some sense of control. Ultimately, the greatest healing has come from surrendering all of this to God and also embracing, with gratitude, every bit of healing I experience, each and every good moment, each and every blessing and wonderful relationship in my life, and each and every fork in my path that has led to the (imperfect) place of where I am today.

I recognize that my suffering has been meaningful and I'm grateful for this opportunity to share my story—but, more importantly, to attempt to raise awareness and provide more patient and provider information about MCAS. Within this process I'm continuing to learn that this book will never be perfect or feel like it's complete. I'm sure you'll find many flaws within it, and I hope that you will overlook them with kindness, as my aim all along has been to provide healing resources for others.

At the end of the day, I hope that my story helps other patients feel less alone and perhaps even gives them confidence that their future can include more answers and improvements in chronic MCAS symptoms. We are facing an era of widespread, chronic, and debilitating "mystery" illness, massive exposure to toxins, and a medical system that turns down the flame without putting out the original fire. In spite of these challenges, there is still great reason to have hope. I believe that the future depends on uniting mainstream and natural medicine approaches to provide patients with the tools that they need to find long-lasting healing from chronic disease. One step at a time, let's keep this hope alive.

Chapter Two

The Mast Cell

MAST CELL OVERVIEW

Before diving into mast cell activation disease specifics, it's useful to have a basic understanding of the physiological role of the mast cell in the human body.

Researchers Walker and colleagues describe mast cells (MCs) as the "jack-of-all-trades immune cells" that have the ability to interact with and modulate the function of many different cells throughout the entire body.[1] They have also been called "Yin Yang" modulators in allergic responses because they possess the ability to both suppress and add inflammation; likewise, mast cells can contribute to both remission and exacerbation of symptoms.[2]

Mast cells are a type of white blood cell that serve as an important part of the body's immune system. Mast cells are present in nearly all types of tissue. Researchers often suggest that mast cells are akin to immune system watchdogs. Ryan and colleagues note, "In keeping with the long-standing theory that mast cells evolved as a means of protection from parasitic infection, these cells seem to be quite important as early sentinels of immune activation."[3] Without them, we would not survive.

Mast cells have the ability to amplify the activation levels of their neighboring immune cells.[4] Compared with other innate immune cells, mast cells can release a substantially higher number and diversity of substances.[4] Mast cells tend to congregate around nerves, blood vessels, and lymphatic tissues. Mast cell mediators gain quick access to the bloodstream due to the locations of mast cells in tissues.[4]

St. John and Abraham discuss a "dual role of mast cells (MCs), both as *sentinels for invading pathogens* and as *regulatory cells* throughout the course of acute inflammation, from its initiation to resolution. This versatility is dependent on the ability of MCs to detect pathogens and danger signals and release a unique panel of mediators to promote pathogen-specific clearance mechanisms, such as through cellular recruitment or vascular permeability."[4]

One of the most "primal" roles of mast cells lies in the attack of parasitic invaders. Mast cell chemical mediators such as histamine regulate the mucus production that leads to parasite expulsion. Communication between mast cells and neurons may assist in other factors like gastrointestinal motility, which aids in the process of parasite removal from the body. Mast cells also recruit other cells, including eosinophils, to the site of parasitic infection.[4] Mast cells and histamine have been found to play a role in a number of different infectious disease scenarios, including malaria transmission and pathogenesis.[5]

It appears that mast cells can promote both beneficial and harmful responses in the same systems and tissue types. For example, mast cell proteases traditionally break down toxins and microbial virulence factors in tissues. In some cases, however, they can have the opposite effect on toxins and intruders. St. John and Abraham note, "Although prompt and localized MC activation during infection usually is beneficial, systemic and sustained MC activation, typically associated with chronic or severe systemic infections, may not be. MCs (mast cells) may also promote chronic infections and exacerbate associated pathologies depending on the pathogen species and load, the site of infection, or any preexisting inflammatory disease."[4] One example of this is *Helicobacter pylori* infections in patients with chronic gastritis. These types of negative effects of mast cells are more commonly noted in cases where the pathogen load is high and widespread.[4]

While the literature is sparse in terms of studies that have directly examined mast cell interactions with viruses, there are some examples. Marshall and colleagues note "substantial evidence of direct mast cell infection and mast cell cytokine and chemokine responses" in the context of dengue virus and HIV-1 infection. Influenza A and Sendai viruses have been found to interact with mast cells and are associated with mast cell proliferation in affected patients. Respiratory Syncytial Virus (RSV) is a common cause of lower respiratory infections in at-risk populations such as young children, and its etiology is not completely understood. Some research indicates that RSV is connected to mast cells.[6]

A 2003 review concluded that "the location, range of mediator production and receptor repertoire of mast cells makes them ideal targets of infection for a number of viruses. Moreover, mast cell responses to infection or viral products could be key to host defense and/or disease pathogenesis."[6]

Treatment to kill mast cells is generally not an option when someone has overactive mast cells or too high of a load, because they are critical pieces of human physiology and promote many important processes that are needed to function. It appears that, physiologically, it's all about balance. With mast cell activation disease (MCAD), the fine line between a healthy functioning system and an excess release of chemicals is crossed dramatically.

Mast cells develop from "parent" cells in the bone marrow known as hematopoietic (blood-forming) progenitor cells. They are created in response to stem cell factor (known as *KIT*-ligand) binding to the c-*KIT* receptor called CD117.[7] CD117 is a receptor protein that influences and regulates the growth, survival, migration and effector functions of mast cells.[7] Mast cells spend about four days in the bone marrow before leaving to mature in the peripheral tissues.[8]

The "parent cells" necessary for this process migrate into various tissues, such as the lungs, skin, ocular tissue, and gastrointestinal system. They are found in all tissues, including the brain, endocrine system and even adipose (fat) tissue.[9,10] Mast cells are especially prominent in "boundary" tissue that is located near the external world, such as the skin, lung mucosa, digestive tract, eyes, nose, and mouth. They are found interstitially in the bone marrow, liver, spleen, and lymph nodes.[11] They are present in most tissues that surround blood vessels and nerves. They are very similar to basophils, another type of white blood cell.[12] Once mast cells have migrated into peripheral tissue, they typically remain relatively immobile, with a lifespan of several months to a few years.[8]

MAST CELL MEDIATORS

Mast cells contain granules that they release when signaled, and these granules contain compounds that stimulate other processes to occur. *Compounds* or *mediators* are essentially biologically active chemical molecules that are released by mast cells. The release of these mediators is a normal occurrence when the body perceives a threat, but it's the *excess number* of mast cells releasing granules at once (mastocytosis) or the *degree of sensitivity to which the cells are getting triggered* to release granules (mast cell activation syndrome) that ultimately creates problems.

Degranulation refers to the process of mast cells releasing compounds into the circulatory system. *Preformed mediators* are stored inside secretory granules in mast cells, ready to be released. Examples of well-known preformed mediators include proteases (including tryptase), histamine, serotonin and heparin. Nearly 500 preformed secretory granules are stored in mast cells.[13] Preformed mediators are released within seconds to minutes of mast cell stimulation.

They are typically what are responsible for acute "attacks" of symptoms such as hives, swelling of the face, throat constriction, and changes in blood pressure.[14,15]

Once a mast cell releases chemical mediators, it can re-create additional vesicles to start the process over again. Refractory periods are recovery windows of time that have been noted between cycles of degranulation due to depletion of intracellular granule stores or desensitization following repeated challenges.[4]

There are also compounds that are created in the moment that degranulation occurs, and these are called *newly formed lipid mediators*. Prostaglandins, leukotrienes, platelet-activating factor, and thromboxane are all examples of newly formed lipid mediators.[14,15]

Cytokines and chemokines make up a third category of mediators that mast cells release, though they can also be classified as prestored (chemokines) or newly synthesized (cytokines). Examples of cytokines include most of the interleukins and tumor necrosis factor-alpha. Interleukin-8 is an example of a chemokine.[14,15] Cytokines and chemokines from mast cells act as neuromodulators and have roles in stress, body temperature/fever regulation and the sleep-wake cycle via interactions with the hypothalamic-pituitary-adrenal axis.[16-19]

Mast cells immediately release histamine, heparin, proteases and tumor necrosis factor-alpha in response to a stimulus. Over the next several minutes, the release of prostaglandins and leukotrienes is generally observed. Over the next several hours, cytokines and interleukins (specifically, interleukin-4 and interleukin-13) add to the inflammatory cascade.[7]

It appears that there are different types of mast cells that, depending on their anatomical location, may be more likely to express certain types of interleukins. Mast cells in connective tissue, the peritoneal cavity, and the skin contain tryptase and express interleukin-5 and interleukin-6.[20] In contrast, mast cells in the gastrointestinal tract and respiratory mucosa contain tryptase and chymase and express interleukin-4.[20]

These subtle differences across tissue location are further influenced by the ability of certain chemical mediators to self-regulate aspects of mast cell function. Interleukin-3, interleukin-4, interleukin-9 and transforming growth factor beta one (TGFB1) have been found to influence mast cell mediator content and the overall number of mast cells in the body.[21,22] This example highlights one important mechanism of mast cells: Mast cells have the ability, via chemical mediators, to influence both the reaction to triggers and the subsequent self-regulation of mast cell-associated baseline activity in the body.

Stem cell factor appears to play a central role in the mechanisms that underlie mast cell regulation. Mast cells and their progenitors are drawn to target tissues from the bone marrow by the "scent" of a chemical attractant called stem cell factor (SCF). According to Okayama and colleagues, "SCF also elicits cell-cell and cell-substratum adhesion, facilitates the proliferation, and sustains the survival, differentiation, and maturation of mast cells. Therefore, many aspects of mast cell biology can be understood as interactions of mast cells and their precursors with SCF and factors that modulate their responses to SCF and its signaling pathways."[23]

Mast cells also have the ability to secrete mitochondrial DNA and release exosomes that are capable of delivering DNA and micro RNAs to other cell types. Thus, they not only "dump chemicals" but they also affect the endocrine and energy system by their DNA secretion.[7] Mast cells mediators are unique in that they have both *autocrine* and *paracrine* function, meaning that they exert hormonal effects on other surrounding cells as well as on themselves. Mast cells are affected by most hormones and neurotransmitters.[9] Mast cells express receptors for hormones, neurotransmitters, neuropeptides, pathogens, and allergens, and they also have the ability to synthesize and release endorphins, leptin, melatonin, substance P, vasoactive intestinal polypeptide, corticotropin-releasing hormone, adrenocorticotropin hormone, and many other neurohormonal triggers.[9]

Mast cells are able to *selectively release proinflammatory mediators* without degranulation occurring when their Fc receptors (cell surface proteins) are bound by non-IgE immunoglobulins, cytokines, neuropeptides and anaphylatoxins.[24] Examples of this include stress-induced corticotropin-releasing hormone, which triggers the selective release of vascular endothelial growth factor, and interleukin-1, which can trigger the selective release of interleukin-6.[25] As another example, in response to pathogens, bacteria bind to mast cell toll-like receptors which can cause selective release of interleukins and tumor necrosis factor without the release of histamine and tryptase.[26] Serotonin and eicosanoids (such as prostaglandins and leukotrienes) also have evidence of selective release without degranulation.[24]

Corticotropin-releasing hormone (CRH) has been theorized to play a big role in chronic inflammation. CRH is set off by nonimmune triggers, including acute stress, and it binds to receptors on mast cells and sensory nuclei.[24] This results in the release of a number of chemical mediators that increase the permeability of the blood-brain barrier.[24] This CRH cascade has been connected to a number of chronic conditions including multiple sclerosis and other neurological diseases, skin conditions, joint inflammation, bladder conditions, cardiopulmonary inflammation, and gastrointestinal complications.[24]

While testing for mast cell activation syndrome (MCAS) relies on a small number of very specific mediators, it's important to remember that mast cells, from a physiological perspective, have evolved to be extremely far-reaching, and allergen responses encompass one small aspect of their role within the human body.

CHEMICAL MEDIATOR SPECIFICS

Some sources estimate that there are over 200 identified mast cell mediators that are released in response to different triggers.[27] This is one of the reasons that it's difficult to "catch" or diagnose mast cell activation disease (MCAD) based on blood or urine samples; there are many mediators released and every patient is a little bit different in regards to which chemical mediator may be high at a given time, depending on the day and a multitude of external and internal factors. Each mediator has its own specific response down the chain, which can explain the wide range of symptoms experienced by patients.

Table 1 shows some of the responses to the release of certain mast cell mediators. While there's a multitude of potential chemical mediators released by mast cells, this chapter will go more in-depth on a few of the mediators that are most commonly associated with mast cell activation syndrome (MCAS) in the literature or "easily" tested in the blood or urine.

Table 1. Common Mast Cell Mediators: Actions and Symptom Correlation[15,28]

MEDIATOR	ACTION	SYMPTOMS TRIGGERED WHEN IN EXCESS
Histamine	Vasodilation, angiogenesis, mitogenesis, pain, bronchoconstriction	Headache, low blood pressure, redness, swelling, itching, intestinal cramping, diarrhea, increased gastric acid, urticaria, activation of leukocytes, throat symptoms
Tryptase	Tissue damage, inflammation, pain; level indicates mast cell numbers, not severity of disease	Leads to low HDL ("good") cholesterol and high LDL ("bad") cholesterol (even in patients with good diets), degrades tissue, causes inflammation
Prostaglandin D2	Bronchoconstriction, vasoregulation, pain	Constriction of airways, flushing, itching, low blood

		pressure, runny nose/mucus secretion, arrhythmias, low bone mineral density
Leukotriene	Vasoconstriction, pain	Narrowing of blood vessels, constriction of airways, increases in vascular permeability and contractibility
Heparin	Angiogenesis, nerve growth factor stimulation	Swelling, anaphylaxis, inflammation, inhibited clotting; long-term effects decrease bone mineral density
Serotonin	Vasoconstriction, pain	Raises blood pressure, increases breathing rate and heart rate, intensifies mood, increases appetite, suppresses insulin release from pancreas

Histamine

Histamine is perhaps the best-known mast cell mediator in the MCAS patient population, and it's been the source of recent attention in terms of its role in the development of "histamine intolerance." A more in-depth conversation about the role of histamine in MCAS patients and a look at the theory behind histamine intolerance and a low-histamine diet will be featured in Chapter 11.

From a physiological perspective, as a chemical mediator, histamine is a potent vasodilator that exerts widening effects on blood vessels, which can cause the systemic blood pressure to drop. This is commonly seen during anaphylactoid reactions.[29] Elevated histamine-related symptoms are also observed in the premenstrual window.[30] Histamine is broken down in the body by either diamine oxidase (DAO) or histamine N-methyl transferase (HNMT).[29]

While other cells do produce histamine, it's been shown that up to 50% of total brain histamine is synthesized by mast cells; 90% of histamine in the thalamus comes from mast cells.[31,32] Histamine appears to work in conjunction with other chemical mediators released by mast cells. Histamine-induced vasodilation helps facilitate the movement of certain molecules toward target organs (even in tissues that lack active degranulation).[3]

There are four types of histamine receptors. Most patients are familiar with histamine 1 (H1) and histamine 2 (H2) receptors, which have over-the-counter medications available as anti-allergy (H1) and acid-reducing (H2) functions.[29]

Histamine 3 (H3) receptors control the synthesis and release of histamine in the central nervous system. Researchers believe that the development of H3 receptor-targeting medications may provide improvements in cognitive dysfunction, memory difficulties, obesity, nasal congestion, Alzheimer's disease, narcolepsy, some forms of epilepsy, and attention deficit hyperactivity disorder (ADHD), though these claims warrant further investigation.[29]

Histamine 4 (H4) receptors are a more recent discovery, and they control immune functions including the chemotaxis of cells (including mast cells and eosinophils) and interleukin-6 release from lymphocytes, similar to the function of H2 receptors. Due to the role of eosinophils in airway inflammation, the development of H4 receptor-targeting medications may provide future assistance for patients with asthma.[29] There are also preliminary indications that future H4-targeting medications may benefit the rheumatoid arthritis population.[29]

The symptomatic effects of histamine may be strongly dictated by which type of receptor is activated. Histamine is commonly associated with increased anxiety levels. Interestingly, a 2008 review noted that, based on several studies, "histamine has been assigned both anxiolytic (anxiety-reducing) and anxiogenic (anxiety-generating) effects, with opposing roles attributed to H1 versus H2 receptors."[16]

Histamine release is associated with numerous physiological reactions and physical symptoms that are associated with its neurotransmitter properties. Within seconds to 24 hours of exposure, patients may experience skin reactions, anaphylactoid-type episodes, gastrointestinal symptoms (including pain, diarrhea, vomiting, bloating, and constipation), fatigue, flushing, eye and visual issues, anxiety, numbness and tingling, blood pressure drops, environmental chemical reactions, shortness of breath, urinary symptoms, auditory problems, muscle weakness and bone pain, chest pain, sinus problems, temperature sensitivities and intolerances, and poor tolerance to exercise.[33,34]

Histamine-associated symptoms may also be experienced as part of a delayed reaction.[34] Histamine has been connected to poor sleep regulation, gastrointestinal issues, headaches, neurological conditions, difficulty with memory and learning, impaired libido, and dozens of other symptoms experienced on a chronic basis.[33,34]

Histamine levels have been associated with difficult/painful menstruation (dysmenorrhea). Dysmenorrhea has long been associated with prostaglandin levels, but it also appears that histamine plays a role. Some women experience a drop in diamine oxidase (DAO) levels with a significant spike in histamine prior to menstruation, which may be responsible for dysmenorrhea.[35] Histamine has a strong contractile effect on the myometrium, and patients with dysmenorrhea may experience increased uterine contractility due to the activation of uterine H1 receptors.[35] Jarisch noted the clinical observation that usage of an H1 blocker on the first day of menstruation appeared to alleviate cramping pain.[35] Histamine levels have been found to be high at the time of ovulation and may also be connected to estrogen/estradiol levels.[35]

Histamine testing via blood and urine samples is widely commercially available and is an important test to include when evaluating a patient for MCAS.

Tryptase

Tryptase is a protein serinase that is specific to secretory granules in mast cells. Tryptase has been deemed by researchers to be the "most abundant protein product of human mast cells."[36] It's been estimated to comprise 20% of the total protein found in mast cells.[37] Out of all the mast cell mediators, it's the one that is most widely accepted and tested by mainstream medical doctors when a patient presents with signs of MCAD.

Tryptase is perhaps most notorious for its role in anaphylactic reactions. Tryptase has been associated with increased vascular permeability and skin microvascular leakage and bronchoconstriction. Tryptase also has the ability to stimulate the release of histamine.[36] Tryptase is more likely to be elevated in non-food-triggered cases of anaphylaxis such as exposure to Hymenoptera venom (bee, wasp, yellowjacket or hornet stings).[38]

On a chronic basis, it appears that tryptase also coordinates a number of very important ongoing physiological processes. Tryptase plays an important role in angiogenesis, or the growth of new blood vessels. Blockage of tryptase specifically may cause a 73%-88% decrease in vascular tube formation.[39]

Tryptase may also serve as an overall regulator of baseline mast cell activity. Tryptase appears to function as an amplification signal for mast cell activation of neighboring cells, and its blockage may reduce overall mast cell activity.[36]

Tryptase is generally believed to be a better indicator of overall *mast cell load* than activation. The blood test is useful for identifying patients with systemic mastocytosis (and some MCAS patients), but it is not the only test that should be used when evaluating for MCAD.

Prostaglandins

Prostaglandins are hormone-like chemicals called eicosanoids that come from fatty acids. They play numerous roles in the body, from blood vessel dilation and smooth muscle contraction to actions that are both inflammatory and anti-inflammatory. Unfortunately, they tend to be more heavily attributed to inflammatory reactions in patients with MCAD. The swelling, stiffness, flushing, and warmth experienced with inflammatory reactions are often attributed in part to prostaglandins. Prostaglandins may also play a role in body temperature regulation, sleep and pain.[16,40-43]

With the female menstrual cycle, some attest that prostaglandins are in higher concentration in the follicular phase. The follicular phase begins on the first day of menstruation and ends with ovulation. The increase in cramping, bloating, headache and joint symptoms that many women experience at this time in their cycle may be attributed to prostaglandins, regardless of whether they have MCAD. Mast cells with low granule content (indicative of degranulation) have also been found during the premenstrual phase in the endometrium.[44] Additional sources support that prostaglandins have preovulatory and premenstrual peaks that may be responsible for increased symptoms in these time frames.[45]

Prostaglandins are believed to play a large role in atherosclerosis, or the thickening of blood vessel walls that can lead to heart problems.[46] Prostaglandins have been linked to arthritis, cancer, strokes, and neurological conditions.[46] The initial inflammatory response following their release is a beneficial event that can restore tissue structure and function, but over time the chemical can contribute to tissue damage and scarring, decreased organ function, and autoimmune characteristics.[46]

Prostaglandins are generated by the COX enzymes from arachidonate. Elevated prostaglandins are often treated with aspirin (for those with MCAD who can tolerate it), and their biosynthesis is blocked by nonsteroidal anti-inflammatory drugs including selective COX 2 inhibitors.[46] (Keep in mind, however, that not all patients with MCAS tolerate aspirin products well.)

There are several different prostaglandins in the human body: Prostaglandin E2 (PGE2) is involved with the immune response, blood pressure regulation, GI integrity, fertility, and inflammation.[46] Prostacyclin (PGI2) mediates edema and pain and regulates cardiovascular function, including roles with vasodilation, clotting and generation of vascular smooth muscle.[46] The increased risk for ulcers when taking NSAIDS is attributed to the disruption of PGE2 and PGI2 pathways, which play protective roles in the integrity of tissue in the stomach

64

and intestine.[46] PGI2 is mainly synthesized in the heart and blood vessels.[47] PGE2 is mainly synthesized in the kidneys, heart, and spleen.[47]

Prostaglandin D2 (PGD2), the third type, is the most widely known with MCAD for its "ease" of measuring in the laboratory and its role in allergic reactions. PGD2 plays a role in inflammation and homeostasis and is made in the tissues as well as the central nervous system.[46] On the tissue level, its release can be triggered by an acute allergic response.[46] Its role in the brain is connected to sleep regulation, headaches, and pain perception. PGD2 has also been connected to acute asthmatic reactions, including bronchoconstriction and eosinophil infiltration in the airway.[46] It may be a more potent bronchoconstrictor than histamine in humans.[48] In the heart, it has been expressed in coronary plaques with severe narrowing. PGD2 is capable of activating multiple signaling pathways in the body at once, since different receptors bind to it and since it is synthesized all over the body.[46]

Prostaglandin F2a (PGF2a) and 9a,11b-PGF2a are metabolites of PGD2. PGF2a tends to test high in both acute and chronic inflammation and is also connected to elevated calcium concentration within the cells.[46] This prostaglandin is most associated with playing important roles in ovulation and uterine contraction in childbirth. Elevated PGF2a is also seen with conditions such as kidney disease, heart disease, brain injury, glaucoma, tachycardia, rheumatoid arthritis, and other types of arthritis.[46] PGF2a is mainly synthesized in the kidneys, heart and spleen.[47]

PGD2 or its metabolite 9a,11b-PGF2a may be ordered in a 24-hour urine sample for patients with suspected MCAS.

Leukotrienes

Leukotrienes are eicosanoid lipid mediators that are derived from arachidonic acid, the precursor to prostaglandins; they are functionally and structurally similar to prostaglandins.[49] Leukotrienes play a role in inflammation and a number of homeostatic mechanisms in the body. The most notable roles of leukotrienes in the MCAS patient lie in airway constriction and the regulation of blood vessels.

Leukotrienes have the ability to attract eosinophils into the bronchioles, which is associated with smooth muscle twitchiness and general bronchial hyperreactivity. It appears that leukotrienes play a role in the triggering of both acute asthma attacks and more chronic long-term hypersensitivity of the airway in patients with asthma.[50]

There's a great body of research surrounding the role of leukotrienes in patients who experience respiratory symptoms, including the asthmatic patient. Leukotriene receptor antagonist medications are frequently used in this patient population. A 2015 meta-analysis confirmed that leukotriene receptor antagonists are effective when compared to placebo for the treatment of asthma in adults and adolescent patients.[51] These medications are sometimes also prescribed for patients with MCAS who have airway inflammation, and leukotrienes remain a useful mediator to have tested in the diagnostic process for MCAS.

Heparin

Heparin is a naturally occurring anticoagulant that is found in mast cells and basophils and tends to be released at blood vessel sites that have damaged tissue. In addition to influencing clot formation, heparin plays a role in immunity against foreign invaders.

In normal circumstances, heparin acts as a blood thinner. Elevated levels of heparin may cause noticeable symptoms such as the tendency to bleed or bruise easily, nosebleeds, and, in more severe cases, blood in the urine or stool.

In the case of excess heparin in the blood, antibodies may mistakenly cause an immune response to heparin, which can lead to inappropriate platelet activation, low platelet counts (known as thrombocytopenia) and the formation of blood clots.[52] Excess heparin levels can be caused by anticoagulation therapy where patients are prescribed heparin, and in theory a similar scenario could occur if mast cells are releasing excess heparin.[52]

Heparin has a short half-life, and while it's an excellent indicator of mast cell activation, it can be somewhat difficult to get accurate test results due to issues with temperature and time delays in testing. (More information on heparin testing suggestions will be shared in Chapter 6.)

Chromogranin A

Chromogranin A is a protein that has a profound impact on the endocrine system and hormones. It has been called the "on/off switch that alone is sufficient to drive dense-core secretory granule biogenesis and hormone sequestration in endocrine cells."[53] Endocrine and neuroendocrine cells are influenced by hormones. The thyroid and sexual organs (testicle, ovary and placenta) are the areas most associated with the endocrine system, but it also includes the pancreas, pituitary gland, thymus, parathyroid gland, pineal gland, hypothalamus, and adrenal glands.

These glands control everything from metabolism to sleep regulation to energy levels and mental health (and much more). The hormones that regulate these processes are synthesized in an area called the rough endoplasmic reticulum before they are transported to the Golgi complex. From there they undergo a complex sorting process where they are "packaged" into a vesicle that allows them to be transported to their target area. Chromogranin A is a key player in interactions that occur in the control center, driving the packaging of the granules within the cells so that they can be utilized in the tissues.[53]

Chromogranin A likely plays other roles. The mediator is currently under investigation in regards to its role in gastrointestinal symptoms and irritable bowel syndrome.[54] While it may test high in MCAS, elevated levels of Chromogranin A have also been associated with neuroendocrine tumors and heart and kidney issues.

There is some debate as to the utility of Chromogranin A in testing for MCAS. A 2017 study determined that Chromogranin A was associated with proton pump inhibitor use but *not* with mast cell burden or activation.[55] However, that study was more specific to mastocytosis and has yet to be replicated.

Chromogranin A currently remains on the list of recommended mediators for MCAS testing according to some experts.[56]

Serotonin

Serotonin is *not* a mediator that is considered diagnostic for MCAS, but it may have some connections with mast cells and mental health. Serotonin is a neurotransmitter most known for its influence on mood and anxiety, but it also plays a number of additional biological roles. Serotonin influences memory, nerve growth, appetite, aggression, and emotions.[16,57-59] Serotonin also influences tissue regeneration, mast cell adhesion and chemotaxis, tumor growth, and cell growth and development.[60] Serotonin influences cell proliferation, migration, and death.[61] It has been associated with regulation of body temperature, sleep cycles, and learning.[61]

Low serotonin levels may be associated with anxiety and depression in patients with MCAS. A 2008 review noted that "selective serotonin reuptake inhibitors increase serotonin signaling and decrease anxiety; therefore, a lack of mast cell derived serotonin may result in an increase in anxiety-like behaviors."[16]

There are several connections that explain the mechanisms that influence serotonin. Tryptophan is a neurotransmitter that regulates mood, and it is a precursor to serotonin.[62] Tryptophan is partly regulated by cortisol, the stress hormone, and elevated levels of stress may contribute to low levels of serotonin.[63] Low levels of serotonin and high levels of cortisol are associated with mood symptoms.[63] The mechanisms between serotonin, tryptophan and cortisol have complex inter-relationships; decreased dietary tryptophan or increased emotional stress appear to be the greatest potential factors that may contribute to the regulation of serotonin.[64]

Genetic mutations likely contribute to predisposition to low serotonin levels. Research indicates that subjects who have genetic mutations affecting tryptophan hydroxylase-2 have decreased serotonin synthesis.[65] Additional mast cell mediators (such as tumor necrosis factor, interleukin-2, and interleukin-6) increase the body's breakdown of serotonin, which can more quickly deplete its circulating levels, also contributing to depression/mood symptoms.[66]

In contrast, *elevated* serotonin levels have been associated with carcinoid tumors and abdominal pain in patients with inflammatory bowel disease and irritable bowel syndrome.[67,68] Ingested sources of serotonin do not influence the brain or cross the blood-brain barrier (unlike other molecules such as histamine).[69] While some sources maintain that it's questionable whether intestinal mast cells release serotonin,[70] others assert that the majority of mast-cell derived serotonin is found in the gastrointestinal tract,[68] where it is released during meals. According to senior scientist/molecular biologist and mast cell disease subject matter expert Lisa Klimas, irritating foods may cause the body to release more serotonin to speed up their passage through the GI tract, which can sometimes result in vomiting and excess release of serotonin into the bloodstream.[69]

A 2007 study noted discrepancies in serotonin levels in patients with mastocytosis in a manner similar to a bimodal distribution pattern, where some patients had very high serotonin levels and others had very low levels.[60] The study evaluated 27 patients with mastocytosis and found that about 37% of patients had serotonin levels considered "low" below 50 ng/ml, but about 33% of patients had serotonin levels above the cut-off of 210 ng/ml.[60]

A follow-up study in 2008 performed by the same authors noted the same trend in bimodal distributions of serotonin levels for 29 mastocytosis patients.[71] Low serotonin levels were associated with fatigue, flushing, headaches, diarrhea, abdominal pain, bone pain, and psychiatric symptoms.[71] No correlations were made between serotonin and the number of platelets, level of tryptase, or liver function test results.[71] Low serum serotonin was correlated with neurological and gastrointestinal dysfunction in mastocytosis patients.[71] Based on the findings of both studies, authors concluded that there's likely a subgroup of patients with mastocytosis who present with low serotonin levels that could be contributing to systemic symptoms.[71]

However, despite the findings of these two studies, another source found normal serotonin levels in MCAD patients. In 2011, researchers Butterfield and Weiler evaluated 36 patients with MCAD; 25 patients had systemic mastocytosis, six patients had cutaneous mastocytosis, and five patients were diagnosed with MCAS.[72] No abnormalities in whole blood serotonin levels were noted for any patient in the study.[72] According to the authors, all patients had less than 330 ng/ml serotonin measured, though the criteria for the "low" cut-off was not available for interpretation.[72]

In summary, it appears that serotonin has been recorded to be normal, elevated and lowered in patients with MCAD, with no clear trend. Abnormally low levels *may be* associated with anxiety or depression, fatigue, flushing, headaches, diarrhea, abdominal pain, and bone pain. Abnormally high serotonin levels *may be* associated with gastrointestinal symptoms and carcinoid tumors. Other cells synthesize and release serotonin, so serum measurements are *not* useful for the diagnosis of MCAS.

THE ROLE OF THE MAST CELL IN IMMUNITY

Mast cells play a crucial role in many important bodily processes that occur continuously, including the generation of new blood vessels, the body's ability to repair wounds, the function of the blood-brain barrier, and the immune system's reactions and defenses against intruders. While the immunomodulatory and antimicrobial functions of mast cells can help the body, the autoimmune and neuroinflammatory functions of mast cells (which are in place to protect us) can arise as a slippery slope.[7,73,74] For example, in terms of bacterial and fungal infections, it appears that mast cells are able to either promote host resistance, or they contribute to the dysregulated immune responses that can increase host morbidity and mortality.[75]

Mast cells are unique in that they are effector cells that receive input from immune cells, and they are also regulators of immune cells via exchange of signal molecules and the release of mediators. Thus, they are considered part of both innate and adaptive immunity.[76] Mast cells are active players in both immediate allergic reactions and delayed hypersensitivity reactions. Immediate hypersensitivity reactions are associated with Immunoglobulin E (IgE) antibodies, and delayed hypersensitivity reactions are associated with Immunoglobulin G (IgG) antibodies.

In the 2016 book "Traditional Chinese Medicine, Western Science, and the Fight Against Allergic Disease" Li and Ehrlich elaborate on this concept. "As part of *innate immunity*, mast cells confront infectious agents and ignite a rapid, potent inflammatory response through the release of a soup of mediators. After an initial exposure to an antigen, *acquired immunity* kicks in."[77] The immune system creates IgE antibodies to particular triggers as part of *acquired immunity*. An allergic reaction is triggered when an allergen binds to IgE antibodies on the surface of the mast cell.

Antibodies are y-shaped proteins that are made mainly by plasma cells that identify and neutralize perceived threats. Perceived threats that can result in mast cell activation as part of the body's defense system include contact with bacteria, viruses, fungi, heavy metals, venoms and parasites.[7,78] This process allows for fast recognition of particular invaders or "repeat offenders," allowing the mast cells to react quickly to identify substances and eliminate a threat before it spreads.

When the body recognizes a repeat offender, the IgE molecule binds to receptor sites on the mast cell, which triggers the degranulation process. This by-product of adaptive immunity allows mast cells to rapidly respond to the first hint of a threat before it can spread. In the cases of certain infectious diseases, this is crucial and important for our survival. IgE receptor site binding also explains the rationale for introducing potentially dangerous invaders to the system via vaccine so that the immune system is well equipped to mount a response in the case of future exposure. Li and Ehrlich note, "In the case of smallpox, say, or measles, this is a good thing, and is the rationale for vaccination. Unfortunately for allergic people, they can also become sensitized to otherwise harmless antigens such as pollens and certain food proteins."[77]

When a person becomes sensitized to harmless food or environmental allergens that are wrongfully perceived as toxic to the body, this can translate to unnecessary and misguided mast cell activation. When there's "too much of a good thing," as in the case when mast cells are over-triggered, oversensitive, or overpopulated, excess allergic reactions and anaphylaxis can become a persistent reality.

Chemical mediators released during degranulation are what cause the allergic response symptoms. These mediators have both vasoactive (blood vessel diameter-altering) and proinflammatory effects systemically on the body.[7] The vasoactive effects of chemical mediators are one of the mechanisms associated with chronically abnormal blood pressure and/or acutely altered blood pressure during reactions in patients with MCAS.

Mast cells are involved in allergen sensitization, in theory, at least partly due to their role in controlling the permeability of epithelial barriers. Mast cell mediators influence the recruitment and migration of other cell types, drive further IgE production, and even have the ability to store allergens in lysosomes that have been phagocytosed (engulfed and ingested) within the mast cell following IgE reactions.[2,79]

During the process of allergen sensitization, the neurological system can also be influenced. Based on guinea pig research, during hypersensitivity reactions associated with food allergies, chemical mediators from mast cells provide signals to intrinsic and extrinsic nerve networks in the gut wall, which result in a defensive response.[70]

An increase in the ability of chemicals to cross from the gut to the rest of the body plays a role in allergic reactions. According to Horowitz, "Inside the gastrointestinal tract, an allergic food can come into contact with IgE on the surface of a mast cell and cause an inflammatory reaction that releases histamines as well as inflammatory cytokines. These chemicals can increase intestinal permeability and allow allergens to move into the bloodstream and throughout the body, causing widespread inflammation that leads to anaphylaxis and shock."[80]

A wide variety of immune and nonimmune factors can influence mast cells, and the breadth of these complex pathways reaches far beyond the traditional "allergic reaction" model. On the cellular level, mast cells can be activated by complement, cell-to-cell contact, cytokines, IgG antigen complexes, pathogen-associated molecular patterns, hormones, drugs and physical activation factors, in addition to the "classic allergy" cross-linking of the high-affinity IgE receptor.[1]

The reference to a mast cell-associated "allergic reaction" in this book is referring to the classic *IgE-mediated* response. *IgG reactions* are similar in that the immune system can create specific antibodies that bind to receptors and trigger a response. However, IgG reactions are delayed (sometimes up to three days) and are more implicated in autoimmune-type inflammation than in acute allergic reactions. IgG reactions are mediated in part by basophils (another type of cell), which release inflammatory chemical mediators and cytokines similar to the mechanism of mast cells.[80]

The role of mast cells in IgG reactions has been less widely accepted but is gaining some support in the literature. According to researchers Malbec and Daeron, "The engagement of mast cell IgG receptors by immune complexes may or may not trigger cell activation, depending on the type of mast cell. The contribution of human mast cell IgG receptors in allergies remains to be clarified. Increasing evidence indicates that mast cells play critical roles in IgG-dependent tissue-specific autoimmune diseases."[81]

Focusing only on the allergic aspects of mast cells may be a limitation in clinical practice. Some MCAS experts theorize that allergists may miss the diagnosis of MCAS because they are primarily focused on the adaptive or acquired immune system and focus on testing for *IgE-mediated* mast cell disorders.[77] If a clinician zooms out to look at innate immunity, they may be more likely to adequately pick up on the big picture of MCAS in certain patients. Innate immunity involves a more widespread group of processes that occur via the formation of a physical and chemical protective barrier, the complement system, the orchestration of a number of different types of cell activity, neural regulation, and the global inflammation process that includes recruitment of chemicals such as cytokines to certain areas.

Maitland uses the analogy, "The immune system is like the Bible. It has an Old Testament and a New Testament. Studying only IgE-mediated mast cell activation is like studying the Bible only through the lens of the New Testament."[77] It's evident that not all patients with MCAS present with acute anaphylaxis or allergy-like symptoms. Not all patients with MCAS have the presence of IgE-mediated measurable reactions in the allergist's office. Viewing MCAS solely through the lens of allergic disorders will likely only reveal the tip of the iceberg and may miss out on identifying patients with MCAS. A systemic approach to evaluating patients with potential MCAS appears to be the most fruitful, as explained in Chapter 6.

MAST CELL TRIGGERS

There are numerous stimuli that can induce mast cell activation on the cellular level.

Examples of triggers reported to induce mast cell activation include[7,82,83]:

- physical stimuli (pressure and temperature changes)
- pharmaceutical drugs
- physical or emotional stress
- certain foods
- extreme temperatures (in the air or in water submersion, like a hot tub)
- invasive medical/surgical procedures
- radiocontrast media
- chemical toxins found in cleaning supplies, swimming pools, etc.
- ingredients in personal health and beauty products (such as nail polish, shampoo, deodorant, lipstick, sunblock, etc.)
- mold and water-damaged buildings
- airplane or car travel
- fevers, bacterial infections, the influenza virus, fungal infections, parasites and other viruses
- direct sunlight

- mechanical vibration (such as vibration experienced while sitting on a bus)

- food additives/preservatives such as carrageenan, citric acid, and "natural flavor"

- pesticides and other food source contamination

- caffeine

- alcohol

- secondhand smoke

- radiation and exposure to electromagnetic fields

- surgical implantations and hardware

- insect stings/bites

- occupational environmental factors

This list is certainly not all-inclusive. Triggers tend to vary between patients and will sometimes vary within the same patient over time. "Typical" culprits like pets, dust, and seasonal allergens may or may not be frequent triggers.

Many patients experience spontaneous reactions to food; often, food that they've considered "safe" in the past will suddenly trigger a reaction. Foods that are high in histamine, oxalates, sulfur or salicylates can be problematic for some patients.

Some of the many medications connected to mast cell activation include: NSAIDs (nonsteroidal anti-inflammatory drugs), morphine, muscle relaxants, vancomycin, estradiol, and adenosine.[7] Hormonal medications including combined estrogen-progestin birth control pills and contraceptive injections may be triggers for some patients. ACE-inhibitors interact with mast cells through influence on the angiotensin/renin system, and beta-blockers may increase the risk of anaphylaxis.[84] (Further medication associations and recommendations for this patient population are available in Chapter 9.)

Surgical implantations have been cited as a potential source of increased reactivity. Mast cell activation is associated with reactions to foreign bodies, including biomaterial implants, which may be partly due to fibrin deposits and subsequent edema.[85]

Emotional stress has been cited as the most common trigger in patients with mastocytosis[86] and also appears to play a substantial role in the MCAS population. The mechanism associated with emotional stress may be connected to the release of corticotropin-releasing hormone, which triggers mast cell activation.[7]

CHAPTER KEY POINTS

- Mast cells are a type of white blood cell that are present all over the body and engage in complex interactions with their environment. They are an important type of immune cell that can both suppress and add to inflammation, depending on the circumstances.

- Mast cells have receptors for allergens, pathogens, neurotransmitters, neuropeptides, and hormones.

- Mast cells contain chemical mediators in vesicles that are released when signaled, a process called degranulation. Some of these chemicals are preformed and waiting to be released, while others are synthesized when signaled.

- These chemical mediators influence a vast number of processes throughout the body, and when in excess, can lead to system-wide symptoms. Tryptase, histamine, leukotrienes, and serotonin are examples of well-known mast cell mediators.

- Mast cells are part of innate and adaptive immunity, and contribute to both immediate allergic reactions and delayed hypersensitivity reactions.

- Mast cell triggers are patient-dependent and generally tend to include environmental toxins, dietary factors, exposure to an "invader" (like insect venom or a virus), medications, and physical/emotional stress.

- While over 200 types of mediators exist, laboratory testing for patient diagnosis is limited to a handful of mast cell mediators.

Chapter Three

Mast Cell Activation Disease

THE LINGO

ast cell activation disease (MCAD) is an umbrella term that refers to a group of disorders characterized by[1]

- The accumulation of pathological mast cells in potentially any or all organs and tissues and/or
- The aberrant (abnormal) release of variable subsets of mast cell mediators

In other words, MCAD involves either *too many abnormal* mast cells around the body, and/or the *abnormal release* of too many chemicals by mast cells. Using the analogy of a college party, things can get out of control when a low-key shindig suddenly has 1) too many people show up and the house is jam-packed with rowdy and inebriated individuals or 2) a normal number of people show up, but those folks are all lightweights with sensitive systems that cause them to vomit after one drink. (Let's face it, either scenario is not ideal!)

The term MCAD is sometimes (incorrectly) used interchangeably with **mast cell activation syndrome (MCAS).** MCAD describes the physiological state of disruption in different mast cell properties; MCAS is *one of the several types of MCAD.* In the above example, the house that is too crowded is akin to mastocytosis, a cancer-like condition of concentrated accumulation of too many mast cells. The example of the scenario with a normal number of houseguests who are unusually sensitive to alcohol is an analogy for MCAS, or patients who tend to have normal quantities of mast cells that behave abnormally or in an extra-sensitive way to their environment. MCAS, mastocytosis, and certain types of cancer are all types of MCAD.

"Mast cell activation" is sometimes abbreviated "MCA" in the literature, and describes symptoms of mediator release, but is *not* the same as a *diagnosis* of MCAS or MCAD. Symptoms of mast cell activation can occur with a large number of conditions and issues.

Colloquially, some patients will say "I have mast cell," but this shortened version spoken as a diagnosis does not clarify exactly what distinction of MCAD they may be referring to. Giving the full "mast cell activation syndrome" or "systemic mastocytosis" distinction is more helpful when educating others on the condition and the different subtypes of MCAD.

THE EXPERTS

Who are the experts on mast cell activation disease (MCAD)? Throughout this book, hundreds of sources will be referenced. However, there are a handful of prominent MCAD specialists quoted from time to time with whom readers should be familiar.

Brigham and Women's Hospital in Boston has a Center of Excellence for Mastocytosis (and MCAD). Historically, Brigham and Women's facility has focused more on mastocytosis than MCAS, though it appears that they do accept patients with MCAS. A number of clinicians are associated with the hospital and its center.

Dr. Cem Akin is an allergist-immunologist clinician and researcher who established the Center of Excellence for Mastocytosis at Brigham and Women's Hospital. He has an impressive background of research on mast cell disorders and anaphylaxis. *Dr. Akin has relocated from Boston and currently practices in Michigan.*

Dr. Mariana Castells is a physician who is faculty at Harvard School of Medicine and is part of the mastocytosis team at Brigham and Women's Hospital. She conducts laboratory research and has been involved with over 100 publications in the areas of allergies, anaphylaxis and mastocytosis.

Dr. Norton Greenberger and **Dr. Matthew Hamilton** have led the way in the gastroenterology specialty aspect of the mastocytosis center at Brigham and Women's Hospital in Boston and are also active in research publications. *As of summer 2018, it appears that Dr. Greenberger retired from clinical practice, but Dr. Hamilton continues to see patients.*

Dr. Gerhard Molderings is Associate Professor of Pharmacology and Toxicology at University Hospital in Bonn, Germany. He works at the University of Bonn Institute of Human Genetics and is a leading expert on clinical immunology and mast cells. He has been part of nearly 200 research studies and frequently provides updates on MCAS management in the literature.

Dr. Lawrence Afrin is a hematologist/oncologist who recently relocated from Minnesota to New York, joining Dr. Tania Dempsey at her Armonk Integrative Medicine practice to pursue a mast cell activation syndrome (MCAS) specialty practice. Dr. Afrin is considered one of the beginning pioneers in clinical identification of MCAS, and his book "Never Bet Against Occam: Mast Cell Activation Disease and the Modern Epidemics of Chronic Illness and Medical Complexity" is the sole physician authority on MCAS that's available in book form. Dr. Afrin also has an extensive record of peer-reviewed publications and speaks regularly in educational settings, in addition to guiding patients and fellow doctors alike in the identification, diagnosis, and treatment of mast cell activation syndrome.

Dr. Theoharis Theoharides is Professor of Pharmacology and Internal Medicine, as well as Director of Molecular Immunopharmacology and Drug Discovery, in the Department of Immunology at Tufts University School of Medicine in Boston. Dr. Theoharides' curriculum vitae is astounding. He's been studying mast cells for over 30 years. He has published three textbooks and over 400 peer-reviewed scientific papers and is in the top 5% of authors most cited in immunological and pharmacological journals. He is well known for his research in autism and inflammation, but also has an impressive background of mast cell-specific research and, in particular, natural substances that may help stabilize mast cells, such as quercetin and luteolin.

All of these specialists are extremely passionate about research in the field, patient care, and raising awareness of MCAD. They frequently speak at conferences and events and the majority of these experts graciously donated their time for interviews for this book.

There are a number of additional practitioners who are considered experts in MCAS, but the above serves as an introduction to some of the more prominent figures in research and education, as opposed to an all-inclusive list of providers who see patients with MCAS.

There's an interesting division between the leading groups in terms of their approach to the diagnosis and treatment of MCAS. This book won't get too much into the associated politics, but it's something to keep in mind when evaluating the literature and searching for a care provider. Certain topics like the clinical diagnostic criteria for MCAS, the utility of tryptase testing, and treatment options are considered controversial. Without a governing board or universal clear-cut guidelines, as of 2018, a gray area remains within this relatively new field. This book aims to present the entirety of the differing professional opinions on topics relating to MCAD.

SYMPTOMS OF MCAD

Symptomatic Episodes

Mast cell activation syndrome is a relatively new diagnosis that has only been in the (hushed) limelight for about a decade or so. It's a condition that involves multisystem inflammation and a wide spectrum of dysfunction of varying complexity. Throughout the course of mast cell activation syndrome, patients tend to experience rises and falls in symptomatic baseline, which are sometimes precipitated by stressful life events.

Some patients tend to suffer more than others in the "allergic" aspect of the disease, and, similarly, some patients tend to suffer more than others in the abnormal tissue growth aspects of the disease.[2] The physiological reach of mast cells is nearly limitless, as mast cells are present in tissues and systems throughout the body, which adds further complication in terms of diagnosis and treatment.

When a thorough patient history is evaluated, mast cell-associated symptoms are often traced back to the early years in patients who have MCAS. Molderings and colleagues note, "Symptoms often initially manifest during adolescence or even childhood or infancy but are recognized only in retrospect as MCAD-related."[1]

The response to degranulation can vary widely among patients. Acutely, most patients experience an individual and unique spectrum from a mild reaction to a full-blown anaphylactic response that requires epinephrine and other drugs alongside an emergency room visit. Acute episodes that fall somewhere in the middle will typically include flushing or redness of the face, itching with or without hives on the skin, blood pressure drops, difficulty breathing, abdominal cramping, nausea, vomiting or diarrhea, nasal and eye symptoms, throat tightness or soreness, and headaches.

On top of these episodic symptoms, patients with MCAD typically experience dozens of problems that fall into their symptom list on a chronic, continual basis—a sort of baseline of instability. And many have strange symptoms that tend to wax and wane for no apparent reason. Both sporadic and chronic symptoms are attributed to the fact that mast cells are present across multiple tissue types and are activated by multiple types of signals.[3] Thus, many patients face challenges of having chronic issues plus a "sprinkling" of anaphylactic-spectrum episodes that can range from the rare episode (a few times a year) to the severe cases of multiple episodes of anaphylaxis per day. There are extreme and rare cases where patients need to be hospitalized and treated with continuous intravenous mast cell stabilizers and monitored constantly due to persistent anaphylaxis.

Signs and symptoms of MCAD can include virtually any body system or area. What further complicates accurate diagnosis is the fact that for many patients, the symptoms seem to flare and remit in various time frames, to be triggered by previously benign factors for no apparent reason and to migrate around the body.

Symptoms by System

The symptoms of MCAD have been listed by numerous authors and studies and can be summed up by one word: "everything!" In all seriousness, most patients have a history of multisystem comorbidities or puzzling ailments, regardless of which type of MCAD they have (with the exception of the form of mastocytosis which affects the skin, which does not always have systemic symptoms).

Examples of symptoms experienced by those with MCAD[4]:

Cardiovascular signs: tachycardia (high heart rate), blood pressure irregularity (both high and low blood pressure), flushing (especially of the face), syncope (fainting) or pre-syncope (near-fainting), heart racing and blood pressure responses to positional changes, heart disease, intermittent chest pain

Commonly attributed to[4]: CRH (corticotropin-releasing hormone), chymase, histamine, interleukin-6, PAF (platelet-activating factor), renin, TNF (tumor necrosis factor), tryptase

Respiratory signs: asthma-like symptoms, sinus inflammation, shortness of breath, cough, rhinitis (nose mucous inflammation), frequent upper respiratory infections and/or pneumonia, shallow breathing patterns, impaired use of diaphragm muscle for breathing

Commonly attributed to[4]: histamine, interleukin-6, CysLTs (cysteinyl leukotrienes), PAF (platelet-activating factor), PGD2 (prostaglandin D2)

Gastrointestinal signs: bloating, diarrhea and/or constipation, nausea, vomiting, abdominal pain, intestinal cramping, abdominal distention, heartburn, malabsorption of nutrients, delayed gastric (stomach) emptying, *H. pylori*-negative gastritis (stomach lining inflammation), oropharyngeal burning pain (in middle part of the throat), aphthae (ulcers on the mouth or tongue), ileocecal valve (valve separating small and large intestine) dysfunction, non-cardiac chest pain, food sensitivities, median arcuate ligament syndrome or "MALS" (structural compression of the celiac artery and possible neural structures resulting in abdominal ischemia and pain), microbiome bacterial issues including SIBO (small intestinal bacterial overgrowth)

Commonly attributed to[4]: CRH (corticotropin-releasing hormone), histamine, interleukin-6, neurotensin, PAF (platelet-activating factor), PGD2 (prostaglandin D2), serotonin, TNF (tumor necrosis factor), tryptase, VIP (vasoactive intestinal peptide)

Neuropsychiatric signs: difficulty with memory and concentration, anxiety, depression, insomnia (difficulty sleeping), lightheadedness, vertigo (sensation of the room spinning), headache and/or migraine, neuropathic pain (abnormal nerve-related pain sensations), polyneuropathy (degeneration of peripheral nerves), lower attention span, organic brain syndrome (decreased brain function due to a medical disease), tinnitus (ringing in the ears)

Commonly attributed to[4]: CRH (corticotropin-releasing hormone), histamine, interleukin-6, neurotensin, PAF (platelet-activating factor), PGD2 (prostaglandin D2), TNF (tumor necrosis factor)

Ophthalmologic signs: conjunctivitis (pink eye), difficulty focusing with vision, increased floaters in eye, intermittent blurred vision, general eye irritation and redness, decreased oxygen to optic nerve resulting in decreased ability to differentiate between contrasting shades

Organ Signs: hepatic splenomegaly (enlargement of liver and spleen), hyperbilirubinemia (elevated bilirubin in the blood), elevation of liver transaminases, hypercholesterolemia (high cholesterol in the blood), splenomegaly (enlarged spleen), lymphadenopathy (lymph nodes enlarged, abnormal consistency or abnormal number)

Cutaneous Signs: urticaria (rash), flushing, hives, efflorescence (spots on skin) with/without pruritus (itching), telangiectasia (red lines on skin from small blood vessels), flushing, angioedema (swelling of the lower layer of the skin), abnormal bleeding, frequent bruising, delayed skin healing from injury, abnormal sweating, abnormal body odor, hair loss

Commonly attributed to[4]: interleukin-8, interleukin-33, PAF (platelet-activating factor), PGD2 (prostaglandin D2), TNF (tumor necrosis factor), tryptase, CRH (corticotropin-releasing hormone), histamine, interleukin-6

Musculoskeletal Signs: muscle pain and aches, osteoporosis/osteopenia (decreased bone mineral density), bone pain, migratory arthritis, fibromyalgia

Commonly attributed to[4]: interleukin-6, PGD2 (prostaglandin D2), RANKL (receptor activator of nuclear factor-κB ligand), TNF (tumor necrosis factor), tryptase

Other Signs: fatigue, asthenia (feeling weak), fever, environmental sensitivities (odors, chemicals, vibration, animals, etc.), interstitial cystitis (bladder pain and increased urinary frequency), unexplained weight loss or gain, poor tolerance to exercise, idiopathic anaphylaxis, sensitivity to sunlight and/or extreme cold and heat, odd reactions to insect stings, difficult menses (females), thyroid and adrenal issues, poor tolerance to medications or anesthesia, poor tolerance to alcohol, poor tolerance to fermented foods and/or processed foods, poor tolerance to foods high in histamine

Fatigue, malaise and weight loss commonly attributed to[4]: CRH (corticotropin-releasing hormone), histamine, interleukin-6, TNF (tumor necrosis factor)

The above-mentioned list of symptoms and associated chemical mediators is certainly not comprehensive. Afrin's book "Never Bet Against Occam: Mast Cell Activation Disease and the Modern Epidemics of Chronic Illness and Medical Complexity" includes a number of case studies that show just how different each patient with MCAD can present. Interestingly, not all of his case studies presented with anaphylaxis or allergic reaction symptoms.[5]

As a general observation, it seems from reading Afrin's case studies that each patient has 1) multisystem symptoms that don't make sense when attempted to be labeled with other diagnoses and 2) a certain area or a few areas that are particularly problematic, such as recurrent strokes or heart problems, gastrointestinal complaints, pulmonary findings, genitourinary concerns, etc.[5] In other words, it seems that each individual has a certain body area (which could include *any* body system) that stands out above the others in terms of dysfunction, but that area is not their only symptomatic spot.

Many patients with MCAS note that they feel susceptible to issues like low blood sugar (even in the absence of measurable changes) and may experience extra irritability as glucose and hormone levels fluctuate. Many also report symptoms of narcolepsy and respiratory depression following meals, exposure to sunlight, vibrations from car rides and other triggers. Histamine and prostaglandins are two mediators that have been theoretically connected to these phenomena.[6,7]

The plethora of varying clinical presentations and characteristics leads one to conclude that there's really no "hallmark" set of signs and symptoms for mast cell activation disease. Some experts believe that the wide array of manifestations is dependent upon which chemical mediator or mediators seem to be driving the symptoms in a particular patient. Some point to genetics and epigenetic factors. Problems with detoxification and mast cell reactivity to different viral and bacterial loads may also be the key to why this condition presents in so many different ways. Patient-specific comorbidities (presence of other diseases), the variety of organ sites that can become infiltrated with mast cells, the wide range of triggering stimuli, local- and organ-specific factors, and the magnitude of the release reaction are all factors that impact the unique patient picture.[8]

CLASSIFICATION OF MCAD

Within mast cell activation disease, there are several subcategories of diagnoses: mastocytosis, mast cell activation syndrome (MCAS), and mast cell leukemia (MCL) or mast cell sarcoma (very rare). The symptoms and clinical presentation of MCAS and mastocytosis are often identical, so testing is important to help identify the precise diagnosis.

Figure 1. Proposed Classification of Mast Cell Activation Disease[1]

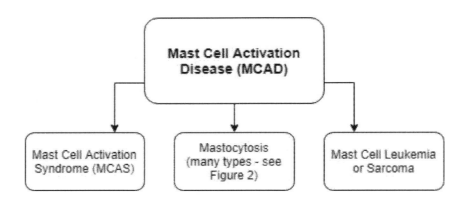

The majority of this book will focus on mast cell activation syndrome (MCAS), but it's important to have an overview of the other types of mast cell activation disease in order to be fully prepared for all possibilities as well as for conversations with physicians, colleagues, and/or fellow patients.

MASTOCYTOSIS

Mastocytosis in a Nutshell

Mastocytosis is defined by abnormal clonal mast cell expansion and accumulation in various tissues. In essence, mastocytosis is a type of myeloproliferative neoplasm, which is a disease of the bone marrow where too many mast cells are produced. There are two broad categories for mastocytosis: systemic mastocytosis (SM) and cutaneous mastocytosis (CM). Within each diagnosis, there are several subgroups.

Figure 2. Types of Mastocytosis, Based on the World Health Organization Classification Scheme for Mastocytosis[9] (2016)

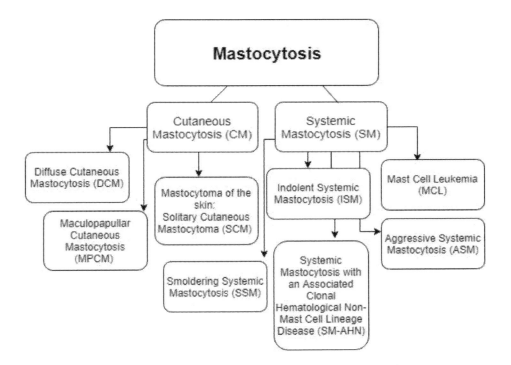

Cutaneous Mastocytosis (CM)

The cutaneous type is classified by mast cell infiltration limited to the skin. Cutaneous mastocytosis is typically diagnosed in the first few years of life. Patients present with a rash and may or may not have additional systemic symptoms, such as fever, gastrointestinal distress, and anaphylaxis, even in the absence of bone-marrow mast cell abnormalities. Diagnosis is made via a biopsy of the skin. The biopsy will also look at the possibility of a mastocytoma, which is a benign tumor on the skin that is typically found in small children. Most cases (60%-80%) of cutaneous mastocytosis are caused by a mutation to the *KIT* gene.[4]

Cutaneous mastocytosis is more common than systemic mastocytosis.[10] Approximately 80% of cutaneous mastocytosis cases that arise before age 2 will resolve before puberty.[11] With onset after age 2, the disease does not tend to resolve and often progresses to systemic mastocytosis.[11]

It's also possible that some cases of CM may fully resolve clinically only to reemerge systemically in later years. Experts have noted that some cases of childhood cutaneous mastocytosis will resolve completely but the same patient may eventually present with MCAS later in life.[12]

Subtypes of cutaneous mastocytosis

- maculopapullar cutaneous mastocytosis (MPCM) – also called urticaria pigmentosa (UP)
- solitary cutaneous mastocytoma (SCM)
- diffuse cutaneous mastocytosis (DCM)
- telangiectasia macularis eruptive perstans (TMEP) – very rare; *this type is *not* included in the 2016 WHO Classification of cutaneous mastocytosis

Systemic Mastocytosis (SM)

The systemic type of mastocytosis is characterized by too many mast cells accumulating in tissues such as the gastrointestinal system, liver, spleen, and bone marrow. This proliferation of mast cells in certain areas can lead to complications like anemia and bleeding disorders, bone fractures, ascites, thrombocytopenia, gastrointestinal inflammation, frequent anaphylaxis, skin reactions, and enlargement of the spleen, liver, and lymph nodes.[13] Flushing, urticaria pigmentosa, gastrointestinal cramping, and hypotensive events are common in the majority of patients with SM. Most people develop SM in adulthood, and the disease is usually linked to a mutation of the *KIT* gene (80% of patients with systemic mastocytosis).[14] This mutation is commonly encountered at codon D816V.[4]

Indolent systemic mastocytosis (ISM) is the most common variant and patients typically experience a normal life expectancy, with very rare likelihood of the disease progressing to aggressive systemic mastocytosis (ASM).[4] ASM tends to have a greater degree of systemic damage and dysfunction.[4]

Diagnostic Criteria for Systemic Mastocytosis

The World Health Organization (WHO) published diagnostic criteria for systemic mastocytosis in 2008. The WHO Classification of mastocytosis was updated in 2016 to include smoldering systemic mastocytosis (SSM) as its own category.[15,16] The prognosis of patients with SSM is less favorable compared with ISM but favorable compared with ASM or MCL.[9]

Subtypes of indolent systemic mastocytosis (ISM)

- isolated bone marrow mastocytosis
- well-differentiated systemic mastocytosis

Subtypes of smoldering systemic mastocytosis (SSM)

- BM mastocytosis (clinically relevant provisional type in updated classification)

Subtypes of aggressive systemic mastocytosis (ASM)

- ASM in transformation

Subtypes of SM with an associated clonal hematological non-mast cell lineage disease (SM-AHN)

- SM-acute myeloid leukemia
- SM-myelodysplastic syndrome
- SM-myeloproliferative neoplasm
- SM-chronic myelomonocytic leukemia
- SM-chronic eosinophilic leukemia
- SM-non-Hodgkin lymphoma
- SM-multiple myeloma

As evident, there are many different variations of SM. Diagnosis of SM is typically made via a combination of blood tests, bone marrow biopsy and/or a biopsy of other organ tissue.

The prognosis for patients with mastocytosis varies depending on the type. Researchers Austin and Akin conclude, "in general, patients with cutaneous or indolent systemic mastocytosis have excellent prognosis comparable to age matched general population. Those with aggressive mastocytosis or other associated hematologic disorders indicative of mutations elsewhere in the development pathway have poorer prognosis."[17]

Major criterion:

1. Multifocal, dense aggregates of mast cells (15 or more in aggregates) in sections of the bone marrow and/or other extracutaneous tissues, confirmed by tryptase immunohistochemistry or other special stains

Minor criteria:

1. Atypical morphology or spindled appearance of at least 25% of the mast cells in the diagnostic biopsy or bone marrow aspirate smear
2. Expression of CD2 and/or CD25 by mast cells in the marrow, blood, or extracutaneous organs
3. *KIT* codon 816 mutation in the marrow, blood, or extracutaneous organs
4. Persistent elevation of serum total tryptase >20 ng/ml

Diagnosis of SM made by either (1) the major criterion plus any one of the minor criteria or (2) any three minor criteria

Systemic mastocytosis has long been recognized by the medical community with relatively clear-cut diagnostic criteria, unlike MCAS. Bone marrow biopsies have long been the diagnostic "gold standard." One bone marrow biopsy does not ensure accurate results, and *anecdotally* some patients report needing a high number of biopsies prior to confirmation of the diagnosis of SM. For this reason, the minor criteria are useful. Most physicians won't perform a bone marrow biopsy unless they have high suspicion of mastocytosis, such as an obviously elevated tryptase level in conjunction with clinical symptoms.

Patients who present with mastocytosis, as a general trend, tend to have a sudden life event that triggers expression of the disease. (This is not always the case, of course.) Often, patients with SM report to the emergency room with anaphylaxis as their initial suspicion of the disease. In contrast, patients with MCAS may have triggers that initiate a change in severity of symptoms but generally tend to have a long-standing history of undiagnosed ailments.

Mast Cell Leukemia

Some people consider mast cell leukemia to be a subgroup of mastocytosis.[9,15] Mast cell leukemia is a very aggressive form of acute myeloid leukemia. A very small percentage of cases can evolve from systemic mastocytosis. This condition is very rare and has a poor prognosis, with typically rapid progression to multi-organ failure within 6 months to one year.[18] The World Health Organization Diagnostic Criteria for Mast Cell Leukemia is a 20% prevalence of neoplastic mast cells in bone marrow and a 10% prevalence of immature mast cells in the peripheral blood.[4,19] These patients typically also have elevated tryptase, a confirmed *KIT* mutation, and elevated histamine levels in blood and urine.[20]

Mast Cell Sarcoma

A mast cell sarcoma is an extremely rare tumor that can lead to mast cell leukemia. A 2016 review article noted 23 cases of reported mast cell sarcomas between 1984 and 2014.[21]

MAST CELL ACTIVATION SYNDROME (MCAS)

Early Presentation

"My health definitely changed around age 20, but when I really look back at my youth, I realize that the signs were there all along."

This is a common sentiment upon deeper reflection for many patients with mast cell activation syndrome (MCAS). By contrast, systemic mastocytosis (SM) is a distinctly different condition where symptoms tend to arrive suddenly and violently, often in adulthood. With MCAS, most patients can identify several concrete large "triggers" and points in time where things changed dramatically, but also have memories of multi-system dysfunction that has been humming in the background all along. Patients with MCAS become experts at ignoring certain symptoms, powering through each day while feeling on the brink of despair and sometimes "forgetting" the less intense symptoms when others become predominant and overbearing.

Symptoms tend to wax and wane, to migrate, and are generally very hard to nail down and diagnose. Most patients have a bitter chip on their shoulder from the (likely) thousands upon thousands of dollars of medical bills, time spent with doctors investigating one of their symptoms under a narrow lens, and the inevitable labeling as a "hypochondriac" or person who has somatization of symptoms (multiple or recurrent medical conditions with no discernible cause).

Many patients feel disrespected and belittled from their experiences with mainstream medicine when doctors have insinuated that their confusingly recurrent ailments (that repeatedly test negative for distinct diagnoses) are all in their head. And when you add in skeptical family members and friends, MCAS can quickly wear a patient down and become very depressing and isolating.

MCAS Overview

MCAS is an immunological condition in which the body has a normal amount of mast cells, but they are inappropriately degranulating or releasing chemical mediators into the blood and abnormally signaling certain physiological processes to occur. In the earlier example, these were the lightweights who were sensitive to alcohol and vomiting at the house party. Mast cells are hyper-responsive to their environment in someone who has MCAS.

In sticking with the party metaphor, one can also think of the condition in terms of birthday party balloons. With mastocytosis, there are way too many balloons bunched together that take over the room, and even if they are responding as one would expect to triggers, their sheer volume can create problems. In patients with MCAS, there's a normal-sized bunch of balloons, but they show up to the party being popped by things that should not pop them (i.e., triggers in the environment). The popping causes a release of chemical mediators into the blood, which can signal the body to respond with a sudden change in blood pressure, swelling of the airways or skin, or other acute allergic reaction signs. Normally benign influences like blades of grass are interpreted by the body as dangerous tacks that trigger the balloon-popping responses more frequently and severely than in a "normally functioning" mast cell response.

When this occurs chronically over time, symptoms can also manifest into chronic gastrointestinal, neurological, cardiovascular, respiratory, and dermatological problems. Symptoms tend to wax and wane and affect multiple systems of the body in an inflammatory manner. Essential systems that govern the immune response, fight or flight sympathetic reactions, hormonal balances, and many other processes in the body become unbalanced due to chronically abnormal levels of the mediators that affect the homeostasis of those systems. Virtually every body system can be affected with this silent disease that often looks normal to the eye and is very difficult to diagnose.

According to Molderings and colleagues, "Symptoms observed in patients with MCAS are little, if any, different from those seen in patients with systemic mastocytosis."[1] This is because the same cell type is involved with both conditions, even though the exact underlying mechanism is slightly different in nature (and specifically, in number).[1,22]

In order to be diagnosed with MCAS, one generally has a clinical picture of multisystem symptoms and the failure to meet the diagnostic criteria for mastocytosis; other potential conditions must all be ruled out. (See proposed diagnostic criteria, below, and the list of differential diagnoses at the end of this chapter.)

Signs of MCAS are typically traced back to the patient's early childhood years, and the condition is currently believed to be lifelong with no cure. However, most people attribute certain types of trauma or moments in time to an increase in their symptom baseline level. Stressful life events such as car accidents, grieving the loss of a loved one, physical or mental abuse, and stressors associated with starting a business or moving states are common triggers. Others can pinpoint an increase in baseline symptoms to a time frame when they changed certain environmental factors, such as moving into a house or office space that they later discovered had a mold issue. When most patients are pressed to reflect on what was going on around the time symptoms worsened, there is typically some type of big or small stressful trigger that they can identify, although some patients cannot recall any triggers.

The lifespan for those with MCAS appears to be normal, but the quality of life can range from mildly impaired to severely uncomfortable, often to the point where patients are homebound and unable to work.[23]

Female Predominance

According to an article by Picard et al., "MCAS affects predominantly women in whom no mast cell abnormality or external triggers account for their episodes of mast cell activation."[24] Studies consistently report more females than males with MCAS diagnoses. A 2011 study by Hamilton and colleagues noted that 89% of patients with MCAS were female.[25] Research conducted in 2012 noted a 75% female predominance in patients diagnosed with MCAD.[26] Similarly, a 2013 study of mixed patients (both MCAS and SM) had a 74% predominance of females.[27] In 2016, Afrin and colleagues found that 69% of their patient sample size of 413 patients with MCAS were female.[28] Research conducted in 2018 reported a 94% female population of allergy clinic patients with MCAS.[29]

In animal studies, in response to passive systemic anaphylaxis, female mice had increased clinical scores, poorer temperature regulation, and elevated serum histamine levels when compared to male mice.[30] Specifically, the mast cells in female subjects had greater physiological sensitivity to stress and increased responses of chemical mediators when compared to their male counterparts.[30]

Preliminary research suggests that the higher prevalence of MCAS in females *may be* explained by cellular gene expression innately tied to gender differences in the mast cell itself. A 2016 study found an increased vulnerability to allergies, anaphylaxis, and irritable bowel syndrome in women compared to men due to over 8,000 differentially expressed genes found in female mast cells.[30] Gender-specific hormonal factors may also be connected to the disparities.

The Diagnosis of Mast Cell Activation Syndrome (MCAS)

One challenging aspect of the differential diagnosis between mastocytosis and MCAS is determining whether symptoms are due to dysfunctional mast cells (in a normal quantity) or an excess number of mast cells proliferating abnormally. Li and Ehrlich present a soldier analogy to help explain the different types of MCAD. "Mast cells can become dangerous if a subset of them 'goes rogue or mast cells are being great soldiers but following bad orders.'"[31] In this analogy, going rogue refers to the rare case of mastocytosis, and the soldiers that follow bad orders reflect mast cells that react to IgE targeting harmless substances or allergens, as is seen with MCAS.

This is *not* a distinction that can be made based on severity or type of clinical symptoms. (One study found that patients with MCAS experience more severe symptoms than patients with SM.[32] However, currently there is no clear trend on this factor to guide clinical decisions.)

Prior to 1991, systemic mastocytosis and urticaria pigmentosa were the main conditions taught in medical school relating to mast cells.[3] Mast cell activation syndrome (MCAS) was first recognized in 1991, expanded to include the title monoclonal mast cell activation syndrome (MMCAS) in 2007, and in 2008 was further categorized to the concept of mast cell activation disease (MCAD).[3,33,34]

The *original* published diagnostic criteria for MCAS (which was only specific to one primary type of MCAD, monoclonal mast cell activation syndrome, or MMCAS) did not include other mast cell mediator levels (besides tryptase) in its diagnostic consideration.[3] The years 2010-2012 reflect an evolution of clinical diagnostic criteria as several papers were published recommending updates to factor chemical mediators *besides tryptase* into the picture and recognition of other types of MCAS beyond primary monoclonal MCAS.

There have been several groups who have proposed updated diagnostic criteria since 2010. There are small nuances between the different criteria, but as a whole they contain similar key components. For the sake of being thorough, the most widely recognized proposed diagnostic criteria are presented below. There are two sets of recommendations that are currently utilized by clinicians, and because neither has an official name, they will be referred to as "Criteria X" and "Criteria Y" throughout this book.

"Criteria X" Development

In 2010, researchers Akin, Valent and Metcalfe published a set of recommended criteria for MCAS diagnosis.[35]

"Criteria X", initial version published by Akin, Valent and Metcalfe[35] (2010):

1. Episodic symptoms consistent with mast cell mediator release affecting ≥ 2 organ systems evidenced as follows:

    a. Skin: urticaria, angioedema, flushing

    b. Gastrointestinal: nausea, vomiting, diarrhea, abdominal cramping

    c. Cardiovascular: hypotensive syncope or near syncope, tachycardia

    d. Respiratory: wheezing

    e. Naso-ocular: conjunctival injection (eye redness), pruritus, nasal stuffiness

2. A decrease in the frequency or severity or resolution of symptoms with anti-mediator therapy: H1- and H2-histamine receptor inverse agonists, anti-leukotriene medications (cysteinyl leukotriene receptor blockers or 5-lipoxygenase inhibitor), or mast cell stabilizers (cromolyn sodium).

3. Evidence of an increase in a validated urinary or serum marker of mast cell activation: documentation of an increase of the marker to greater than the patient's baseline value during a symptomatic period on ≥ 2 occasions or, if baseline tryptase levels are persistently >15 ng/ml, documentation of an increase of the tryptase level above baseline value on one occasion. Total serum tryptase level is recommended as the marker of choice; less specific (also from basophils) are 24-hour urine histamine metabolites or PGD2 or its metabolite 11-β-prostaglandin F2.

4. Rule out primary and secondary causes of mast cell activation and well-defined clinical idiopathic entities.

"Criteria X" - Updated Version

Shortly thereafter, these same authors—with the assistance of a group of additional colleagues—published another set of MCAS diagnostic criteria that are mostly the same, with a few minor updates. Specifically, they changed the tryptase criteria from >15 ng/ml to an episodic "20% above baseline plus 2 ng/ml" which makes it easier to capture within-individual changes in tryptase levels.[8]

Secondly, they changed some of the symptoms listed; namely, they *removed* vomiting, diarrhea, tachycardia, abdominal cramping, eye redness, and syncope and *added* throat swelling and headache. Like the 2010 criteria, they (somewhat begrudgingly) included mention of histamine and prostaglandins as other potential mediators for testing to be acceptable in the context of a "transient increase of another established mast cell mediator."[8]

The updated version, *below*, is one of two sets of recommendations currently used to guide clinicians today (in 2018).

"Criteria X", updated version published by Valent and colleagues[8] (2012):

Major Criteria:

1. Absence of any known disorder that can better account for symptoms

2. Typical clinical symptoms (flushing, pruritus, urticaria, angioedema, nasal congestion, nasal pruritus, wheezing, throat swelling, headache, hypotension, diarrhea)

3. Increase in serum total tryptase by at least 20% above baseline plus 2 ng/ml during or within 4 hours after a symptomatic period OR transient increase of another established mast cell mediator

4. An objective response of clinical symptoms to anti-mediator drugs, such as histamine receptor blockers or 'mast cell targeting' agents, such as cromolyn*

All major criteria must be satisfied to meet diagnosis.

Note: The study with the above criteria was published in the *International Archives of Allergy & Immunology* in 2012, available online in 2011, and discussed extensively at a global conference in 2010. For the sake of this book, this set of recommendations will be referred to as "Criteria X."

*In regards to an objective response of symptoms to mast cell-targeting medications, the authors of "Criteria X" agreed that histamine receptor antagonists (H1/H2 blockers) are most specific to mast cells and thus should be the medications of choice for fulfilling this criterion of MCAS. Other types of medications, such as leukotriene inhibitors and corticosteroids, impact other cell types and would be less specific to rule in MCAS.[8]

"Criteria Y"

Amid the process of revising the above criteria, Molderings and colleagues, a second group of researchers and clinicians, published a separate set of guidelines for MCAS diagnosis in 2011.[1]

"Criteria Y", initial version published by Molderings and colleagues[1] (2011):

Major Criteria:

1. Multifocal or disseminated dense infiltrates of mast cells in bone marrow biopsies and/or in sections of other extracutaneous organ(s) (e.g., gastrointestinal tract biopsies; CD117-, tryptase- and CD25-stained)
2. Unique constellation of clinical complaints as a result of a pathologically increased mast cell activity (mast cell mediator release syndrome)

Minor Criteria:

1. Mast cells in bone marrow or other extracutaneous organ(s) show an abnormal morphology (>25%) in bone marrow smears or in histologies
2. Mast cells in bone marrow express CD2 and/or CD25
3. Detection of genetic changes in mast cells from blood, bone marrow, or extracutaneous organs for which an impact on the state of activity of affected mast cells in terms of an increased activity has been proven
4. Evidence of a pathologically increased release of mast cell mediators by determination of the content of
   a. tryptase in blood
   b. *N*-methylhistamine in urine
   c. heparin in blood
   d. chromogranin A in blood
   e. other mast cell-specific mediators (e.g., eicosanoids including prostaglandin PGD2, its metabolite 11-β-PGF2α, or leukotriene E4)

The diagnosis mast cell activation syndrome is made if both major criteria or the second major criterion and at least one minor criterion are fulfilled.

"Criteria Y" - Updated Version

Since 2011, multiple papers published by the same authors have discussed slight modifications to the above criteria for MCAS diagnosis. Minor criteria 1 and 2 (above) are the same thing as two of the minor criteria for the WHO diagnosis of systemic mastocytosis, so the diagnostic criteria may be encountered with slightly different wording but ultimately continues to reflect the same guidelines for those two criteria. Publications since 2016 have reflected a change that moves major criterion 1, "multifocal or disseminated dense infiltrates of mast cells in bone marrow biopsies and/or in sections of other extracutaneous organ(s)," into a minor criterion role, leaving "unique constellation of clinical complaints as a result of a pathologically increased mast cell activity (mast cell mediator release syndrome)" as the *sole major criterion*.[36]

This change is reflected in shifting the guidelines to *the presence of the major criterion and one minor criterion OR three minor criteria* as diagnostic.[36] The authors also added an additional minor criterion to reflect a medication response (see minor criterion 6, below).[36] The revised criteria are shared below; these recommendations by Molderings and colleagues will continue to be referred to as "Criteria Y."

"Criteria Y", updated version by Molderings and colleagues[36] (2016):

Major Criterion:

1. Unique constellation of clinical complaints as a result of a pathologically increased mast cell activity (mast cell mediator release syndrome)

Minor Criteria:

1. Multifocal or disseminated dense infiltrates of mast cells in bone marrow biopsies and/or in sections of other extracutaneous organ(s) (e.g., gastrointestinal tract biopsies; CD117-, tryptase- and CD25-stained)
2. Mast cells in bone marrow or other extracutaneous organ(s) show an abnormal morphology (>25%) in bone marrow smears or in histologies (minor criterion 1 for SM)
3. Mast cells in bone marrow express CD2 and/or CD25 (minor criterion 2 for SM)
4. Detection of genetic changes in mast cells from blood, bone marrow, or extracutaneous organs for which an impact on the state of activity of affected mast cells in terms of an increased activity has been proven

5. Evidence of a pathologically increased release of mast cell mediators by determination of the content of tryptase in blood, *N*-methylhistamine in urine, heparin in blood, chromogranin A in blood, or other mast cell-specific mediators (e.g., eicosanoids including prostaglandin PGD2, its metabolite 11-β-PGF2α, or leukotriene E4)

6. Symptomatic response to inhibitors of mast cell activation or mast cell mediator production or action (e.g., histamine H1 and/or H2 receptor antagonists, cromolyn)

Diagnosis of MCAS made by either (1) the major criterion plus any one of the minor criteria or (2) any three minor criteria.

Needless to say, the different criteria, separate research groups, and time frames are a bit confusing. Appendix 1 contains a simplified summary of the most recently published diagnostic criteria.

Criteria Comparison

Both "Criteria X" and "Criteria Y" are used clinically, and there are pros and cons to utilizing either recommendation. There are some similarities between the two research groups: both include in their criteria the mention of 1) clinical signs and symptoms of MCAD, 2) evidence of one abnormal mast cell mediator level to count as part of the diagnosis decision, and 3) the presence of a symptomatic response to mast cell-targeting medications.

There are several fundamental differences between the two groups who have suggested the separate diagnostic criteria. "Criteria X"[8] list a *limited number* of clinical symptoms that could be considered consistent with mast cell activation. As evidenced earlier in this chapter, that list is *usually significantly longer and more varied in a typical MCAS patient.*

The changes in specified symptoms from the 2010 to 2012 publications of "Criteria X" (by the same authors) appear somewhat arbitrary. However, they actually based the change of those specific symptoms off an international conference (the 2010 Working Conference on Mast Cell Disorders) where doctors came together to discuss the symptoms they most commonly encountered in patients with MCAS.[8] This group of faculties included experts in MCAD from Austria, France, Poland, Italy, Germany, Spain, and the United States.[8]

The consensus statement revealed that clinicians agreed 100% that no *one* symptom is specific for mast cell activation disease, and that a number of different symptoms are typically observed.[8] While interesting, it appears that the 11 symptoms they published were anecdotal and not based on specific case reviews.

Specifically, flushing and hypotension (low blood pressure) achieved a 95% consensus level *among doctors at the conference as symptoms consistent with MCAS*.[8] Pruritis (itching), nasal congestion, nasal pruritis, headache, and diarrhea achieved a 90% consensus level among the doctors present.[8] Throat swelling and urticaria each achieved a consensus level of 85%; angioedema (75%) and wheezing (70%) rounded out the list of top symptoms consistent with MCAS based on doctor opinions at the event.[8]

While it's clear that the changes reflected the *consensus majority opinion of physicians* that were present at the conference, the conference attendees did not include all of the MCAS experts in the global field and, perhaps more importantly, the 2012 authors did *not* appear to base their symptom inclusion from scientific literature.

"Criteria X"[8] have also been scrutinized for item 3, the tryptase requirements. Some argue that patients with MCAS may never have a truly "asymptomatic baseline" to conduct the math calculation from. In addition, it's difficult to get a tryptase level measured within 4 hours of an episode both logistically and also because many emergency room staff simply refuse to do so, even with a piece of paper in hand that specifies test orders. There's a very narrow window of time to ensure accuracy (due to the half-life of tryptase) and patients are often unable to get to the clinic during the correct time frame while experiencing an attack. Also, the "20% + 2" criteria makes it possible for people with especially low baseline levels to be diagnosed with the disease even if their level rise slightly but stay within a normal-range limit.

While it's important to make sure one is not missing anything when it comes to differential diagnosis (as is suggested by "Criteria X"),[8] it's also possible to encounter patients whose co-morbidities could very well explain some of their symptoms—but not all of them. One example is someone who first tested positive for Lyme disease. Some of the symptoms of Lyme disease overlap with MCAS, such as fatigue, flushing/fevers, insomnia, and joint pain. It's very possible that Lyme disease could be the underlying root cause of secondary MCAS; indeed, one study found that Lyme bacteria induce mast cell degranulation.[37]

It's also possible that the patient has had MCAS their entire life and was exposed to Lyme disease at some point, leading to the eventual expression of more Lyme disease symptoms at a certain stressful point in their life. With this example, if the doctor followed these guidelines and blamed everything on Lyme disease, the first condition that was discovered, the patient might never reach an accurate/complete diagnosis that would lead to their full healing potential. Therefore, the criterion from "Criteria X"[8] stating "absence of any known disorder to better account for symptoms" can be tricky to determine.

On the other hand, "Criteria Y"[36] did not include the first clause about the absence of any known disorder that could account for the symptoms. This is an aspect that has received some criticism; however, that factor could be inferred as an underlying assumption, and the authors of "Criteria Y"[36] have since explained that they do wish that they had been more explicit about stating the differential diagnosis aspect. Indeed, it is important that all medical professionals who diagnose and treat this condition complete a thorough differential diagnosis process before labeling anyone with MCAS.

One other interesting difference between the two groups is that the researchers of "Criteria Y"[36] made it possible for three minor criteria to fulfill a diagnosis. So, a patient who does not present with a clinical history suggestive of MCAS can still be diagnosed with the condition if they have concrete lab evidence (with positive chemical mediators and tissue biopsy results). This could be useful in the case of a child, elderly adult, or person who has a disability or cognitive impairment who may not be able to articulate or recall their symptoms clearly.

It's also possible that patients can be poor historians or may not yet be aware of multisystem dysfunction. The example of a severe reaction to a bee sting can prompt allergists to investigate for the possibility of the presence of MCAD, which may help capture at-risk patients early on before they might reach the point of seeking medical care for chronic illness. Thus, it appears that the ability to diagnose patients even in the absence of certain symptoms may be a positive thing when factoring in special scenarios that could occur.

Another key difference between the two published criteria is that "Criteria Y"[36] include aspects of test results that are only possible through either a bone marrow biopsy and/or other tissue biopsy sample, and "Criteria X"[8] do not mention this type of testing. One of the four minor criterion options from "Criteria Y"[36] includes chemical mediator levels that can be tested in the blood or the urine, so in the event that a patient is symptomatic with signs consistent with mast cell activity, *a biopsy is not mandatory in order to make the diagnostic decision*, as long as the patient has evidence of an abnormal chemical mediator.

Thus, if utilizing "Criteria X"[8] it's possible to achieve a diagnosis of MCAS without the patient undergoing a bone marrow biopsy or extracutaneous organ biopsy. So, from one perspective, it can eliminate some time and cost in the diagnostic process. But the same "Criteria X"[8] do not account for patients who may have normal blood and urine samples but abnormal tissue biopsy samples, which is one limitation to following those standards.

One special utility of "Criteria Y"[36] is that patients who may have had a prior biopsy of tissue can have post-procedure tissue analysis performed (even several years later) in the event that the blood and urine testing is not easily accessed in their geographical area. Failure to include mast cell-specific tissue biopsy tests, and instead focus on a reliance of capturing abnormal chemical mediators in one snapshot in time, could possibly miss the chance to identify patients with MCAS.

Lastly, both the updated version of "Criteria Y"[36] and "Criteria X"[8] require an objective clinical response to symptoms before a diagnosis can be made, which seems a little bit backwards. Many patients encounter hurdles to acquiring certain medications (like cromolyn) with their insurance companies and would have to pay out of pocket if they did not have the appropriate insurance diagnostic code. Most patients with MCAS have frequent reactions to most oral medications and have to use caution in trialing a new drug. It's not a quick process to determine whether one medication is effective; rather, it's a slow, trial-and-error methodological approach. Patients may require painstaking efforts in terms of trying every version of each medication (i.e., generic vs. brand name) and a variety of dosages before deeming a medication effective or not.

Furthermore, most patients require months, if not years, of trial and error with medications to find the right combination in the event that they require more than one medication. So, in some opinions, requiring a successful medication response for diagnosis can be a hindrance to this patient population. In addition, certain medications target cells other than mast cells, so a response to one out of a variety of mast cell medications may not be highly specific.

While it's clear that the revised diagnostic criteria recommendations are not perfect, they are what's currently available for this relatively new diagnosis, and they *have* come a long way from the initial approach that mainly focused on tryptase.

PROPOSED CLASSIFICATION SCHEMES
Primary, Secondary and Idiopathic MCAD

In 2010, literature was published by Akin and colleagues that recommended that diseases associated with mast cell activation be broken down into categories.[35] Keep in mind that "MCAD" refers to an umbrella term of diseases encompassing MCAS, mastocytosis, and mast cell leukemia; MCAS is one type of MCAD.

The <u>subgroups of MCAD</u> were suggested as follows:

- Primary MCAD (encompassing mastocytosis and monoclonal mast cell activation syndrome "MMCAS")
- Secondary MCAD
- Idiopathic MCAD

In order for MCAD to be considered primary, the authors recommended an individual patient classification dependent on the mechanism of the disease, serum tryptase level, and bone marrow biopsy findings.

Figure 3. Proposed Classification of Diseases Associated with Mast Cell Activation, based off suggestions from Akin, Valent & Metcalfe[35] (2010)

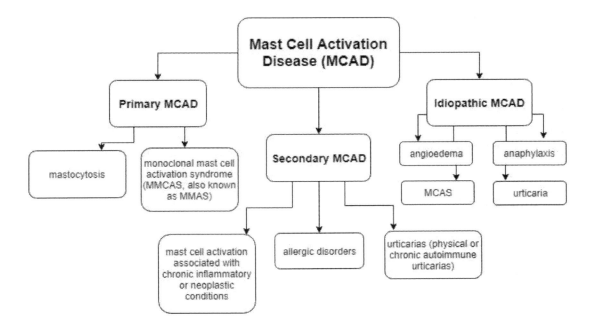

Primary MCAD

As presented in Figure 3, the proposed classification of primary MCAD includes mastocytosis and MMCAS.[35] Specifically, to have primary MCAD most experts agreed that the patient must have the presence of an inherent genetic defect in the mast cells or their progenitors that presumably results in a reduction in their activation threshold.[3] These patients have evidence of both the MCAS criteria and mast cell monoclonality proven via the c-*KIT* and/or CD25 analysis. MMCAS typically presents with one or two minor criteria, such as the c-*KIT* mutation or CD25 expression on bone marrow analysis, but not the complete criteria for diagnosis of systemic mastocytosis.

Patients who have MMCAS often have normal baseline tryptase levels that may raise to abnormal levels in symptomatic episodes. According to Soderberg, another hallmark is that patients with MMCAS present with less than 15 mast cells per high-powered field and the mast cells are hypogranulated and spindle-shaped, whereas patients with mastocytosis will have numbers greater than 15 per high-powered field.[3]

MMCAS can be thought of as mastocytosis' baby sister—many things look alike and they both have the same "clonal" background, but there are some fundamental differences in the laboratory findings that distinguish the two.

Secondary MCAD

The proposed category of secondary MCAD includes allergic disorders, mast cell activation associated with chronic inflammatory or neoplastic conditions, and urticarias (physical or chronic autoimmune urticarias).[35] These patients meet the diagnosis of MCAS and also have clinical diagnoses for an underlying type I allergy or other medical condition that can induce mast cell activation. This category covers a broad range of root causes and there are many descriptions of secondary MCAD in the literature.[3]

Secondary MCAD could be considered the cousin of primary MCAD. They are related and some things look alike, but they were raised in a different household and the secondary folks have some unique factors that appear to be the true root of the symptoms.

Idiopathic MCAD

The proposed category of idiopathic MCAD includes the subgroups of anaphylaxis, angioedema, urticaria, and MCAS.[35] Idiopathic (or "without a known origin") is a more puzzling category from a clinical diagnostic perspective. These patients also meet the criteria for MCAS, but there is no discernable clonality or secondary cause found. In other words, the idiopathic group is where patients are placed if they display no type I allergy, no underlying condition that can explain the symptoms, and no monoclonal mast cells or skin mastocytosis. Patients with idiopathic MCAS have an absence of clonal markers (like the c-*KIT* mutation or CD25 expression).[3]

Idiopathic MCAD could be considered that favorite wild aunt who shows up to family events unexpectedly. She's unpredictable, often unexplainable, and still very much a real and powerful presence.

Distinction Considerations

It's important to note that patients can have the coexistence of both primary MCAD and a true allergy at once. Patients may also shift between idiopathic and secondary diagnoses from different points in time and testing.

Some patients or physicians feel that simply identifying that a patient's mast cells are overactive is enough to explain the symptoms and justify diving into pharmacological treatment. However, other experts believe it's important to avoid taking shortcuts here, as the primary/secondary/idiopathic categorization could have important implications for treatment approaches. The distinction of primary, secondary and idiopathic MCAD is not widely accepted across the board by specialists, but these terms are sometimes used in the literature and it's important to have an understanding of what theoretically distinguishes each subgroup.

Updated Classification

Shortly after *MCAD* was recommended to be classified according to the three subgroups (primary, secondary, and idiopathic) in 2010,[35] some of the same authors proposed an updated classification scheme in the 2012 consensus proposal[8] with a slightly different method of organization. The 2012 version included the primary/secondary/idiopathic terminology in reference to *MCAS* (and not MCAD). Additional aspects of the 2012 recommendations vary slightly from what was published in 2010. Some consider these recommendations controversial and it's unclear whether the proposed classification(s) will become widely accepted.

Figure 4. Proposed Global Classification of Mast Cell Disorders and Pathological Reactions by Valent et al.[8] (2012)

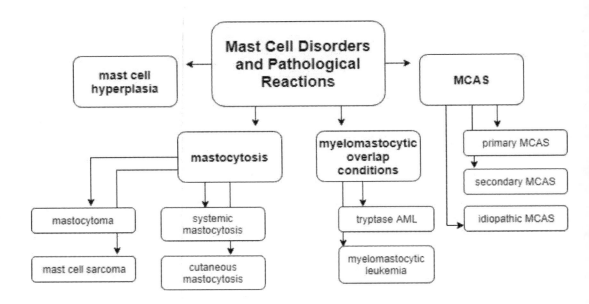

Valent et al. recommended a few changes to the current World Health Organization classification of mast cell-associated disorders, as outlined above.[8] The suggestions appear to stem from concern about the potential overdiagnosis of MCAS. Specifically, the authors mention overlaps between MCAS and other diseases seen in internal medicine, including allergic disease, mastocytosis, autoimmune disease, and skin conditions, as well as diverse neoplasms.[8]

The 2012 consensus suggested that a new classification include the following four categories: mast cell hyperplasia, MCAS, mastocytosis, and myelomastocytic-overlap conditions.[8] They included four conditions as subgroups of mastocytosis: systemic mastocytois (SM), cutaneous mastocytosis (CM), mastocytoma, and mast cell sarcoma.[8] The theoretical primary, secondary, and idiopathic terminology for MCAS are not currently applied *universally* in clinical practice.

The authors noted that "In order to count as co-criterion of mast cell activation (MCA), these symptoms need to be recurrent or permanent, cannot be explained by other known disorders/conditions (other than MCA), and require a therapeutic intervention. Moreover, apart from these symptoms, additional clinical and laboratory criteria have to be fulfilled for the condition/reaction to be considered as MCA."[8] They also commented that the likelihood of systemic mast cell activation increased when two or more organ systems show such symptoms at the same time.[8]

Mast cell hyperplasia typically occurs in the absence of MCAS, though some patients do present with both conditions. Criteria for diagnosis include an increase in tissue (non-clonal) mast cells with the absence of mastocytosis on testing, the absence of c-*KIT* genetic mutation, and no signs of neoplastic conditions.[8] Mast cell hyperplasia is thought to be a reactive state more so than a distinct disease process. This can be caused by autoimmune conditions, chronic infections, cancer, bone marrow suppression states, and lymphoproliferative disorders, and may also occur following stem cell factor administration and with other chronic inflammatory reactions.[8]

Myelomastocytic-overlap conditions refer to a mast cell lineage involvement in the presence of myeloid neoplasms.[8] Myeloid neoplasms by definition include therapy-related myelodysplastic syndrome or therapy-related acute myeloid leukemia. These conditions are thought to be due to long-term consequences of cytotoxic (cell-killing) treatments for another disease, including chemotherapy for cancer and other drugs for autoimmune conditions. Tryptase AML and myelomastocytic leukemia are examples of diagnoses that fall into this category of classification by Valent and colleagues.[8] These conditions are tricky to diagnose. While they are rare and the WHO does not recognize them as official mast cell-origin diseases as of 2018, they do exist along this spectrum.[8]

Regardless of which classification or diagnostic scheme may be accepted and utilized, it's crucial to determine the root issue(s) triggering MCAS. If an allergic disorder or infectious disease is at the root of the mast cell activation, pinpointing the underlying mechanism is essential in order to move forward in a timely manner with appropriate treatment. Patients with secondary or idiopathic presentations ought to have other factors evaluated with scrutiny to determine what underlying issues may be triggering symptoms. Patients with primary mast cell activation issues (as evidenced by monoclonality or mastocytosis) would also benefit from a thorough examination of the factors that may exacerbate the condition.

Physical therapists typically attempt to identify the root issues contributing to an injury in patients, and failure to do so can lead to further injury down the road. Complacency with the label of MCAS without further investigation into the underlying factors could lead to more chronic debilitative issues and a suboptimal "Band-Aid" approach to treatment. It's evident that while recommendations have been published and subsequently updated, the field lacks a universal consensus for clinical practice in this area.

Monoclonal MCAS Clarifications

Clonal mast cell disease ("primary MCAD" in the classification) includes either mastocytosis or monoclonal mast cell activation syndrome (abbreviated MMCAS or MMAS, depending on the author). *Anecdotally*, there is some debate about whether MMCAS is actually a premature form of systemic mastocytosis (SM), or perhaps it is truly SM but has not yet been detected diagnostically. (After all, multiple bone marrow biopsies may be performed over time in order to capture the SM diagnostic criteria.)[38,39]

Clonality in a Nutshell

The distinction of "clonality" is traditionally focused predominantly on whether a proven *KIT* (D816V) mutation is identified.[40] However, other tests are also used to confirm clonal mast cell disease. According to Austen and Akin, "Patients with clonal mast cell disorders generally have varying degrees of expansion of the mast cell compartment derived from a progenitor with a *genetic defect that presumably reduces the cell's threshold for activation*. These patients may have elevated serum tryptase levels, carry c-*KIT* mutations (most commonly D816V) in lesional mast cells, or have other markers of mast cell clonality such as aberrant CD25 expression."[17]

As discussed later on in this chapter, MCAS and MMCAS and SM *all* have evidence of genetic mutations that likely contribute to the disease process, but the *KIT* mutation at codon D816V is much more common in patients with clonal disease, including SM and MMCAS.

Molderings argues against the concept of somatic mutations in *KIT* as a key to definitive diagnostic criteria of clonality, adding that "until whole genome sequencing becomes routine, the term 'undetermined clonality' may be more accurate."[40]

It's important to note that there's a discrepancy between testing for clonality in the research laboratory versus in the commercial laboratory. For most patients with suspected MCAS, the investigation into potential clonality classification may prove futile, as it appears that only a small minority will actually test positive for signs of clonality in the currently available commercial lab techniques. According to Afrin and Khoruts, "Although MCAS appears usually clonal in the research laboratory, most commercial laboratories today assess MC (mast cell) clonality only by *KIT* mutation analysis at codon 816 (via polymerase chain reaction) or by MC CD25 or CD2 expression (by flow cytometry). As these signatures appear rare in MCAS, diagnosis presently rests on finding elevated MC mediator levels and excluding differential diagnoses."[41]

Biopsy Test Interpretation

Diagnostically, a patient with clonal disease at current guidelines must present with certain evidence of traits of SM without achieving the full criteria for SM. The presence of a cluster or group of identical mast cells made visible with special staining tests is one possible aspect of a clonal diagnosis and is one factor that can help confirm this label of clonality. The other traits of SM, determined by bone marrow or other tissue biopsy, include: infiltrates or groupings of mast cells in higher numbers than average with special staining (but not high enough to be considered SM), and/or expression of CD2 and CD25, and/or abnormal morphology (shape), and/or detection of genetic mutation(s). The literature consistently states that monoclonal MCAS occurs when *one or two of the characteristics of SM* are met, without the presence of all diagnostic criteria for SM.

Based on wording, some interpret the clonality diagnosis as the presence of any type of abnormalities on biopsy, which could include a genetic mutation but could also include abnormalities in mast cell shape or other characteristics that are found in SM (without the confirmation of a c-*KIT* mutation). A 2015 review paper indicated that monoclonality (in the absence of SM) is diagnosed in terms of an "either/or" scenario between genetic mutations and other biopsy findings.[3]

However, a 2010 paper by Akin and colleagues specified that *both* the c-*KIT* mutation and aberrant CD25 expression on bone marrow mast cells are considered hallmark of clonality.[35] A 2013 paper by Valent clarified that in order for MCAD to be primary (clonal), *KIT* D816V clonal mast cells must be found, and usually these mast cells express CD25.[42]

On the contrary, a 2012 consensus paper by the same authors (and subsequent publications) defined mast cell monoclonality as "CD25+ mast cells and/or *KIT* D816V."[8,43] By definition, "clonal" refers to a colony or group of organisms that have identical genetic traits. So, this begs the question, what about a patient who has abnormal CD25 expression but tests negative for the *KIT* mutation? Is this still considered clonal disease? *Anecdotally*, there appears to be some confusion among patients regarding how to properly classify this scenario and interpret the wording cited in different studies.

CD25 is regarded as a reliable immunohistochemical marker for the discrimination between neoplastic mast cells and normal mast cells.[44] Research consistently shows that the majority of patients with SM test positive for CD25. In a 2004 study, 98.6% of 73 patients with SM had CD25 expression;[44] 100% of 26 patients with SM tested positive for CD25 expression in a more recent (2015) study.[45] Other 2017 research also noted that 100% of 19 patients with SM expressed CD25 on bone marrow testing.[46]

It appears that CD25 is also a sensitive marker for SM in other tissue biopsies beyond bone marrow. Seventeen gastrointestinal biopsy samples in patients with SM were all determined to test positive for CD25 expression, whereas in the same study, over 200 biopsies from patients with other conditions (urticaria pigmentosa, irritable bowel syndrome, inflammatory bowel disease, parasites, eosinophilic gastroenteritis, and other gastrointestinal diagnoses) were used as the control group and *all tested negative* for CD25 expression.[47]

CD25 and mutations in *KIT* D816V generally appear to go hand-in-hand in patients with SM. The mutation can be multilineage or can be restricted to bone marrow mast cells. However, research has noted that about 20% of patients with SM do not test positive for the c-*KIT* D816V mutation.[14]

In 2012, researchers Morgado et al. evaluated the sensitivity and specificity of the CD25 and CD2 tests to determine the diagnosis of systemic mastocytosis.[48] Based on 886 bone marrow biopsies and 153 other (non-bone marrow) tissue samples, they determined that mast cell CD25+ expression *alone* had a stronger diagnostic accuracy (100% sensitivity and 99.2% specificity) than combined CD25+ and/or CD2+ expression for SM in bone marrow.[48] Prior studies reported similar values for combined CD25+ and/or CD2+ expression sensitivity and specificity.[49,50]

The recorded sensitivity and specificity of the research by Morgado and colleagues is indicative of a near-perfect diagnostic test. When put another way, if the CD25 test was negative, they could *rule out* the diagnosis of SM in 100% of patients. If the CD25 test was positive, they could *rule in* the diagnosis of SM in 99.2% of patients.[48]

The authors recommended that the World Health Organization (WHO) change the "CD25+ and/or CD2+" minor criterion to a "CD25+ expression" major criterion for the diagnosis of SM.[48] However, the subsequent WHO updated diagnostic criteria for SM did not reflect these recommendations in 2016.

A different research group in 2012 also evaluated the sensitivity of CD25+ and CD2+ mast cells by using a testing method called flow cytometry utilizing CD117 staining.[50] They found a sensitivity of 95% for both tests and determined that flow cytometry is more accurate than morphological analysis for these particular tests in order to evaluate for SM.[50]

A 2013 study evaluated 25 patients with suspected SM and found that 11 patients had the clinical diagnosis of SM, two patients had the clinical diagnosis of monoclonal MCAS (MMCAS), and two patients had the clinical diagnosis of MCAS.[51] All of the patients with SM had CD25+ expression on mast cells, and 10 of the 11 diagnosed with SM had evidence of the *KIT* mutation.[51]

Out of the patients that were diagnosed with monoclonal MCAS, one patient had a positive CD25+ expression test and a positive chemical mediator test plus signs and symptoms consistent with MCAD.[51] *However, this patient tested negative for the KIT mutation at D816V—and was still diagnosed with monoclonal MCAS based on the CD25 positive test.*[51] The other patient diagnosed with MMCAS had a positive *KIT* mutation and positive CD25+ expression test in the absence elevated mast cell mediators, also presenting with signs and symptoms consistent with MCAD.[51] Thus, both patients in this study had CD25 positive testing but only one had a *KIT* mutation; both patients were labeled with monoclonal MCAS.

The two patients with (non-clonal) MCAS had positive chemical mediator tests, but their CD25 and KIT tests were normal.[51] *The authors concluded that if less than three minor criteria were fulfilled for SM and patients exhibited clinical signs of MC degranulation, CD25 expression on mast cells was indicative of the presence of monoclonal MCAS.*[51]

A subsequent 2017 study also diagnosed patients with monoclonal MCAS based off CD25+ findings even in the absence of *KIT* mutations.[46] Though utilizing a small sample size, the study found that only *half* of patients with monoclonal MCAS had bone marrow evidence of the *KIT* D816V mutation, whereas *all* of the same patients with monoclonal MCAS had positive mast cell CD25 expression (via flow cytometry).[46]

In conclusion, based off the available literature, it appears that one can be clinically diagnosed with monoclonal MCAS in the absence of a proven *KIT* mutation, presuming they meet other inclusion criteria. Furthermore, the expression of CD25 on mast cells appears to be an especially useful indicator of clonality and may also suggest the presence of SM.

Clinically, Dr. Hamilton has noted the scenario where some mast cell-specific staining tests (specifically, CD25) are positive on colonic or gastric biopsies while others are negative.[52] He asserts that anytime a clonal mast cell disorder is suspected, such as the scenario when CD25 on the intestinal biopsies is positive, that patient should have bone marrow biopsy testing performed.[52]

Does Monoclonal MCAS lead to Systemic Mastocytosis?

Patients with primary (clonal) MCAS may or may not be *symptomatically* different from secondary and idiopathic cases of MCAS, and their tryptase levels are not always elevated. However, they tend to report more severe manifestations of anaphylaxis such as a drop in blood pressure or fainting.[17] Logically one could speculate that the primary (monoclonal) MCAS subgroup of patients is predisposed to developing the proliferative mast cell patterns of mastocytosis later on in life.

Anecdotally, some experts label the subgroup of patients with evidence of monoclonality as a "Pre-SM" patient population.[53] Senior scientist/molecular biologist Klimas explains, "Monoclonal mast cell activation syndrome is borderline for proliferation, meaning the body is thinking about making too many mast cells or is just starting to."[53] According to Austen and Akin, "The long-term natural course of monoclonal mast cell activation syndrome is not known, but a subset of patients may progress to systemic mastocytosis. Life threatening anaphylactic reactions may be encountered in a non-clonal setting or in all patients with underlying clonal mast cell expansion."[17]

Austen and Akin published a summary paper in 2016 in the Oncology Section of the Clinical Pain Advisor that addressed this theoretical possibility. They wrote, "While one might speculate that MMAS (monoclonal mast cell activation syndrome) may simply be a precursor to systemic mastocytosis, several lines of evidence suggest that this is not the case. First, follow up data available so far do not indicate progression to systemic mastocytosis in most patients with MMAS. Second, not all patients with systemic mastocytosis go through a phase with mast cell activation symptoms before developing signs or symptoms of tissue mast cell expansion. Finally, molecular studies of various hematopoietic cell lineages in patients with clonal mast cell disorders indicate that the c-*KIT* mutation is limited to the mast cell compartment in MMAS, whereas multilineage involvement in non-mast cell lineages is common in systemic mastocytosis."[17]

A literature search was unable to locate any follow-up data that tracked this patient subgroup over time. Thus, it appears that the jury is still out; there is a lack of ample evidence supporting or denying the development of SM from patients who originally presented with monoclonal MCAS.

Pitfalls to Current Diagnostic Scheme

Molderings and colleagues comment on the cons to following a black and white test-dependent diagnostic scheme with this subgroup of patients. "It remains unsettled in professional opinion of whether demonstration of an elevation of mast cell activity markers is absolutely necessary for diagnosis of MCAD because (1) many conditions (e.g., degrading enzymes, complexing molecules, tissue pH) may attenuate or impede spill-over of exocytosed mediators from tissues into the blood, (2) only a handful of the more than 60 releasable mast cell mediators can be detected by routine commercial techniques, and (3) mediator release syndrome may be due to an amplification cascade of basophil, eosinophil, and general leukocyte activation induced by liberation of only a few mast cell mediators which, again, may not be detectable by present techniques."[1] The currently available mast cell mediator testing and diagnostic schemes are far from perfect.

Furthermore, the decision of whether to perform a bone marrow biopsy does not currently appear to have a universal standard. Clinical considerations for the bone marrow biopsy decision-making process are discussed at length in Chapter 6.

The two different sets of recommended diagnostic criteria ("Criteria X" and "Criteria Y") are confounded by differing classification schemes—with no universally agreed-upon approach—and the poor sensitivity of blood and urine tests, which explains some of the variability in physician approaches to MCAS diagnosis. Some doctors will choose to perform the bone marrow biopsy without evidence of elevated mediators, and some doctors trial certain medications such as H1 and H2 blockers prior to confirmation of the diagnosis. Some doctors will label a patient with MCAS even in the absence of positive tests, while others will require two different positive tests across two different points in time before discussing MCAS with the patient.

At current, there is no *universal* set of agreed-upon criteria to guide clinical decision-making for the large number of patients walking into clinics with signs of MCAS. This challenge is a major pitfall in the advancement of MCAS awareness and acceptance in the medical community, and hopefully the future will provide greater uniformity and clarity for the diagnosis of this condition.

Differential Diagnosis

Critics argue that MCAS is largely overdiagnosed. An important aspect of clinical judgment lies in ruling out other potential differential diagnoses that may mimic or be associated with mast cell activation. Table 1 lists some of the conditions that experts recommend for consideration when a patient presents with signs of MCAS.

Table 1. Differential Diagnosis Considerations for MCAS, based on recommendations from Molderings and colleagues[1] (2011) and Theoharides and colleagues[4] (2015)

Endocrinological Disorders	diabetes mellitus
	Morbus Fabry
	pancreatic endocrine tumors (gastrinoma, insulinoma, glucagonoma, somatostatinoma, VIPoma)
	parathyroid tumor
	porphyria
	thyroid gland disorders
Gastrointestinal Disorders	eosinophilic esophagitis
	eosinophilic gastroenteritis
	GERD (gastroesophageal reflux disease)
	gluten enteropathy/celiac disease
	H. pylori-positive gastritis
	infectious enteritis
	inflammatory bowel disease (Crohn's disease, ulcerative colitis)
	intestinal obstructions
	irritable bowel syndrome
	microscopic colitis
	parasitic infections
	primary lactose intolerance
	vasoactive intestinal peptide-secreting tumor
Immunological / Neoplastic Diseases	autoinflammatory disorders such as deficiency of interleukin-1–receptor antagonist
	carcinoid tumor/syndrome
	familial hyper-IgE syndrome
	hereditary angioedema
	hypereosinophilic syndrome
	intestinal lymphoma
	pheochromocytoma
	primary gastrointestinal allergy

	vasculitis
Neurological and Psychiatric Conditions	anxiety
	autonomic dysfunction
	chronic fatigue syndrome
	depression
	headaches
	mixed organic brain syndrome
	multiple sclerosis
	somatization disorder
Skin Conditions	angioedema
	atopic dermatitis
	chronic urticaria
	scleroderma
Other Conditions	coronary hypersensitivity (Kounis syndrome)
	cholelithiasis
	fibromyalgia
	hepatitis
	hereditary hyperbilirubinemia
	POTS (postural orthostatic tachycardia syndrome)

Many of the conditions in Table 1 can mimic MCAS in some way. However, it's important to note that in some cases, patients may present with true clinical diagnoses of MCAS and one or more of the above conditions. For example, many patients with MCAS also have clinical diagnoses of POTS, irritable bowel syndrome, anxiety, and/or depression. Guidance from a skilled medical practitioner is important to ensure not only the validated presence of MCAS, but also that no other condition(s) are being missed in the MCAS diagnostic process.

Disease Spectrum

It's unclear exactly what percentage of patients with MCAS experience more serious or life-threatening complications of the disease. However, it's very clear that there is a wide spectrum of the disease, ranging from mild intermittent symptoms and intolerances to severely impaired organ function, continual anaphylaxis and other complications.

Molderings and colleagues note, "Clinical features and courses vary greatly and range from very indolent with normal life expectancy to highly aggressive with reduced survival times."[1]

Aggressive mast cell infiltration on the systemic level can sometimes lead to impaired organ function in patients with MCAS (not just SM or MCL). According to Molderings et al., "Organopathy due to mast cell infiltration is indicated by findings termed C-findings: (1) significant cytopenia(s); (2) hepatomegaly with impairment of liver function due to mast cell infiltration, often with ascites; (3) splenomegaly with hypersplenism; (4) malabsorption with hypoalbuminemia and weight loss; (5) life-threatening impairment of organ function in other organ systems; (6) osteolyses and/or severe osteoporosis with pathologic fractures. Urticaria pigmentosa-like skin lesions are usually absent."[1] This can occur even when the bone marrow smear shows less than 20% mast cells, which is the cut-off for MCL.[1]

The potential for a wide disease spectrum is reflected in the clinical decision-making algorithm (in Chapter 6), which highlights the need for considerations like organ evaluation and bone mineral density testing during patient examination.

Prevalence of MCAS

Historically, MCAD has been thought to be a rarity and has been infrequently recognized as a diagnostic option. The prevalence of mastocytosis in the general population was estimated to be 1 case per 10,000 persons by a 2014 study by Cohen and colleagues in Denmark.[54] While mastocytosis itself may indeed be that rare, it's becoming more and more theorized by specialists that the larger subgroup of patients with MCAS makes up a much larger proportion of the population than modern medicine may realize.

Since 2006, numerous studies have been published that link pathological mast cells to irritable bowel syndrome, inflammatory bowel disease, asthma, infectious disorders of the gastrointestinal tract, interstitial cystitis, and fibromyalgia, to name a few.[1,55-58] (Future chapters will elaborate more on these research areas.) The question is, how many people out there are simply living undiagnosed?

In 2012, German researchers conducted a study evaluating 120 patients (102 with MCAS and 18 with systemic mastocytosis) and a control group of 258 subjects in order to determine 1) familial aggregation within MCAD and 2) the prevalence of MCAD within the general population.[26] The study found that 75% of patients in the MCAD group had at least one first-degree relative with systemic MCAD, suggesting a heritability component.[26]

Researchers also found that the actual prevalence of systemic MCAD in first-degree relatives of patients with MCAD was 33%, compared to *14% in the general population.*[26]

112

However, one limitation to the study was that the control group was assessed using a survey and MCAD prevalence was determined through a checklist and differential diagnosis exclusion process, whereas the MCAD group prevalence was determined by an actual clinical diagnosis based on laboratory criteria for MCAD diagnosis.

The same German research group of Molderings and colleagues completed a second study evaluating the prevalence of MCAS and familial heritability in 2013. They determined *the general population prevalence of MCAS to be 17%.*[27] Thus, based on the two existing studies, it appears that 14%-17% of the general population *may be* walking around with (largely undiagnosed) cases of MCAS or other types of MCAD.

It's clear that more epidemiological research needs to happen in this area on a larger scale, with more stringent methodology in terms of the clinical criteria utilized for diagnosis, and in other geographical locations. That being said, the true prevalence will possibly be underestimated until mainstream medicine gets more on board with acknowledging and diagnosing the condition.

Physical therapists and other professionals who are afforded longer time frames to get to know patients may serve as important gatekeepers to 1) detect patients who may be presenting with chronic "mysterious" ailments consistent with MCAS, and 2) refer patients to providers who can perform all of the appropriate testing.

Regardless of the exact prevalence of each type of mast cell-related disease, experts agree that MCAS is the most common class of MCAD. Research published in 2014 noted that MCAS was most prevalent, followed by cutaneous mastocytosis, indolent systemic mastocytosis, systemic mastocytosis with associated clonal hematologic non-mast-cell lineage disorder (SM-AHNMD), aggressive systemic mastocytosis, and then mast cell leukemia.[23]

Figure 5. Visual Depiction of Prevalence of Mast Cell Activation Disease by Type[23]:

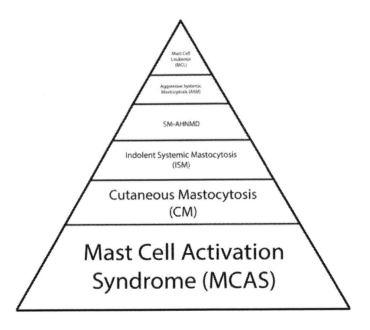

CHAPTER KEY POINTS

- Mast cell activation disease (MCAD) is an umbrella term for several diseases including forms of mastocytosis, mast cell leukemia, mast cell sarcoma, as well as mast cell activation syndrome (MCAS).

- Patients with MCAD typically have multi-system symptoms and a generalized widespread inflammatory pattern. Symptoms are often noted in the skin, eyes, major organs, gastrointestinal, respiratory, genitourinary, neuropsychiatric, and musculoskeletal systems. Patients may or may not present with signs of acute allergic reactions/anaphylaxis.

- Both MCAS and mastocytosis involve symptoms triggered by chemical mediators released by mast cells. The chemicals released by overactive (or high quantities of) mast cells create a wide array of acute and chronic symptoms.

- Mastocytosis is a rare disease that involves the presence of too many mast cells, often reflected in an elevated tryptase level, and is typically diagnosed with a bone marrow biopsy. Most patients with mastocytosis have a c-*KIT* mutation at codon D816V.

- MCAS is a disease that involves a normal number of mast cells that are "misbehaving" or reacting inappropriately to a wide range of triggers. MCAS is typically diagnosed by the presence of elevated chemical mediators in blood and/or urine testing, and/or the presence of abnormalities on tissue biopsy. Factors including a thorough differential diagnosis, the presence of mast cell-associated symptoms, and a clinical response to mast cell-targeting medications are also utilized in the diagnostic process.

- Monoclonal MCAS (MMAS or MMCAS) is a disease where the patient does not meet all of the criteria for systemic mastocytosis but does have measurable sign(s) of clonality on the tissue biopsy exam.

Chapter Four
Special Topics in MCAD

WHAT CAUSES MCAS?

This is the million-dollar question. Currently there is evidence supporting a relationship between MCAS development and genetic factors. There is great debate over other conditions that appear associated with MCAS (such as Lyme disease or Ehlers-Danlos syndrome) and whether MCAS makes one susceptible to these conditions, or vice-versa. There are theories about immune system function, emotional trauma, and other factors that may also be causative or contributory that will all be discussed at length in this book.

MCAS & Autoimmunity

Some research indicates that mast cells may participate in immune responses to self-antigens and may contribute to autoimmune pathologies.[1] Researchers have noted that IgG receptors and the complement system appear to be involved in autoimmune-type mast cell mechanisms.[2] But it still remains somewhat cloudy: technically, is MCAS an autoimmune disease?

According to Afrin, "The answer is, we really don't know. An autoimmune disease is a disease where the immune system has inappropriately and erroneously generated antibodies that target one tissue or another, one cell or another, that leads to dysfunction of that cell or tissue... A classic example is the anti-nuclear antibody (ANA) and lupus and other rheumatological diseases. There are a small number of autoantibodies that seem to have potential for causing abnormal activation of the mast cell. But it is far from clear that it is autoimmunity that is at the root of the improper mast cell activation in most patients who have MCAS."[3]

According to Afrin,[3] the main theories at present are that:

- MCAS is due to a primary activation process,* ie) genetic mutations;
- MCAS is due to a secondary activation process (normal mast cells responding to some trigger); and
- MCAS is due to autoantibodies playing a role in an autoimmune process.

*Afrin notes that the best presently available preliminary research data regarding the roots of MCAS strongly suggest that it is a primary process, i.e., a mutationally driven process, in the vast majority of patients. He adds, "But these mutations, present just in the mast cells, are presently detectable only in research laboratories, not clinical laboratories."[4]

Inflammation and autoimmunity have been extensively studied and linked to mast cell activation.[5] Autoimmune diseases of the skin, joints, and brain have been associated with mast cell activity, and some authors believe that mast cells may be part of the complex cellular chain that leads to autoimmunity.[6]

Cross-talk between mast cells and other cells like neurons, lymphocytes, and glial cells has been associated with a number of inflammatory and autoimmune conditions.[7] Inflammatory diseases involving mast cells are well-documented and include asthma, osteoarthritis, fibromyalgia, atopic dermatitis, chronic rhinitis, chronic prostatitis, coronary artery disease, migraines, interstitial cystitis, and others.[8]

Gregory and colleagues published a paper on mast cells and autoimmunity in 2008 and noted that mast cells and other allergic components (such as IgE) have been implicated in autoimmune mechanisms.[9] Studies have connected mast cells to the pathology of autoimmune conditions such as rheumatoid arthritis, multiple sclerosis, Graves' Disease, type I diabetes, systemic lupus erythematosus, and bullous pemphigoid, to name a few.[9,10]

In a review on the potential autoimmune-like characteristics of mast cells, Walker and colleagues note that there's a growing body of evidence connecting mast cells to autoimmune disease exacerbation.[10] They comment that the immune responses in autoimmune disease are very similar to what is observed with allergic responses.[10] In many diseases, mast cells recruit other cells like neutrophils to the area of autoimmune destruction.[10] Mast cells also influence the activity of T regulatory cells, B cells, and central nervous system cells in autoimmune conditions.[10]

Several mediators are beginning to be researched in terms of their roles in autoimmunity.[10] Some are more familiar suspects, such as substance P, an inflammatory mediator that has been

118

widely associated with a number of different pathological conditions.[10] Substance P can contribute to the release of tumor necrosis factor (TNF) by mast cells, which is believed to contribute to multiple autoimmune diseases.[10]

Other mediators, such as osteopontin, are lesser known and offer interesting theories for future research direction. Osteopontin is a protein that has been implicated in both multiple sclerosis and experimental allergic encephalomyelitis.[10,11] Mast cells are one type of cell that release osteopontin. Walker and colleagues note, "Although there is no direct link between mast cell expression of osteopontin and MS (multiple sclerosis), the presence of mast cells at sites where this protein is highly expressed in inflammatory CNS (central nervous system) plaques and its ability to modulate mast cell function is intriguing."[10]

The 2012 review[10] noted that, based on the literature,[12] Guillain-Barré syndrome, Graves' ophthalmopathy, pemphigus vulgaris, systemic lupus erythematosus, and Sjogren's syndrome are other diseases that have *potential* mast cell-autoimmune connections, as evidenced by mast cell activation during the disease or responses to mast cell-targeting medications.[13]

On the contrary, there are some who believe that MCAS results in overall immunosuppression. One theory is that the distinction between immune system suppression and over-activation may depend on which type of chemical mediator is being released. Interleukin-10 released by mast cells has been associated with an overall suppression of the immune system response.[14]

St. John and Abraham note, "MCs (mast cells) initiate proinflammatory cytokine production, but they also inhibit these responses when a situation warrants such action. MC-directed responses *may also promote immunity in one context while having a suppressive function in another*. Thus, MCs may have widely divergent proinflammatory or immunosuppressive effects depending on the cell types that they recruit to, or encounter within, an inflammatory milieu."[15]

Kinet has an interesting evolutionary theory on the shift of mast cells from a protective role to inflammatory (and potentially autoimmune) agents. He discusses the question, "Are mast cells conducting the orchestra, or simply blowing the trumpet?"[16] Kinet asserts that while many other cells are involved in inflammatory responses, mast cells play a central role in conducting the orchestra.[16] Mast cells are associated with numerous inflammatory diseases, play a role in innate immunity as well as in anti-inflammatory processes, and were arguably one of the first primitive cells from an evolutionary perspective.[16]

According to Kinet, "The real question, then, is whether mast cells are still necessary and essential as a protective shield in our Westernized societies, which show the highest prevalence for many inflammatory diseases such as asthma and multiple sclerosis. One could hypothesize precisely that because mast cells are no longer needed to play a protective role, they now are dominant in orchestrating the inflammatory reactions leading to these diseases."[16] The hygiene hypothesis suggests that individuals who were protected from exposure to infectious substances go on to develop hypersensitivity to minor or harmless agents, which could be associated with chronic inflammatory and/or autoimmune conditions. Perhaps mast cells play a pivotal role in this physiological process, as Kinet suggests.

Other researchers question whether autoimmunity is truly the body "attacking itself" or whether it's a normal immune process that is occurring as the body encounters and reacts to the presence of chronic viruses, bacterial infections or other causes. Proal and Marshall note that when the theory of autoimmunity originally developed, the body was considered a sterile playing field, and antibodies in ill patients were not tied to persistent pathogens, birthing the term "autoantibody."[17] However, recent evidence of a vast internal microbiome (consisting of viruses, bacteria, fungi, and other organisms) in humans challenges the conceptual basis of autoimmunity. "Autoantibodies" could actually be normal antibodies that are created in response to pathogens in the microbiome.[17]

While the available theories are intriguing, it's clear from MCAS experts that no concrete answer is presently available to justifiably label MCAS as an autoimmune disease; likewise, the consensus is currently unable to state with confidence that mast cells are causative agents in autoimmune diseases. And it's also plausible that the modern medicine label of a disease as "autoimmune" is faulty in itself as an explanation for what is occurring physiologically. In light of the role of the microbiome, microorganisms could act as pathogens in an immunosuppressed host, resulting in widespread inflammation, as suggested by Proal and Marshall,[17] though this book will not dive too deep into this debate.

Genetics: The c-KIT Mutation and Systemic Mastocytosis

One of the major hallmarks in genetic research for MCAD was the identification of the somatic mutation *KIT* D816V in patients with systemic mastocytosis (SM). For a while after this discovery, research then narrowed in on mutations of tyrosine kinase *KIT* in the bone marrow and peripheral blood (a criterion to determine "clonality") as the main focus of genetic and clinical testing. Recent publications state that "Expressed 10-fold brighter in MCs (mast cells) than in any other human cells, transmembrane tyrosine kinase *KIT* is the dominant MC regulator."[18,19]

The spindle-shaped morphology of mast cells, the overproduction of tryptase, their expression of CD25 (the appearance of a certain protein that is never seen on the surface of a "normal" mast cell), and the presence of mast cell clusters are all consistent with a c-*KIT* mutation at codon 816 and the World Health Organization's clinical diagnosis of mastocytosis (previously presented in Chapter Three).[20] Experts in MCAS agree that the "classic" mutation at codon D816V as well as other *KIT* mutations in exon 17 should both count as signs of monoclonal mast cells.[21]

However, not all research supports the utility of *KIT* to determine severity of MCAD. A 2013 study evaluated 48 patients with Indolent Systemic Mastocytosis (ISM) to determine whether clinical severity correlated with *KIT* D816V mutation-positive findings. Researchers found that the presence or absence of the *KIT* mutation had no association with the presence of symptoms, severity of symptoms, bone mineral density status, or presence of absence of anaphylactic episodes.[22]

Recent research has noted that somatic mutations in epigenetic regulator genes have been associated with SM, particularly those involved with DNA methylation and the regulation of chromatin modification.[23] Specifically, researchers have noted mutations in TET2, DNMT3A, IDH2, ASLX1, SRSF2, and EZH2. TET2 has been correlated with a more aggressive progression of SM, and one study found that it was present in 39% of patients with SM.[23]

In the SM population, mutations have also been noted in genes that encode proteins of other cellular pathways and genes that encode RNA splicing proteins.[23] Interestingly, it appears that some of these mutations play a bigger role in the *initial* proliferative clonal phase of SM only. TET2 and SRSF2, for example, are labeled "founder mutations" because they typically occur prior to a mutation in *KIT*.[23] Thus, *KIT* may be more of a "driver" in disease progression than an instigator of the disease itself.[23]

Research published in 2015 noted that over 20 single point *KIT* mutations are also possible, in addition to mutations with familial inheritance in patients with MCAD.[24] The same authors also confer that additional mutations in genes such as TET2 and ASXL1 are detectable in the presence of mast cell monoclonality, particularly in patients with associated hematologic disorders.[24] Afrin noted in a 2017 presentation on MCAS that there are now "more than 50 mutations (mostly heterozygous, but still functionally dominant) found scattered across all domains of *KIT*."[25] Thus, multiple research groups agree that a plethora of identified mutations have been confirmed, and that the *KIT* D816V is not the only pathogenetic factor associated with mastocytosis (and potentially clonal cases of MCAS).[23-25]

Molderings et al. further elaborates on this concept in an article published in 2011.[20] "Another aspect that limits the diagnostic value of this mutation is that during progression of SM the *KIT* mutant D816V may disappear.[20,26] Taken together, the recent genetic findings[2,27-29] suggest that the clinically different subtypes of MCAD (encompassing SM, MCL, and MCAS) should be more accurately regarded as varying presentations of a common generic root process of mast cell dysfunction than as distinct diseases."[20]

There are other physiologic factors that could play a role in the etiology or progression/outcome of mastocytosis, and the c-*KIT* mutation has also been found in an asymptomatic population, which raises questions to the underlying mechanism behind mastocytosis.[20] Some researchers theorize that mutations in certain receptors and enzymes (such as Src-kinases, JAK2, histamine H4 receptor, c-Cbl-encoded E3 ligase, and others) could also be a possible link to the disease.[20] In addition, somatic mutations to the gene FIP1L1-PDGFR-alpha are now connected to mastocytosis.[20,30]

Clearly there is a (potentially) much more complex role of genetic mutations in patients with SM that expands far beyond the *KIT* mutation at D816V. This is one example indicating that current knowledge about SM and genetic influences is likely just the tip of the iceberg; and yet, SM is a diagnosis that has been around for a long time. Logically, one would expect that research will find increasing genetic mutation connections to MCAS over the next several decades. MCAS etiological findings are simply in the "infancy" stage of knowledge.

Genetics and MCAS: The Simplified Version

The theorized difference between SM and MCAS genetic mutation expression in testing, based on multiple studies, is that MCAS typically does not involve altered morphology of mast cells or readily detectable mast cell accumulation with staining, even though both conditions involve aberrant mediator release and production.[23]

Molderings' team in Germany is leading the way with research about genetic findings in the MCAS population. Molderings and colleagues noted that the *KIT*-specific mutations in the majority of patients with MCAD were somatic rather than germline in nature.[23] *Somatic mutations* are not inherited and are generally acquired early on in life. While somatic mutations do not get transferred to offspring, *germline mutations* by nature do get transferred to offspring.

Afrin comments, "It's increasingly evident that most MCAS patients have mutations in one or more of the regulatory genes in their dysfunctional mast cells. These mutations are almost never inborn (i.e., 'germline,' or inherited, mutations) and instead are almost always acquired

122

('somatic' mutations), typically at a relatively early age (in some patients perhaps even in utero)."[31]

Multiple somatic mutations in *KIT* D816V have been identified in *some* patients with MCAS. A 2010 study by Molderings and colleagues examined 20 patients with MCAS and 20 age-matched healthy volunteers and found that 13 out of 20 MCAS patients (65%) presented with tyrosine kinase *KIT* mutations, compared to one person out of 20 (5%) in the non-MCAS group.[28]

Research conducted in 2013, also by Molderings and colleagues, determined a 46% prevalence of MCAS in relatives of MCAD patients (based on symptomology).[32] When compared to the 17% percent estimated prevalence of MCAS in a German population, it appears that the 46% familial connection is not due to chance. Molderings notes that "although familial occurrence due to shared environmental factors cannot be ruled out, a significant genetic contribution to this family occurrence is likely."[23]

That same study found that 75% of patients with some type of MCAD (SM or MCAS) had at least one first-degree relative with MCAD.[32] The researchers explained, "Our findings observed in the three pedigrees together with recent reports in the literature suggest that, in familial cases (i.e., in the majority of MCAD), mutated disease-related operator and/or regulator genes could be responsible for the development of somatic mutations in *KIT* and other proteins important for the regulation of mast cell activity."[32]

According to Afrin, "The particular set of these mutations present in any one patient (their 'mutational profile') is usually different from any other patient's mutational profile. Even in families affected by MCAS, the disease may not affect every member of the family, and the mutational profiles of the different MCAS-affected members of the family are usually different. This goes a long way toward explaining why the clinical presentation/behavior of the disease can be so different from one member of an affected family to the next affected member of an affected family, in turn making it difficult to recognize the infiltration of the disease throughout the family."[31]

Afrin theorizes that perhaps each mutation results in the abnormal release of a certain set of mediators, and that patients with MCAS may have multiple mutations, which could explain the multiple mediators released, leading to multisystem comorbidities and clinical heterogeneity noted in this patient population.[25]

As an example of this theory, perhaps one particular, single mutation is responsible for excess prostaglandin synthesis/release (which results in a particular group of symptoms) and another specific single mutation is responsible for excess degranulation of heparin. Perhaps the

123

reason that patients with MCAS may present so differently—despite the same diagnosis—lies in which particular combination of mutations are present, how they interact with each other, and the resultant barrage of chemical mediators in the body. Indeed, research has already focused on connections to specific genetic mutations that may be responsible for elevated histamine and tryptase, supporting the idea of chemical mediator-specific anomalies.[33-36]

Recent research has shifted to next-generation sequencing techniques in testing, which has led to the identification of mutations in other genes for patients with MCAS, including germline mutations (the type that *do* get transferred to offspring).[23]

A 2017 study also based out of the research group in Germany evaluated 25 different genes of patients with clinical diagnoses of MCAS; genes were selected based on published genetic research in cohorts of patients with SM.[37] The study found 67 different germline mutations present in patients with MCAS.[37] Researchers concluded that these findings "may be functionally relevant and explain familial aggregation."[37] They encouraged independent replication studies to follow.

While these findings are exciting, as a whole there's inadequate research regarding the influence of somatic and germline mutations in the MCAS patient population, and future replications of research utilizing cohorts from other geographical locations will hopefully provide more clarity.

The implications of continued developments in this area could be far-reaching. Improved detection of MCAS via genetic testing could transform the management of MCAS, saving patients time and money in the process. Determination of mutations specific to chemical mediators could also have implications for the pharmacological management of MCAS. Thus, further research in this area is extremely important.

The Role of Epigenetics in MCAS

Epigenetics may play a bigger role than somatic or germline mutations in MCAS. According to Afrin, "Current thinking suggests that perhaps something really is getting inherited in MCAS-afflicted families, but it's not the genetic mutation which is being inherited. Instead, it may be epigenetic mutations which are being inherited."[31]

The concept of epigenetics is embedded in a normally occurring ebb and flow within the body that influences the way that cells interpret genes. Epigenetics involves changes in the way genes are expressed without them undergoing structural changes in the underlying DNA sequence. Epigenetics dictate whether genes are active or inactive, which can influence molecular processes such as the migration of cells (or, in unfortunate cases, cancer). Epigenetic changes can be influenced by factors like disease state, age, and lifestyle.[38] Epigenes, whether normal or mutated, can be passed on to offspring.

There are multiple systems in place that are able to initiate and sustain epigenetic changes, and methylation is one of them.[38] Methylation is the process by which methyl groups are added to the DNA molecule. This is an epigenetic process that modifies the function of genes. It's responsible for many of our vital functions and processes on a cellular level and is well known for its influence in the body's ability to remove toxins, repair DNA and reduce inflammation levels.[39]

There's certainly signs of epigenetic factors in the etiology of MCAS. Molderings notes an association between MCAS and mutations in splicing proteins, as well as alterations in DNA methylation.[23] Molderings and other researchers conclude in multiple papers that "epigenetic processes appear to make a substantial contribution to the transgenerational transmission of MCAS."[23,40] A 2015 review on MCAS also concluded that "most MCAD-associated mutations appear somatic, but familial MCAD appears common and may be an epigenetic phenomenon."[19]

In summary, the search for *KIT* mutations at D816V may identify patients with systemic mastocytosis, but when it comes to MCAS, there's (currently) no such single gene that explains everything. The potential genetic or epigenetic mutations for MCAS come along sometime in utero or after birth; they may or may not be copied and passed down, and individual specific genetic mutations are likely different from those of family members, even if all family members have MCAS. (Ironically, family members may not recognize they have MCAS because of the different presentations and manifestations of the disease, which may be regulated by different chemical mediators.) Along the way, depending on the environment, individuals may "turn on" the expression of certain epigenetic factors that influence physiologic efficiency (or "methylation"), which could play a role in the subsequent symptom level.

MCAS and the RCCX Theory

Dr. Sharon Meglathery is board-certified in psychiatry and has noted a high percentage of her patients suffering from chronic illness, including mast cell activation syndrome (MCAS). She devised a hypothesis called the "RCCX Theory," which aims to explain the connections between a wide range of chronic overlapping medical diagnoses.[41] Specifically, she theorizes that mutations along the RCCX gene module (specifically, CYP21A2, TNXB, and C4 genetic mutations) are responsible for predisposition in individuals and families to psychiatric illness and medical illness.[41]

Meglathery notes that "unlike contiguous gene mutations in other parts of the genome, these genetic mutations are often inherited together, conferring vulnerabilities to multiple genetic issues at one time."[41] The RCCX Theory associates changes in the CYP21A2 gene with vulnerability to an altered acute stress response, changes in the TNXB gene with tissue characteristics seen in hypermobility of the joints, and changes in the C4 gene with a variety of autoimmune diseases, immunodeficiency states, and changes in dendritic branching in the brain.[41] Meglathery states that "CYP21A2 mutations are between 10-20% of the population… TNXB and C4 mutations are also extremely common."[41]

Mutations to the RCCX gene region are not the epigenetic/SNP types that are commonly discussed with methylation, but are rather a *copy number variation* type of mutation. RCCX mutations are not identified in commercial "over-the-counter" genetic testing like 23andMe. Currently, testing for the RCCX gene is not readily available to most patients.[42] The three areas of RCCX need *not* be affected simultaneously in order to trigger illness. Some patients may have mutations of all the RCCX genes, while others may have a single mutation in one area.[42]

Not all patients with MCAS have RCCX mutations, and not all patients with RCCX mutations have MCAS. Meglathery believes that MCAS is one of the many physiological states that can occur as a downstream side effect from a CYP21A2 RCCX genetic mutation.[42]

Meglathery connects genetic mutations of CYP21A2 to conditions such as postural orthostatic tachycardia syndrome (POTS), MCAS, hypermobile Ehlers-Danlos syndrome, fibromyalgia, chronic fatigue syndrome, Lyme disease, Epstein Barr infection, and mold toxicity, as well as a spectrum of psychiatric conditions including autistic features and high intelligence.[41] Her website lists a great number of conditions that are often comorbid with the MCAS population, such as adrenal fatigue and thyroid disorders, interstitial cystitis, gastrointestinal findings such as small intestinal bacterial overgrowth, candida overgrowth, fungal infections, temperature dysregulation, Raynaud's disease, connective tissue irregularities, and much more.[41]

CYP21A2 Mutation – RCCX Gene Module

The RCCX Theory maintains that the presence of one or more mutations at CYP21A2 may be enough to trigger an aberrant stress response in utero and in infancy that "wires the brain for danger" and results in chronic problems with cortisol and post-traumatic stress disorder (PTSD)-like responses due to epigenetic stress effects.[42] When people with CYP21A2

126

mutations are exposed to prolonged stress, known elevated corticotropin releasing hormone (CRH) turns on inflammatory cascades and stimulates mast cells, which can trigger a clinical picture of MCAS.[42]

Acute stress emerging from factors like exposure to mold or Lyme bacteria via CYP21A2 mutations also appears to lead to the same inflammatory cascades and activation of mast cells in the brain and in the body.[42] Meglathery notes that viruses like Epstein-Barr, strong bacterial infections, or physical trauma could indeed be strong enough to "flip" a CYP21A2 mutation carrying population into chronic illness.[42]

Meglathery believes that there are two groups of MCAS patients[42]:

- Patients who likely have CYP21A2 RCCX genetic mutations driven by stress who tend to be very "unique psychologically," and
- Patients who have MCAS without RCCX mutations who lack the psychological profile

Specifically, Meglathery notes that a large subgroup of patients that have a CYP21A2 RCCX genetic mutation exhibit unique psychological characteristics like elevated intelligence levels or other special abilities.[42] These patients tend to be empathic, highly reactive, and sensitive to the environment. Patients in this category may have clinical symptoms of PTSD, many without significant trauma. She believes that patients with mild CYP21A2 mutations (not requiring treatment at birth) have a resulting neuropsychiatric profile with the brain wired for danger by the age of 5, which she terms "CAPS" or the psychological profile "CYP21A2 associated neuropsychiatric spectrum."[42] Patients with CAPS tend to have enlarged limbic structures that correspond to increased emotions and fear, high levels of stress arousal, sensory sensitivities, and intersex tendencies, and some meet the criteria for autism spectrum disorders.[42] They may have clinical diagnoses of conditions such as Asperger's or bipolar disorder, but often have no clear psychiatric diagnosis.[42]

CYP21A2 codes for a crucial enzyme called 21 hydroxylase that is involved with stress reactions. Initially, patients with a CYP21A2 mutation have elevated cortisol in response to stress and low basal cortisol.[42] In response to prolonged or strong stressors, 21 hydroxylase becomes blocked, which can transition the patient into a more chronic illness state, where cortisol is actually low and orthostatic stress and POTS may potentially develop.[42] This pathway can then lead to elevated corticotropin-releasing hormone, which increases norepinephrine and mast cell activation and decreases stomach acid, leading to dysbiosis.[42]

127

Basal cortisol decreases more dramatically with inappropriately low stress cortisol and high cholesterol, and progesterone and androgens can develop.[42] According to Meglathery, the elevated progesterone can lead to a number of symptoms and can also trigger an increase in mast cell activation.[42]

The resulting inflammation from CYP21A2 RCCX mutations may be tied to a variety of neuroimmune symptoms. Epigenetic stress wiring in the brain pushes toward increasing danger responses in the form of fight or flight, freeze and shutdown.[42] Initially, most patients exhibit fight or flight sympathetic nervous system activity, characterized by elevated heart rate and blood pressure, increased sweating, and decreased gut motility.[42]

Over time, many patients move toward the freeze phase in response to perceived danger, where they tend to experience a lower heart rate, breath holding, muscle tension (especially in the shoulders, neck, and back), hearing changes, and sometimes immobility.[42] The freezing state is triggered by neural memory networks from PTSD and can result in a catatonic or dystonic state.[42] Shutdown can also occur when there is opiate dumping preparation in addition to freezing.[42] Patients may predominantly experience one side of the nervous system spectrum but can also shift between states over the course of time.[42] Pseudoseizures are sometimes observed with CYP21A2 mutations and may be associated with the danger response and PTSD wiring.[42]

Patients with CAPS tend to experience various phases of dysautonomia-associated stress responses. Meglathery explains that there is a "wired for danger scale" dependent on factors in-utero that appears to determine whether a person will be more of an extroverted thrill seeker or more fearful and anxious.[42] Likewise, she notes that patients with presumed CYP21A2 RCCX mutations tend to be either more of an empath or more of a narcissist; both personality types tend to read people well.[42]

TNXB Mutation – RCCX Gene Module

TNXB gene mutations increase levels of TGF-beta in the system, which can lead to slow, gradual changes in the extracellular matrix that influence collagen, joint mobility, and orthostatic stress. If a patient has abnormal connective tissue from a TNXB mutation, the body is more predisposed to dysfunctional movement and chronic overuse issues with a greater inflammatory cascade in the tissues. Clinically, this could present as something like myofascial pain or joint issues noted in patients who have the hypermobile type of Ehlers-Danlos syndrome. Meglathery notes that as the body responds to an increasing danger response, more stooped and twisted postures often develop.[42]

128

"Additionally, TNXB mutations increase orthostatic stress due to floppy blood vessels with resultant blood pooling in the extremities contributing to the stress load which activates the CYP21A2 mutation-associated issues. Further, TNXB mutations are associated with TGF beta signaling abnormalities which can result in fibrotic and inflammatory conditions as well."[42] TNXB mutations may trigger changes in the extracellular matrix that influence factors like lymphatic function and glial cells, among others.[42]

C4 Mutation – RCCX Gene Module

If a particular patient also has a mutation at C4, the inflammatory responses may be more severe, and the patient may also go on to develop autoimmune problems or immunodeficiencies and abnormal dendritic branching patterns in the brain.[42] Specifically, C4 gene mutations influence the development of autoantibodies, which are associated with the development of autoimmune conditions as well as POTS.[42]

Patients with C4 mutations tend to have slower onset symptoms that wax and wane-—often across the lifetime—but may experience a sudden deterioration or collapse associated with stress.[42] Meglathery believes that some patients with immunodeficiencies like CVID and IgG issues are likely carrying C4 mutations.[42] They tend to present with longstanding immunodeficiency-associated problems, like difficulty clearing Epstein-Barr virus.[42]

RCCX Theory Conclusions

It appears that variations in symptom onset may be related to the type of RCCX mutation present, as well as presence of stressors. Certain downstream effects of CYP21A2 mutations develop slowly (like PTSD/danger wiring and rises in norepinephrine) while others (like drops in cortisol and mast cell activation) can develop suddenly and intensely.[42] In contrast, TNXB mutations lead to slow, gradual changes and C4 mutations tend to have an underlying current of dysfunction that can go overboard with sudden severe stress.[42]

According to Meglathery, additional subgroups are emerging that appear to have certain tendencies. For example, some people with presumed CYP21A2 mutation without TNXB mutations experience 21 hydroxylase block with stress, endocrine issues, chronic illness, mast cell activation issues, and psychological manifestations without exhibiting hypermobility.[42] In addition, some patients with CAPS seem to have a normal immune system prior to becoming sick and once ill with MCAS, they demonstrate a highly functioning system where they never get the common cold but suffering recurrent herpes and fungal infections.[42]

Meglathery supports the relationships postulated in the Driscoll Theory (discussed in Chapter 7) regarding intracranial pressure and acquired cases of Chiari malformation from the brain getting pushed down in the skull.[42,43] She notes that factors like elevated progesterone, mast cell activation, neuroinflammation, and low cortisol (resulting from the cascade of influences of RCCX genetic mutations) can elevate intracranial pressure.[42]

Meglathery notes that, based on Dr. Naviaux's research,[44] mitochondrial shutdown can occur in these types of patients. Mutations to any or all three RCCX genes may shut down the mitochondria—the energy powerhouse of the cell—which can contribute significantly to chronic fatigue, the cell danger response, and lack of healing.[42,44]

Meglathery comments, "Over time, it became clear to me that there seems to be a frequently disabling epidemic involving a large number of syndromes/symptoms/diseases with overlapping symptoms affecting mainly young, vibrant, talented people (predominantly women) and if you look, many, but not all, have joint hypermobility (double jointedness, ligament laxity)."[41] She adds, "There are still many people who believe that these chronic illness conditions are completely separate in pathophysiology, e.g. all of the symptoms associated with EDS are solely caused by a genetic defect of collagen, all of the symptoms of Lyme disease are caused by *borrelia burgdorferi*, all symptoms of CIRS are caused by the inciting agent, etc. But, every day, it is becoming more clear that these conditions all go down a common pathway. There are just too many very specific overlapping symptoms for it to be any other way."[41]

Like MCAS, the breadth of issues and potential triggers is enormous, and there is no single hallmark clinical picture for patients with RCCX genetic mutations. The RCCX Theory supports that MCAS is *one of many* physiological changes that can occur as a result of genetic mutation(s) coupled with the right environmental factors, as opposed to pointing a finger of blame at mast cell activation as the trigger for comorbid conditions.

Meglathery is the first to note that despite compelling indicators of these connections, the RCCX Theory is (currently) just that: *a theory*. Hopefully research will focus in on this particular gene module in the future.

THE TRYPTASE CONUNDRUM

Despite the MCAD algorithms and classifications that have been widely published, chances are patients have already encountered allergists or other medical professionals who simply want to order one test: tryptase. *Anecdotally*, many patients become frustrated that so many practitioners continue to rely heavily or solely on tryptase levels before they are willing to further pursue additional diagnostic testing or move forward with care. The focus on tryptase is particularly frustrating in light of literature that supports that tryptase is a poor indicator of MCAS.

In 2017, Afrin and colleagues evaluated and published the laboratory values of approximately 400 patients with a confirmed diagnosis of MCAS.[45] They found that the average serum tryptase level was 5.77, and only 16% of patients in the study had elevated tryptase levels.[45] (Depending on the laboratory, tryptase levels greater than ~11.4 ng/ml may be considered elevated.) Further, only 3.9% of this patient population had tryptase levels above 20 ng/ml, the typical cut-off level for consideration of systemic mastocytosis.[45] The authors concluded that "relative utilities of mast cell mediators for diagnosis in our patients were similar to a recent report[46] and further suggest serum tryptase—while still a good screen for mast cell neoplasia—poorly reflects mast cell activation."[45]

In 2014, Zblewski and colleagues evaluated tryptase levels and symptoms reported by patients as a comparison between patients with MCAS and (various types of) SM.[47] The research utilized the Mastocytosis Symptom Assessment Form (MSAF) which has 20 items totaling a maximum score of 200 points, plus additional scoring depending on the frequency (per week) of flushing and the frequency (per month) of attacks with or without a loss of consciousness. Fifty-three patients were studied, and the patients with SM had a median symptom score of 47, compared to a median symptom score of 127 in patients with MCAS.[47] (Higher scores indicate greater symptom severity.)

When broken down by system, patients with MCAS had a statistically significant higher severity of symptoms in all areas except genitourinary and respiratory symptoms, which were similar in both patient populations.[47] Patients with MCAS had an average symptom score that was most debilitating in the neuropsychological, musculoskeletal, cutaneous, and constitutional symptom categories.[47]

In the same 2014 study, patients with SM had a median tryptase level of 48.4 ng/ml, and four of those patients (14%) had a value *less than* 20 ng/ml (the traditional cutoff for diagnostic consideration of SM).[47] The median tryptase level for patients with MCAS was 12.7 ng/ml, and only about one-third of MCAS patients presented with levels *higher* than 20 ng/ml.[47] According to the authors, "serum tryptase level had limited if any correlation with symptom scores."[47]

This single study indicates that patients with MCAS may be more symptomatic than patients with SM[47], though it was unclear which patients, if any, had adequate symptom control due to medications. (The testing was performed on patients "at referral," indicating that none of the studied patients had been counseled prior on MCAD treatment with medications.)

Furthermore, the study confirms that 1) serum tryptase is a laboratory test that does not appear to be associated with symptom severity, and 2) relying solely on tryptase as a chemical mediator is not sufficient to capture the majority of patients with MCAS.[47]

While elevated tryptase levels are certainly not tell-tale for MCAS, it's possible that a *small subgroup* of MCAS patients have a genetic predisposition to elevated tryptase. Research indicates that 4%-6% of the general population may have elevated tryptase levels.[48-49]

Lyons and colleagues have been evaluating the concept of *familial hypertryptasemia* for a number of years. In 2014, their research team from the University of Cincinnati evaluated connections between high tryptase levels, connective tissue issues, atopy, and mast cell symptoms.[50] They evaluated nine patients with hypertryptasemia who had evidence of non-clonal mast cell activation and atopic (skin or asthma) signs and noted that multiple family members of each patient shared these characteristics.[50] In addition, all nine families had evidence of an autosomal dominant inheritance pattern for elevated tryptase.[50] The additional findings showed some interesting characteristics, including that 30% of subjects from six families reported history of anaphylaxis.[50] One subject had a history of anaphylaxis to Hymenoptera venom despite a normal tryptase level.[50] Out of those with elevated tryptase levels, nearly 70% had connective tissue abnormalities, approximately 94% had atopic symptoms, 30% had autonomic dysfunction with the diagnosis of POTS, and over 87% had gastrointestinal symptoms.[50] However, one limitation to the study was the very small sample size.

A 2016 study by the same group of researchers indicated that a certain subgroup of patients with mast cell issues, connective tissue abnormalities, dysautonomia, and irritable bowel problems had more than one copy of a gene that influences tryptase production.[51] The gene TPSAB1 was associated with elevated basal serum tryptase in a retrospective study that evaluated tryptase levels in 35 families.[51] Upon further questioning, many of these patients revealed histories of symptoms consistent with MCAS and its common comorbidities, though they were not always official diagnoses.[51]

Research from Sabato and colleagues in 2014 described cases of familial hypertryptasemia "with associated mast cell activation syndrome," and evidence of some of the patients in these families who met the clinical diagnosis of MCAS.[52] By definition, the presence of such symptoms plus the presence of an elevated mast cell mediator (including tryptase) in light of a differential diagnosis rule-out and a response to mast cell medications meets the diagnostic criteria for MCAS by both of the currently utilized diagnostic criteria discussed in Chapter 3.

In 2018, Sabato and colleagues identified a patient with an increased (quintupled) copy number of the inherited TPSAB1 gene who also tested positive for clonal mast cell disease (with a somatic *KIT* mutation), suggesting that a link exists between mastocytosis and hypertryptasemia.[53]

Based on the available literature, it appears that a small subgroup of patients with MCAS (and a larger subgroup of patients with other types of MCAD including mastocytosis) may have a specific genetic influence that contributes to high tryptase. The research into the concept of familial hypertryptasemia is in the early stages, and this diagnostic label has not been integrated into the MCAD classification scheme.

In addition to capturing patients who may be genetically predisposed to elevated tryptase, the utility of tryptase testing may be supported for certain special scenarios. It's possible that serum tryptase can be a clinical tool to capture certain populations who would not otherwise be especially symptomatic yet. For example, Austen and Akin recommend screening all of patients who present to the clinic with anaphylaxis to Hymenoptera venom, even if patients don't express a primary concern for MCAD symptoms.[54] They suggest that patients with tryptase levels over 12 ng/ml undergo a further work-up that includes CD25 and D816V c-*KIT* testing.[54]

That being said, the majority of patients with MCAS do NOT present with high tryptase or an allergy to Hymenoptera venom. While tryptase is an easy, relatively cheap test with clinical value in patient screening, it should not be the only "line drawn in the sand" for diagnostic consideration. This is a common frustration point for many patients who end up having to argue with their doctor in order to have other mast cell mediator tests ordered. It may be useful to print out the study by Afrin and colleagues[45] showing the poor association between MCAS and tryptase to present to one's doctor. If a practitioner is unwilling to consider other mediators, that may also signify that it's time to go doctor shopping. Persistence definitely pays off in this area of self-advocacy.

HISTAMINE INTOLERANCE VS. MCAS

"Do you experience unexplained headaches or anxiety? What about irregular menstrual cycles? Does your face flush when you drink red wine? Do you get an itchy tongue or runny nose when you eat bananas, avocados, or eggplants? If you answered yes to any of these questions, then you could have a histamine intolerance."[55]

This excerpt came from a popular website, and it seems that histamine intolerance (also known as histaminosis) is becoming a more widely known concern in the chronic illness community.

Many patients are initially drawn in the direction of MCAS investigation after first learning about histamine intolerance from a medical practitioner or website. Histamine is one of the more "famous" mast cell mediators that is a notorious culprit in the production of certain distinct allergy-like symptoms, but it is only *one of the many* chemicals released by mast cells.

Are histamine intolerance ("HIT") and MCAS the same thing? The short answer is no, but it's very possible that patients who have signs of histamine intolerance actually have an underlying case of MCAS, and it's also possible that certain patients with MCAS struggle with histamine issues more so than with other chemical mediators.

Histamine intolerance is believed to be linked to certain genes that may contribute to an individual's difficulty processing histamine, specifically HNMT, DAO, MAO, PEMT, and NAT2.[56]

If any of these genes or the particular enzymes, B vitamins, or minerals that support them aren't working properly, the individual may experience a build-up or overload of histamine that can trigger a number of symptoms. Gastrointestinal issues, hormones, and a deficiency in the DAO enzyme are also tied to HIT.[57] Common triggers are ingested foods and beverages and sometimes exercise. Patients may experience many symptoms of MCAS, including headaches, fatigue, swelling, hives, difficulty breathing, nasal congestion, flushing, abdominal symptoms, anxiety, fast heart rate, difficulty sleeping, and high blood pressure.[57]

Some patients with HIT report the majority of symptoms related to food triggers that may last for several hours after eating, and some do experience chronic issues or a "ramping up" of symptoms as their "histamine bucket" gets fuller and fuller. *Anecdotally*, patients with a true histamine intolerance will struggle with low-level (non-anaphylactic) reactions to fermented foods, leftovers, and high-histamine dietary culprits like alcohol, aged cheeses, and cured meats. Some people with HIT find that a trial of a low-histamine diet may be helpful. Some people also report relief with supplementation of the DAO enzyme.

Patients with MCAS may note some initial symptomatic improvement with a low histamine diet (discussed later in Chapter 11), but this change is not typically sufficient to counteract the root issue of inappropriate mast cell degranulation to non-food triggers on a chronic basis, as occurs with MCAS. For patients with MCAS, the symptom chronicity, triggers, intensity, and wide scope of problems look distinctly different from HIT because MCAS involves a number of different chemical mediators—not just histamine—that are perpetually reacting inappropriately to factors beyond the narrow lens of diet.

For insurance coding, histamine intolerance as a diagnostic label tends to fall under "other adverse food reactions, not elsewhere classified." This is clearly different from the description of MCAS, which expands far beyond the realm of diet.

One cannot assume that all patients with MCAS have issues with the breakdown or degradation of histamine. Thus, the current belief is that HIT and MCAS are caused by two distinct physiological mechanisms. One is an innate issue within mast cells resulting in the release of a whole bunch of chemical mediators, and the other has to do with poor methylation and the reduced efficiency of chemical reactions relating to histamine alone. Both issues are theorized to be associated with different genetic mutations. While they do have some overlapping symptoms, the two conditions are distinct.

MCAS AND HYMENOPTERA VENOM

The subject of a specific patient subgroup with severe reactions to insect stings has been studied fairly extensively. Numerous studies have noted episodes of idiopathic anaphylaxis and anaphylaxis as the result of a sting by an insect in the Hymenoptera order (such as wasps, bees, hornets, and yellowjackets) to be more prevalent in patients with systemic mastocytosis than in the general population.[24,58-60]

A 2009 study found that out of all patients who had allergic reactions to Hymenoptera venom, nearly 14% were found to have underlying mastocytosis or mast cell activation syndrome.[61] More recent research estimated that clonal mast cell disease is at the root of up to 10% of patients who experience systemic reactions to insect stings.[54]

In patients who have Hymenoptera venom allergies, a tryptase level of less than 11.4 ng/ml was found to be indicative of non-clonal disease, and patients with tryptase levels above this threshold tended to test positively for a primary MCAD (either mastocytosis or monoclonal MCAS). Specifically, a 2009 study found that 29 out of 31 patients with allergies to Hymenoptera venom also had tryptase levels above 11.4 ng/ml.[61]

However, the presence of high tryptase as a sort of "inclusion criteria" for the suspicion of mastocytosis in patients who present with severe allergies to Hymenoptera venom may be faulty. A 2015 study evaluated 22 undiagnosed patients who presented with anaphylaxis to Hymenoptera venom, documented low blood pressure during reactions, normal tryptase levels (*less than* 11.4 ng/ml) and the absence of urticaria pigmentosa.[62] They performed bone marrow biopsies and found that 16 of the 22 patients (73%) had the diagnosis of MCAD; out of the patients with MCAD, 15 patients had indolent systemic mastocytosis and one patient had monoclonal mast cell activation syndrome.[62] Also, 25% of the patients with MCAD had osteoporosis on further imaging.[62] The patients with MCAD had slightly higher baseline tryptase levels compared to the non-MCAD patients (a median of 8.6 vs. 7.1 ng/ml), still well below the 11.4 ng/ml cutoff.[62] In this study, the patients with MCAD rarely experienced angioedema or urticaria during their hypotensive anaphylactic events.[62]

Thus, conflicting evidence is out there on whether the tryptase cutoff of 11.4 ng/ml is an appropriate starting point for raising suspicion of an underlying monoclonal mast cell disorder in patients who present with severe reactions to insect venom.

When it comes to the association between high mast cell load and Hymenoptera venom-induced anaphylaxis, a study published in 2013 indicates that the relationship may not be entirely linear.[59] A group of researchers in the Netherlands found that in a population of patients with existing mastocytosis, the association between high mast cell load and Hymenoptera venom anaphylaxis risk is more of a bell-curve shape.[59] It appears that the higher tryptase levels and increased mast cell load initially pose a gradually increasing anaphylaxis risk up to the 50th percentile, at which point the risk actually turns to trend toward a decreased risk with increasing mast cell loads.[59] Thus, the relationship between tryptase/high mast cell burden and Hymenoptera venom-induced reactions is complex and not entirely predictable in patients with MCAD.[59]

Ruling out MCAD should be a rapid priority in patients with severe reactions to Hymenoptera venom. Experts recommend prompt diagnosis of clonal mast cell disease for patients with normal tryptase levels and severe reactions to Hymenoptera venom so that complications including osteoporotic fractures and fatal sting reactions can be prevented. Limitations in the tests themselves may complicate matters; quantitative reverse transcriptase polymerase chain reaction (RT-PCR) testing is recommended to enhance sensitivity of identifying a *KIT* mutation.[62]

For patients who have clonal disease and experience Hymenoptera venom sensitivities, it's theorized that a combination of both IgE and genetic mutation-associated factors initiate anaphylaxis.[54] The exact mechanism behind this reaction in a subgroup of venom-reactive patients is still unclear. According to researchers Theoharides et al., "It is not known how the presence of clonally expanded mast cells might lead to increased susceptibility to anaphylactic reactions to certain triggers, such as Hymenoptera venom. Perhaps perivascular mast cells can rapidly deliver vasoactive mediators into the intravascular compartment, venom may have direct effects on clonal mast cells, or dysregulated signal-transduction pathways downstream of mutant *KIT* molecules may be involved in mast-cell activation."[24]

Research conducted by Austen and Akin in 2016 noted that about 30% of patients with mastocytosis experience signs and symptoms of severe anaphylaxis (including drops in blood pressure with fainting).[54] Out of these patients, about half tend to react primarily to Hymenoptera venom as an IgE-mediated trigger, suggesting an approximate 15% prevalence of Hymenoptera venom allergies in the mastocytosis population.[54] The prevalence of Hymenoptera venom allergies in patients with MCAS in undetermined.

Special considerations with Hymenoptera venom allergies in patients with suspected MCAD may over-ride traditional decisions about bone marrow biopsies. Zanotti and colleagues note, "As a speculative aspect, we can hypothesize that patients with no skin involvement, normal serum basal tryptase levels, and anaphylaxis with ascertained hypotension and loss of consciousness caused by Hymenoptera stings should undergo a bone marrow examination to detect a possible clonal mast cell disorder."[62]

It's important to note that patients who have both mastocytosis and Hymenoptera venom allergy are recommended to continue venom immunotherapy (allergy shots) indefinitely, since systemic reactions have been reported after stopping that treatment.[63] Additional information on venom immunotherapy is shared in Chapter 10.

CURRENT CONSIDERATIONS FOR MCAS
Bridging the Gap

Why has the medical community been seemingly "slow" to accept this condition? Why are there so few practitioners who specialize in MCAS in the United States (and beyond)? Some theorize that the disease is simply still too new, and it needs time before it becomes integrated into medical school education and sees widespread continuing education recognition. Ample studies are out there on the disease, yet they don't seem to be getting into the hands of many doctors.

Today there is still much controversy about diagnosis of MCAS in the allergist clinical setting. Li believes that her fellow allergists miss the diagnosis of MCAS because they are primarily focused on the adaptive or acquired immune system and focus more on testing for IgE-mediated disorders like atopy.[64]

Anecdotally, countless fellow patients who have MCAS experience frustrating interactions with doctors and allergists about their condition. Some doctors deny the condition altogether, and others get fixated on tryptase levels. Others appear unsure of what to do with patients and may either under- or over-medicate. There also seems to be a large discrepancy in whether bone marrow biopsies or other tissue biopsies are considered and/or ordered. Some practitioners believe that MCAS describes a bunch of symptoms that are entirely secondary reactions to other triggers.

There are dozens of conditions out there deemed "controversial" in mainstream medicine, and MCAS is certainly one of them, right alongside Lyme disease and mold illness. There seems to be a communal "black and white" bias approach by many doctors. They may recognize acute Lyme disease but scoff at post-Lyme syndrome. They may acknowledge mastocytosis but have never heard of, or do not believe in, MCAS.

It could be that the testing for these more chronic, hidden diseases is more complicated and subject to debate. In a perfect world, there would be bright, glaring "POSITIVE" results on tests that rule in the condition with extreme confidence. Most chronic conditions only have subtle tangible test results, at best.

Another key to the discrepancy in disease acknowledgement may lie in the nature and design of the American medical system, where doctors are so specialized that they may have tunnel vision on one very narrow differential diagnosis possibility list. Likewise, patients may only mention symptoms related to one body area that is of the greatest concern at one moment in time, therefore omitting pertinent system-wide information that could guide the doctor to look outside of their specialty.

The key to bridging this gap is to gently share, advocate, and educate in a professional manner. As a patient and even a colleague, it can be difficult not to harbor some resentment at the medical practitioners who seem unwilling to open their eyes to the possibility of these chronic conditions. Medical professionals have a duty to keep up with the literature and to alter one's practice as more information becomes available. It's unproductive to angrily blame mainstream medicine practitioners for the education and training they've received, the narrow field of expertise in their specialty, or the lack of awareness on the latest information out there. That will simply create more of a division.

One does not need to look far to find academic papers that support the fact that MCAS, as a diagnosis, is underestimated and clinically "neglected." Researchers Hamilton et al. from Brigham and Women's in Boston, one of the top centers for mast cell disease in the U.S., noted in a 2011 study that "...We have classified these patients as having MCAS. We believe this is a unique and underrecognized population of patients who might be encountered in various medical specialty clinics, especially allergy, immunology and gastroenterology clinics."[65]

Likewise, Molderings and colleagues also noted in 2011, "Mast cell activation disease is now appreciated to likely be considerably prevalent and thus should be considered routinely in the differential diagnosis of patients with chronic multisystem polymorbidity or patients in whom a definitively diagnosed major illness does not well account for the entirety of the patient's presentation."[20] One can only hope that with time, medical professionals will begin to "zoom out" when patients experiencing a variety of systemic symptoms arrive at their door.

The MCAS Slippery Slope

When one finally receives a diagnosis of MCAS, it's tempting to blame *everything* on the new diagnosis. However, it's important to avoid the slippery slope of attributing every condition on one's medical "resume" to MCAS. When MCAS is diagnosed on top of other conditions, it doesn't mean that the other condition is not necessarily there. While there are good odds that dysfunctional mast cells are contributing to the etiology of prior diagnoses, and adequate treatment of MCAS will likely improve other conditions, this doesn't mean that one should discontinue treatment or medications for other preexisting diagnoses.

It's also essential to avoid the temptation to associate every new symptom or problem that pops up with MCAS immediately. According to Afrin, it's important to seek a standard diagnosis and therapy for other problems that may arise. For example, a patient with MCAS may develop a type of cancer that ought to be funneled through a mainstream medical approach, but they may ignore the symptoms for a long time under the assumption that they are due to MCAS.[66]

Afrin adds another example, "Don't assume that your chest pain is MCAS! Go to the emergency room. Even if your EKG was normal the last 99 times and the medical staff just roll their eyes at you…"[66] Indeed, patients with MCAS, like any others, are not immune to experiencing a true heart attack or other medical comorbidities, regardless of whether such problems are ultimately attributable to MCAS or not.

Patient Characteristics

Researchers at Brigham and Women's Hospital conducted a 2011 study that aimed to determine the clinical presentation of patients with diagnosed mast cell activation syndrome.[65] They prospectively evaluated 18 patients who had been symptomatic for a mean of 4.6 years (range was 1 to 9 years) prior to diagnosis.[65] The study patient population was limited to patients seeking consultation to rule out mastocytosis, or patients seeking gastroenterology specialist care. Approximately one-third of the patients studied had an abnormal baseline tryptase level.[65] While all patients had at least one abnormal mast cell mediator level confirmed, interestingly, only 2 of the 18 patients tested positive for *both* high 24-hour urinary prostaglandins and histamine levels.[65] In the study, 67% of patients underwent an endoscopy and abdominal imaging before their eventual referral and diagnosis of MCAS.[65] It's important to note that none of the patients in this study had an abnormal number of mast cells on biopsies, nor did they present with clonal signs such as a c-*KIT* mutation or CD25-positive staining.[65]

The researchers found that 94% experienced abdominal pain, 89% experienced flushing, 89% experienced dermatographism, 83% experienced headaches, 67% experienced difficulty concentrating, 67% experienced diarrhea, 39% experienced asthma, 39% experienced naso-ocular symptoms, and 17% experienced anaphylaxis.[65] Also, 72% of patients experienced at least one allergy to a medication, and 67% of patients experienced increased symptoms with alcohol consumption.[65]

The researchers then followed these patients for 1 to 4 years (average 2.8 years) and monitored their symptoms as they underwent pharmacological treatment using a "standard" approach to treating MCAD.[65] They were prescribed H1 and H2 blockers, and depending on their response to treatment, other medications were eventually added if needed to include monteleukast sodium (Singulair), and mast cell stabilizers including oral cromolyn sodium (Gastrochrome).[65] Two years into the study, they added aspirin to the regimen for patients who tested with high prostaglandin levels.[65]

The researchers found that all of the patients reported some degree of positive response to the treatment; one-third of patients had a complete regression of symptoms, one-third had a major regression (an improvement in symptoms greater than 50%), and one-third had a partial regression when revisited.[65] They were unable to find any particular characteristics that predicted whether a patient would achieve partial or full regression of symptoms. The most impressive response was noted in regards to abdominal pain, where 14 of the 17 patients that initially presented with abdominal pain responded to treatment.[65] In addition, 12 of the 15 patients with headaches responded positively with fewer or no symptoms at follow-up.[65] They also found that the majority (17 of 18 patients) had a sustained response to anti-mast cell mediator medications.[65] One limitation to this study was the small sample size.

A study published in 2017 by Afrin and colleagues[45] evaluated a large group (over 400 patients) with the diagnosis of MCAS (as per Criteria Y[20]). The majority of patients were

Caucasian (75%) and the authors reported that virtually all of the rest were African-American.[45]

Their retrospective and prospective combined analysis determined that 83% of patients reported fatigue, 76% experienced dermatographism, 75% reported fibromyalgia-type pain, and 71% experienced syncope or pre-syncope.[45] The median number of comorbidities was 11 and the median number of symptoms was 20.[45] Thirty-five percent of patients were diagnosed with GERD, 29% had clinical hypertension, and 23% had multiple/atypical drug reactions.[45] The median time from symptom onset to diagnosis was 30 years, with a range from 1 to 85 years.[45] Breast cancer (26%) and atherosclerosis (21%) were the most common family medical problems in this patient cohort.[45]

The authors noted that 72% of the patients appeared to be chronically ill, and the majority of patients had a history of routine but modest lab abnormalities present for years prior to their diagnosis.[45] Many patients noted that they had been told that their diagnosis was somatic in nature and they had "learned to live with it."[45] In routine hematologic and serum testing, 66% of patients had anemia, 38% had elevated ALT (alanine transaminase), 34% had elevated alkaline phosphatase, and 75% had high glucose levels.[45] Authors estimated that their findings were likely *underestimated* since the majority of data (72%) were assessed retroactively.[45]

In 2018, researchers evaluated the medical records of 56 patients at the University of Wisconsin Allergy Clinic who were diagnosed with MCAS.[67] They determined that approximately two-thirds of patients had a positive mast cell mediator lab test.[67] Allergic disease (67%), hypothyroidism (31%), depression (31%), Ehlers-Danlos syndrome (24%), POTS (24%), anxiety (24%), and gastroesophageal reflux disease (24%) were the most common co-morbidities.[67] Foods, medications and stress/anxiety were the triggers most frequently reported by patients.[67]

In 2018, Weiler and colleagues compared 45 patients with systemic mastocytosis and 44 patients with MCAS to see if there were differences in symptoms reported.[68] Systemic mastocytosis was more associated with syncope, forgetfulness, weight loss, reflux disease, depression, anemia, lymphopenia, eosinophilia, osteopenia, bone fractures, adenopathy, and enlarged organs.[68] MCAS was more associated with urticaria, angioedema, hypotension, dermatographia, bloating, belching, hiccups, rhinorrhea, sneezing and wheezing.[68]

In 2018, The Mastocytosis Society published the second section of a large patient survey of approximately 420 patients with MCAD (SM, MCAS and other MCAD).[69] Based on patient survey responses, 22.9% of patients reported a possible mast cell disease presence in family members.[69] Out of patients surveyed, 31.4% reported osteopenia or osteoporosis confirmed by a bone scan or bone density scan (dexascan), and 13.9% of patients reported a history of cancer.[69] (Additional survey findings are available in online publications.)

Survey of Patient Needs

The same international group that published the 2012 consensus statement of MCAD classification also included a pilot project that examined patient perspectives for those residing in the United States and Europe.[21] Patients suggested their most important or urgent concerns, and the top 10 most common concerns were compiled together.[21]

Top 10 issues raised by MCAD patients in the U.S. and E.U.[21]:

United States:

- Better access to care from physicians knowledgeable in MC disorders and more specialized centers
- Definitions and criteria for MCAS (clonal and non-clonal variants)
- Curative rather than symptomatic therapy
- Education and awareness of physicians and health care professionals in recognition of symptoms of MC disorders
- Practice parameters of diagnosis and therapy incorporating commonly available methods
- Better access to and assistance in obtaining medications
- More recognition of gastrointestinal manifestations of MC diseases
- Better holistic care plans to address symptoms such as anaphylaxis, fatigue, bone pain, brain fog, pain, and neuropsychiatric symptoms
- More research into familial occurrence
- New treatment options for cutaneous disease, aggressive SM, and MCL

Europe:

- Improved knowledge of all doctors in various disciplines relevant to MC disorders
- ID card for all patients and countries in Europe
- New better therapeutic agents
- More specialized centers in various countries in the EU
- Improved knowledge and definition of mediator-associated symptoms

- More Mastocytosis specialists
- Improved diagnostic methods
- More information to patients
- Further development of existing classifications of MC disorders
- More information to patients via commonly accessible media

Interestingly, across both geographical areas, the number one concern of polled patients was the access to medical professionals knowledgeable about MCAD.[21] This is, unfortunately, an area that will take time to improve. In the United States, there are currently very few specialists in the field of MCAD. If nearly 20% of the population has underlying MCAD, the current infrastructure is unprepared for a surge in patients seeking care in this relatively unrecognized specialty. Some clinics only accept patients who have already had a bone marrow biopsy performed with concrete signs of mastocytosis present, while others will accept patients for consideration of MCAS.

Anecdotally, patients have a number of other concerns that are not being addressed.

Patients have expressed the following topics in support groups as current widespread areas of need:
- additional training for emergency room staff and allergists
- inclusion of more information about MCAS in medical school
- "more research and less politics"
- more provider education about the many presentations of anaphylaxis
- general MCAD awareness that expands beyond tryptase levels and systemic mastocytosis
- patient access to resources for modifications to employment and disability resources
- increased awareness and research on the concurrence of Ehlers-Danlos syndrome and POTS with MCAS
- more constructive ways for physicians to interact with patients in place of the "it's in your head" mentality
- more education on the high prevalence of MCAS
- more education within the medical field regarding the dangers of indoor chemical and fragrance exposure for this patient population

This is a small smattering of the topics that are regularly discussed within the MCAS patient population, highlighting the vast array of facets to patient management that are currently appearing to fall short.

Challenges in Where We Are Today

The comment about "less politics" is an interesting one. There are several areas of internal battles in which the topic of MCAS invokes debate among those best versed in the condition. There are several distinct groups of leading clinicians and researchers who have devised slightly different diagnostic criteria and who differ on key areas such as the role of genetic influences, the proper way to test for MCAS, and the focus on mastocytosis vs. MCAS. There's debate about the etiology of MCAS and the appropriate patient classification; the medical community lacks clear clinical guidelines for this patient population. The research is still in its infancy in terms of defining a clear picture of MCAS etiology, the role of genetics, and treatment options. And *much* more research is needed in other areas. One can make speculations based on studies about the role of mast cells in certain tissues and in conjunction with certain diseases, but there are still many holes and gaps in the understanding of the disease.

Outside of the few practitioners considered specialists in the disease, there's a general lack of uniformity in decisions for things like lab testing and whether to perform a bone marrow biopsy, or when to start a patient on something above and beyond the first line antihistamine blockade. In general, a discrepancy sometimes is present between the management of patients by allergists as opposed to true MCAD specialists, and yet there are so few specialists in the United States, each with lengthy waitlists and barriers in terms of insurance coverage. Globally, there's a huge void of knowledge and acceptance of the condition in mainstream medicine, similar to the struggles of other conditions that are difficult to diagnose, like Lyme disease.

There's a need for the development of better diagnostic testing, reinforced lab protocols, and training of lab technicians to increase testing accuracy. There's a need for better clinical screening tools, questionnaires and the development of clinical prediction rules that could be more based on history and physical exam to assist in raising the index of suspicion of the disease. There's a need for specialty centers that provide holistic care.

In certain countries it's difficult to gain proper insurance coverage for MCAS, making it difficult to find adequate treatment and access to necessary prescriptions. Some medications are not available at all and others are available only for outrageous costs. This is true for many diseases and some of what is needed as a MCAS community is unfortunately dictated by the overarching medical system.

144

One hope for the future is that telemedicine regulations will improve to allow for more access to care for MCAS patients, which would save travel costs and time for patients and their families. Currently, in the United States there are many barriers to practicing telemedicine because of the necessity for practitioners to have a medical license for each state that they see patients in.

The Role of Primary Care and Other Providers in MCAS

There are differing opinions on the topic of which type of provider is best suited to see patients with MCAS. Dr. Hamilton acknowledges that there's currently a lack of professionals who are well-versed in MCAS, and the existing experts are spread thin.[70] Mast cell experts often have wait times of one year or longer to be seen for a new patient consult.

Hamilton encourages other providers to start seeing patients with MCAD but notes that many doctors are hesitant to do so, perhaps due to the medical complexity and inherent challenges in testing and finding the right treatment for patients.[70] Hamilton notes, "In an ideal world, allergists and immunologists are the professionals best suited to take care of patients with mast cell activation. It will be important to continue to train and educate specialists to be able to recognize, diagnose, and treat this disorder. These may include specialties where MCAD patients are likely to present, including dermatology, pulmonology, cardiology, gastroenterology, among others."[70]

Dr. Afrin asserts that "MCAS is so prevalent that, for the most part, it needs to be the province of primary care providers."[66] Afrin believes that the key to improving patient care in this area is *not* solely to identify more names of well-versed "specialists" to see this patient population, as these existing few resources are currently bombarded with unrealistically large patient caseloads and not enough waking hours in the day to get to everyone.[66] Afrin asserts that the key in expanding care for the MCAS population lies in *patients searching for doctors who are open-minded and willing to learn more*, as opposed to increasing the burden on the few existing practitioners who are "experts" in the condition.[66]

Even with these types of efforts, many doctors will remain resistant to change, and patients should be prepared to be persistent advocates for their rights. It's an uphill battle when the system is not set up to allow for adequate time for a thorough medical history to assist in MCAS diagnosis.

There is an immense need for more access to specialists in this area, but there is also a large need for 1) existing primary care doctors to expand their scope to recognize and diagnose MCAS, 2) allergists to acknowledge and test for MCAS, and 3) additional professionals (like

145

physical therapists, nurse practitioners, nutritionists, occupational therapists, mental health specialists, and others) to learn more about MCAS in order to improve recognition and refer patients to physicians knowledgeable in MCAS testing and treatment. Naturopaths and functional medicine doctors often tend to be well-versed in MCAS and are an important aspect of a patient care team.

Rheumatology practices may also be a future specialty area that could help capture the diagnosis of MCAS, as there is a tendency for hypermobile patients to be referred to rheumatology clinics, and a potential correlation between MCAS and joint hypermobility in rheumatology patients.[71]

Afrin agrees that physical therapists and other medical "ancillary" professionals should have an important role in the initial spark of recognition with this patient population.[72] An initial non-MD recognition model of MCAS suspicion may be better equipped for success, because professionals who have more regular interaction with patients may be afforded a substantial amount of quality time with each patient over the course of several treatment sessions. If anyone is going to pick up on the many puzzle pieces that may increase suspicion of MCAS, it's the people who build a continual rapport with patients over time and begin to recognize patterns.

Physical therapists (PTs) are one example of professionals who may pick up on MCAS in a patient over time. If while following the idea of this initial non-MD recognition model a patient fits the profile, the PT (or other medical professional) should suggest MCAS as a *possibility* to the patient, who should then *seek an MD who is willing to test them and learn with them in the process*. This suggestion is a big challenge in itself because, speaking from experience, PTs don't like to mention something new to patients unless they have a specific specialist in mind who can carry the torch forward in the diagnostic process.

In the majority of communities, a direct referral won't be possible yet due to the limited knowledge of this disease. There must be excellent communication between the PT (or other professional), the patient, and the subsequent MD that they visit with a goal of discussing MCAS. *The more that the PT (or other professional) advocates for the patient and communicates with their primary care provider, the more likely a given doctor who has never heard of MCAS will be willing to test for it anyway.* It's important to encourage the patient to keep fighting to find a professional who can order the tests, even if it means seeing multiple doctors in a row.

As patients, we ought to inspire greatness in the medical professionals we encounter. We can encourage the special ones who are open to learning more about MCAS to become the experts in the field. We can patiently become advocates for our own care and the care of our peers suffering with the disease. We can work together to increase awareness about MCAS.

As medical professionals, we have a duty to share this knowledge. Even if we ourselves are not in the position to order the testing for MCAS, we can still create positive working relationships with professionals in the local area who have knowledge about MCAS as referral sources. We can team up with them to make sure that this patient population is being recognized, diagnosed, and heard.

The Future of MCAS

What's in the future of MCAS? The future is bright for an increase in the number of medical professionals and patients knowledgeable in MCAS. Though it may seem like a slow process, MCAS awareness and advocacy is gaining momentum.

The future of research provides hope for the ability to minimize the trial and error in the diagnosis and treatment of MCAS. The future may also bring more clarity to classifying subgroups of patients with the disease or perhaps providing a universal grading system and diagnostic criteria for MCAS.

The future provides hope for a more stable prognosis and access to treatments that may improve the quality of life in patients with MCAS. One of the silver linings to chronic illness is that the pharmaceutical companies need little convincing to jump on board. Additional mast cell stabilizing medications and histamine receptor antagonists are currently in development, and the natural supplement world also offers promising future options and research.

Functional medicine doctors and naturopaths have many tools to help uncover root issues in this patient population and could have a very powerful impact on the diagnosis and treatment of MCAS in the years to come.

CHAPTER KEY POINTS

- Research supports the possibility that MCAS has underlying somatic (acquired) and/or germline (inherited) mutations that contribute to disease etiology. Epigenetic factors also likely play a role.

- The RCCX Theory by Dr. Meglathery offers a potential genetic explanation for the connections between a certain subgroup of patients who have MCAS (and its common comorbidities) plus unique psychological characteristics.

- A recent study estimated that MCAS has a prevalence of 17% in the general population – nearly one in every five people!

- Histamine intolerance is not the same thing as MCAS, although some patients with MCAS do exhibit symptoms of histamine intolerance.

- A subgroup of patients with primary (clonal) MCAD exhibit serious reactions to insect stings, and there's mixed research regarding whether tryptase testing helps capture this patient population.

- Patients with MCAS frequently report experiencing abdominal pain, dermatographism, fatigue, headaches, fibromyalgia-type pain, fainting or near-fainting, difficulty concentrating, and allergies to a medication.

- There are many barriers for the newly diagnosed and those who suspect they have the disease, and patients in the U.S. and in Europe have identified a large need for specialization centers and more physicians trained in disease management.

- Functional medicine doctors, naturopaths, primary care doctors, physical therapists, and other healthcare professionals are poised to play an important role in capturing patients with chronic multisystem ailments who may need to consider the diagnostic possibility of MCAS.

Chapter Five

Many Systems, One Diagnosis

THE MANY FACES OF MCAS

I t's difficult to convey how all-encompassing MCAS can be, and some physicians may have a narrow view of the condition as an allergic-type phenomenon. However, MCAS can also present as predominantly chronic and systemic debilitative symptoms, or some combination between that and a sliding position on the allergic spectrum. What seems to be uniform across the board, however, is that most patients experience confusing symptoms in multiple systems at once. Some patients end up being diagnosed with or evaluated for many other conditions. And the day-to-day realities can be extremely challenging.

This chapter is *not* meant to alarm patients, nor is it an all-inclusive guide to possible symptoms that could be attributed to mast cell activation. Rather, it's a summary of some of the more common findings noted in the literature that *may be* associated with MCAS.

"Correlation does not assess causality" was one of my most memorable phrases as a doctoral student. This chapter aims to share observations from literature searches and connect the dots between mast cell activation/infiltration and pathologic conditions. The presented information is superficial in terms of depth and *does not indicate a cause and effect relationship* but, rather, highlights the areas of potential mast cell influence on complex physiological systems.

Unfortunately, the majority of the available research has small sample sizes, numerous confounding variables, and other methodological flaws. Systematic reviews and meta-analyses are few and far between, particularly in terms of MCAS-specific research. Thus, this chapter more accurately notes *associations* that should be further researched in the years to come.

CARDIOVASCULAR AND CIRCULATORY SYSTEM

Anecdotally, a common area of concern for the MCAS patient lies in the cardiovascular system. Many patients with MCAS have experienced chest pain or heart palpitations with normal EKG and imaging analyses. Some have unexplained symptoms that can mimic a heart attack, while others have true changes in their arterial system that do indeed produce cardiovascular events such as myocardial infarctions. Aggressive atherosclerosis and aneurysms have been noted. The venous system may also have abnormalities (such as hemorrhoids or venous insufficiency in the legs).

Mast cells have been deemed "pro-atherogenic" by several researchers. Bot and colleagues discuss human histological observations and findings from mice studies that provide evidence that "mast cells are more than just bystanders in the process of atherosclerosis, and that there are multiple mechanisms by which these cells contribute to the progression of this disease."[1] Specifically, tryptase, chymase, histamine, cytokines, chemokines, and growth factors secreted by mast cells may be more closely associated with cardiovascular conditions and the development/destabilization of plaques.[1] The complement system, and in particular activated C5a receptors on mast cells, may also be tied to the development of atherosclerotic plaques.[1]

Plasma cholesterol levels are typically chronically high, even in patients with proper diet and exercise, and one study found that 75% of patients with MCAS had high cholesterol.[2] Mast cells in the brain have been found to exacerbate stroke pathology in mice, and mast cells have extensive documentation in regards to the release of proinflammatory mediators that can increase the risk of stroke and heart attack.[3]

Most patients with MCAS have a blood pressure abnormality, and it can be either high or low (or both, depending on the moment and whether the patient is experiencing anaphylaxis or varying degrees of mast cell degranulation). Anaphylactic shock typically involves a dramatic drop in blood pressure. Near-fainting or fainting episodes may be tied to the cardiovascular system in patients with MCAS. Mast cell mediators may play a role in the blood vessel vasodilation that occurs with a subsequent drop in blood pressure during degranulatory episodes. While drops in blood pressure are more often associated with anaphylaxis, it appears that a subgroup of patients (nearly 13%) experience high blood pressure during anaphylaxis.[4]

The hyperadrenergic variation of postural orthostatic tachycardia syndrome (POTS) also appears to be common in the MCAS population.[5] This condition predominantly affects females and is characterized by a chronic (>6 months) increase in heart rate (30 beats or more) *without a significant drop in blood pressure* with a change in position to upright posture.[6] POTS will be discussed in depth in Chapter 7.

Raynaud's disease is a circulatory condition that primarily affects the hands, feet, and nipples. *Anecdotally*, Raynaud's disease appears to be more common in the MCAS population. Vasoconstriction of the vessels, typically triggered by a change in temperature, wind, or emotional stress, leads to a lack of blood circulating distally at the hands and feet. The skin turns white and is numb, lasting from minutes to hours, and when the blood eventually returns to those areas, it can be quite painful. Rarely, some patients with severe Raynaud's may experience tissue death and neurological damage after prolonged episodes. Episodic migratory edema has also been noted.

Variances in the body's blood clotting system are also noted in MCAS. Some patients seem to stray toward the bruising and bleeding end of the spectrum, whereas others may have unexplained excess clotting problems. Excess bleeding with the menstrual cycle (menorrhagia) and excess nose bleeds (epistaxis) are also commonly reported.[7]

The more serious cardiac conditions that have been noted in patients with MCAS include congestive heart failure, Kounis syndrome, and Takotsubo syndrome.[7] Kounis syndrome and Takotsubo syndrome are theorized to be connected to mast cell activation. Kounis syndrome involves the spasm of normal, plaque-free arteries, which is thought to be triggered by mast cell activation. This syndrome can affect the arteries that feed the heart, as well as the arteries in the brain and in the abdomen. Takotsubo syndrome is a more rare condition that involves acute heart failure that is typically preceded by an acute physical or emotionally stressful event.

DENTAL HEALTH

Dental and periodontal (gum) deterioration is a common finding in patients with MCAS, despite patients typically reporting proper oral hygiene techniques. Afrin notes, "Teeth 'crumble' years prematurely. As with just about every aspect of MCAS, we are far from knowing the particular abnormal mast cell mediator 'soups' that cause each of these problems."[7] Patients who have gastrointestinal problems may have a higher propensity for dental issues, particularly those who vomit often, as the acidity can affect the teeth and gums.

A 2004 review noted that chronically inflamed gingival tissue, such as that found in patients suffering with chronic marginal periodontitis (CMP), tends to exhibit higher numbers of mast cells than what's found in normal gum tissue.[8] Preformed cytokines may be responsible for some of the accelerated deterioration noted in patients with MCAS and/or CMP.[8] In addition, matrix metalloproteinases, which are enzymes released by mast cells, have been shown to degrade the gingival extracellular matrix.[8]

It's also been indicated that heparin, histamine, nitrous oxide, and tumor necrosis factor-alpha released by mast cells may contribute to tissue destruction and bone loss in chronically inflamed oral gum tissue.[9] Mast cells play an important role in attacking "bad" bacteria in the mouth and promoting healing, so perhaps *in theory* the patients who suffer from persistent and chronic gum and dental issues comprise the patient population who have an underlying MCAS mechanism that results in a flooding of too many chemical mediators to the area (which subsequently increases inflammation).

Visits to the dentist can be particularly difficult for patients with MCAS, and premedication may be advised by the patient's medical team. It's important to explain the MCAS condition to all dental staff, as sensitivities to gloves, numbing medications, injections, pressure/vibration, and ingredients in the flavored cleaning agents can all occur. Patients with MCAS may also react chronically to filling ingredients, and the discussion of pulling a tooth vs. filling a cavity may be relevant for some individuals in this patient population.

DIABETES SPOTLIGHT

Type II diabetes is a condition where the body develops resistance to insulin, the hormone that controls blood sugar, resulting in hyperglycemia, or high blood sugar. Risk factors for type II diabetes include obesity, high blood pressure and cholesterol, genetic factors, and lifestyle factors such as improper diet and lack of exercise. Fluctuations in blood sugar level despite adherence to a healthy diet are reported in patients with MCAS. Prediabetes, high triglycerides, and diabetes have been reported in this patient population, though it's unclear whether the prevalence differs from that of the general population.

It's theorized that mast cells could be involved in the pathophysiology of both obesity and type II diabetes, and there are links between a high mast cell number and the increased inflammatory and fibrotic characteristics of white adipose tissue.[10] Diet-induced obesity, metabolic syndrome, insulin resistance, and type II diabetes have been connected to mast cell activity, though exact mechanisms are not clear yet.[11] Inflammation, including mast cell-mediated cytokine and chemokine release, is believed to contribute to the pathogenesis of type II diabetes.[12]

Diabetes has been associated with systemic and chronic inflammation that contributes to impaired wound healing, and in understanding the role of mast cells in the disease, one must remember that a certain amount of mast cell degranulation is healthy and important. Wound healing is an important topic to address with the diabetic population, since poorly healed ulcerations can lead to infections and amputations.

A 2016 study found increased mast cell degranulation in the skin of humans and mice with both type I and type II diabetes.[13] However, following a wound on the skin, the diabetic mice did not have the normal degranulation response crucial for mounting an acute response to foster healing.[13] Mast cell-deficient mice displayed similarly impaired wound healing.[13] It appears that the mechanisms between diabetes, mast cells, insulin, and wound healing are complex.

Type I diabetes, which is less common, involves the autoimmune destruction of B cells in the pancreas and is typically diagnosed at a younger age. Activated mast cells have an influence on T cell activity and migration, which appears to influence the development of type I diabetes.[14] When mice with type I diabetes predisposition were treated with the mast cell stabilizer cromolyn sodium, type I diabetes onset was significantly delayed, further supporting the theory that diabetes etiology may be closely tied to mast cell overactivity.[14]

However, additional evidence suggests that there are differences in mast cell mechanisms between type I and type II diabetes. Atopy, or the tendency to be "hyperallergic" (as is observed in allergic rhinitis, asthma, and conditions like atopic dermatitis), is *inversely* associated with type I diabetes.[15] In other words, patients with asthma and allergic conditions appear *less likely* to have type I diabetes. This may be due to a protective effect of low insulin in type I diabetes that appears related to reduced mast cell activation in the initial inflammatory process that would normally trigger acute reactions.[16] Animal studies have supported that type I diabetic rats may be less likely to experience anaphylaxis following exposure to antigens, though this may be modulated by the influence of glucocorticoids.[17]

Further research is certainly needed to better understand the exact mechanisms between mast cells and the development of both type I and type II diabetes.[14]

EARS, EYES, AND NOSE

Tinnitus (ringing in the ears) and hearing loss are commonly reported in the MCAS population. Non-infectious inflammation may present in the form of inner ear inflammation that is often diagnosed as an ear infection and treated accordingly with antibiotics, which may not resolve the symptoms.[7] Otosclerosis (abnormal bone growth near the middle ear) is connected to hearing loss. It's possible that mast cells and their mediators may impact auditory nerve fibers, or the hair cells in the semicircular canals.[7]

Benign paroxysmal positional vertigo (BPPV) has been reported *anecdotally* in conjunction with MCAS. Hairlike sensors monitor the rotation of the head and help the body to have a sense of what position it's in. BPPV involves floating crystals that are dislodged (for reasons unknown) and end up in a part of the semicircular ear canal where they shouldn't be, confusing the sensors and resulting in symptoms of severe vertigo. This condition is fairly easily resolved with repositioning maneuvers that help to move the crystals back into the proper part of the ear canal. The treatment can be performed in a doctor's office, and physical therapists are also trained in how to diagnose and resolve this condition, often in one to two sessions.

Meniere's disease is another inner ear-related condition that involves dizziness, vertigo, and nausea. Unlike BPPV, which tends to occur in response to changes in position and movements, Meniere's disease is a typically constant presence of disabling vertigo. Most sufferers have difficulty with walking, driving, and most other daily tasks. The exact cause of Meniere's disease still remains a mystery. Interestingly, there has been one case report of a patient presenting with both Meniere's disease and cutaneous mastocytosis (CM) who, after starting omalizumab (Xolair) therapy for CM, had a complete resolution of Meniere's disease symptoms.[18] It's quite possible that a number of vestibular and inner ear conditions could be connected to MCAD and the chemical mediators released by mast cells, though more research is needed to investigate this theory.

The concentration of mast cells in the ocular (eye) tissue in undisputedly high.[7] Eye irritation, intermittent blurred vision or loss of visual focus, eye "twitching" or blepharospasm, and eye dryness and burning are commonly reported symptoms in patients with MCAS. "Floaters" in the eye and idiopathically elevated eye pressure are also reported *anecdotally*. Afrin also notes that occasionally a patient will experience inflammation and (unprovoked) bleeding that occurs in the whites of the eyes, and his theory is that heparin could be released by ocular mast cells to cause such phenomena.[7]

Afrin[7] also notes that in his experience:

- Virtually everybody with MCAS has some eye-related issues.
- Virtually nobody with MCAS has a life-altering, serious eye-related issue—but the few who do are why the word "virtually" is used to modify "nobody."[19]

This does give patients with MCAS some piece of mind, particularly as they often are told by their ophthalmologist that their eyes are "normal" despite suffering regularly with symptoms.

IgE-mediated mast cell activation in the eyes occurs following the release of both preformed mediators (like histamine and proteases) and de novo formation of cytokines and lipid-derived mediators that contribute to the inflammatory cascade on the surface of ocular tissue.[20]

Glaucoma has also been associated with higher numbers of mast cells in conjunctival tissue.[21] Mast cell activity has been connected to eye scarring that can occur in disease processes as well as post-operatively.[21]

Mast cells have been associated with autoimmune uveitis. Uveitis is an inflammatory condition that induces eye swelling and can lead to tissue damage and vision loss. In particular, it's believed that mast cell mediators have a direct contribution to the development of this connection via their influence on inflammation and immune regulation and/or their potential role in the blood-retinal barrier breakdown with this condition.[22]

Nasal irritation in the form of dryness, nosebleeds, congestion, and post-nasal drip are common complaints when experiencing seasonal allergies, so it's not surprising that these symptoms are quite common in patients with MCAS. Chemical mediators such as histamine are connected to nasal drip.

Frequent or chronic sinusitis is also common in this patient population. Some report relief of symptoms with antibiotics (or perhaps with the passage of time), but *anecdotally* most report frequent relapses and resistance to antibiotics when attempting to resolve the symptoms of inflammation in the sinuses. *Anecdotally,* many patients eventually connect these symptoms to the presence of resistant fungal infections or chronic mold exposure, with the help of naturopaths or functional medicine doctors.

ENDOCRINE SYSTEM

Mast cells and their relationship with the thyroid gland have been investigated since the early 1980s, where it was determined that mast cell activity impacted thyroid-stimulating hormone (TSH) secretion.[23] It's possible that histamine released by mast cells plays a particularly influential role in the physiological regulation of TSH.[23]

Hashimoto's thyroiditis, Graves' disease, hypothyroidism, and hyperthyroidism have all been noted in patients who have MCAD. Afrin notes that many of his patients with thyroid gland dysfunction do not tend to stabilize well when only on thyroid medications, further raising suspicion of mast cell activation roots in the disruption.[7] Pituitary and sex hormone abnormalities have also been noted.

Research has noted that the thyroid hormones may regulate the *number* of mast cells in the brain, thereby impacting the release of histamine and other chemical mediators.[24] Recent studies suggest that the brain mast cell population may be closely regulated by the pituitary-thyroid axis.[24]

A scarcity of literature exists evaluating autoimmune thyroid problems and MCAD. A few existing case reports are available describing patients with MCAD who had coexisting autoimmune thyroid issues.[25,26] It also appears that mast cell-derived prostaglandins and cytokines may play a role thyroid eye disease.[27,28]

Both hyperthyroidism and hypothyroidism have been associated with chronic urticaria.[29] Idiopathic chronic urticaria and angioedema have been associated with a higher prevalence of thyroid autoimmunity, and a small subgroup of patients who had thyroid-targeting treatments had a significant response in other (mast cell-driven) symptoms in one study.[30] However, some authors have concluded that the presence of anti-thyroid antibodies and chronic idiopathic urticaria are associated parallel events lacking pathogenic connections.[31]

It's been theorized that histamine and thyroid hormone function may influence each other.[32] Research indicates that histamine-receptor antagonist medications may alter iodine and thyroid function in animal studies.[33] However, as a whole, there is still insufficient information on exact pathways/mechanisms and potential causality between thyroid problems and mast cell-associated disorders.

Mast cell infiltrates have been associated with tumor promotion in patients with thyroid cancer.[34] Specifically, mast cells were found to stimulate thyroid tumor growth and vascularization, an effect which was "reverted" once the mast cell stabilizer cromolyn sodium was administered.[34]

The adrenal glands produce a number of hormones, such as cortisol and adrenaline. The hypothalamic-pituitary-adrenal axis regulates a number of hormones including cortisol, the "stress hormone," and research has shown that cortisol is activated when brain and nasal mast cells are stimulated in animal research.[35] Isolation and social stress increased the number of mast cells in the brain in animal studies.[36-38] Thus, stimulation of mast cells appears to increase cortisol, and stress appears to increase the number of brain mast cells, creating a potentially debilitating vicious cycle for patients with MCAD.

Corticotropin-releasing hormone is released by mast cells in the hypothalamus in response to stress. This increases cortisol levels to help the body combat the stressful trigger. Specifically, this hormone has been identified to contribute to the flushing and low blood pressure response seen with mast cell degranulation.[39]

There are a number of disorders connected to the adrenal system that have been noted in patients with uncontrolled MCAS. Addison's disease involves insufficient production of cortisol, which also has roles in metabolism and immune system suppression. Cushing's syndrome involves high production of cortisol. *Anecdotally*, both conditions have been noted in patients with MCAD. Many patients with MCAS note disruptions in their adrenaline levels, such as sudden surges in the "fight or flight" mechanism for no apparent reason or in response to trivial triggers. This may be connected to the adrenergic form of POTS, previously described in the Cardiovascular and Circulatory Section of this chapter.

GASTROINTESTINAL SYSTEM

A 2011 study noted that 94% of patients with MCAS reported gastrointestinal symptoms, specifically "abdominal pain."[40] It's not surprising that most patients with MCAD suffer from some sort of GI distress, given the amount of mast cells that tend to reside in the GI tract as one of the body's primary defense zones from initial intruders.

Mast cell mediators including histamine are classically more often associated with diarrhea and cramping, particularly during acute episodes, but chronic constipation is not uncommon in this patient population. Nausea, vomiting, abdominal distention, intestinal obstructions, aerophagia (swallowing of air) that leads to distension, and gastroparesis are also reported in patients with MCAS. In fact, pain anywhere along the gastrointestinal tract, from the mouth to the anus, is often reported. Gastroesophageal reflux disease (GERD) is a common finding.

Malabsorption is fairly common in patients with MCAS, which is why a nutrient panel analysis is beneficial to acquire at baseline. *Anecdotally*, some patients report unexplained weight loss, while others struggle with puzzling weight gain for no apparent reason.

Irritable bowel syndrome (IBS) is a common diagnosis prior to detection of MCAS. Research has found an increased number of mast cells in the intestinal mucosa of patients with IBS.[41] The severity of abdominal pain sensations is correlated with the degree of mast cell activation and mast cell location in proximity to nerve fibers in the gastrointestinal tract. Due to these findings, mast cells have been theorized to have a role in visceral hypersensitivity and pain perception with IBS.[41]

A number of factors are theorized to be responsible for mast cell infiltration and activation in the GI system. Genetic factors, food allergies, prior history of infectious gastroenteritis, bile acid malabsorption, changes in the microbiome and increased intestinal permeability ("leaky gut") are postulated to be responsible for mast cell activation.[42] Acute stress is also noted to be a "powerful trigger for intestinal mast cell activation."[41]

IBS has been theorized to be caused by small intestinal bacterial overgrowth (SIBO), another common finding in patients with MCAS. This condition is characterized by excess methane- or hydrogen-producing bacteria that inappropriately reside in a part of the intestine that is normally free of bacteria. SIBO can lead to debilitating chronic gastrointestinal pain, gas, bloating, constipation, and/or diarrhea. Food allergies and multisystem inflammation, including the presence of gastrointestinal dysfunction *plus* interstitial cystitis ("painful bladder"), have been reported in patients with SIBO.[43]

Anecdotally many patients with MCAS report gastroparesis. Gastroparesis is a delayed gastric emptying in the absence of any type of obstruction and is characterized by pain, nausea, bloating, vomiting, and early satiety. It appears that the etiology of this condition is complicated and multifactorial. Prostaglandins released by mast cells appear to play a role in mediating gastroparesis, both in diabetic and non-diabetic patients.[44,45] A 2013 study looking at patients with Parkinson's disease found that the use of the H2 (histamine) blocker nizatidine significantly reduced the gastric emptying time in this patient population.[46] It's possible that mast cells, histamine, prostaglandins, and other mediators play a role in the etiology of gastroparesis, the interactions with the migrating motor complex, and other factors that influence this debilitating condition.

Mastocytic enterocolitis is a condition that is associated with chronic diarrhea and inflammation. Research indicates that higher numbers of mast cells in the gastrointestinal tract (greater than 20 mast cells per high-powered field) are associated with the majority of cases of mastocytic enterocolitis that have chronic intractable diarrhea, whereas patients with other diagnoses that trigger diarrhea tend to have normal numbers of mast cells on biopsy.[47]

Mast cells are believed to be an important element in the pathogenesis of inflammatory bowel disease (IBD) including Crohn's disease and ulcerative colitis.[48] Specifically, mast cell mediators are associated with the stimulation of nerve endings that influence intestinal permeability, intestinal motility, and inflammation modulation in these patients.[48]

Eosinophilic esophagitis is a chronic atopic disease that involves a higher than average number of eosinophils on biopsy that contribute to inflammation. Difficulty swallowing, heartburn, and vomiting can occur. When unmanaged, it can lead to esophageal stricture and food impaction.[49] The condition does not typically occur in isolation, is usually accompanied by atopic dermatitis, food allergies, or asthma,[49] and is reported *anecdotally* in the MCAS patient community.

Mast cell activity has been implicated in the etiology of eosinophilic esophagitis.[50] Specifically, elevated levels of proteases and stem cell factor released by mast cells are

158

associated with eosinophilic esophagitis, and these patients show a higher density of mast cells when compared to controls.[50] Similarly, mast cells decrease in number with disease remission, which can sometimes be achieved with dietary treatment.[50] The preliminary research provides some compelling links between mast cells and eosinophilic esophagitis, though more research is certainly needed.

It's clear that MCAS can have a profound impact on the gastrointestinal system and can produce very intense and real symptoms in this area even in the absence of abnormalities on diagnostic imaging. The chemicals released by mast cells appear to alter the bacterial balance and intestinal permeability, which is theorized to increase susceptibility to small intestinal bacterial overgrowth, co-infections, and parasites. These conditions in turn can stimulate further mast cell degranulation, food sensitivities, and autoimmune-like degradation of intestinal tissue, creating a vicious cycle.

A more in-depth analysis of the gastrointestinal comorbidities associated with MCAS is located in Chapter 7.

GENITOURINARY SYSTEM

The genitourinary tract is another area of the body with connections to the "outside" world, thus making it a bigger target in terms of the consequences of increased mast cell activity. Vaginal inflammation, painful urination, frequent urination, urinary urgency, difficulty initiating urination, and urinary incontinence are common in patients with MCAD. Swelling of the urethra can occur. *Anecdotally*, many women report frequent symptoms of urinary tract infections (UTIs) over the years, often with negative cultures.

Some researchers believe that the high pain experienced with endometriosis may be attributed to mast cells.[51,52] Specifically, the cross-talk between mast cells and neurons could be responsible for endometriosis-related chronic and neuropathic pain.[53] Endometriosis is a condition where tissue that normally grows in the uterus is found growing in other areas, typically the peritoneum, the membrane that forms the lining of the abdominal cavity. This can lead to fibrosis, inflammation, pelvic pain, and infertility.

Mast cells are increased in number and highly activated in biopsies of patients with endometriosis.[54] Adhesions are known to recruit mast cells to the peritoneum, and research has found that women with adhesions have higher levels of histamine in their pelvic fluids.[54]

The close proximity of mast cells to the blood vessels of endometrial cysts supports that they play a role in the development of adhesions and fibrosis in patients with endometriosis.[55] A 2018 research study investigating endometriosis-associated dysmenorrhea found that elevated estrogen concentrations appear to be a key factor for mast cell recruitment and degranulation in ovarian endometriomas.[56]

Interstitial cystitis, or "painful bladder syndrome," is another chronic, debilitating condition that has been connected to mast cell activation, and part of the treatment plan typically involves antihistamines. According to French and Bhambore, "The activation of mast cells results in a cycle of neuronal hyperexcitability leading to secretion of neurotransmitters and triggering further mast cell stimulation and degranulation. This process appears to contribute to the chronic pain, urgency, and frequency experienced by (the interstitial cystitis) patient."[57]

A 2015 review article by Ratner discusses the role that MCAS may play in interstitial cystitis and painful bladder syndrome.[58] Specifically, the number of mast cells on bladder biopsy may be high, or if they are normal in number, it's also possible that the mast cells may be hyper-responsive and degranulate more frequently with triggers.[58] Ratner also notes that mast cells release inflammatory mediators *selectively* without degranulation occurring in the urinary system.[58] "The inflammatory mediators, once released into the bladder could initiate urgency, frequency, supra-pubic pressure and pain of varying degrees."[58]

Ratner describes the process of trans-granulation that can occur between mast cells and the neurological system in the bladder that could explain the pain experienced with interstitial cystitis.[57] "Mast cells can both degranulate as well as trans-granulate via the formation of filipodia (thin, finger-like projections) that attach directly to the neuronal membrane. Trans-granulation has been shown to occur in the normal bladder. Via trans-granulation, mast cell inflammatory mediators are taken up directly by the nerve via endocytosis and released into the cytoplasm of the nerve, or found in membrane-bound organelles within the nerve. This could trigger pain fibers in the bladder and the electrical impulses would then travel via the ascending pain pathway from the bladder to the spinal cord and on to the central nervous system (CNS), targeting the limbic system, thalamus and cortex."[58] It's possible that this trans-granulation process could also occur in other areas of the body, and it likely plays a role in non-infectious inflammatory bladder pain experienced by many MCAS patients.

Several sources note that diencephalic (brain) mast cells increase in quantity during mating activity in animals.[35,38] Research supports that the gonadal hormone fluctuations that occur with mating are responsible for increasing both mast cell number and activation in the brain.[59-61] Painful sexual intercourse, alterations in libido, and infertility have also been associated with mast cell activation disease.[7] *Anecdotally*, some women with MCAD report allergic reactions with semen contact and/or allergies to condoms.

Histamine is implicated in aspects of arousal-related sexual behavior.[62-64] Oxytocin receptors are present in uterine mast cells, and oxytocin appears to influence sexual behavior through serotonin mechanisms.[65-67] According to Theoharides and Stewart, "Interestingly, anecdotal information indicates that female patients with mastocytosis or mast cell activation syndrome may have increased libido. Preliminary evidence also suggests that MCs may have olfactory receptors. MCs (mast cells) may, therefore, have been retained phylogenetically not only to 'smell danger,' but to promote survival and procreation."[67] However, reports of decreased libido are not uncommon in this patient population, either.

Human mast cells have estrogen, progesterone, testosterone, and gonadotropin receptors and are influenced by sex hormones. It appears that estrogen, estradiol, leutinizing hormone, and follicle-stimulating hormone all increase mast cell degranulation, while activation of progesterone and testosterone receptors may have the opposite (inhibitory) effect.[67]

According to Afrin, mast cell disease has been associated with decreased sperm count (oligospermia) that can be reversed in some cases to result in pregnancy once mast cell medications have been initiated.[7] It's also widely accepted that mast cells are commonly associated with chronic prostatitis.[68]

Prostaglandins and other chemical mediators have been connected to the concept of premenstrual syndrome or "PMS" with the female menstrual cycle, and the symptoms of bloating and cramping may be associated with mast cell degranulation.[69] Estrogen also directly causes mast cell degranulation,[70] so the phases of the menstrual cycle that have higher levels of circulating estrogen may be more symptomatic, such as the start of ovulation.

HEMATOLOGIC FINDINGS

MCAD is considered hematologic in nature due to the fact that mast cells originate in the bone marrow. A variety of blood abnormalities have been uncovered in patients with MCAD, though this is not always the case, which can be puzzling and create controversy around clinical findings for patients. Some patients with MCAS have normal blood counts, while others may express chronic abnormalities, and still others may have abnormal values one day, only to have normal results on subsequent retesting.

Afrin notes that, just like many other systems of the body, a wide range of blood-related issues emerge in MCAS with seemingly no rhyme or reason and no predictable pattern. He's treated patients with MCAS who have polycythemia (too many red blood cells) and anemia (too few red blood cells).[7]

Polycythemia Vera (PV) is a cancerous condition that is sometimes mimicked by a benign version of the disease in patients who have MCAS. It's possible that the cancerous version may also be connected to MCAD. PV is characterized by an increase in red blood cell mass, which is accompanied by increased white blood cell and platelet production. Pruritis (itching) of the skin is common and significantly impacts the quality of life for these patients. A 2014 study found massive accumulations of mast cells in the skin of mice with PV, and further investigation found higher mast cell counts in the bone marrow, peripheral blood, and the peritoneal (abdominal) cavity.[71]

A 2013 study indicated that mast cell activation is a contributing factor to the pain experienced with sickle cell anemia (SCA), as it contributes to the release of substance P and subsequent neurogenic inflammation in animal models.[72] Furthermore, mice pretreated with the mast cell stabilizer cromolyn sodium had improved pain levels, and the inhibition of mast cells with the drug imatinib was effective in reducing cytokine levels and pain in mice with SCA.[72]

Afrin has noted clinical associations between SCA and MCAS. In a 2014 paper, he presented 32 patient cases with SCA that had "poor phenotypes" who also met the diagnostic criteria for MCAS.[73] The "poor phenotype" patients make up a group of SCA patients that tend to "disproportionately present with crises and other SCA complications."[73] Inflammation and genetic abnormalities have been hypothesized to account for the widespread issues encountered in this subgroup of patients with SCA.[73]

In the study, 38 original patients met the inclusion criteria for the SCA "poor phenotype," which included at least three emergency department visits or hospitalizations per year for the previous five years, and/or treatment of hydroxyurea or chronic red cell transfusions.[73] of these 38 patients, 32 patients (84%) ended up testing positive for MCAS.[73] Elevated heparin levels and elevated prostaglandin D2 levels were positive in the majority of the patients.[73]

All of the cases that followed up responded at least partially to treatment targeting MCAS, and nearly 20% experienced complete improvement.[73] Afrin noted that the utility of the drug hydroxyurea in a subgroup of SCA patients may be attributed to the treatment of underlying (previously unrecognized) MCAS.[73] While more research is needed, it appears that there are some compelling connections between MCAS and SCA.

Problems with too many platelets (thrombocytosis) and too few platelets (thrombocytopenia) have been noted in patients with MCAS.[7] The role of platelets in allergic reactions has been a topic of much research. Mice deficient in mast cells can still experience anaphylaxis, leading researchers to suspect that other cells such as platelets may play a role in severe allergic reactions. A 2004 study found that the role of mast cells in allergic reactions may be tissue-specific, as allergic reactions *of the skin* were predominately governed by mast cells when exposed to triggers.[74] In the same study, increased vascular permeability and leukocyte recruitment via granules released from platelets occurred in *muscle tissue* of mast cell-deficient mice, which led to anaphylactic shock.[74]

Another review described platelets as a factor during anaphylactic reactions and noted the trend of a drop in platelet numbers immediately following anaphylactic shock.[75] Platelets have been connected to hypersensitivity to acetylsalicylic acid (aspirin) and to anaphylactic episodes in patients who received injected contrast for radiologic imaging.[75] Platelets have also been implicated in part of the anaphylactic response in patients who have allergies to Hymenoptera venom.[75] Thus, it's clear that platelets can influence allergic reactions and potential chemical mediator release, though the relationship between platelets and mast cells in terms of MCAD still needs much research.

There are patients with MCAD who have too much blood clotting (hypercoagulability) and too little blood clotting (bleeding issues).[7] Too many white blood cells (leukocytosis) and too few white blood cells (leukopenia) are also reported.[7] Myelodysplasia is a disordered blood cell development that is also anecdotally noted in some patients with MCAD. Red blood cells may also exhibit size abnormalities, both large and small.[7]

Idiopathic CD4 lymphopenia is a rare disorder of the immune system characterized by low levels of CD4+ T cell, a type of white blood cell. Recent research indicates that T cell dysregulation in patients with idiopathic CD4 lymphopenia may be responsible for secondary mast cell activation, though more research is needed to confirm the association between MCAS and CD4 lymphopenia.[76]

MCAD is so unpredictable in terms of what side of the hematologic spectrum is problematic, as evidenced by the wide range of blood-related findings reported in patients. This variability is certainly a barrier to universal acceptance of the disease in the medical community, as the "common findings" are not entirely predictable. However, considering the fact that mast cells have the potential to release such a wide range of different mediators and are acted upon by many epigenetic factors, the discrepancy in clinical findings in this area, like so many others, makes sense.

According to Afrin, "Bone marrow (hematologic) malignancies are some of the most common malignancies seen in MCAS patients."[7] There are some types of hematologic malignancies where the cause is universally undetermined, and Afrin suspects that some of these may be strongly connected to MCAS.[7] One such example is multiple myeloma, a cancer of abnormal plasma cells. Plasma cells are a type of white blood cell that produce antibodies. When the plasma cells are abnormal, thick blood and kidney problems can result. This can also lead to masses formed in bone marrow. Before patients are diagnosed with this cancer, they are often diagnosed with the precursor called monoclonal gammopathy of undetermined significance (MGUS), which is characterized by high levels of certain antibodies and high blood calcium levels.

A 2015 study found that mast cell density in bone marrow was correlated with the proliferation of multiple myeloma. Specifically, the study authors determined that mast cells influence the growth of the disease via cytokines and the induction of angiogenesis.[77] Mast cells and their chemical mediators have also been implicated in the bone complications that occur with multiple myeloma, and another study affirms that patients with the disease have a higher density of mast cells that correspond linearly to the stage of the disease.[78] A 2010 case report described associations between systemic mastocytosis and multiple myeloma in a patient who presented with urticaria as the primary complaint.[79]

Mast cell mediators interleukin-6 and tryptase have been studied and determined to play a large role in the proliferation of certain cancers, as well as the degradation of bone leading to osteoporosis in hematologic disease.[78,80] Hopefully more research will be conducted to determine if MCAS is indeed connected to the development of MGUS and subsequent multiple myeloma and other hematologic conditions.

INTEGUMENTARY SYSTEM

The integumentary system encompasses the body's barrier with the outside world—the skin, teeth, hair, and nails. It's no surprise that the mast cells are especially active in these areas, since they serve as the body's first defense line and alert system for foreign intruders.

Patients with MCAS commonly present with one type of skin-related ailment, or even several. Afrin notes a plethora of different types of rashes and skin lesions in this patient population; urticaria (hives) and telangiectasia are common.[7] Telangiectasis is the presence of spider-like blood vessels near the surface of the skin. Cherry angiomas are small cherry-red spots on the skin. Migratory redness (erythema) and flushing are other common findings.[7] Patches of small open sores occur in some patients, often with scabs.[7] Livedo reticularis are prominent vein-related patterns on the skin that may be noted. Acne-like folliculitis is also reported.[7] Patients harboring a high burden of comorbid bacterial and viral infections may have a sluggish liver with noticeable yellowing of the skin.

Anecdotally, poor or delayed healing time is also commonly reported, even with smaller wounds or scratches. Hair loss is another common complaint, although it's not always severe or visibly recognized by others. Nails often develop ridges, bumps or lines, or may break easily.

Some patients tend to have slower wound healing, while others appear to have issues with too much scar tissue. Mast cell mediators such as tryptase and chymase play important roles in tissue repair and wound healing, but in excess these mediators can also contribute to the formation of keloid and hypertrophic scarring.[81]

Mast cells have been implicated in the etiology of a number of immunological skin diseases, such as contact dermatitis, scleroderma, atopic dermatitis, chronic graft-vs.-host disease, and immunobullous disease.[82,83] Research also supports that mast cells play a key role in the development of psoriasis and rosacea.[83,84]

Skin mast cells express interleukin-22 and interleukin-17, two proinflammatory compounds that are believed to be responsible for the skin conditions psoriasis and atopic dermatitis.[83] Mast cells appear to be the predominant producers of interleukin-22, whereas other cell types such as T cells produce the majority of interleukin-17.[83] C-*KIT* positive mast cells and greater numbers of mast cells in the upper dermis have also been shown to accumulate in skin lesions in patients with psoriasis.[85,86]

Urticaria pigmentosa causes discolored skin lesions, typically accompanied by itching. The majority of urticaria pigmentosa associated with cutaneous mastocytosis (CM) presents in young children, but it has been found in older children and adults as well. If a patient has persistent skin issues such as urticaria pigmentosa, it's important to make those issues known to the patient's specialist in order to determine if a skin biopsy for CM is a relevant part of differential diagnosis.

LYMPHATIC SYSTEM

The lymphatic system, part of the circulatory system and the immune system, is composed of organs and tissues that help the body to get rid of toxins and waste naturally produced by cells in the body. The lymphatic system is immunoregulatory in nature and functions via the transport of lymph, the fluid that contains white blood cells. As part of the "clean-up crew," the lymphatic system goes hand in hand with mast cells, the "emergency response team," and tends to be affected in some way in patients with MCAS.

The lymph nodes may be enlarged in patients with MCAS. According to Afrin, "Rarely do they markedly enlarge (as might be seen in lymphoma or infection), and rarely do they continuously enlarge (if they do, lymphoma needs to be ruled out)."[7] Lymph node enlargement may be painless or tender to the touch.

The spleen works as a blood filter and functions as an important part of the lymphatic system. Spleen enlargements sometimes occur in patients with MCAD. Intermittent splenitis (inflammation of the spleen) is a common cause of left upper quadrant pain in the MCAS patient population, according to Afrin.[87]

Epstein-Barr virus (EBV) is responsible for acute cases of mononucleosis, or "mono," a viral condition which usually results in swollen neck lymph nodes in addition to a sore throat, fever, headache, and rash. Mono can also cause enlargement of the spleen to the dangerous point of rupture. It's believed that chronic EBV infection can lead to a number of systemwide problems, and *anecdotally* this condition appears common in the MCAS community.

When lymph nodes are enlarged or abnormal, they may be biopsied. Afrin notes that the lymph node biopsy can often lead to confusion within the medical team as it's common for patients with MCAS to have "abnormal but inconclusive" findings.[7] He also comments that in his clinical experience, some patients with lymphatic cancer diagnoses and poor prognoses or poor response to traditional treatment may achieve full resolution of symptoms once they address their underlying MCAS.[7]

Indeed, mast cells and their mediators have been indicated in the etiology of certain lymphatic cancers, such as Hodgkin's lymphoma.[88] Increased mast cell density or numbers are associated with tumor development and progression in this disease.[88]

It appears that mast cell activity contributes to the immunological phenomenon where lymph node cells pause in activity based on the presence of environmental triggers. According to a 2010 review, "MC (mast cell) derived TNF-alpha has been shown to further promote inflammation by enhancing T cell activation and inducing cytokine release from a variety of cell types, and is thought to play an important role in lymph node 'shutdown' which temporarily prevents lymphocyte departure from draining lymph nodes to enhance adaptive immune responses."[70] This downregulation of the lymph nodes is similar to the response that occurs with vaccines and is theorized to "buy time" for antigen-based cell activity to arrive.[89]

MENTAL HEALTH

Depression, anxiety, and bipolar disorder are frequent diagnoses among patients with MCAD, *anecdotally*. Sadly, it may never be entirely clear how many suicides have been inherently connected to this disease. Additional psychological conditions, such as autism, dementia/Alzheimer's disease, and schizophrenia may also be connected to MCAD. Research is emerging that continues to support the involvement of mast cells in all of these conditions.

Research by Theoharides supports the natural flavonoid luteolin, a mast cell inhibitor, as a potential tool in the treatment of autism spectrum disorders (ASD) and other neurological conditions.[90] The incidence of ASD has been determined to be nearly seven times higher in patients with MCAD (specifically, mastocytosis) and their immediate family members when compared to the general population.[38] In children, this number was measured at one in every 10 cases![91] (ASD is discussed in greater detail in Chapter 7.)

Mast cells have an undeniably influential presence in brain tissue. Natural and pharmacological triggers can induce the release of cytokines, neurotransmitters, proteases, and chemokines by mast cells in the brain.[92] Elevated levels of mast cell mediators in the brain have been associated with influential forces on blood-brain barrier permeability, neurogenesis, and neurodegeneration.[92]

Serotonin is a well-known neurotransmitter released by a number of cells (including mast cells) that acts in both the central and peripheral nervous systems. Many patients with depression have been treated with SSRIs, or selective serotonin reuptake inhibitors. These medications block the reabsorption of serotonin so that the levels of serotonin in the brain are increased. Some studies have reported low serotonin levels in patients with systemic mastocytosis and MCAS, while others have found no discrepancies.[93]

Acute stress has been shown to increase histamine levels in the diencephalon area of the brain. The diencephalon area impacts sleep regulation, heat and cold regulation, the autonomic nervous system, skeletal muscle movements, sensory and motor function, memory, emotions, behavior, olfaction (smell), and other important functions.[94]

Chronic stress is associated with increased histamine in the nucleus accumbens and striatum areas of the brain.[94] The nucleus accumbens and striatum play a role in both motor and reward systems. Specifically, brain functions including learning, decision-making, motivation, impulsivity and processing of fear, and the encoding of new motor programs are all connected to this area.

Antihistamine medications, particularly H1 blockers, are theorized to reduce anxiety and depression in patients.[94] Hydroxyzine, an antihistamine prescription medication, is also used as an anti-anxiety medication, although it has some potential side effects like drowsiness.[95]

There are a large number of neurotransmitters and chemical mediators beyond histamine and serotonin that impact brain function, and it's clear that stress and the subsequent degranulation of chemical mediators by mast cells have a powerful impact on mental health.

METABOLIC SYSTEM

Many patients with MCAD present with metabolic abnormalities on testing that don't seem to add up. *Anecdotally*, abnormal iron and magnesium levels are sometimes noted. However, Afrin notes that in his clinical experience, magnesium is usually normal in his MCAS patients, but severe magnesium deficiency can be found in a very occasional MCAS patient.[19]

Vitamin D deficiency appears to occur in some patients. Mild transient increases in liver function tests may be noted, and some patients have chronic electrolyte, vitamin, and mineral imbalances.[7]

Metabolic syndrome, also common with MCAD, involves the presence of a cluster of several risk factors for cardiovascular disease, diabetes, and stroke. The National Institutes of Health defines metabolic syndrome by the presence of three or more of the following: high body mass index (BMI), high blood pressure, low "good" HDL cholesterol, high triglycerides, and elevated fasting blood sugar.[96]

MUSCULOSKELETAL SYSTEM

Joint pain is a frequent complaint in patients who have MCAD. The joint pain may or may not have swelling and sometimes migrates around the body. Generalized bone pain is also common. Certain patients have a history of osteoporosis or osteopenia (low bone mineral density) despite their younger age, well-balance diet, and adequate calcium intake. The research confirms that an increased number of mast cells and the by-products of mast cell degranulation are associated with accelerated bone loss in patients with MCAD.[97,98] According to Johansson and colleagues, "Mast cells release a number of vasoactive substances, including histamine which promotes osteoblasts and heparin and prostaglandin D2 which induce bone resorption by activation of osteoclasts."[98]

Patients who have mastocytosis tend to present with an especially high risk of spine fractures, and bisphosphonates are first-line treatment for this patient population, which could also potentially be appropriate for certain patients who have MCAS and osteoporosis or osteopenia.[99] Others may exhibit abnormal bone solidifying issues, termed osteosclerosis, though this appears to be less common than bone loss issues.

An autoinflammatory bone disease called chronic recurrent multifocal osteomyelitis is characterized by sterile inflammatory patterns that have been linked to increased mast cell density and degranulation.[100]

True osteoarthritis and seronegative rheumatoid arthritis are also commonly noted in the MCAD population. Tryptase released by mast cells has been shown to activate the protease-activated receptor 2 (PAR2), which contributes to cartilage damage.[101] A 2015 study from a group of researchers in the Netherlands found that the presence of increased mast cells in knee synovial joint fluid was significantly higher in patients with osteoarthritis and was linearly associated with the presence of structural damage in this patient population.[101] Femoral acetabular impingement (FAI), a painful and disabling hip cartilage condition, has also been associated with a higher number of mast cells in the joint space.[102]

Mast cells may play a role in nerve-mediated back pain and sciatica. Increased mast cell proliferation and inflammatory mast cell mediators (including prostaglandins, tumor necrosis factor-alpha, and interleukins) have been associated with sciatic nerve inflammation and intervertebral disc herniation injuries.[103-105]

It's been theorized that mast cells play a causative role in low back pain by contributing to the growth of blood vessels and nerves in injured tissue.[106] The intervertebral discs in the spine are typically avascular (with no or limited blood supply) and aneural (with no or limited nerve innervation), but production of nerve growth factor and mast cell-induced angiogenesis may explain some of the aberrant findings in symptomatic patients,[106] though the research is still inadequate to fully confirm this theory. Mast cells and their mediators also appear to contribute to other areas of nerve-based orthopedic pain, peripheral nerve fibrosis, and myelin destruction via other pathways.[107-109] Clinically, complex regional pain syndrome (CRPS) and thoracic outlet syndrome (TOS) have also been associated with mast cell activation disease.

Muscle pain and tendon irritation may be especially pronounced in patients with MCAS, and chronic inflammatory-patterned "overuse" injuries may appear with little provocation. According to Li & Ehrlich, "Patients with connective tissue disorders appear to have mast cells that are following bad orders, but we just haven't figured out where these bad orders are coming from."[110] In patients with signs suggestive of connective tissue disorders, research has found an increase in chymase-positive mast cells in the skin.[111]

Biopsies of patellar tendons in patients with a history of chronic patellar tendon inflammation (tendinopathy) show an increased density of mast cells compared to controls.[112] Studies have noted the same finding of increased mast cells present locally in the tissues of symptomatic cases of shoulder rotator cuff inflammation, as well as in the Achilles tendon.[113-114] Mast cells in tendons release excess amounts of prostaglandin E2, which reduces the production of new collagen, a crucial element in healing.[112]

Ehlers-Danlos syndrome (EDS) is a group of connective tissue disorders that's also commonly noted in patients with MCAS. Patients suffering with certain types of EDS typically have a number of inherent orthopedic concerns, such as neck and spine instability, temporomandibular joint (TMJ) issues, shoulder dislocations or subluxations, hand and wrist issues, and lower extremity joint injuries, in addition to inflammatory concerns with tendons and muscles. The hypermobile type of EDS is a relatively common finding in patients seeking physical therapy who also experience chronic health issues, and in many cases the condition has not yet been recognized or diagnosed. (EDS will be further discussed in Chapter 7.)

Fibromyalgia and polymyalgia rheumatica appear to have mast cell connections in their symptomology. Polymyalgia rheumatica involves moderate to severe muscular pain and stiffness that typically affects the neck, shoulders, and hips. Fibromyalgia is characterized by widespread pain and heightened tenderness to pressure in certain areas, often with clinical signs of excessive trigger points and myofascial tension, plus a plethora of other symptoms.

Fibromyalgia has been linked to abnormalities in the hypothalamic-pituitary-adrenal (HPA) axis, as well as elevated corticotropin-releasing hormone (CRH) and substance P (SP) in cerebrospinal fluid and elevated serum interleukins.[115-116] Increased numbers of mast cells have been found in skin biopsies in patients with fibromyalgia.[117] It's been theorized that in these patients, mast cells are activated by the release of CRH and SP from nerve endings, which triggers mast cells to release substances that contribute to inflammation and hyperalgesia, such as interleukin-6, interleukin-8, and tumor necrosis factor, which may then stimulate the release of additional CRH, creating a vicious cycle.[116]

A 2014 randomized controlled trial evaluated the treatment of fibromyalgia patients with ketotifen (2 mg twice a day) compared to placebo and found no significant differences between groups.[117] However, the study duration was only eight weeks, and authors concluded that future research should evaluate higher doses of ketotifen (a mast cell-targeting medication) with this patient population.[118]

Substances that decrease mast cell activation such as flavonoids like quercetin may be suitable as potential treatment options for patients with fibromyalgia, according to research conducted by Theoharides and Bielory.[119]

Anecdotally in the physical therapy clinic, low back pain, neck pain, and headaches are often associated with patients presenting with multisystem symptoms, multiple comorbidities, and the presence of chronic pain or chronic fatigue reminiscent of the clinical picture of MCAD. Case reports have found that some patients with proliferative mast cell pathology may initially present with primary concerns over acute and chronic low back pain,[120] further highlighting the importance of educating physical therapists and occupational therapists who are especially likely to regularly encounter patients with underlying MCAD.

NERVOUS SYSTEM AND BRAIN

Theoharides and colleagues postulate that mast cells are the "immune gate to the brain," having the ability to regulate the permeability of what enters the brain via the blood-brain barrier.[39,121] A large number of neurological-associated conditions are considered common among patients who have MCAS.

Mast cell degranulation has been connected to headaches and memory deficits. Patients with MCAS report difficulty with memory and cognition, word-finding, and poor concentration, often referred to as "brain fog." Migraines are also frequently noted. Paresthesia (numbness and tingling), chronic muscle weakness, neuropathy, seizure disorders, changes in muscle tone including spasticity and hypotonicity, and alteration in sensations (particularly taste, hearing, smell, and vision) are reported.

Systemic mastocytosis appears to have an association with epilepsy, and it's been suggested that mast cells play a role in the etiology of seizure disorders. A 2017 case study reported a nine-year-old patient who presented with urticaria pigmentosa (since age one) and seizures.[122] After gaining complete control of her MCAD via cromolyn, monthly omalizumab injections, and high-dose antihistamines, the patient no longer experienced seizure activity.[122]

Acute stress-induced seizures have also been reported in a child with cutaneous mastocytosis.[123] Similarly, adults with different types of mastocytosis have been reported to experience different types of seizure activity.[124-126] A case report of a mastocytoma (mast cell tumor) presented initially as an epileptic disorder, further supporting the role of mast cells in neuroinflammatory symptoms.[127]

Seizure disorders appear high *anecdotally* in the MCAS population, though the exact prevalence of this comorbidity is unknown. It's plausible that epilepsy induces mast cell activation, and mast cell activation may be able to trigger seizure activity, which could lead to a vicious cycle between abnormal neuronal function and mast cell activation.

In 2011, Theoharides and Zhang published a paper in the *Journal of Neuroinflammation* discussing potential connections between epilepsy, autism, mast cell activation, neurological inflammatory factors, and the blood-brain barrier (BBB).[128] According to the authors, "Local activation of brain mast cells could lead to focal disruption of the BBB, permitting focal neuroinflammation that could become an epileptogenic site."[128] Specifically, mast cell mediators such as interleukin-6, tumor necrosis factor, vascular endothelial growth factor, and mtDNA likely contribute to the development of inflammation, autism, and seizures.[128]

Histamine may also play a role. One study found that histamine-1 receptors have the ability to increase seizure activity.[129] A 2015 study found that histamine was released in the hippocampus area of the brain during seizures.[130] The histamine was associated with damage to neurons and these effects were diminished in animals that were pre-treated with sodium cromoglicate (a mast cell stabilizer).[130] Furthermore, the subjects who received the mast cell stabilizing medication prior to *status epilepticus* had an increased latency before developing seizures and lower numbers of brain mast cells following the induced seizures.[130]

Dystonia is the presence of involuntary muscle movements that often involve sharp twisting or jerking movements that can be slow, rapid, or rhythmic. Dystonia is theorized to be connected to the basal ganglia part of the brain that is responsible for initiation of motor control. *Anecdotally,* dystonia appears to be a common concern for some patients with MCAS. Preliminary research suggests that dystonia may be associated with mast cell mediators including histamine.[131-132] A 2018 case report discussed a 17-year-old female who presented with systemic mastocytosis and dystonia who achieved symptom elimination with the use of antihistamines including diphenhydramine.[133]

Sleep disorders and insomnia are common among MCAS patients. Histamine is believed to regulate the sleep-wake cycle[134] and high levels have *anecdotally* been connected to sleep difficulties in patients with MCAS. More histamine is naturally released in the late evening around 10 p.m., which may contribute to insomnia. Certain antihistamines tend to have the opposite effect, making one drowsy. Histamine drops during the day, which could be connected to the extreme drowsiness or narcolepsy that some patients report during daytime hours.[135]

Narcolepsy was originally thought to be due to loss of orexin/hypocretin neurons, but research has recently found that patients with narcolepsy also have significantly higher number of neurons that produce histamine.[135] Researchers theorize that the dramatically higher number of histaminergic tuberomammillary nucleus (TMN) neurons may be a compensatory mechanism to make up for the decrease in the other neuron type; they are likely responsible for the hallmark problem of fragmented nighttime sleep and severe drowsiness during the day experienced by sufferers of narcolepsy.[135] Whether patients with MCAS have a true narcolepsy neuronal issue, or simply an imbalance in circulating histamine levels, it can be very difficult to get adequate sleep to promote healing.

Prostaglandin levels may also contribute to sleep-wakefulness cycle abnormalities in MCAS patients, and symptoms may be dependent on the type of prostaglandin(s) in excess.[136] Animal studies frequently use prostaglandin D2 as a sleep-inducing substance,[137] but prostaglandin E2 may be more associated with wakefulness.[136] It's clear that mast cell mediators have a complex (and likely underestimated) role in circadian rhythm regulation. Patients who have adrenal issues may also experience difficulties in sleep due to their abnormal circulating levels of hormones.

Theoharides and Cochrane describe a number of ways that mast cells may be involved in the pathogenesis of neurodegenerative conditions including multiple sclerosis (MS).[138] They describe a cycle in which mast cells damage myelin, the connective sheath around nerves, and promote increased secretion of tryptase, which further increases inflammation and demyelination.[138] The authors note, "Mast cells have been reported in MS plaques and could participate in demyelination directly."[138] Theoharides and colleagues also suggest mechanisms by which other chemical mediators influence T cells and macrophages, which perpetuate the chronic neurodegenerative properties noted in MS.[39]

In 2018, Haenisch and Molderings reported similar alterations in brain white matter in patients with MCAS compared to what's been observed in patients with systemic mastocytosis.[139] They were unable to confirm a causal relation between neurological symptoms and white matter abnormalities in patients with MCAS, but urged researchers to conduct further investigation into the prevalence of such abnormalities in patients with MCAD.[139]

It appears that the vagus nerve may exert an influence over a number of physiological factors associated with MCAD. Specifically, patients with MCAS who experience POTS, headaches associated with chiari malformation or intracranial pressure issues, digestive problems, and other issues connected to sympathetic nervous system activation may be affected by the interplay between the vagus nerve and other systems. More in-depth information on these potential connections will be presented in Chapter 7.

OROPHARYNGEAL FINDINGS

Burning mouth syndrome (BMS) is quite possibly linked to MCAD, though Afrin noted in 2016 that the evidence up to this point was purely anecdotal.[7] Patients may present with excruciating pain and sometimes constant burning sensations along the GI tract anywhere from the mouth to the anus. Afrin noted a correlation with an increased number of mast cells in the GI tract in his first case, with a profound response to antihistamines and NSAIDs.[7]

Afrin published a case study in 2011 that describes three patients with BMS who had subsequent clinical evidence of MCAS.[140] All three patients went on to respond well to mast cell-targeting medications (including antihistamines and NSAIDs) for relief of their BMS symptoms.[140]

Patients presenting with BMS plus chronic inflammatory involvement of other system(s) may benefit from consideration of MCAS if other causes have been ruled out. As of 2017, Afrin has reported that every subsequent case of idiopathic burning mouth syndrome seen in his office since his first case has tested positive for MCAS.[141] High-level clinical research is certainly needed targeting this subgroup of patients.

Patients may also present with ulcerations, sores, white patches (leukoplakia), and scarring in the mouth.[7] The tongue may exhibit abnormalities in color and texture, which could be a reflection of imbalanced gastrointestinal bacterial flora or the presence of a yeast (candida) fungal infection.

Throat irritation is common, and it's important to ascertain whether the throat is truly "irritated" or actually "swollen" as part of an anaphylactic reaction. Throat swelling (particularly when accompanied by episodes of swelling in other areas) should also be evaluated to rule out hereditary angioedema. Throat irritation and vocal cord dysfunction will be discussed in the Respiratory System section.

OTHER MAJOR ORGANS

It's clear that MCAD can affect some or all of the vital organs. Mast cells in the heart, lungs, brain, and gastrointestinal system were already presented, and it's becoming apparent that MCAS can also impact the function of additional organs such as the liver, gallbladder, pancreas, and kidney.

Approximately half of patients with MCAS may have some sort of liver abnormality.[2] Patients may be first clued in by routine lab blood values that are high, such as elevated liver enzymes like alkaline phosphatase or transaminases. Mast cells are known to especially proliferate to the liver in patients with MCAD. A 2009 study found that 44% of patients with MCAS had elevated liver enzymes (by at least two-fold), 36% had bilirubin in the blood, 15% had a fatty liver, and 34% had an enlarged liver or some sort of liver shape alteration.[2] Cirrhosis and/or ascites (fluid in the abdomen) are possible and are more often associated with mastocytosis compared to MCAS, though they can occur with MCAS as well. According to Afrin, "Idiopathic ascites also is quite infrequently seen in both SM and in MCAS. It may be seen with or without portal hypertension but, when present, is often massive and difficult to manage."[142]

Hepatic portal hypertension (high venous pressure between the intestines and the liver) has been associated with higher mast cell densities in animal studies,[143] and it appears that mast cells regulate the inflammatory responses present in this condition.[144] Hepatic portal hypertension has been reported in patients with MCAD, and it can lead to esophageal varices and swelling of the spleen.[145-146]

In 2009, researchers also found that 14% of patients with MCAS had elevated amylase or lipase, indicating pancreatic dysfunction.[2] Chronic pancreatitis appears to be regulated by mast cells.[147] Experts have linked the role of the mast cell mediator histamine to pancreatitis and pancreatic cancer.[148] The local and systemic inflammation associated with early phases of acute pancreatitis appear to be caused by mast cells, and the mast cell stabilizer cromolyn sodium was able to reduce the inflammation in active cases of pancreatitis in rats.[149] However, Theoharides notes that cromolyn is weakly absorbed in humans and is likely not sufficient as a treatment option for pancreatic cancer.[150] It appears that there is a void in effective mast cell stabilizers that could selectively inhibit pro-tumor factors without inhibiting the other chemical mediators that may be beneficial to fighting pancreatic (and other types of) cancer.[150]

There are a large number of different heavy metals, chemicals, physiological factors, infections, and chronic/autoimmune diseases that have been linked to kidney damage and dysfunction. The potential role of mast cells in kidney disease is a bit cloudy. Kidney problems are noted in some patients with MCAS, and increased mast cells have been associated with renal fibrosis.[151] However, the presence of mast cells in the kidneys is not always pathologic and may be protective in some instances; mast cells contribute to the ability to restore homeostasis and induce repair and remodeling following kidney injury.[152] Different types of allergic disease have been associated with idiopathic kidney disease, though this may be more mediated by the stimulation of IgE responses via interleukin-13.[153]

Gallbladder referral pains and gallbladder inflammation have been associated with mast cell activation. Symptomatic cholelithiasis (gallstones) and biliary dyskinesia (motility disorder affecting the gallbladder) are associated with a nine- to twelve-fold increase in mast cells in the gallbladder walls when compared to controls.[154] Gallbladder spasms have been linked to histamine and leukotrienes, two common mast cell mediators.[155-156]

A 2011 study examined patients with both symptomatic cholelithiasis and biliary dyskinesia and found that they were associated with a higher mast cell density and a moderate to high level of mast cell activation, though the gallbladder ejection fraction was not correlated with mast cell findings.[157] Mast cell activation was determined by electron micrographs taken in control subjects compared to those of symptomatic subjects, which showed empty granule chambers in mast cells in the symptomatic group.[157] Interestingly, piecemeal degranulation was noted, which means that certain mediators were selectively part of the degranulation process by mast cells in the chronic inflammatory group with confirmed gallbladder pathology.[157]

Mast cell density may influence response to gallbladder removal surgery. In patients with biliary dyskinesia, a lower level of epithelial mast cell density was correlated with a complete clinical response following laparoscopic removal of the gallbladder, whereas other patients with higher concentrations of mast cells had partial response or no relief.[157] More research is certainly needed to investigate this area.

RESPIRATORY SYSTEM

The upper and lower respiratory tracts represent a large environmental interface within the body, and they present with relatively more mast cells than most other places in the body.[7] Patients may report hoarseness, a chronic cough, laryngitis, wheezing, and shortness of breath.[7]

Many patients complain of sore throats and excess post-nasal drip that irritates the throat.[7] It's important to differentiate throat soreness from throat swelling. *Throat swelling* that occurs with angioedema and an allergic reaction more commonly involves difficulty swallowing and breathing, since the airway is narrowed. Throat swelling is an emergency medical situation that may necessitate medications and/or epinephrine. Throat soreness, on the other hand, is usually distinct, and *anecdotally* patients with MCAS report frequent signs of strep throat or other viruses with negative bacterial cultures.

Some patients experience a chronic, dry (unproductive) cough of unknown origin. Many patients note intermittent hoarseness and the frequent urge to clear their throat.[7] Vocal cord dysfunction (VCD) is another common finding in patients with MCAS. VCD involves the inappropriate closing (partial or full) of the vocal flaps during inhalation and sometimes exhalation. The exact cause is unknown but could be connected to the pattern of inflammation commonly encountered with MCAS.

Anecdotally, many patients have carried around the diagnosis of asthma since youth, despite the fact that no treatments seem to be effective at reducing symptoms. Pulmonary function testing may also be "normal" despite the report of significant breathing difficulties, but it can also present as true asthma in some patients. The roots of clinical asthma have been theorized to be connected to mast cell activation.[158]

According to Theoharides and Kalogeromitros, "the role of mast cells in asthma is undisputed."[158] Higher levels of cytokines have been measured in the baseline exhaled breath of patients with asthma compared to "normal" subjects.[159] Bacterial and viral toll-like receptors (TLRs) on mast cells have been associated with the release of inflammatory compounds including interleukins.[158] TLRs play a role in the adaptive immune responses associated with asthma. Viral infections appear to worsen asthmatic symptoms, and activation of mast cell TLRs from contact with a virus may explain this connection.[158]

There's no shortage of research regarding the pharmacological management of asthma. Omalizumab (Xolair) is a medication that inhibits the binding of IgE to high-affinity receptors, preventing the development of subsequent allergic reactions. Multiple systematic reviews support the efficacy of Xolair in the asthmatic population for the treatment of asthma in children,[160] the long-term management of severe allergic asthma,[161] and the reduction of corticosteroid medications needed to control symptoms.[162] Xolair is one treatment option for patients with MCAS, and it's believed to alleviate asthma-type symptoms in this patient population.

According to Afrin, another common respiratory system complaint is brief spells of difficulty with getting a deep breath, despite no noted abnormalities on pulmonary testing (usually performed days or weeks after the last such spell).[7] Short-lived episodes of inflammation, bronchoconstriction, or edema caused by mast cell degranulation may be responsible for this transient symptom. Afrin has noted "patchy ground-glass infiltrates" consistent with inflammation on lung imaging in patients with MCAS, and some doctors may incorrectly diagnose patients with pneumonia even in the absence of fevers consistent with a true infection.[7] True bacterial pneumonia may also be present in an MCAS patient with a weakened immune system.

Studies with mice have found that mast cells are an important part of the body's response to and recovery from mycoplasma pneumonia infection.[163] However, if mast cells are dysfunctional, it's possible that their response to this bacterium is altered or can wreak more havoc. Mycoplasma pneumonia releases a toxin called CARDS, which is associated with an increase in asthma-type symptoms.[164] It's plausible that MCAS patients who have been historically exposed to mycoplasma pneumonia are more at risk for chronic airway inflammation and mast cell degranulation consistent with intermittent asthma and other respiratory symptoms.

Chronic obstructive pulmonary disease (COPD) and pulmonary fibrosis are two more serious conditions that have been linked to mast cell activation. COPD is an umbrella term that encompasses diseases like emphysema and chronic bronchitis, sometimes attributed to smoking or second-hand smoke. COPD causes obstructed airflow and chronic inflammation in airway tissues; most patients experience shortness of breath on a regular basis. Environmental pollutants and respiratory illness tend to be a big trigger with this condition. According to the Mayo Clinic, 20%-30% of smokers eventually develop COPD.[165] *Anecdotally,* most patients with MCAS tend to avoid cigarette smoke, so it's likely that other mechanisms are triggering the issue. One theory is that the excess release of proinflammatory mediators triggers a response in MCAS that is similar to the inflammation triggered by smoking in "healthy" subjects.

Pulmonary fibrosis is a condition that involves the scarring and thickening of lung tissue. This process makes it difficult for the lung tissues to expand normally, and patients have difficulty breathing. Mast cells have a clear proliferative role in the initial and chronic response to injury signals and are theorized to be linked to the scar formulation process in this disease.[166] Stem cell factor from mast cells appears to play an important role in pathological pulmonary fibroblast function.[167] Mast cell-associated stimulation of fibroblasts in lung tissue can lead to alveolar tissue destruction and poor blood oxygenation in patients with idiopathic pulmonary fibrosis.[167] The disease is fast-progressing with a poor prognosis. Mast cell-targeting agents have been the topic of recent research consideration for cases of idiopathic pulmonary fibrosis.[167]

MCAS AND CANCER

Thus far, research connections between mast cells and thyroid tumors as well as hematologic malignancies (including multiple myeloma and Hodgkin's lymphoma) have been discussed. There's an abundance of additional research that examines the potential role of mast cells and their proliferation on other types of cancer. Interestingly, the literature shows mast cells appear to have both a protective and proliferative role in cancer.

A number of literature findings support a theoretical association between mast cells and cancer. The interpretation of findings of a higher number of mast cells present in cancerous areas can be tricky. After all, mast cells as part of the immunoregulatory "first response" system will naturally be drawn to any "invader" or infection and thus would be expected to be naturally higher in concentration in cancerous areas. The theories lead back to the ever-common question of "which came first, the chicken or the egg?"

Regardless of whether the increased mast cell activity is due to true MCAS or simply the body's natural defense system in a "normal host," compelling evidence suggests that the presence of mast cells in the vicinity of cancerous tissue can often be problematic. So, by logical *assumption*, the presence of a potential cancer source could *possibly* be especially detrimental in patients who already have MCAS. One such *theory* is that patients who have too much mast cell activity (and a likely subset of genetic and environmental predispositions) are the ones who go on to develop cancer. Others theorize that the total exposure to toxic and infectious burden levels influence cancer the most, and these factors also influence the rate of mast cell activity.

One retrospective study has been conducted that investigated the prevalence of cancer reported in the past medical history in patients with MCAS. Molderings and colleagues conducted a study in 2017 that evaluated the prevalence of solid tumor forms of cancer in 828 European (German) and American MCAS patients.[168] In the study, 68 patients (8.2%) of the total reported the development of a solid tumor prior to their diagnosis with MCAS.[168]

As a whole, MCAS patients presented with a higher prevalence of lung, thyroid, bladder, breast, and reproductive organ (cervical, ovarian, testicular, uterine) cancers and melanoma than the general population.[168] The German group had a higher rate of melanoma than the U.S. group;[168] melanoma has been associated with SM and theorized to be connected to cytokine production and the presence of tyrosine kinase *KIT* genetic mutations.[169-172] The German MCAS study population also appeared to be at higher risk of testicular cancer and breast cancer than the American MCAS patients.[168] The U.S. MCAS group had a higher prevalence of ovarian and thyroid cancer when compared to the German MCAS group.[168] Both MCAS groups had higher than average rates of lung cancer and bladder cancer when compared to the general population.[168]

In MCAS patients, many of the sites found to have a higher prevalence of cancer are areas of physiological interface between the body and the outside world—places that are known to be higher in mast cell concentration. The authors concluded that mast cells *may contribute to malignancy*.[168] They also *theorized* that the treatment of MCAS could potentially reduce the risk of neoplasia, and mast cell-targeting treatment while also undergoing treatment for existing cancer may be a potentially beneficial intervention for this patient population.[168]

A limited age range was available for analysis with the MCAS patient cohort compared to what was used to determine general population statistics, which is one limitation to this study. Interestingly, the results of a higher prevalence of cancer, and particularly melanoma, in MCAS patients appear similar to what's been noted in the systemic mastocytosis patient population.[173]

A 2017 study by Afrin and colleagues noted that a family history of breast cancer and brain cancer were reported in 26% and 5% of patients with MCAS, respectively.[174] The authors concluded, "The data in this study suggest the families of MCAS patients bear various cancers at much higher rates than the general population, raising the question of whether MCAS underlies significant portions of the populations with at least some types of cancer. The outcome of cancer treatment has long been recognized to improve when comorbid mastocytosis is recognized and concurrently treated."[174]

In 2018, Molderings and colleagues described a case report of a 58-year-old woman who presented with a MCAS-associated infiltration of mast cells visible on MRI that mimicked breast cancer.[175] They noted that mast cell specific staining of breast biopsy samples may prove useful as a way to differentiate between mast cell infiltrations and cancerous masses in women with existing MCAD, and may prevent unnecessary surgeries and false-positive breast cancer testing.[175] Thus, it's also possible that mast cells contribute to physical masses that may mimick cancerous tumors, and patients with MCAS *may be* more likely to experience such infiltrations, though more research is needed.

In a review of mast cells and their immunoregulatory functions, researchers Ryan et al. noted, "If chronic inflammation promotes oncogenesis, the mast cell is a logical participant in this process."[176] Mast cells have the ability to elicit migration of other types of cells to certain areas, specifically via inflammatory cytokines like tumor necrosis factor (TNF) and the four types of vascular endothelial growth factor (VEGF) that they can secrete.[176]

TNF has been associated with tumor growth, cancer metastasis, and an increase in the growth of new blood vessels around growing tissue.[176] An inflammatory cascade can be triggered by the interactions stemming from tryptase, COX activity, and prostaglandins, which in turn increase VEGF production in mast cells.[176] VEGF may enhance migration of cancerous cells and also contributes to the vascular supply that fuels tumor survival and growth.[176]

Additional mediators (such as histamine and leukotrienes) simultaneously increase vascular permeability and contribute to the process of leukocyte migration.[176] In addition, it appears that there's cross-talk between mast cells and tumor cells that results in a positive feedback loop that increases inflammation and potential progression of malignancies.[176] Ryan and colleagues note, "Mast cells have also been shown to be pivotal in the angiogenesis of several murine (rodent) tumors."[176] It appears that bidirectional interactions between mast cells and eosinophils also influence a number of physiological mechanisms that occur in cancerous and inflammatory conditions.[177]

A review in 2011 by Schor noted that mast cell proliferation and/or density is associated with the development and/or progression of the following cancers: rectal cancer, melanoma, squamous cell carcinoma of the mouth and lip, Hodgkin's lymphoma, multiple myeloma, endometrial cancer, pancreatic cancer, gastric cancer, thyroid cancer, non-small cell lung cancer (NSCLC) adenocarcinomas (conflicting evidence), and follicular lymphoma (except diffuse B-cell lymphoma).[88]

Schor concluded, "Mast cells appear to have two very different actions in regard to cancer, and it appears to vary with cancer type. Mast cells appear to promote the growth of several tumor types, especially increasing angiogenesis through generation of VEGF and other cytokines. This seems especially true in rectal cancer, pancreatic cancer, and melanoma. Yet there are other cancers—breast, prostate, and ovarian—that appear to be hindered by mast cells and high mast cell counts would seem to improve survival of these patients."[88]

What further confounds these types of findings is the fact that, in some types of cancer, mast cells appear to simultaneously both contribute to cancer development and improve patient outcome. For example, in colorectal cancer, mast cells appear to play a role in the adenoma to carcinoma development, yet in preliminary research their higher densities are associated with more favorable outcomes.[178]

Schor cites research that suggests that the mast cell stabilizer cromolyn sodium appears to be a useful treatment in pancreatic cancer and breast cancer.[88] So, with breast cancer as an example, it appears that high mast cell counts actually help improve survival, but yet the cancer is improved with mast cell stabilizer medication… such contradictory findings! And then with pancreatic cancer, high mast cell densities seem to be a bad thing, and logically cromolyn sodium appears to be especially helpful. These reported findings are confusing; however, it's important to remember that cromolyn sodium is not a systemic drug, and this is just preliminary research.

The proliferative vs. protective roles of mast cells in tumor development also appear to have mixed results in the literature. Increased angiogenesis, or the formation of new blood vessels, is typically observed alongside areas of tumor growth, in addition to a heightened inflammatory response.[179] Mast cells are considered "critical regulators of inflammation and the immunoregulatory response in the tumour microenvironment."[179] However, studies of mast cell proliferation and mediators reflect both protective and pathological contributions to tumor development and growth, depending on the different clinical and experimental contexts.[179]

Benign and cancerous polyps appear to have increased mast cells and greater levels of mast cell activation. According to a literature review by Menzies et al., "a 7-fold increase in activated MCs has been found in endometrial polyps compared with normal endometrium. MCs (mast cells) are also increased in benign nasal and colonic polyps compared with normal tissue, suggesting that MC increases may be a common feature of polyps."[180]

Theoharides has noted that some cancers, like pancreatic cancer, secrete chemo-attractants that lure mast cells into the area of existing cancer.[150] He explains, "Many mast cell mediators that could be considered 'protumor' include heparin, metalloproteinases, platelet-derived growth factor, and vascular endothelial growth factor (VEGF). However, mast cells also release molecules that could participate in tumor death and be considered 'anti-tumor.'"[150]

In many instances, the literature notes a seemingly bipolar connection between mast cells/their mediators and cancer. It's possible that the presence of an increased number or increased sensitivity of mast cells could very well be the difference between adequate protection in a "MCAS-free" population and the "on" switch for unfortunate cancer proliferation, as is the case in other non-cancerous conditions where mast cells gone awry appear to contribute to dysfunction on the cellular level.

It's plausible that individual chemical mediator discrepancies in MCAS patients may play a role, and perhaps certain patients have a predominance of select chemical mediators that contribute to whether the subsequent effects on the cellular level and protective or harmful.

It's also possible that other (non-mast cell) factors are more predominant in the outcome in terms of cancer proliferation, and mast cells could be simply the "innocent bystanders" that migrate to the area. The research seems to support that they indeed play an important role, but the human body is complex and obviously many other factors have been identified to play a role in cancer development and progression.

Hopefully time and additional research will provide more information on the relevance of mast cells in oncologic disease. Fortunately (or unfortunately), there is more financial motivation for cancer research than research focused on MCAS alone, so this could be the area that continues to spread more limelight onto the condition.

OTHER POTENTIAL CONNECTIONS

Restless leg syndrome (RLS) is an irritating phenomenon of leg aching and the strong urge to move the lower extremities. Many patients theorize that restless leg syndrome is connected to histamine overload or mast cell activation, with *anecdotal* reports that the antihistamine diphenhydramine is effective at immediate cessation of restless leg syndrome. RLS seems to be (*anecdotally*) worse after the consumption of wine or following physical exercise for many patients.

A large number of conditions have been connected to RLS in the literature, including inflammatory bowel disease, SIBO, iron deficiency, neuropathy, immune system disorders, and inflammatory conditions.[181] One theory states that increased levels of vasoconstricting cytokines (such as what occurs with exercise, and mast cell degranulation) results in decreased oxygenation to tissues, causing the urge to move one's legs.

Multiple chemical sensitivity (MCS) is a condition that is predominantly experienced by women (80%).[182] The underlying mechanism of MCS is unclear and it's generally regarded as an idiopathic condition.[183] Is it possible that these patients actually have underlying MCAD?

Patients with MCS experience a chronic sensitivity—often to triggers that are undetectable or non-irritable to their peers—to the same repeated triggers and typically react to a large number of different substances. Symptoms can include difficulty breathing, burning in the eyes, difficulties with memory and concentration, fatigue, throat and sinus problems, skin rashes, sensitivity to light and noise, gastrointestinal issues, and muscle and joint pain. Symptoms tend to improve when the trigger has been removed.

Heuser postulates that a chemical injury can trigger a mast cell disorder which may then cause the patient to experience MCS.[184] He notes limbic, hypothalamic and brain stem changes on PET scans in patients with MCS, similar to what is observed during seizure activity, which may explain some of the emotional instability during chemical reactions in these patients.[184] Clinically, Heuser has also begun to test patients with MCS for MCAD and notes a surprising number of positive cases for either systemic mastocytosis or other types of MCAD.[184] It's quite possible that the conditions are related, though research is needed to dig deeper into the connections.

Summary

Do mast cells cause the initiation or progression of the diseases and conditions discussed in this chapter? Or is something else causing an underlying process that recruits extra mast cell activity in the area? Hopefully more time and research will tell. The take home message in all of these areas is that more research is definitely needed!

CHAPTER KEY POINTS

- Mast cells have been implicated to play a major role in a number of diseases and conditions across virtually all body systems. Research has noted increased volumes of mast cells and high concentrations of mast cell mediators in chronic and acute inflammatory conditions.

- While interesting, the associations in existing literature often lack clear mechanisms and causality cannot be inferred. Further, in many conditions (such as cancer) it's difficult to determine which came first: the chicken or the egg?

- Many patients with MCAS present with multiple comorbidities. Though many associations have been made, there is still a need for more research before causal relationships can be determined.

Chapter Six

Clinical Considerations for Diagnosis

This chapter provides additional insight into currently available recommendations for the diagnostic process for patients presenting with signs of MCAS.

CONSIDERATIONS FOR CLINICAL DECISION-MAKING

Patient History

Most doctors do not have adequate time for a lengthy history, which may lead patients to focus on a few of their biggest concerns without painting a full picture of what they are experiencing. This phenomenon is only exacerbated by the American medical system's specialty-based organizational hierarchy. It's evident that patients suffering from long-standing cases of MCAS symptoms can become so adapted to their symptoms over the years that they often do not mention everything that may be relevant.

Accurate history sharing is often further complicated by the waxing and waning nature of the symptoms. For example, a patient may not mention that they were tested for multiple sclerosis because they are no longer experiencing those same neurological symptoms like they were a decade ago, because they've learned to ignore those symptoms, or because the condition was previously ruled out.

Another possibility creating varied clinical presentation is that certain symptoms could be (falsely) attributed to other ideas or explanations that make sense to the patient and therefore could be omitted from the history. For example, one may blame difficulty breathing and near-fainting episodes with exercise on a childhood diagnosis of asthma. Other patients sometimes describe flushing episodes as "fevers" even in the absence of a truly elevated body temperature due to a lack of familiarity with the term "flushing."

And yet another perspective is that there are certain symptoms that patients refrain from sharing intentionally with a new doctor for fear of being labeled a certain way. Once a patient has been told that their problems are all in their head, a large gaping canyon of distrust emerges, and patients may teeter on the edge of the cliff until they find a practitioner who exhibits openness or instills confidence in them before they are willing to come forward with certain information.

Dr. Diana Driscoll, a Texas-based optometrist and Clinical Director of POTS Care, explains, "When patients struggle with as many as 100 symptoms, they 'learn' to be afraid to share these with any doctor, for fear of being labeled as mental cases. As such, patients try to hide symptoms in order to keep doctors on their team. Patients are often 'on their best behavior' during medical exams, and the extent of their suffering can be underestimated."[1]

Therefore, it's important to keep in mind that by the time a patient is in the office of someone knowledgeable in MCAD, they may accidentally omit details from their history, or they may do it intentionally because of prior bad experiences with the medical system. Further probing and a thorough checklist of questions is strongly encouraged, alongside a complete history that encompasses the patient's entire lifespan. Above all, a non-rushed and empathetic history-taking will enhance the likelihood that patients will provide information for a complete clinical picture.

MCAS is a tricky condition to diagnose, even when the patient's history points to mast cells. Diagnosis rarely comes easy. Lab tests often come back normal or slightly positive for vague inflammatory markers and radiologic tests.[2] Or, tests may come back positive one month and then suddenly be negative the following check-up, baffling doctors and putting the patient into even more despair at the countless false hopes and misdiagnoses.

Patients with MCAS are often labeled as hypochondriacs, told that the symptoms are all in their head, or agonized by naïve commentary from peers or even doctors—"But you look normal!" Chronic fatigue and fibromyalgia are often present and blamed as the culprits, though some believe these conditions are merely labels describing clusters of symptoms without an identified cause. Stress is another commonly labeled "diagnosis." Stress can certainly trigger mast cell degranulation, but it's extremely frustrating to be told repeatedly by doctors that stress is *the* problem.

There's a vicious cycle that many patients experience prior to their diagnosis of MCAD (or other chronic unexplained illness) that is just as damaging mentally as it can be physically. This cycle includes fluctuating between relentless searching for answers and a sense of shame or depression when concerns are brushed aside by doctors (or when testing comes back inconclusive, without a "real" diagnosis, or with a misdiagnosis that is later revoked). Then the patient typically decides to mentally resolve to be tougher and try harder to push through the symptoms until they can't handle it anymore, and then they're back in the doctor's office again.

Without a socially accepted "diagnosis," the patient lacks validation for what they are experiencing, which often plunges them into the depths of despair, self-loathing or self-doubt. In addition, the patient then lacks adequate information to move forward proactively into some type of a treatment approach, creating a damaging pattern of continual suffering, frustration, hopelessness, and despair.

Many patients experience this for several years or even decades before they get their true diagnostic answer. The importance of a thorough and lengthy history cannot be emphasized enough. Patients ought to seek out practitioners who are able to schedule longer initial appointments for that first history; it's wise to call ahead to verify when in doubt. For practitioners who simply cannot afford an hour for a new patient visit, perhaps there are ways to get around the time constraints. It may be feasible to schedule more than one session up-front in order to have adequate time for the patient history, broken into two separate visits. Chances are, if the rationale is presented to the patient in the right way, they will jump at the opportunity to share their history with someone who is willing to be that thorough, even if it's more time and money for them. Practitioners willing to take that time with patients are few and far between.

Challenges in Differential Diagnosis

A mainstream approach that focuses on one system or type of symptom is *not always irrelevant* in patients with suspected MCAS. In general, by the time the patient is considering MCAS, they've most likely had the more common conditions ruled out by system (such as inflammatory bowel disease for patients who have chronic gastrointestinal issues). But one should *never assume* that this is the case.

It's also crucial to keep in mind that not all patients have had the rare "zebras" considered. Due diligence is needed when evaluating MCAS, and though it may be tempting to jump immediately to one broad explanation for everything, true comorbidities can and do occur.

Generally, patients with potential MCAS will share symptoms that are their biggest concerns or complaints that stand out above the others. One example of this may be reported in patients who present with severe flushing as a main symptom. Rosacea is a common diagnosis for flushing of the face. Mast cell activation most certainly can cause flushing of the skin, and it may also present as part of anaphylaxis or part of menopause.[3] However, more serious diagnoses such as carcinoid syndrome, pheochromocytoma, and mastocytosis should be considered. Experts also recommend that the rarer causes of flushing, such as renal carcinoma, medullary carcinoma of the thyroid, and pancreatic cell tumors be considered.[4] This is one example of a glimpse into the clinical diligence necessary when evaluating a patient with multisystem symptoms.

Algorithms for Clinical Decision-Making

Just as there is no one set of universal recommendations for criteria for the diagnosis of MCAS, there is no *universally agreed-upon algorithm* to guide clinicians in a step-by-step manner through the process. Researchers in the same two groups that proposed the original *similar but different* recommendations for MCAS diagnosis in 2011 and 2012, referred to as "Criteria X" and "Criteria Y" in this book,[2,5] (See Chapter 3) have since both published *similar but different* algorithms for clinical decision-making.[6,7]

The algorithms serve as useful tools for clinicians and may be important resources for patients to bookmark and share with medical practitioners who are not familiar with MCAD and MCAS. The *main* differences between the two algorithm approaches lie in the order or sequence of testing, the particular mast cell mediators considered useful in testing, the search for secondary causes of MCAD, and the focus on exon 17 c-*KIT* mutations.

Clinicians are strongly encouraged to reference the original articles that contain the algorithms directly to ensure full understanding and accuracy. The clinical decision-making algorithms published in 2013 and 2014 are both available in full text for free online.[6,7] A listing of recommended diagnostic algorithm resources is available in Appendix 2.

Validated Mast Cell Mediator Release Syndrome Questionnaire

The 2014 algorithm for clinical decision-making is more specific in terms of which exact chemical mediators and other laboratory tests should be performed. It also includes mention of a validated questionnaire (see Appendix 2) that can assist the clinician in a quantitative analysis of their index of MCAD suspicion based on both concrete clinical findings as well as pertinent information from the patient history.

The questionnaire was created by Dr. Molderings and colleagues in Germany and is referred to as "Mast Cell Mediator Release Syndrome Questionnaire" with no other designating title. It appears that the questionnaire is the first published and validated tool of its kind for this patient population. The tool was modified from an earlier version and has been validated twice, upon its initial design and in 2013, by biometrics using logistic regression in a large number of patients.[7-9]

There are a few important things to remember about this particular tool. First of all, the questionnaire is *not* necessarily required for making the diagnosis. According to Molderings, "If the diagnosing physician is sufficiently familiar with MCAD, he/she will also be able to recognize the various affected systems of the body without the questionnaire, and thus the constellation of findings of the mast cell mediator release syndrome. On the one hand, the questionnaire serves as a memory aid for those who are inexperienced with the disease and, on the other hand, for any scientific evaluations as a standardized, validated basis for assessment. However, the evidence for the presence of a mast cell mediator release syndrome is the major criterion to diagnose systemic mast cell activation disease."[8]

Secondly, it is inappropriate to examine the different items in the questionnaire individually, as they lack specificity when isolated. According to Molderings, "It is about recognizing whether several systems of the organism, at least four or five, simultaneously have symptoms that can then be attributed to one underlying disease."[8]

The questionnaire is utilized internationally and is organized by categories including clinical signs, triggering factors, laboratory parameters, imaging methods, and medical history. Some of the items are logical and seem to be "common knowledge" among MCAS sufferers—e.g., "histamine-containing food (red wine, cheese, tuna)" is listed as a triggering factor. Other questionnaire items, such as "anal pruritic and/or anal eczema," "fasting for 24 hours" or "low titers of antibodies" seem arbitrary, random, or less publicly known compared to other information on the tool. In viewing the questions, therefore, it's important to heed Dr. Moldering's advice about avoiding dissecting the individual items. Instead, the questionnaire should be viewed as a tool that functions as a whole package.

The questionnaire has certain tests that have a range of scoring based on findings. For example, a patient with gastroscopy and biopsies from the stomach and duodenum may score 1 point if they show "minor signs of inflammation," or 10 points for that item if they show "clusters of mast cells and/or a considerable number of spindle-shaped mast cells and/or CD-25 positive mast cells."

Twenty-eight of the items are based off the patient history and a basic office examination, for a combined section maximum of 33 possible points. Three of the items are based off biopsy testing or surgical history, for a combined section maximum of 21 possible points. Five of the items are based off blood or urine laboratory tests, for a combined section maximum of 25 possible points. Two of the items are based off bone and organ imaging methods, for a combined section maximum of 2 points. Cumulatively, the tool has 38 different items in question, with a maximum score of 81 points.

Fourteen points is the main cut-off score. According to the questionnaire developers, a score of 14 or higher (17.2%) is indicative that a systemic mast cell mediator syndrome is present.[9] Scoring of 9-13 points indicates a pathological activation of mast cells.[9] If a clinician were to utilize the tool based on history alone for a patient who had not had any prior testing, the maximum score a patient could achieve (presuming they said "yes" to all history questions) would be 33/81 points, or just under 41%.

The questionnaire appears to be more designed as a final diagnostic assessment score as opposed to a pretesting screening questionnaire that predicts likelihood of MCAD. While the 2014 algorithm[6] describes use of the questionnaire as a tool to help *establish suspicion* of MCAD, as the first step in the diagnostic algorithm, much of its conclusions depend on testing that is designated to occur in the subsequent steps (*initial testing* or *additional mast cell mediator testing*). Thus, the questionnaire appears less useful for the patient who has not undergone testing yet, though it's still possible to achieve the cutoff score of 14 based on history alone.

As is the scenario with many topics related to MCAD, it's not perfect, but it's all that's available! In a perfect world, there would be separate tools: 1) a validated screening questionnaire for the patient to complete that could serve to raise the index of suspicion for MCAS based on patient history; 2) a validated clinical tool or clinical prediction rule factoring in the physical examination, laboratory, and biopsy testing findings to assist in the MCAD diagnosis; and 3) a validated outcome tool to be completed by the patient (at diagnostic baseline and periodically over time) to track progress in functional tasks and quality of life, so that the clinician could determine efficacy of the treatment plan in a more objective manner.

Currently, the questionnaire tool that is available attempts to combine subjective and objective information in order to raise suspicion of a systemic mast cell mediator syndrome, and it covers a wide variety of tests and factors. The questionnaire assigns more weight in its scoring scheme to concrete evidence from testing as opposed to being based solely on the patient history. It was *not* designed as a tool to measure outcomes/success with treatment, nor does it predict prognosis. The questionnaire may be a useful starting point to assist in clinical diagnosis considerations, particularly for practitioners who may not be entirely familiar with the condition. (See Appendix 2 for a link to the questionnaire.)

A completely separate patient questionnaire, the Mastocytosis Symptoms Assessment Form (MSAF), was created by J.C. Kluin-Nelemans at the University Medical Center Groningen. This questionnaire is shorter and measures the severity of symptoms as well as the impact of fatigue on daily activities and relationships. It appears to be designed specifically as a way to develop a score to track progress in symptoms for patients with mastocytosis.

For the systemic mastocytosis patient population, the MSAF and Mastocytosis Quality of Life Questionnaire (MQLQ) were reported to be valid and reliable tools for use in clinical research.[10] A tool called the Advanced Systemic Mastocytosis Symptom Assessment Form (ADVSM-SAF) was under development for clinical use in 2016, but it's unclear whether the tool would also be appropriate and valid for use in patients with other types of MCAD, such as MCAS.[11]

PUTTING IT ALL TOGETHER: A STEPWISE DIAGNOSTIC APPROACH

It's important to note that, in terms of billing options for insurance in the United States, ICD-10 codes now include "MCAS nonspecific" as a diagnostic option, in addition to codes for "monoclonal mast cell activation syndrome," "idiopathic mast cell activation syndrome," "secondary mast cell activation," and "other mast cell activation disorder."[12]

When assessing all of the available approaches in the literature, there are some mainstays to the clinical diagnosis decision-making process that remain intact across different publications: the raising of clinical suspicion based on patient history, the testing of certain mast cell mediators, the consideration of tissue biopsies depending on the scenario, the differential diagnosis process, the classification of the type of MCAD present, and the testing of medications. While small nuances exist between the approaches of different authors and the sequence that they recommend for testing, they generally follow similar guidelines in terms of the big picture.

Below is a nine-step process that combines suggestions from the literature into one concise decision-making process, *with my own additions italicized*. In the instance where certain recommendations differed between authors, I included all of the options. For example, some authors recommended that only tryptase, prostaglandins, and histamine should be tested in blood and urine, whereas other authors recommended additional mast cell mediators be considered. In this case, I included *all* of the mediators suggested by the experts, since there was no universal consensus available.

The following nine-step process (Table 1) is based on written recommendations by Molderings and colleagues (2011),[2] Afrin and Molderings (2014),[6] and Picard et al (2013).[3]

Table 1. Example of a Nine-Step Process for MCAD Diagnosis

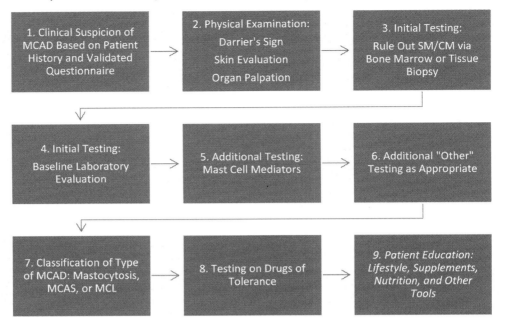

1. Clinical Suspicion of MCAD Based on Patient History and Validated Questionnaire	2. Physical Examination: Darrier's Sign / Skin Evaluation / Organ Palpation	3. Initial Testing: Rule Out SM/CM via Bone Marrow or Tissue Biopsy
4. Initial Testing: Baseline Laboratory Evaluation	5. Additional Testing: Mast Cell Mediators	6. Additional "Other" Testing as Appropriate
7. Classification of Type of MCAD: Mastocytosis, MCAS, or MCL	8. Testing on Drugs of Tolerance	9. Patient Education: Lifestyle, Supplements, Nutrition, and Other Tools

Step 1: Clinical Suspicion of MCAD Based on Patient History

Unfortunately, there is no one telltale sign or symptom that helps alert clinicians for suspicion of MCAD. MCAD can manifest itself throughout multiple systems, in multiple manners, and as noted in Chapter 7, alongside many true comorbidities. Some patients present with low blood pressure, while others may present with high blood pressure. (And, some patients have a see-saw variation of the two.) Some patients are chronically constipated, while others have chronic diarrhea. (Others may fluctuate between both extremes.)

The consensus article for MCAS criteria by Valent and colleagues identified these as the most common symptoms from the patient history: flushing, pruritis, urticaria, angioedema, nasal congestion, nasal pruritis, wheezing, throat swelling, headache, hypotension, and diarrhea.[5] Other authors argue that this list is insufficient to capture the wide array of clinical presentations for MCAD. This is where a review of the MCAD symptoms listed in Chapter 3 may serve as a reference.

It's important to note that some patients display signs of both MCAS and mastocytosis. Patients with mastocytosis do not always display signs of mast cell activation.[13]

The questionnaire created by Molderings and colleagues can also help clarify whether a patient's symptoms are consistent with MCAD.[9] As previously mentioned, some aspects of the questionnaire may not be relevant if the patient has not previously had certain laboratory or tissue biopsy tests done. Nonetheless, there's a great number of items on the questionnaire that are based entirely off the history that can help assist the clinician in whether to proceed with testing for MCAD. The tool may be something that is begun at the first visit and held onto for subsequent updates in scoring if the patient has more tests ordered.

An important part of the initial process lies in noting whether the patient has 1) signs of mastocytosis, 2) signs of mast cell activation, 3) indicators that a prior diagnosis is inadequate to fully explain what the patient is experiencing (as evidenced by signs and symptoms that don't add up), and 4) indicators that treatment for a prior diagnosis has been unsuccessful.[6] It's important to note that *not all patients* with MCAS are going to present with anaphylaxis or a high level of "allergic" symptoms. Many may present with chronic multisystem issues that are non-allergic in nature.

The recognition of two "meta-patterns" can assist in raising the index of suspicion for MCAS: 1) multiple chronic inflammatory illnesses that have a poor response to treatment, and 2) a previously acquired definitive diagnosis that does not seem to fully explain the symptoms and test results.[14] That being said, there is no silver bullet to confirm suspicion, so logically even the *slightest* suspicion could easily lead a clinician to step 2 (a quick physical examination).

The clinician should most certainly exercise caution in jumping to the conclusion of MCAS without a careful screening for other potential conditions that may mimic MCAS and other conditions that may be true undiagnosed comorbidities. A list of suggested differential diagnoses can be found in Chapter 3.

Step 2: Physical Examination

The physical exam is often the aspect the receives the least clinical time, but it can be especially important in this patient population. It's important that the patient is in a gown so that cutaneous signs can easily be assessed during a full head-to-toe exam.

Darrier's Sign

- This test looks for the presence of dermatographism, or a change in the skin's appearance as a result of the release of inflammatory granules and histamine from mast cells in the skin. A light stroking of the skin with pressure (typically performed on the patient's back) can cause a raised, red, itchy, and possibly swollen or blister-like mark in the case of a positive test. This reaction should be observed in the first few minutes after the test, and again 10 to 20 minutes later to assess the reactivity of the mast cells. Is this diagnostic in itself? Certainly not... but Afrin asserts that long-standing dermatographism is not normal.[14]

Skin Evaluation

- There are a number of dermatological characteristics noted in patients with MCAD, and the trunk, extremities, head, and neck should all be examined. Dermatological findings may include cherry angiomas, varicose veins, eczema, flushing or redness in areas, itching, sores/lesions, hair loss, swelling or angioedema, decreased skin sensation, and other rashes. Some patients with MCAS have rashes on the groin and chest that they may fail to mention or expose, so it's important to examine or at least verbally assess these areas as well.

- Chronic urticaria, a skin rash with red, raised, and typically itchy bumps, is one of the most common skin findings with MCAS. Keep in mind, "urticaria" alone is not the same thing as "urticaria pigmentosa." Urticaria pigmentosa (UP) consists of brownish lesions on the skin, typically with overpigmented or dark lesions. True UP reflects an increased number of mast cells present in the skin.

- One reason to perform the skin examination is to determine if the patient has areas of urticaria pigmentosa that were not mentioned in the patient interview. According to a 2016 paper by researchers Austen and Akin, "Approximately 80% of patients with mastocytosis present with cutaneous involvement, most commonly urticaria pigmentosa. Therefore, a careful skin exam is necessary in all patients with suspected mast cell activation disorders. Urticaria pigmentosa is not found in patients with monoclonal mast cell activation syndrome or non-clonal mast cell activation disorders."[15]

- Urticaria pigmentosa can certainly move a clinician to order biopsies and have a higher suspicion of Primary MCAD, but the more commonly encountered dermatological findings will be typically be less pronounced than urticaria pigmentosa in the patient with MCAS.

Organ Palpation

- Reports of an enlarged liver or spleen typically precede abnormal enzyme levels in blood work.[9] Hepatosplenomegaly (liver and spleen enlargement) is common enough in this patient population that it's important to take the time to palpate the abdominal cavity on initial examination. Likewise, lymphadenopathy (abnormal size, number or consistency of lymph nodes) can be present in the lymph tissue in the head and neck as well as other areas of the body with MCAD. It's important to document all palpation findings.

Other Clinical Tests

- The above three tests (Darrier's sign, skin evaluation and organ palpation) were recommended by the authors in the article by Molderings and colleagues.[2]

- *From a physical therapist perspective, this is the part of the process where I would also consider adding a few additional simple clinical tests.* Many patients with MCAD have Ehlers-Danlos syndrome (EDS) and postural orthostatic tachycardia syndrome (POTS) as comorbidities. (More information on these conditions is located in Chapter 7.) If a patient history included signs of either of these conditions, I would also add in testing for the hypermobility type of EDS and tilt table testing for POTS, time permitting.

- While these tests for EDS and POTS do not assist in making the diagnosis of MCAD, they can provide additional valuable information that is especially pertinent to a patient's plan of care. These tests are relatively quick to do in clinic and don't necessarily require additional laboratory testing, though some patients may need referrals for genetic testing or blood work. The diagnosis of either of these conditions does not signify that the patient has a higher likelihood of having MCAS, though the three conditions do appear to have some associations in the literature (further explained in Chapter 7).

- Addressing these other conditions may be a crucial aspect of care that could impact the management of MCAS, and vice versa. Note that these italicized "other" suggestions are mine and are not reflected in the literature. Since physical therapists are generally unable to order lab work or biopsies, a more in-depth physical exam provides useful information for the future referral source who will carry on the diagnostic evaluation from this point forward.

Step 3: Initial Testing: Rule Out Systemic Mastocytosis and Cutaneous Mastocytosis, if Applicable

According to the recommendations by Molderings and colleagues,[2] Step 3 may be omitted for many patients, depending on their history, physical examination, and tryptase levels. They recommend that patients with *urticaria pigmentosa* undergo a skin biopsy for evaluation of cutaneous mastocytosis. They also recommend that patients who have a *persistent tryptase level of greater than 20 ng/ml* have a tissue biopsy (bone marrow and/or other) to rule out systemic mastocytosis.

The gold standard for MCAD diagnostic clarity is to look at mast cells from a bone marrow or other tissue sample. Bone marrow biopsies have been the classic test for looking more closely at genetic factors and mast cell characteristics, but in recent years other types of tissue samples are also being analyzed with mast cells-specific testing. For patients who present with gastrointestinal distress, samples from an endoscopy and/or colonoscopy can be useful. Most laboratories store tissue biopsies from prior procedures for many years, so it may be possible to order the appropriate tests on old biopsy samples, thus reducing the cost of a new diagnostic procedure for the patient and eliminating the risks associated with a bone marrow biopsy.

However, if the patient's baseline tryptase is above 20 ng/ml, many doctors would rather do a bone marrow biopsy to have the likelihood of gaining the most information about the mast cells, since they originate in the bone marrow. Keep in mind that due to the typically patchy distribution of mast cells in bone marrow, false negatives and repeated testing are common.

Even though the concentration of mast cells in bone marrow is typically higher than that of peripheral blood or other tissue samples, bone marrow biopsies are sort of like shooting in the dark. The needle removes tissue from one small area and the hope is that the randomly selected spot reveals clusters of mast cells for analysis. Many specialists perform bilateral biopsies at one time in order to increase the likelihood of capturing groupings of mast cells, which tend to be patchily distributed.[16]

A wide variety of average numbers of bone marrow biopsies have been performed to diagnose patients with systemic mastocytosis (SM). A 2013 study evaluated 50 patients with SM who had a history of anywhere from two to 14 bone marrow biopsies, with a group median of four.[17] The bone marrow biopsy is generally considered useful for the diagnosis of SM but does not appear to be useful for monitoring progress or symptomatic response in patients with SM, so it's mainly performed as a diagnostic test.[17]

There's some confusion about why the tryptase level is set at 20 ng/ml and what different test results signify. A 2017 review clarified interpretation of the cutoff: "It needs to be stressed that a normal serum tryptase level does not exclude MCAS. Furthermore, levels above 20 ng/ml do not exclude MCAS, and levels below 20 ng/ml do not exclude SM. Persistence of

196

the serum tryptase level above 20 ng/ml makes SM more likely, necessitating marrow examination to exclude mastocytosis. Even if the serum tryptase level is persistently below 20 ng/ml, consideration of SM may need to be made if the patient's history of illness is more consistent with SM (i.e., sudden onset of symptoms in middle or older age in contrast to MCAS's usual history of symptoms dating back to adolescence or childhood)."[18]

Afrin factors in the tryptase level with other clinical features. He notes that most of the patients who have underlying mastocytosis will have evidence of being perfectly fine and healthy until a sudden abrupt onset of symptoms in middle or older age. Thus, the patient history can also give clues to whether a bone marrow biopsy may be warranted. It appears that, in general, patients with mast cell disease who have had chronic underlying symptoms since infancy or youth tend to be diagnosed with MCAS and not mastocytosis.[19]

To Biopsy or Not to Biopsy?

"To biopsy or not to biopsy" appears to be an area of discrepancy among clinicians/researchers. Experts recommend that patients be further classified correctly with MCAS, monoclonal MCAS, or mastocytosis once clinical suspicion of MCAD has been determined, and biopsy testing can help rule in/out clonal (Primary) disease.

Special scenarios may warrant that mast cell-specific testing is ordered on biopsied tissue samples, even when urine or serum mediator testing has not been performed. The analysis of non-bone marrow tissue biopsies may be useful for patients who live in rural areas and don't have access to a lab equipped to perform the chemical mediator testing with accuracy or under the appropriate temperature and time guidelines.

Most experts agree that the presence of a tryptase level of 20 mg/nl or greater mandates a bone marrow biopsy to rule out mastocytosis. According to a 2015 summary paper by Soderberg, "A baseline tryptase level of >20 ng/ml or those who have syncopal/ hypotensive episodes (regardless of tryptase levels) should have bone marrow biopsies. If a patient presents with urticaria or angioedema, bone marrow biopsy probably would not be a consideration (urticaria and angioedema are rarely seen with … mastocytosis)."[20]

When it comes to ordering the bone marrow biopsy, it appears that the majority of doctors are on the more conservative side and will only consider a bone marrow biopsy if baseline tryptase levels test high, or if certain symptoms are present that are more consistent with clonal disease. Each leading group has published different opinions on what criteria should rationalize a bone marrow biopsy.

Bone marrow biopsy decision-making recommendations in the literature:

- Picard and colleagues[3] recommended that a bone marrow biopsy be considered in cases of:
  - baseline tryptase levels of 20 ng/ml, or
  - unexplained anaphylaxis, or
  - the presence of urticaria pigmentosa in adults, or
  - abnormalities in complete blood count testing (cytopenias, thrombocytosis, or leukocytosis) for patients with existing MCAD, or
  - the presence of unexplained osteoporosis, hepatomegaly, or splenomegaly in patients with existing MCAD
- Austen and Akin[15] recommended the following criteria for a bone marrow biopsy:
  - tryptase of 20 ng/ml, or
  - patients who have a history of Hymenoptera venom reactions and tryptase >12 ng/ml and hypotensive syncope (low blood pressure-associated fainting) or presyncope (near-fainting) without the presence of urticaria (skin rash) and angioedema (swelling)
- Soderberg and colleagues[20] recommended the following criteria should affirm the bone marrow biopsy decision:
  - a baseline tryptase level of 20 ng/ml, or
  - patients who has syncopal (fainting)/hypotensive (low blood pressure) episodes (regardless of tryptase levels)
- Theoharides and colleagues[13] recommended a bone marrow biopsy if the patient has mildly elevated tryptase levels plus the presence of:
  - osteoporosis (particularly in males)
  - unexplained episodes of syncopal hypotension
  - splenomegaly
  - lymphadenopathy
  - blood count abnormalities
- And, as already shared, the 2011 article by Molderings et al.[2] presented in this chapter recommended a bone marrow or tissue biopsy in the presence of:
  - urticaria pigmentosa consistent with mastocytosis, or
  - persistently elevated tryptase levels above 20 ng/ml

What basis guides clinicians toward these particular factors? A 2010 study evaluated characteristics in patients that may help predict the presence of clonal MCAD prior to bone marrow biopsy testing.[21] Specifically, based on an 83-patient sample size, they determined that male sex, baseline serum tryptase levels greater than 25 ug/nl, the presence of syncopal or presyncopal episodes, and the absence of urticaria and angioedema were statistically significant factors that best predicted the presence of underlying clonality.[21]

Many experts agree that patients would probably not be considered for a bone marrow biopsy if they have regular urticaria or angioedema, since these characteristics are very rarely encountered with mastocytosis.[20] Angioedema is defined as swelling in the lower layers of the skin, often presenting in the face, hands, feet, groin, and abdomen, though it can occur anywhere.

Why do researchers frequently mention syncope/presyncope and hypotension as more consistent with clonal disease/SM and angioedema and urticaria as symptoms more consistent with MCAS? One theory is that the presence of the c-*KIT* mutation at codon 816 is the key to the clinical manifestations and differences between MCAS and monoclonal disease.

In 2016, Austen and Akin noted that activation of *KIT* reduces the activation threshold of mast cells (to both IgE- and non-IgE triggers), which influences the rate of anaphylaxis and dictates the typical characteristics of symptoms.[15] According to the researchers, clonal mast cell disease appears to be accompanied by the cardiovascular manifestations of anaphylaxis including hypotension, tachycardia, presyncope, and syncope—all hallmarks of an "expanded pool" of mast cells.[15]

In contrast, the non-clonal MCAS cases tend to involve an allergen binding to IgE as a mechanism that induces angioedema, urticaria, and difficulty breathing.[15] Based on these characteristics, a clinician may be more likely to pick out patients who have clonal vs. non-clonal disease in order to make the bone marrow biopsy decision, although it appears to be an imperfect art. *Anecdotally*, many patients with non-clonal disease on testing report experiencing cardiovascular manifestations during anaphylaxis.

In a 2017 review, experts noted that while it's important to rule out SM, there's not a significant benefit to ordering a tissue biopsy with the sole purpose of distinguishing what could be monoclonal cases of MCAS from MCAS.[18] "When MCAS seems more likely than SM, marrow examination is usually *unhelpful.* Even if MMCAS is found on flow cytometric or mutational testing, at present there are no known differences in prognosis of, or the therapeutic approach toward, MMCAS versus MCAS."[18]

Thus, it appears that the main priority for tissue biopsy should be to rule out SM, and it may occasionally be used to help confirm MCAS or MMCAS. Tissue samples from prior procedures (like a past colonoscopy/endoscopy) that were already done (even up to several years ago) offer lower risk of side effects/complications when compared to scheduling a new bone marrow biopsy and may be preferred when the main purpose is to confirm MCAS.

Technically, MCAS can be diagnosed with negative urine and blood work when in the presence of abnormalities on tissue biopsies. The 2017 review by Seneviratne noted that "If mediator testing is unrevealing, the Molderings diagnostic criteria[2] provide an alternative path to diagnosis of MCAS, namely, finding increased mast cells (MCs) in extracutaneous tissue, most commonly gastrointestinal (GI) or genitourinary (GU) tract mucosal biopsies."[18]

What to Look for in Tissue Biopsies

Regardless of which type of tissue biopsy is performed or used, tests are typically ordered to determine whether any of the following signs of mastocytosis are present:

- Multifocal disseminated or dense infiltrates of mast cells (bone marrow biopsy or extracutaneous organ) as determined by staining for CD25, CD117, and tryptase
- >15 dense mast cells in aggregates is considered diagnostic for mastocytosis*
- Bone marrow smears or histologies show more than 25% abnormal morphologies (bone marrow or extracutaneous organ)
- Mast cells express CD2 and/or CD25 (bone marrow)
- Detection of genetic changes in any mast cell tissue sample, including c-*KIT* mutation in tyrosine kinase at codon 816

*some sources cite 20 mast cells per high powered field[18]

Austen and Akin describe the specifics that tissue biopsy testing should encompass: "The bone marrow biopsy should be stained immunohistochemically for tryptase to visualize mast cells. CD25 staining should be employed by immunohistochemistry or flow cytometry to look for aberrant expression of this molecule, which is a very sensitive marker of clonal mast cell disease. Mast cell morphology should be examined carefully for aberrations in morphology including spindle shapes, hypogranulation, eccentric, or multilobated nuclei which favor clonal disease. A c-*KIT* mutational analysis for D816V mutation should be performed."[15]

At a glance, it's difficult to find clear instructional details for tissue analysis specifics. Laboratories do not routinely order these tests, and it's important that the referring doctor communicate well with the laboratory in order to ensure that the bone marrow or tissue biopsy sample testing is adequately performed. It may be useful to highlight the following section from the 2014 article by Afrin and Molderings[6] to confirm that everyone is one the same page.

Afrin and Molderings recommend the following to be ordered when marrow examination is felt warranted: "Bilateral marrow aspiration/biopsy including mast cell-specific immunohistochemical staining (e.g., CD 117, tryptase, toluidine blue, Giemsa, Alcian blue), multicolor flow cytometry for co-expression of CD117/CD25, CD1117/CD2, and molecular testing for *KIT* mutations as available (PCR for *KIT* D816V at a minimum)."[6]

Real-time quantitative PCR testing for *KIT* D816V appears to be more sensitive than routine PCR testing for the *KIT* mutation in tissue biopsies.[22] A review paper in 2015 mentions an additional blood test looking for the *KIT* mutation.[13] According to Theoharides et al., "For patients with unclear symptoms that are not attributable to another disease entity or for patients with slightly elevated serum tryptase levels, screening with highly sensitive polymerase-chain-reaction (PCR) techniques for *KIT* D816V transcripts in peripheral-blood leukocytes has been introduced to the diagnostic algorithm for suspected mastocytosis."[13] The authors state that if the *KIT* mutation is detected in peripheral blood, the bone marrow evaluation (Step 3) is then indicated.[13]

In addition to the above suggestions, experts also recommend considering chymase and CD 30 testing with bone marrow biopsies. "Antibodies against *KIT* (i.e., CD 117), CD 25, tryptase and chymase should be used. Flow-cytometric assessment of co-expression of CD117 together with CD25 and/or CD2, CD 30, and mutational assessment for mutations in *KIT* (in particular, the *KIT* D816V mutation at a minimum) should be done."[18]

A 2017 review noted that on *bone marrow* biopsies, "*KIT* codon 816 mutations and CD117 co-expression with CD25 and/or CD2 in flow cytometry testing are both rare in patients with MCAS."[18] Seneviratne and colleagues report that, based off genetic research, "although one or more mutations are found in almost every MCAS patient, codon 816 mutations (whether D816V or any other) are virtually never found in MCAS."[18]

According to an article on MCAS and bladder pain by Ratner (2015), CD117 staining is the most accurate for viewing mast cells from *bladder/urinary system biopsies*.[23] Additional authors concur that CD 117 testing is more reliable for *gastrointestinal, genitourinary tract, and skin* tissue samples.[18]

Granule-targeting stains are at higher risk of false-negative tests since mast cell contents are more likely to be recently released in patients with MCAD. Examples of granule-targeting stains include toluidine blue, Alcian blue, Giemsa, and tryptase stains. "Granule-targeting stains may miss mast cells that have recently degranulated their contents and result in false negative testing, so CD117 should be considered the standard."[18] CD117 appears to be superior to granule-targeting stains regardless of tissue biopsy type.

Patients with MCAS typically have normal dispersion of mast cells on biopsy, while abnormal aggregates are more indicative of SM. A normal round to ovoid mast cell shape is common in patients with MCAS, whereas abnormalities such as "spindled" shapes are more typical in patients with SM.[18] A good working relationship and ample communication between physician and laboratory technicians are essential for these special tests.

Step 4: Initial Testing: Baseline Laboratory Testing

Magnesium levels, a comprehensive metabolic panel (CMP), and a complete blood count (CBC) with platelet differential are recommended to be ordered at this point in time.[6] Patients who experience delayed healing or frequent infections may also have a Quantitative Immunoglobulin Profile tested.[6] If the patient has a history of clotting events or easy bruising or bleeding, a prothrombin time (PT) or partial thromboplastin time (PTT) may be ordered.[6]

Step 5: Additional Testing: Mast Cell Mediators

The mast cell mediator tests are not likely to be run by local labs and are usually sent out to reference labs. In the United States, certain companies such as LabCorp, Mayo, Quest, ARUP, and Interscience Institute tend to offer MCAD-specific tests. According to Afrin, there's no clear benefit for pursuing testing at any given lab—they all appear to be similar in the quality of the testing they perform.[24]

Baseline mediator levels should be tested to include the following:

- Plasma *tryptase* (baseline measurement while not in a flare; some doctors also order subsequent "stat tryptase" for patients to obtain while flared/within 4 hours of an anaphylactic episode)

- 24-hour urine metabolites: *N-methylhistamine, prostaglandin D2 or F2a.* (These tests MUST be kept cold continuously by the patient and lab for accurate results! It's <u>very</u> important to educate everyone who handles the sample, as even short periods without refrigeration can cause false-negative results. Transport to a lab in another state requires that the sample be frozen.)

- *Heparin* in blood

- *Chromogranin A* in blood

- Other mast cell-specific mediators (i.e., *leukotrienes* in blood or urine)

- Some authors have also suggested testing for histamine in the blood and serum prostaglandin isoform levels, in addition to the urine tests listed above.

- Some experts will also check whether mast cell activity-related eosinophilia, basophilia, or monocytosis in the blood can be observed.[2]

Some tests are more time-sensitive than others. Serum (blood) tryptase is typically measured both at baseline and also within 4 hours of an acute reaction. Tryptase has a short half-life and its levels return to baseline fairly quickly, so it's difficult to catch an elevated level following an acute episode, particularly if episodes occur "after hours" or on weekends when the lab is not open. Emergency room doctors are not always willing to test tryptase levels, even with the lab orders in hand. Tryptase levels appear to peak 15-60 minutes after the onset of symptoms, declining with a half-life of about 2 hours.[5] The length of time that tryptase is elevated depends on the magnitude of anaphylaxis.[5]

The baseline tryptase level provides a good indicator of suspicion for mastocytosis based on overall burden, since in theory an elevated number of mast cells would likely equate to a larger resting proportion of tryptase circulating in the blood. However, this is not always the case and it certainly is not the only diagnostic criteria to factor into the picture. In addition to MCAD, chronic renal failure, myeloproliferative or dysplastic neoplasms, and chronic eosinophilic leukemia can all present with elevated baseline tryptase levels.[15]

Based on the 2012 suggested diagnostic criteria by Valent and colleagues, measurement of acute serum total tryptase level at 20% plus 2 ng/ml over baseline level is considered diagnostic for MCAS.[5] Thus, the calculation is as follows:

Baseline level (0.2) + Baseline Level + 2 ng/ml = Cutoff for MCAS criterion (as part of "Criteria X") via tryptase level during a symptomatic episode

The baseline level needs to be measured at least 24 hours outside of an acute anaphylactic type episode for this formula to be valid. For the example of someone who has a baseline tryptase level of 6 ng/ml, the math equation would look like this:

$$6 \times (0.2) + 6 + 2 = 1.2 + 6 + 2 = 9.2 \text{ ng/ml}$$

Thus, for this patient, if following "Criteria X" for diagnosis, a symptomatic level sufficient to qualify for the tryptase diagnostic criterion of MCAS would need to be 9.2 ng/ml or higher during an acute episode, when compared to a 6 ng/ml baseline level. (Of course, if this is negative there are many other chemical mediators that can confirm MCAS as well.)

One huge drawback in this area is that clearly defined cutoffs for other mast cell mediator levels are not published in regards to MCAS in particular, and most physicians use the widely published clinical norm values as their cutoff for determining a positive test.

Table 2. Common Chemical Mediators Tested in Patients with Suspected MCAD

MAST CELL MEDIATOR	INTERPRETATION OF VALUE	CLINICAL NOTES	REFERENCE FOR LAB VALUES (2018)
24-hour Urine N-methylhistamine (NMHIN)	Normal: Age 0-5: 120-510 mcg/g creatinine Age 6-16: 70-330 mcg/g creatinine Age >16: 30-200 mcg/g creatinine	High levels common with MCAD; Keep sample chilled continuously; Diet can influence histamine level by ~30%; DAO supplementation and anti-histamine medications can affect this test result	Mayo Clinic
24-hour Urine Prostaglandin D2 (PGD2)	Normal: 100-280 ng	High levels common with MCAD; Keep sample chilled continuously; Aspirin and other NSAIDs can affect this test result; Urine more accurate than blood test	Mayo Clinic/ Inter Science Institute

24-hour Urine Prostaglandin 9a,11b-F2 (PGF2a)	Normal: 375-800 ng	High levels common with MCAD; PGF2a is (more stable) metabolite of PGD2 (PGF2a believed to be superior for MCAS detection); Keep sample chilled continuously; Aspirin and other NSAIDs can affect this test result; Urine more accurate than blood test	Inter Science Institute*
Tryptase (serum)	Median normal values: Age <6 months: 6 ng/ml Children & Adults: 3-4 ng/ml High >11.5 ng/ml (or may use formula comparing to baseline level for cutoff)**	High levels sometimes encountered with MCAD; Baseline testing at least 24 hours after acute episode; Acute measurement within 15 minutes to 4 hours of episode; Criterion for consideration of SM: >20 ng/ml	Mayo Clinic
24-hour Urine Leukotriene E4 (LTE4)***	Normal: < or = to 104 pg/mg creatinine	High levels common with MCAD; Keep sample chilled continuously; Zileuton/Zyflo medication May affect this test result; Urine Leukotriene B4, C4, and D4 may also be ordered	Mayo Clinic
Stat chilled Plasma Heparin (PH) via Chromogenic Anti-Factor	Upper reference value: 0.02 to 0.05 anti-Xa IU/ml, depending on lab	High levels common with MCAD; Specific/sensitive mast cell marker but metabolizes quickly even when refrigerated so has to	Vysniauskaite et al, 2015

Assay "Anti-XA Assay"			be centrifuged within 30 minutes and must be kept cold	
Serum Chromogranin A	Normal: < 93 ng/ml (all ages)	High levels common with MCAD; High levels may also indicate heart conditions, kidney problems, or neuroendocrine tumors; Proton pump inhibitors (PPIs) can affect this test result	Mayo Clinic

*The Inter Science Institute norm for *serum* PGD2 is 35-115 pg/ml and for *serum* PGF2a is 80-240 pg/ml.[20]

**Baseline level (0.2) + Baseline Level + 2 ng/ml = Cutoff for MCAS criterion via tryptase level during a symptomatic episode

***Leukotrienes B4, C4, D4, and E4 may be tested[6]

Plasma heparin and chromogranin A testing are becoming more widely tested as part of MCAS diagnosis. Afrin elaborates on the rationale behind the Anti-XA Assay testing for heparin. "Plasma heparin testing yields readings in terms of anti-Factor-Xa activity, and although such testing is more commonly pursued to determine the efficacy of low molecular weight heparin therapy, the same test as applied in individuals not on heparin therapy reveals endogenous levels of heparin, which seems to be a sensitive and specific indicator of MC (mast cell) activation because it is known to be produced in humans only by MCs and indeed was the first MC mediator to be discovered nearly 80 years ago."[25]

Heparin shows promising results in terms of its utility as a mast cell mediator to help identify patients with MCAS. A 2015 study evaluated the sensitivities of different mast cell mediators in a large group (257 patients) with MCAD.[26] In MCAS patients, tryptase, chromogranin A, and N-methylhistamine levels had poor sensitivities (10%, 12% and 22% respectively) compared to higher sensitivities in systemic mastocytosis patients (73%, 63%, and 43%, respectively).[26] (Higher sensitivities indicate the tests has greater ability to rule out diagnoses when the test is negative.)

However, basal plasma heparin levels had a sensitivity of 41% for MCAS patients and 27% for systemic mastocytosis patients.[26] When the heparin test was performed after a test modification that obstructed venous flow locally for 10 minutes (to stimulate mast cell degranulation), plasma heparin sensitivities increased to 59% in MCAS patients and 47% in systemic mastocytosis.[26] The authors concluded that plasma heparin may be more accurate at detecting MCAS than other mediators.[26]

While heparin could *theoretically* be the best diagnostic marker for mast cell activity,[26] plasma heparin tests were originally designed to monitor patients who were receiving heparin therapy so the test is designed to detect the upper limits in the body. Thus, one consideration to keep in mind is that the level of heparin that is found normally (as well as in most cases of MCAS) may not be detectable by standard clinical options that are currently available.[26] In addition, heparin has a short half-life and needs to be chilled and measured immediately. The addition of the modified testing parameter (10-minute blood flow obstruction prior to blood draw) described in the work by Vysniauskaite and colleagues may be a useful consideration to enhance the sensitivity of the serum heparin test.[26]

A 2017 study of 413 patients with the diagnosis of MCAS that met the published diagnostic criteria for at least two elevated mediator level tests (and/or abnormal biopsy tissue tests) had laboratory tests evaluated for all mast cell mediators. The study found that of the patients with *confirmed MCAS diagnoses*, only 15% of tests showed elevated tryptase and 10% of tests had elevated urinary N-methylhistamine levels. *Plasma* histamine, however, was positive in 41% of tests. The best performer, serum chromogranin A, was positive in the most cases, at 48% of tests—still less than half of all patients. (Chromogranin A can be confounded by other variables such as neuroendocrine cancers, the use of certain medications, and kidney or heart failure.) Plasma heparin was the second-best indicator and was positive in 45% of tests. Urinary prostaglandin D2 levels and plasma prostaglandin D2 levels were positive in 41% and 40% of tests, respectively. This study reflects that there is no sole laboratory test that is overwhelmingly accurate for diagnosis in patients with signs and symptoms of MCAS.[27]

Laboratory Instruction Considerations

According to the recommendations by the Mayo Clinic laboratory, all 24-hour urine samples must be continuously chilled or the test may be inaccurate. This is true for urinary prostaglandins, N-methylhistamine, and leukotrienes. Afrin clarifies, "… This means that patients should keep their urine collection bin refrigerated overnight *before* they begin to collect the sample. They should leave it in the fridge at all times, except for when adding urine to it.

They should transport it to the lab on ice and make sure that it is immediately put into a fridge or freezer where they drop it off."[28]

Indeed, meticulous care is advised when patients are conducting mast cell mediator urine tests. Just a few minutes of room-temperature air can alter the test results. Afrin also notes, "Many patients leave the urine aliquots to cool in the refrigerator in a small container for a while before then adding them to the main container, so that the urine being accumulated in the main container is not subject to repeated warmings by the addition of fresh urine."[29]

The laboratory needs to freeze the sample and pack it with ice when they send it off to a specialty lab to complete the testing. (This is almost always the case, because very few labs in the United States do this testing, so chances are they will be sending it elsewhere.) It's not a bad idea to take a permanent marker and write "MUST be chilled continuously" or "keep refrigerated and frozen for transport—please" on the collection bin, just to make sure that nobody in the chain of handling forgets this information. It's also important to have a polite conversation with laboratory staff where the sample is dropped off.

As already mentioned, in terms of the blood (serum) testing, the plasma heparin test is a tricky one. Even if it's chilled, the test needs to be performed right away (within 30 minutes of the blood draw), which is not always possible, depending on the laboratory. Tryptase is more stable than the other chemical mediators, but if it's going to sit around for longer than two days, it may be important to keep it chilled. Tryptase can be refrigerated for up to five days after collection, but if the analysis will happen after a longer period than five days, it ought to be frozen.[30] Keeping the samples chilled won't hurt anything, so sometimes doctors will request that all samples are continuously chilled for continuity's sake to make instructions easier on lab technicians.

Medication Considerations for Laboratory Testing

In the chemical mediator chart (Table 2), certain medications are listed to interact with the laboratory testing for certain chemical mediators. For example, aspirin and nonsteroidal anti-inflammatory drugs (NSAIDs) such as ibuprofen or naproxen may interfere with accurate measurements of prostaglandin levels. Afrin notes that "this applies regardless of the fashion in which the NSAID is taken (for example, orally or as a skin cream)."[28] Supplements that have NSAID-like activity (I.e., inhibition of the cyclooxygenase-1 and/or cyclooxygenase-2 enzymes) should also be avoided in the five days prior to testing.[29]

Proton pump inhibitors impact serum levels of chromogranin A and should be omitted at least five days prior to testing, if possible.[18] Zileuton and Zyflo may impact Leukotrienes. DAO supplementation and antihistamines may alter the measured levels of histamine in the blood or urine.

Antihistamines do not always need to be stopped prior to testing (and in some cases this can trigger life-threatening emergencies, so extreme caution may be warranted). *Anecdotally,* some patients with MCAS may still have positive mediator test results, regardless of whether they discontinue antihistamine medications. This decision should be a case-by-base consideration with one's medical team.

This is where the testing recommendations may become individualized. Some patients are already on a number of medications prior to an MCAS diagnosis in order to stay stable and avoid anaphylaxis. Each patient needs to have a conversation with their doctor about whether or not it's appropriate to alter all of their medications (or certain medications) during the week prior to MCAS testing. *In some cases, it may be too dangerous to remove the medications prior to testing.* In other cases, mild side effects of medication removal may be permitted and justifiable.

Considerations for Testing Following Food-Mediated Anaphylaxis

When patients are having chemical mediator levels tested for the possibility of MCAS, there's some debate about whether the "flare" or "symptomatic" testing should be conducted following food-mediated allergic reactions. The general consensus appears to be that it's valid to measure tryptase within two to four hours of an acute food-induced allergic reaction in patients who are looking to determine their *reactive* non-baseline tryptase level.

Researchers Lin and colleagues evaluated tryptase levels in the emergency room setting with patients presenting with anaphylaxis concerns. They found that the mean tryptase level was higher in patients with a history of prior food reactions who had consumed tree nuts, shellfish, and peanuts (mean of 11.7 ng/ml) compared to other foods.[31] Of course, one major limitation to this study was that they did not provide baseline non-reactive tryptase levels to compare to the emergency room value.

Another study evaluated histamine and tryptase levels following food challenges in children and found that the mean plasma tryptase level was significantly increased at 240 minutes following the food challenge in patients who had immediate reactions.[32] However, plasma tryptase levels were not increased in patients who had non-immediate reactions.[32] The authors concluded that "the elevation of plasma histamine and tryptase in patients with immediate reactions following food challenge indicates mast cell activation."[32]

A 2018 study evaluated patients with peanut allergy and determined that food allergic reactions were associated with a 30% increase in tryptase levels.[33] They noted that the peak reactions tended to occur closer to the two-hour mark following the food allergen ingestion.[33] They concluded that serum tryptase correlates with symptom severity and is a valuable marker in food allergic reactions.[33]

The Diagnostic "Gray Area"

Is one positive chemical mediator enough for diagnosis? Technically, according to "Criteria Y", patients can be diagnosed with MCAS based off one positive chemical mediator test.[2] However, "Criteria X" does specify that two separate mediator measurements are required for diagnosis,[5] and most physician experts (including the authors of "Criteria Y") will state that they prefer to have evidence of two different chemical mediator abnormalities, or two abnormal tests for the same chemical mediator at different times, or a combination of chemical mediator and tissue biopsy abnormalities, in order to confidently diagnose someone with MCAS.

On the other hand, there are physicians out there who will find overwhelming evidence of MCAS on every aspect *except* for laboratory/biopsy testing and may then give the patient the diagnosis of MCAS if they cannot find any other diagnostic possibility. This is referred to as a "clinical diagnosis" as opposed to a "medical diagnosis." I am not saying that this is correct, but it has been known to happen. This remains a controversial topic among the MCAS patient community.

A clinical diagnosis (as opposed to medical diagnosis) doesn't appear to be very common and sometimes depends on the patient scenario. Some patients may need multiple rounds of mediator testing to test positive, but in the meantime, they may be in danger of severe complications and anaphylaxis if they continue to go untreated. Furthermore, a response to mast cell-targeting medications is part of the evaluation, and withholding treatments that could improve a patient's quality of life and stability is not recommended. It's important to make the distinction between going *untreated* or *unassisted* vs. going *undiagnosed*.

Since there is no universal World Health Organization Classification for MCAS, and two different published recommendations currently exist for MCAS diagnosis, this leaves a bit of gray area. Molderings and colleagues comment on this gray area in their 2011 clinical algorithm paper.[2] Commercial testing for chemical mediators is limited, as is the adherence of all parties in the chain of handling of lab specimens. Chemical mediators fluctuate within subjects' bodies and throughout the course of the day, and it's difficult to guess which mediators may be responsible for the typical complexity of symptoms. This is where tissue biopsy samples may be the gateway to more clinical certainty with patients who repeatedly test negative for MCAS chemical mediators in the blood and urine.

Critics question doctors who give out MCAS diagnoses without "laboratory and/or biopsy" evidence, and this remains a very controversial topic. The diagnosis of MCAS can carry heavy lifestyle change implications, but it can also bring a great deal of emotional relief and closure to a patient who has been suffering with mysterious symptoms of MCAS for decades. The diagnosis can also lead to a treatment plan that over time may dramatically alter the patient's quality of life. The diagnosis can change the life of someone who is homebound, unable to work, and struggling to meet the criteria for disability or other types of assistance. It's obvious that labeling someone with MCAS without clinical evidence can be empowering in some ways but can also present as an ethical and moral dilemma.

The experts assert that the diagnosis should be based off *at least* one positive test for the simple reason: What if something is missing? What if the signs of mast cell activation are simply a secondary reaction to cancer or another condition that is going unnoticed in the body? Getting to the root cause must be the priority, as painful as it can be to endure a lengthy, repeated testing process.

This is not to say, however, that patients who have clear signs of mast cell activation issues without a "legitimate diagnosis" should be ignored or untreated. This is mainly a debate about labeling someone with a "diagnosis." All patients should be taken seriously and should be offered assistance with what they are experiencing, regardless of what their ICD-10 codes say (or don't say). Unfortunately, this is not always the way that the medical system works, and once a physician cannot find a clear-cut explanation for symptoms, they may simply shrug their shoulders, say "I don't know what's wrong with you" and abandon the patient.

Instead, the hope is that more and more professionals will say, "We haven't ruled MCAS out yet, but we may need to do another round or two of testing and also look into other possibilities." Patients with clear suspicion of MCAS who have been tested once (with negative results) should not lose hope. In the event that the provider is unwilling to retest, patients should be encouraged to keep searching for someone who "gets it" and is willing to continue investigating. Unfortunately, the reality is that in the American medical system most patients at some point or another have to engage in "battle mode" techniques to self-advocate for access to testing and treatment.

For practitioners who are not licensed to order such tests (such as physical therapists, occupational therapists, etc.), it's important to take the time to establish connections with a local specialist. In many communities, it's hard to find a doctor who is knowledgeable in this condition. Seeking out a local allergist in the area may be a good a starting point, as most are familiar with mastocytosis. Hematologists are another option to network with for this patient subgroup. There are also many professionals in the field of functional medicine and naturopathy who are well-versed in the clinical presentation of MCAD. For a medical professional who is unable to order the laboratory tests directly, the initial process of getting connected with a reputable outside referral source may be arduous, but it is certainly something worth fighting for.

If the above mast cell mediator tests are normal, factor VIII, plasma free norepinephrine, epinephrine, dopamine, tumor necrosis factor alpha, and interleukin-6 are other mediators that are sometimes tested when looking at the possibility of MCAS, but the overall value of these (relatively non-mast-cell-specific) mediators for diagnosing MCAS is questionable.[6,26,29] High norepinephrine and low-normal or low epinephrine may be seen in patients with MCAS.[6]

It's important to educate the patient on the importance of patience in this process. Another take-home message is the importance of educating the laboratory technicians on the necessary parameters for *time and temperature* in the case of certain urine/blood samples.

Step 6: Additional Diagnostic Evaluation, if Appropriate

Molderings and colleagues[2] recommend the following tests be considered when investigating the possibility of MCAD:

- Gastroscopy, coloscopy with biopsy
- Sonography of the internal organs
- Echocardiogram, 24-hour ECG, stress test
- DXA Bone density measurement

These tests can be useful for a number of reasons. In some cases, they can serve as further evidence for mast cell-mediated systemic issues, in the case that the patient has unusual osteoporosis or osteopenia given their age, or in the case that they have enlargement of their internal organs. As already mentioned, tissue samples from gastrointestinal scopes can also give more concrete information about mast cells, and if they haven't been performed in the past and the patient has severe GI issues, they may be ordered at this time. Cardiovascular and organ imaging tests may also assist in determining potential comorbidities commonly associated with MCAS and are useful for differential diagnosis and ruling out other causes of symptoms.

In the absence of the presentations that warrant a bone marrow biopsy, Picard and colleagues[3] also recommend evaluating for secondary MCAS factors, including:

1.   allergens that could cause IgE-mediated mast cell activation (such as insect stings, foods, latex, and drugs)

2.   a thorough assessment of medications to eliminate drugs as potential triggers for mast cell activation

3.   other underlying potential causes of mast cell hyperplasia

Step 7: Classification of Type of MCAD

After following a thorough differential diagnosis reasoning process, according to the MCAS suggested diagnostic criteria ("Criteria X" and "Criteria "Y"),[2,5] clinical symptoms without other explanation that respond to mast cell mediator targeted treatment with evidence of at least one elevated laboratory marker are considered diagnostic. (Again, recent literature affirms that most clinicians follow requirements for positive test results of two separate mediators, one mediator and biopsy confirmation, or the same mediator (collected twice), conducted across two different points in time, for the diagnosis of MCAS.[18])

If it has been determined that the patient does indeed have evidence for MCAD, the next step would be to delineate whether the patient has mastocytosis or MCAS (or the very rare possibility of mast cell leukemia or other neoplastic conditions), and to also tease out whether the MCAS is primary, secondary or idiopathic in nature. (See diagnostic criteria in Chapter 3 to assist with interpreting test results and the criteria necessary to confirm whether the patient may have systemic mastocytosis, monoclonal MCAS, or MCAS.)

According to Afrin, there is currently no way to make a clear distinction, in most cases, between primary and secondary MCAS in the clinic.[34] This distinction is reliant on interpretation of certain laboratory test results in addition to the clinical presentation.

Now armed with a slew of test results (typically several months later), the clinician can move forward with sharing the diagnostic subgroup of MCAD with the patient. Patients who present with primary disease (SM or monoclonal MCAS) may need to be more carefully monitored or may have additional testing done (from Step 6) over time in the event that organ enlargement or bone mineral density issues arise.

If the patient does not meet the criteria for the diagnosis of MCAS, depending on the case, repeat testing of MCAS mediators or subsequent ordering of tissue biopsies may be warranted. Of course, other differential diagnoses should be re-considered and evaluated as well.

The differential diagnosis chart (presented in Chapter 3) should serve as a useful reference in consideration of other conditions that may mimic MCAS. Additional tests may be warranted. For example, in ruling out thyroid tumors or gastrinoma, calcitonin levels, parathyroid levels, and serum gastrin should all be evaluated. Theoharides and colleagues also recommend testing for serum complement C4 and C1 inhibitor levels to rule out hereditary and acquired angioedema that is present without urticaria.[13] They also suggest 24-hour urinary metabolites of serotonin and catecholamines to screen for carcinoid syndrome and pheochromocytoma, respectively.[13]

Can the Diagnosis Change Over Time?

It seems that the answer to this question is still unclear. It appears that patients can slide between the idiopathic and secondary classifications of MCAS over time, as further testing sheds light onto potential underlying mechanisms. Patients with secondary MCAS may eventually be diagnosed with clonal (primary) disease, but it's unclear whether in these cases the clonality was there all along (and missed) or whether there was an actual disease progression or spontaneous genetic mutation. And lastly, patients may shift to different diagnoses within the primary classification of MCAD; monoclonal MCAS patients may eventually be diagnosed with systemic mastocytosis, though the reverse effect (systemic mastocytosis reverting to MMCAS) is not expected. (A discussion on the progression from MMCAS to SM was discussed in Chapter 3.)

Step 8: Testing on Drugs of Tolerance

Patience is required as the patient and provider work together to determine what pharmacological approach is ideal; a lot of what ends up working will be determined by trial and error. By nature, patients with MCAD are highly reactive or intolerant to many medications, so a stepwise approach is very important in determining the correct plan of action with over-the-counter and prescription medications. Introducing too many medications too quickly can often be problematic.

A step-by-step integration of supplements and/or medications is helpful for determining which substances and dosages are most effective and which one(s) a patient may possibly be reacting negatively to. Both the generic and brand-name version of each medication should be trialed, as patients with MCAD often react to the fillers or dyes in the medications and not necessarily the medications themselves. There's often a several-ingredient difference when comparing generic and non-generic over-the-counter and prescription medications. Many capsules contain corn or wheat ingredients in addition to additives, dyes, and preservatives, so it's important to read the labels and utilize a compounding pharmacy when appropriate.

One month is generally enough time to determine if a medication is effective once it's reached the suitable dose.[2] New medications that trigger allergic reactions should be stopped immediately.

Stepwise Prophylactic Medication Suggestions

Picard and colleagues[3] presented a table of suggestions for a stepwise prophylactic treatment approach for patients with MCAS and MMAS. This resource offers a hierarchy for pharmacological management based on symptoms and systems and can be accessed from the link provided in Appendix 2 of this book. This resource is useful for clinicians who may need some initial guidance in determining an appropriate progression of medication trials to help confirm the diagnosis of MCAS. In-depth information on pharmaceutical and over-the-counter drug and supplement options are presented in Chapters 9 and 10.

Step 9: Patient Education: Lifestyle, Supplements, Nutrition, and Other Tools

I added Step 9 because I believe that every medical diagnosis should include a lengthy patient education step that dives into holistic management of the condition beyond the medication aspect before the patient leaves the office with the new diagnosis. Step 9 also circles back to Step 8 often, because most patients with this diagnosis experience an initial several-month to several-year window where they experience trial and error in determining the right combination of prescription medications, over-the-counter medications, supplements, and lifestyle changes to find a more stable baseline for the condition.

It's important to ascertain whether referrals to other specialists could benefit the patient at this time. Many patients with MCAD suffer from anxiety and depression, and it's crucial to address this possibility with every patient and to provide them with the resources that they need moving forward. The initial diagnosis is often a period of euphoria ("Finally, I have answers!") followed quickly by severe depression ("Will I ever feel better again?"). It's the responsibility of the practitioner to address the psychological impacts of the disease and to check in on this aspect of care with each and every visit.

More information about patient resources, lifestyle modifications, nutrition, and supplements are shared in the second half of this book. In addition, I firmly believe that every patient should seek naturopathic or functional medicine care to address any potential underlying issues that may be triggering mast cell activation, as will be discussed in more depth in this chapter.

Lastly, the patient should be educated on how to proceed in the event of minor or major emergencies with MCAS. Considerations for anaphylaxis are further outlined later on in this chapter.

Utility of the Nine-Step Process

The nine-step process example presented in this chapter is a reflection of the current research guidelines but is not intended to be a black-and-white clinical tool, as it does have some limitations. It's important to note that for many patients, certain steps may fall in a different order. For example, Step 3 involves ruling in/out cutaneous mastocytosis, systemic mastocytosis, or other neoproliferative conditions via bone marrow or tissue biopsy. However, most of the provided published criteria for the decision of whether or not to biopsy is based (in part) off one chemical mediator value, tryptase, which is not supposed to be tested until Step 5 in additional testing for mast cell mediators. This consideration at Step 3 is likely based off the assumption that most patients whose cases are suspicious of mastocytosis will have already had their tryptase measured before in order to make the biopsy decision in Step 3, but it's important to note this discrepancy.

In some senses, the steps may defy initial logic. Many are tempted to jump straight to chemical mediator testing, neglecting earlier steps. In clinical practice, some physicians will consider the tissue biopsy step only after chemical mediator testing, but the presented order reflects the fact that for certain patients, an earlier biopsy analysis may be warranted.[6]

When time is an issue, practitioners may be tempted to skip the physical exam or questionnaire. It's very important to include some sort of objective clinical score (Step 1), and a physical examination should not be overlooked as it can provide important information (Step 2).

Patients often come in with a list of tests they've had done over the last several decades, but it's important to ensure that up-to-date basic labs are ordered on day one. This can assist in capturing the bigger picture, which may be useful for differential diagnosis considerations, and

216

"baseline" lab values that may be especially relevant for monitoring potential responses to medication trials.

Step 5 offers concrete suggestions for which chemical mediators to test. Step 6 includes a number of tests that are relevant to determining the severity of MCAS: Are there problems with bone mineral density, organ enlargement/dysfunction, or other systems affected? The physician who diagnoses a patient with MCAS may very well be the first clinician to take them seriously and consider investigation of some of these systemic complications that can occur. Prompt recognition of cardiac, gastrointestinal, and bone mineral density concerns, for example, can lead to improved quality of life on both a short- and long-term basis.

Step 8 serves as a reminder that unlike other conditions, which can be relatively well-managed with bi-annual or quarterly check-ins, MCAS may require much more frequent communication and office visits in the first year or two until an appropriate treatment plan and symptomatic baseline are achieved. And lastly, patient education is a step that may be skipped over due to preformulated assumptions or lack of time, but it's a crucial step to assist the newly diagnosed patient in moving forward safely and with confidence.

ADDITIONAL CONSIDERATIONS AT THE TIME OF DIAGNOSIS

Patient and Family Education: Anaphylaxis

It's important from day one to educate patients, family members, caregivers, and friends on what to do in the event of an anaphylactic reaction. Anaphylaxis is a serious and acute allergic reaction where chemical mediators cause a number of physiological responses. This usually occurs in response to a predictable trigger, such as a bee string, medication, or ingesting a food that's a known allergen, but can also occur "idiopathically" or for unknown reasons. Anaphylaxis can occur very rapidly—in a matter of seconds from exposure to a trigger—so it's crucial that each patient and their families, caregivers, or housemates are aware of what to do in the event of an emergency. Anaphylaxis typically affects multiple body areas and can be life-threatening if proper treatment is not administered. Epinephrine injections are usually necessary to stop the reaction.

It's important to emphasize that one should not rely on waiting for emergency medical services during anaphylactic episodes. Life-saving decisions can come down to a number of seconds, and one cannot assume there will be time to drive to the hospital or wait for an ambulance to arrive.

The signs and symptoms of anaphylaxis[35] can include:

- Respiratory: wheezing, shortness of breath, coughing, clearing throat, hoarseness, pain with swallowing, difficulty swallowing

- Skin: hives, itching, flushing, swelling of mouth or tongue, angioedema

- Eyes: swelling or redness of the conjunctiva, itching or tearing of the eyes

- Nose: runny nose, nasal congestion, sneezing

- Gastrointestinal: crampy abdominal pain, diarrhea, vomiting

- Central nervous system: anxiety/sense of doom, confusion, headache, loss of consciousness, lightheadedness, change in mood in children (quiet or irritable)

- Genitourinary: loss of bladder control, pelvic pain, uterine cramps

- Cardiovascular: low blood pressure*, fast or slow pulse rate

Note: occasionally blood pressure is elevated instead of lowered

The presence of fainting or the absence of hives may be indicative of more serious reactions and a more serious potential underlying condition. Patients with systemic mastocytosis tend to present with syncope during anaphylactic episodes and are less likely to have cutaneous engagement.[21]

The simultaneous presence of multiple cofactors as triggers, in general, seem to contribute to more cases of anaphylaxis in patients with MCAD.[36] The combination of more than one trigger appears to account for reactions in about one-quarter of patients with systemic mastocytosis.[36,37] Food reactions are a common trigger, and idiopathic anaphylaxis also appears common in the MCAD patient population.

Research indicates that the scenarios that are more likely to trigger patients may depend on whether they have clonal or non-clonal disease. A 2010 study found that patients with clonal mast cell disorders (51 patients) were most likely to experience anaphylaxis following an insect sting (Hymenoptera venom), whereas patients with non-clonal MCAS (32 patients) more often had drugs as a trigger preceding anaphylaxis.[21]

NIAID Clinical Emergency Room Guidelines

The NIAID (National Institute of Allergy and Infectious Disease) panel developed clinical emergency room guidelines for anaphylaxis in 2004 that were updated in 2006. Their clinical decision-making guideline for physicians was evaluated in 2012 and found to have a sensitivity of 96% and specificity of 82% for the diagnosis of anaphylaxis. In other words, the guideline below is better for *ruling out* anaphylaxis if someone does not meet the criteria and has moderate validity for *ruling in* anaphylaxis when someone does meet one of the three scenarios.

Anaphylaxis is likely to occur in any of the following three scenarios:[38,39]

1. Acute onset of an illness (minutes to hours) with involvement of: skin, mucosal tissue, or both <u>and at least one of the following:</u> respiratory compromise **or** decreased blood pressure/end organ dysfunction (such as collapse, incontinence, or fainting)

2. <u>Two or more</u> of the following occur rapidly after exposure to likely allergen: symptoms in skin/mucosa, respiratory compromise, persistent gastrointestinal symptoms, decreased blood pressure/end organ dysfunction (such as collapse, incontinence, or fainting)

3. After exposure to known allergen for that patient (minutes to several hours): <u>low blood pressure (BP)</u>

   a. Infants and children: low systolic BP (age specific) or greater than 30% decrease in systolic BP.

      i. Age one month to one year: systolic BP less than 70 mmHg

      ii. Age one-10 years: systolic BP less than (70 mmHg+ [2 x age])

      iii. Age 11-17 years: systolic BP less than 90 mmHg

   b. Adults: systolic BP of less than 90 mmHg or greater than 30% decrease from patient's baseline

The American Academy of Allergy, Asthma & Immunology's most recent guidelines (2014) for management of anaphylaxis includes intramuscular epinephrine injected into the anterolateral thigh as an "immediate intervention."[40] This is the first-line treatment, based on strong evidence.[40] There are no substitutes for epinephrine (with the except of a few special scenarios where epinephrine is contraindicated, discussed below). Antihistamines, breathing treatments, diphenhydramine, steroids and other medications may be used in conjunction with epinephrine, but are *not* considered first-line treatment and do not work fast enough.[40,41] A number of further subsequent interventions are recommended that would take place in a hospital setting.

This information is not intended to diagnose or treat anyone. Anaphylaxis should be discussed with one's medical team and patients should be prepared for what signs could constitute an emergency room visit, a 911 call, and self-administration of epinephrine.

Special Considerations for Anaphylaxis

The main exception to traditional anaphylaxis guidelines occurs if a patient has Kounis syndrome, where inflammatory cytokines released by mast cells lead to coronary artery vasospasms and/or atheromatous plaque erosion or rupture.[42] These patients typically need to avoid certain medications like epinephrine, morphine, and beta blockers to avoid further heart complications; the anaphylaxis management plan ought to be different for this patient population.[42]

Patients who tend to have high resting heart rate and elevated blood pressure may also have special considerations for anaphylactic management. Certain medications—such as beta blockers, ACE inhibitors, and alpha-adrenergic blockers—can interfere with the body's endocrine system and control of mast cells in allergic reactions, which may pose a problem in acute allergic reactions. These medications have been claimed to interfere with epinephrine effectiveness and may not be recommended for patients who tend to experience anaphylaxis.

Patients who do not have cardiovascular disease are generally advised to avoid such medications if they've been prescribed epinephrine. However, according to a 2017 literature review, for some patients, the increase in life expectancy from the reduction of cardiovascular disease risk factors may warrant the continued use of medications like beta blockers and ACE inhibitors in patients prone to anaphylaxis who also have cardiovascular disease, even during periods of venom immunotherapy.[43]

Some researchers also claim that beta blockers and ACE-inhibitor blood pressure medications do not aggravate anaphylactic reactions, as once previously thought, though there are conflicting study findings in regards to different medications.[44] Ultimately, patient decisions in this area should be strongly guided with the help of one's medical team.

Glucagon is sometimes prescribed as an alternative to epinephrine. Seneviratne and colleagues noted, "All patients with systemic MC (mast cell) activation or susceptible to anaphylaxis should be prescribed two self-injectable epinephrine devices and taught how and when this should be used. A glucagon autoinjector may be needed instead if the patient requires beta adrenergic receptor blockade."[18]

Anaphylaxis can be biphasic (recurrent) where symptoms appear to resolve and then resume, typically within 1-8 hours after the initial reaction, but occasionally up to 72 hours later.[45] Multiple doses of epinephrine are necessary in some cases (studies estimate in 16%-36% of episodes).[46] Injection of epinephrine in the anterolateral thigh muscle (vastus lateralis) appears to be have the highest absorption and most rapid plasma levels when compared to subcutaneous sites; no comparisons have been made with inhaled epinephrine, which appears to have more side effects and may not have the same speed for sufficient plasma levels.[46-48]

The shift of intravascular fluid to extravascular space (due to increased vascular permeability) during anaphylaxis is common and can encompass 35% of fluid volume in a matter of 10 minutes.[46] Fatalities related to anaphylaxis are typically related to respiratory compromise and cardiovascular collapse and can occur quickly (10-15 minutes post insect sting or 25-35 minutes following ingestion of offending foods, according to one study).[46] This highlights the importance of the patient and/or family reacting quickly to anaphylactic reactions. Calling 911 (in the United States) and reporting to the nearest emergency room should be advised but should not replace or precede administration of life-saving medications.

A common concern among patients is whether there is a risk when using epinephrine. A 2008 review noted that "rarely, and usually associated with over dosage or overly rapid rate of intravenous infusion, epinephrine administration might contribute to or cause myocardial ischemia or infarction, pulmonary edema, heart arrhythmias, and risk for high blood pressure and stroke. These scenarios typically occur in patients who have high risk factors, comorbidities, are taking certain medications, or engage in recreational drug use. Nonetheless, some patients have survived massive overdoses of epinephrine, with no evidence of myocardial ischemia."[46]

As a whole, the risky outcomes are rare and typically have predictable factors involved. The risk of utilizing epinephrine pales in comparison to the risk of not using epinephrine during suspected anaphylaxis. When in doubt, epinephrine should be used.[41]

Despite the clear advice on management of anaphylaxis, *anecdotally*, some physicians assert that false anaphylaxis can occur in some patients when they experience a small trigger on the physiological level (such as a blood pressure change) and then the mind tricks them into thinking it's anaphylaxis. There are other *anecdotal* patient resources that also maintain that it's possible to calm down an allergic reaction with meditation and lying flat on your back. These are controversial standpoints and do *not* reflect current recommendations for anaphylaxis management.

In contrast, the American College of Allergy, Asthma, & Immunology offers additional suggestions for emergency allergic reaction management. A 2015 panel stated that "epinephrine should be given to patients at risk of an anaphylactic reaction based on a) a previous severe reaction or b) those who have had a known or suspected exposure to their allergic trigger with or without the development of symptoms."[41] These suggestions factor in the patient history and not simply whether certain symptoms are physically present. They also recommended that patients who report to the emergency room always receive a referral for a follow-up with an allergist after discharge from the emergency room.[41]

The take-home message is this: experts maintain that anaphylaxis is a very serious, life-threatening event that should be treated immediately without hesitation. If a patient has doubts about which symptoms constitute anaphylaxis, it's very important to discuss all of this with one's doctor before an episode occurs. If a patient has doubts in the moment of experiencing symptoms, it's best to administer epinephrine if they've been prescribed it, according to the latest guidelines.

It's also important that caregivers and family members are up to speed with what needs to happen in the event of an anaphylactic emergency. Epinephrine prescriptions typically come with a training device that one can practice with in order to avoid accidental self-injection when trying to use the medication on someone else. It's helpful to educate the whole family on the details (such as how to hold the device properly, how many seconds to inject it for, how to monitor vitals, and how often they can repeat injections). It's also important to remind patients that epinephrine, like other prescriptions, has expiration dates and certain temperature regulations.

A 2017 study looking at over 400 children with allergies found that while 65% had experienced an anaphylactic reaction prior, only 36% were administered epinephrine before reaching the emergency room.[49] Administration of epinephrine before reaching the emergency department often results in less severe consequences and less need for hospitalized stays. Only 70% of those with an EpiPen prescription were carrying their medication on them at the time.[49] Children who experienced reactions at school were much more likely to receive epinephrine compared to reactions that occurred at home.[49] This study reflects a great need for caregivers to have more clarity in terms of how to proceed during allergic reactions as well as the importance of carrying an EpiPen at all times.[49]

The Mastocytosis Society has a free downloadable Emergency Room Protocol that's highly recommended for patients who have MCAD, regardless of whether they frequently experience anaphylaxis or not. It's strongly advised that patients with any type of MCAD wear some type of medical alert jewelry that indicates their conditions, allergies, etc. (A full list of suggestions is available in the Emergency Room Protocol packet.) The resource has a list of medications commonly found in hospitals, with suggestions on what to avoid and what can be best tolerated by most patients with MCAS. For example, fentanyl or tramadol are *in general* better tolerated than pain medications like NSAIDs and narcotics in patients with MCAS. The

American Academy of Asthma Allergy and Immunology also has free downloadable anaphylaxis wallet cards and a printable Emergency Action Plan. (See Appendix 2 for the links to these resources.)

Patients and families should be well-educated on signs of anaphylaxis and appropriate responses, and epinephrine, diphenhydramine, and other well tolerated medications (such as antihistamines) should be stashed in several locations in the house, kept in one's vehicle (presuming appropriate temperatures are maintained), and carried with the patient at all times.

Patient-Specific Documents

Another useful tip for the newly diagnosed MCAS patient is to complete written documents, with the help of one's medical team, with clear customized guidelines to what should occur during different potential scenarios so that the emergency plan is clear. Patients who have frequent hospital trips (or the risk of anaphylaxis) should have a standing order document signed by the doctor that includes:

Patient name, symptoms, risk of anaphylactoid reactions, labs to be drawn (before treatment), medications to administer, considerations for pre-medication prior to procedures, drugs to avoid, and instructions for continuation of care.

A standing order document may also benefit the patient who is suspected to have MCAS but does not have laboratory evidence yet in order to enhance the likelihood that symptomatic tests will be ordered by other physicians, and in order to reduce the risk of adverse reactions from exposure to substances more likely to trigger reactions.

Some physicians prefer to delineate three separate patient care documents: one for an outpatient strategy, one for an inpatient strategy, and one that is specific to the emergency room. Regardless of the paper approach, a written format will help keep instructions clear for everyone and should minimize unnecessary stress and anxiety.

THE BIG PICTURE APPROACH

Some practitioners believe that MCAS is another label for something that is part of a much bigger picture of multisystem dysfunction. As noted in Chapter 4, theories exist for genetic explanations that could be responsible for multisystem dysfunction, like the RCCX Theory.

Other experts have attempted to explain the phenomenon of so many patients presenting with large "resumés" of comorbidities by looking at other (environmental) factors.

Survival Overdrive Syndrome or "SOS"

Dr. Aviva Romm is an herbalist and specialist in women's health who describes a commonality she notes in patients who have a large number of seemingly unrelated symptoms that all have one underlying source. She has coined this state "Survival Overdrive Syndrome" or "SOS."[50]

According to Romm, "SOS is what happens when the body becomes chronically overloaded by a number of factors that cause stress to our body. That can be obvious stress like emotional stress or lifestyle stress, but it can also be poor diet, lack of sleep, toxic environmental overload, and chronic viral infections. EBV (Epstein-Barr virus) is commonly picked up or reactivated when we're in SOS. And when we're in SOS, because the immune system is already on overdrive, it's harder for your immune system to kick it."[50]

The concept of "SOS" could be tied to MCAS. If the body is fighting a viral load or attempting to remove toxins, the immune system is working harder, which would naturally induce increased mast cell activation. If the immune system is in overdrive chronically, one could imagine how this could create a vicious cycle of inflammation and immune system strain. Over time, this could lead to new elevated baseline levels of mast cell activity.

In "The Adrenal Thyroid Revolution: A Proven 4-week Program to Rescue Your Metabolism, Hormones, Mind & Mood," Romm suggests a number of important steps to helping the body heal from a state of SOS. These include tips for resting to repair, nourishing with specific foods, supporting for the immune system, addressing the viral load, and reducing stress on the adrenal system.[51]

Multiple Systemic Infectious Disease Syndrome

Similar to the concept of "SOS," Multiple Systemic Infectious Disease Syndrome (MSIDS) is another theorized physiological state that could explain the dozens upon dozens of different symptoms that patients may experience when suffering with chronic illness. MSIDS has many similarities with both MCAS and Myalgic Encephalomyelitis/Chronic Fatigue Syndrome (ME/CFS) in terms of the symptoms reported. The condition was coined by Dr. Richard Horowitz, a prominent Lyme disease specialist and author of "How can I get better? An action plan for treating resistant Lyme and chronic disease."[52]

MSIDS refers to a melting pot of infectious exposure. Lyme disease and tick-borne co-infections, viruses, bacterial infections, parasites, and fungal infections may all be occurring in a single patient, leading to the presentation of a very complex condition with a plethora of root issues.[52] Horowitz notes that detoxification problems, endocrine abnormalities, food allergies, mitochondrial problems, autonomic nervous system dysfunction and postural orthostatic tachycardia syndrome (POTS), dysbiosis in the gastrointestinal microbiome, heavy metals and environmental toxicities, neurodegenerative and neuropsychiatric disorders, nutritional and enzyme deficiencies, liver issues, and sleep disorders are all possible with MSIDS.[52]

MSIDS supports that a secondary mast cell activation could be occurring in patients with multiple high infectious loads going unrecognized.[52] According to Horowitz, "One of the essential problems with the traditional medical model is that doctors are taught that there is generally only one cause for each illness. Yet I believe that instead of looking for one answer, we should be looking for many."[52]

Kryptopyrroluria

Chronic infections and/or emotional trauma may also lead to a physiological state where the blood oxygen levels and subsequent availability of nutrients are affected. Kryptopyrroluria (KPU) is a condition that is also known as the "mauve factor" or "malvaria." It's a condition where a biotoxic substance (hemopyrrollactamuria, or HPU complex) is identified in the urine.[53] High levels are strongly associated with heavy metal toxicity and positive Lyme tests, and are seen in children with autism.[53] Historically, the complex first came to light in research of patients with schizophrenia.[53] It has since been associated with learning disabilities, ADHD, multiple sclerosis, multiple chemical sensitivity, Parkinson's disease, epilepsy, criminal behavior, schizophrenia, Down syndrome, depression, bipolar disorder, and substance abuse.[53]

KPU (sometimes shortened to "pylouria") is believe to be caused or triggered by an inherited condition or environmental factor such as physical/emotional trauma or chronic infections. The HPU complex binds strongly to vitamins and micronutrients which are all excreted in the urine.[54] This results in abnormal heme synthesis and chronic loss of zinc, biotin, vitamin B6, arachidonic acid, manganese, and other nutrients from the body.[54]

Experts note that depression is one of the tell-tale signs of KPU.[53] Poor dream recall and nail spots (leukodynia) are other common signs, though the condition may present with a variety of system-wide symptoms, many of which overlap with MCAS.[53]

Chronic deficiencies in vitamin B6 may be associated with poor sleep and peripheral neuropathy in these patients.[54] A lack of zinc may contribute to impaired detoxification and immune problems.[54] Depletions in biotin levels may be associated with short-term memory loss, skin aging, immune system issues, and detoxification problems.[54] Micronutrient deficiencies are considered secondary complications of KPU by some researchers, where abnormal heme synthesis appears to be the biggest issue, which can lead to mitochondrial dysfunction.

Specifically, it's possible that biotoxins from microbes in chronic infections such as Lyme disease can lead to the blockage of one of the enzymes of heme synthesis, resulting in a loss of key minerals in the body which may contribute to an overall state of immunosuppression and therapy-resistant infections.[53]

Heme is a part of hemoglobin molecule, which is a protein in red blood cells that has an important "carrier" role in the oxygenation of tissues and subsequent removal of carbon dioxide from tissues back to the lungs. A consequence of decreased hemoglobin function on a chronic basis may be low ATP (cellular energy) and low glutathione, leading to fatigue and decreased efficiency of the body's detoxification pathways.[53] With fewer routes for environmental toxins to be eliminated, patients often experience a buildup of heavy metals, mold, and other irritants that can certainly trigger mast cell activation.[53]

Indeed, it appears that patients who are more susceptible to difficulty removing biotoxins such as mold and heavy metals also tend to be harboring KPU.[53] Experts also claim that high KPU levels are associated with high histamine levels.[53] Fructose intolerance, poor dietary tolerance to histamine, and IgG food reactions to gluten, dairy, and eggs are also reported clinically.[55] A recent article suggested that German researchers are now linking KPU with mastocytosis and MCAS, and that treatment of KPU that repairs the heme molecule appears to stabilize mast cells and influence histamine levels.[53]

KPU may also be responsible for increased susceptibility to parasitic infection in the body. It's possible that low levels of zinc may foster a more hospitable environment for parasites in the mucosal layer of the gastrointestinal system.[53] KPU is also clinically associated with elevated levels of histamine in stool samples, leaky gut syndrome, and inflammation in the gastrointestinal tract.[55]

Experts advocate first addressing KPU in order to have more effective remediation of all of the above problems (such as bacterial infections, parasites, or environmental/chemical sensitivity).[53] DHA Laboratory and Health Diagnostics and Research Institute perform testing for "HPL" (hydroxyhemopyrrolin-2-one).[53] Just like many mast cell mediators, the urine test must remain chilled to ensure accuracy. There's also a questionnaire for KPU that can be helpful in determining whether to order the urine test.[53] Treatment for KPU includes very specific dosages of important vitamins and minerals.[53] It's crucial to work with a physician in the diagnosis and treatment process.[53]

KPU offers a possible explanation for why so many patients are becoming chronically ill with an extensive abundance of viruses, bacterial issues, and other infections that thrive in an immunosuppressed host. Perhaps KPU is the glue that connects so many conditions together, including MCAS and its comorbidities?

UTILITY OF FUNCTIONAL MEDICINE AND NATUROPATHIC CARE

Getting at the Root Cause in Diagnosis

Regardless of what one decides to call this phenomenon of immune system dysfunction with multiple chronic symptoms—whether it's SOS or MSIDS or a true diagnosis of Kryptopyrroluria—it's clear that it's a problem that needs to be taken seriously. With the constraints of the current modern medical system, available specialists often lack the time and wide lens necessary to evaluate a patient comprehensively. Functional medicine doctors and naturopaths may be the key to success for this patient population.

A *root mechanism* approach is growing in popularity among some practitioners who treat MCAS, but the approach is still far from being adequately integrated into the mainstream medicine model for patients with chronic illness (including MCAS). According to Driscoll, "If MCAS is secondary to an underlying inflammatory process, treating mast cells will help the patients feel better, but will not 'cure' the patient. If the patient is left to treat mast cells (a secondary response) without treating the primary problem causing MCAS, they will never be free from the presentation."[1]

Therefore, if the patient care team only focuses on antihistamines and other medication options but does nothing to identify underlying factors and remove the triggers, it will have provided a disservice to the patient with a "Band-Aid" approach to symptoms. While medications may play a crucial role in helping the patient to stabilize, identifying underlying issues is the key to a more sustained lower symptomatic baseline.

A *root mechanism* approach is more than just identifying comorbidities. For example, it's important to determine if the MCAS patient has additional factors like Ehlers-Danlos syndrome (EDS) or postural orthostatic tachycardia syndrome (POTS), two diagnoses with distinct sets of symptoms and findings that appear to have a complex relationship with mast cell activation. However, the identification of *root mechanisms* goes even deeper than the concept of correctly identifying additional pertinent labels or diagnoses. It's not necessarily about creating a longer pathology "resumé," it's about *reading between the lines*.

Dr. Joseph Pizzorno, founder of Bastyr University, is one of the world's leading authorities on science-based natural/integrative medicine. According to Pizzorno, "Naturopathic medicine is built on the profound belief that the body has a tremendous ability to heal, if we just give it a chance."[56] In order to facilitate healing, *root mechanisms* are identified that may assist in guiding the patient toward what underlying factors may be triggering inappropriate mast cell activation.

Identification of the root issues is relevant for all patients with MCAD, regardless of whether they have clonal disease or whether their MCAS is deemed idiopathic or secondary. Patients can simultaneously have genetic influences and environmental factors impacting disease, so the environment should always be addressed.

A sole focus on mast cells is akin to addressing one small tip of the iceberg while ignoring the much more complex series of influences hidden underwater. How can a patient expect to reduce inflammation and mast cell activation while living in a moldy environment, harboring a hidden bacterial infection, or consuming a diet of mostly processed foods and artificial sugar? Mast cell-targeting medications may mask the symptoms, but failure to eliminate underlying triggers makes it difficult for the body to find a place of healing and homeostasis.

As a culture, a quick (and easy) fix is desired. Mainstream medicine should not be seen as the enemy; rather, mainstream doctors with an openness to MCAS should be considered a valuable part of the team. Physicians and specialists should not be blamed for practicing medicine in the way they've been taught or under the constraints that dictate their schedules. However, when the system does not deliver all of the answers and resources, it's important that the patient is guided into the hands of someone who can uncover the *root mechanisms*.

Functional Medicine and Naturopathy for the Win!

Naturopathic care, as a field, is largely under-researched in this arena, but it has been shown to reduce chronic allergies and antihistamine dependence in case studies conducted in Australia.[57] A case report in the Pacific Northwest (United States) published in 2016 reflects ample knowledge of MCAS characteristics and the appropriate diagnostic and treatment approaches within the field of naturopathic providers,[58] though it is unclear what proportion of practicing naturopaths are educated about MCAS in their initial schooling. Regardless of whether the naturopath is already well-versed in MCAS, it's most important that the practitioner is open and willing to listen and learn with the patient (just like mainstream doctors should be).

Naturopathic doctors have the advantage that they typically 1) have greater time frames initially with the patient to take a thorough (systemic) history, and 2) are well-equipped to investigate underlying *root mechanisms* that may be responsible, at least in part, for triggering excess mast cell activation that is occurring. Naturopathic care is focused on the body's innate ability to heal itself, and it also incorporates the healing power of nature.[59] Naturopathic doctors focus on removing obstacles so that the body has what it needs to regain health and vitality.[59]

Similarly, functional medicine doctors (FMDs) incorporate the whole-person approach and typically include a longer patient interview and system-wide considerations. However, unlike naturopaths, FMD education is a supplement to original training. The additional scope incorporates aspects of nutrition and herbal/natural therapies, with an ultimate aim to uncover and eradicate underlying microbes that may be contributing to a loss of homeostasis in the body.[59]

It appears that both FMDs and naturopaths share the commonalities of thorough, patient-centered care that addresses the cause and not simply the symptoms. Naturopaths will have a greater length and depth of training in holistic areas compared to FMDs and an approach that is akin to "evaluation of the terrain" as opposed to "eradication of microbes."[59]

The differences seem subtle when compared to the mainstream medical approach, but it's important to realize that patients with MCAS may individually respond better to one method or the other, so trial and error may also apply in the realm of functional medicine and naturopathy. And just like any experience with the medical system, there may also be a trial and error approach needed to find a reputable naturopathic or functional medicine ally. Regardless of which approach is trialed first, some type of approach that evaluates underlying root issues is crucial to the long-term quality of life of the patient with MCAS.

Proposal of a Second-Tier Approach

Once the patient has already completed the important "first tier" tests for MCAD (such as urine or blood testing, tissue biopsies, and other considerations useful in the diagnostic process) and has clarity in their diagnosis, it will be useful to add a functional medicine or naturopathic approach to the care team with additional investigation right away.

Functional medicine doctors and naturopaths generally already have bountiful information regarding the most common root mechanisms that can lead to chronic disease, which can be assessed with an individualized patient history, examination, and further testing. *However, for patients with MCAD in special circumstances who may not have access to such providers, this chapter will conclude with a proposed second-tier checklist that could be useful to review with one's medical team. Ultimately, however, there is no replacement for a high-quality practitioner of holistic medicine who can aim to shine an individualized spotlight on underlying mechanisms of chronic illness.*

In order to maximize holistic management of MCAD, a number of tests/underlying conditions should be considered as part of a complete diagnostic workup for each patient who presents with a MCAD. *The proposed checklist is not all-inclusive and is not meant to replace an individualized, professional-guided approach.* The checklist reflects aspects of published recommendations from a number of prominent naturopathic and functional medicine doctors.

Dr. Nicola Ducharme (previously known as Nicola Mcfadzean), ND is a doctor of naturopathy and the clinical director of RestorMedicine in California. She has authored several books and describes "The Top 5 Tests in Functional Medicine Testing (that won't break the bank)" to be:[60]

- Adrenal and Reproductive Hormone Level Testing
- Heavy Metal Testing
- Food Sensitivity Testing
- Gluten Intolerance Testing
- Lyme Western Blot Test

Ducharme recommends that patients (especially those suffering from long-standing chronic illness) be examined thoroughly and systematically in order to maximize their success potential.[60] That includes ruling in/out certain factors that may significantly impact the management of a condition like MCAS.[60]

The Western Blot Test is not the most accurate test out there, but it can serve as a starting point in the investigation of Lyme disease. Food testing can be tricky and less than accurate in the MCAS patient, and most patients have already had a smattering of testing done with allergists. However, it's important that true allergies (including ones that cause delayed reactions or reactions limited to the GI tract) are identified in some way at the start of a treatment program. Most patients with MCAS already have some awareness of the particular foods that tend to trigger reactions (and should continue to be avoided).

Problems in all five areas can potentially influence patterns of mast cell activation. Many of the symptoms that coincide with dysfunction in those five areas overlap with symptoms experienced by patients with MCAS. Underlying issues with hormones, bacterial infections, toxins, and factors that influence the gastrointestinal tract and mast cell reactivity need to be identified and isolated in order to break the "vicious cycle" of chronic dysfunction and immune system dysregulation.

Ducharme also recommends that a comprehensive functional medicine gastrointestinal investigation include analysis for the following:[60]

- Parasitic Infections
- Bacterial Infections
- Yeast Overgrowth ("candida")

Once parasitic infections have become chronic, they are very difficult to detect with "standard" stool sample tests. H. Pylori is the most commonly seen type of bacterial infection, but others may also need to be ruled out.[60] Bacterial infections such as Mycoplasma pneumoniae and Streptococcus pneumoniae have also been shown to induce mast cell activation[61] and may be especially relevant in the MCAS patient. An unbalanced microbiome can also wreak havoc on the digestive system, and the presence of fungus such as candida can influence this system. Many practitioners believe that gut health is the key to achieving optimal wellness.

Even if patients are asymptomatic or only mildly symptomatic in the gastrointestinal system, it can be especially important to address the gut because of the theory that increased intestinal permeability can lead to increased mast cell degranulation (and vice-versa) if the foods and medications ingested are not properly filtered through the system. Theoretically, medication-based treatment—without addressing the integrity of gastrointestinal health—can lead to suboptimal control of symptoms, improper long-term health management, and impaired cost-effectiveness.

Colorado-based functional medicine doctor Jill Carnahan recommends a diagnostic approach that assesses both toxic and infectious burden in her patients, with a goal to identify and reduce the overall load.[62] She typically focuses her initial evaluation at Flatiron Functional Medicine on blood work (including tests that evaluate for viral, bacterial and tick-borne infections), stool testing, and organic acid testing (including testing for mycotoxins, toxic profile, and glyphosate).[62] Carnahan also includes food allergy testing with some patients, noting that it can be useful to help patients buy into dietary changes.[62]

Licensed nutritionist and herbalist Rebecca Snow also suggests the utility of an organic acid test for patients with MCAS that has the ability to measure dysbiosis, candida, nutritional deficiencies, and toxic load.[63] She supports a comprehensive stool analysis, Spectracell micronutrient panel, toxic metal burden testing, genetic testing, and tests that evaluate inflammation (such as C-reactive protein) in her MCAS patients.[63]

Thus, some of the common threads in comprehensive functional medicine or naturopathic testing entail: 1) "standard" medical tests, 2) a thorough gastrointestinal evaluation, 3) inclusion of tests addressing environmental factors, and 4) other useful tests that help rule in/out certain conditions and shed light onto the role of genetics and epigenetics.

Table 3. Proposed Second-Tier Checklist: A Functional Medicine/Naturopathic Type Approach for Comprehensive Management of Patients Presenting with MCAS

Standard Medical Tests	Gastrointestinal Investigation	Environmental Factors	Other Useful Tests
•inflammatory markers •comprehensive metabolic panel •thyroid function •hormonal profiles	•Stool analysis/ parasitic infection tests •bacterial infection tests (H. pylori, SIBO, etc.) •fungal infection/ candida evaluation •microbiome bacterial balance/ intestinal permeability	•heavy metal analysis •CIRS/mold toxin evaluation •allergy testing* •testing for Epstein-Barr virus and other viruses •Lyme/vector-borne illness testing	•Ehlers-Danlos syndrome consideration •other genetic testing •Spectracell micronutrient panel •celiac disease or gluten sensitivity testing •adrenal function and POTS consideration

*Note: *Anecdotally*, allergy testing may not be recommended for all MCAS patients.

If they've been suffering chronically, many patients will likely already have had a smattering of these tests done before they reach the office of a naturopath or functional medicine doctor. And perhaps they have already been diagnosed with celiac disease, hypothyroidism, adrenal fatigue, chronic inflammatory response syndrome (CIRS) following mold exposure, or others on the list. *It may also be relevant to test for anemia, Chiari malformation, intracranial pressure issues and/or a cerebrospinal fluid leak in patients with MCAS*, depending on their symptoms.

Through compiling a thorough list of the root physiological mechanisms that can be barriers to healing, a comprehensive and proactive plan of action can be developed that targets these root mechanisms. It's helpful to know that the mast cells have "gone awry" so to speak, but only mildly helpful if it's not clear what mechanisms are contributing to the dysfunction for a particular individual. Most likely, findings in the naturopathic realm relate closely to mast cell activation. And even if the identified dysfunctional systems aren't the root cause of the issue, and are potentially more of a consequence, they may still play a role and become a chronic barrier in efforts to help the patient heal.

Thoughts on Allergy Testing

Experts generally maintain the need to rule out the presence of an allergic disease via measurements of total and allergen-specific serum IgE, particularly if the patient's history includes an allergic trigger, and regardless of whether they have SM. However, *anecdotally* many argue that IgE allergy testing may be inaccurate and inconclusive in this patient population.

IgE testing aims to determine allergies for foods and other environmental factors that the patient is currently exposed to. Foods that have been avoided may test (falsely) negative because the body may not have sufficient antibodies for them. Some believe that the testing may also be inaccurate in patients who have dermatographia, even if control areas are utilized. Others assert that food allergy testing may be inaccurate in patients who have a leaky gut, where they tend to test positive to the foods that they consume the most.

Anecdotally, some patients with MCAD react to nearly everything and others appear to have no skin prick abnormalities. Some patients also report that skin prick testing has resulted in symptom flares and anaphylaxis. Some patients with MCAD report that their "true" allergens that consistently trigger anaphylactoid reactions will test negative on skin prick testing and blood allergy testing, while others come back with dozens of IgE-positive "allergies" to previously benign foods. Some patients also report that their IgE-positive tests results are completely different every time they are tested.

Bahri and colleagues noted in 2018, "Conventional allergy tests assess for the presence of allergen-specific IgE, significantly overestimating the rate of true clinical allergy and resulting in overdiagnosis and adverse effect on health-related quality of life."[64] Recent literature indicates that researchers are attempting to develop a specific mast cell activation test to assist in the diagnosis of allergic disease and anaphylaxis that may eventually replace existing food allergy diagnostics.[64]

Allergy testing should be performed with care in this patient population and should be discussed with one's medical team on a case-by-case basis.

Restoring Balance

Following a naturopathic or functional medicine approach to additional testing, with the help of the same practitioner, one can then focus on a list of priorities to restore systemic balance and calm inflammation in order to achieve a more stable "baseline" of reduced mast cell activation. The second-tier testing suggestions may not be all-inclusive, but they provide a good customizable starting point when creating an individualized holistic healing plan for a patient. Many functional medicine and naturopathic care providers include components of detoxification, mitochondrial support, hormone balance, optimization of gastrointestinal health/nutrition, and addressing psychosocial issues as fundamental aspects of holistic care. The latter part of this book dives more into these topics.

Supporting the other systems and giving them what they need to recalibrate, heal, or establish a new baseline is a piece of the puzzle that should impact the quality of life dramatically for someone living with MCAD. Treating the downstream effects of chemical release without removing or addressing something like a moldy environment or heavy metal toxicity will most likely feel like an uphill battle. It's important to note that the patient must be prepared to make drastic lifestyle changes in order to complete the resulting recommendations, particularly if they mean relocating to a new home or making dramatic changes to dietary habits.

It's certainly expensive to order more tests, *but that decision should not be assumed for the patient!* (Most patients meet their deductibles very quickly with the frequent doctor and emergency room visits that tend to accompany MCAD!) At the very least a thorough comprehensive and holistic approach should be *offered and encouraged* for each patient. If cost is a concern, focusing on one test or tier at a time may also be better than nothing.

It's certainly worth taking the time to look into insurance coverage. When one looks at the big picture, they may find that a bigger cost up front with second-tier testing could very well eliminate other tests or treatment costs down the road.

The Risks in Skipping the Second-Tier Approach

Sending a patient home with just the basic blood and urine tests and eventual diagnosis of MCAD is like setting someone up on a paddleboard, but without a life vest, leash, paddle, or fin to help steer! Suddenly, from the vantage point standing above the water, the patient will be able to see the choppy turmoil with greater clarity and awareness, but they'll still most likely feel powerless to control their own level of stability and safety as the waves crash into them.

The patient will be stuck in a reactive approach as opposed to a proactive approach. *In my opinion,* naturopathic and functional medicine are the missing tools to help provide much-needed balance and direction.

As a physical therapist, this scenario reminds me of the classic patient with neck pain who works 40 hours per week in front of a computer. The physical therapist (PT) can label the patient with cervical myofascial pain and throw everything under the sun at them: manual therapy to help the joints move, trigger point release or dry needling to help release myofascial tension, exercises to improve range of motion, strength and endurance training, etc. But if the patient is not provided with education and tools to change their ergonomic setup or alter their schedule to reduce the chronic postural strain, they'll likely be back in the same office several months later.

In this example, perhaps the patient had a car accident or traumatic mechanism that caused the original injury, but the daily postural factors that set up the area for reaggravation or relapse still need to be addressed. The underlying muscles that provide cervical spine stability may not have ever been an issue for that patient before but following trauma they are physiologically altered.

Failing to address both the more recent dysfunction that arises or comes to one's attention (such as comorbidities like POTS and EDS) and the preexisting issues that may now contribute to heightened sensitivity (such as the presence of toxicity buildup or Epstein-Barr virus) are substantially detrimental to the plan of care for the patient with MCAS. Regardless of what physical or mental type of "trauma" was the tipping point for the system's mast cells, addressing "daily postural strain" aspects like nutrient deficits, environmental triggers, and the function of other body systems is crucial to maximize proper effective patient care and prevention of future flare-ups.

Patients should not have unrealistic expectations to be paddling off into the sunset like a pro right away, but with time and the proper guidance from a well-rounded and holistic team, it's possible to identify and address important factors that can help provide a more stable baseline for this patient population.

The take home message is: 1) Consider a second-tier cluster of tests once a diagnosis of MCAS has been made (if the patient has not already gone this route) and refer to a naturopath or functional medicine doctor if needed; 2) Make sure the patient is involved in the decision-making process and rationale for further tests, and 3) Ensure that the patient is prepared for the possibility of lifestyle and dietary changes depending on the results.

Ensure adequate time to educate the patient on putting together all of the test result puzzle pieces and encourage a multidisciplinary team approach for the holistic management of MCAS.

Of course, this should be occurring with concurrent medication and lifestyle management to prevent serious reactions like anaphylaxis. Adding a naturopathic/functional medicine approach should by no means undermine the importance of creating a stable initial baseline for MCAS symptoms. Hopefully, over time, the fruits of this approach will result in the shifting of the patient's baseline to fewer reactions/symptoms and less reliance on medication.

CHAPTER KEY POINTS

- While there is no universal algorithm for clinical decision-making to assist in the diagnosis of MCAS, several algorithms have been published to assist in the process. (See Appendix 2)

- A questionnaire was developed and validated to assist the clinician in establishing suspicion of MCAD. (See Appendix 2)

- There are differing expert opinions on the criteria that necessitate a bone marrow biopsy or other tissue biopsy to rule out mastocytosis.

- The diagnostic process should include the following components: thorough patient history, questionnaire evaluation, differential diagnosis consideration, physical examination, tissue or bone marrow biopsy when certain criteria are met, baseline laboratory tests, specific chemical mediator testing of the blood and urine, consideration of additional imaging or testing if appropriate, classification of the specific type of MCAD, testing on drugs of tolerance, and patient education.

- Screening for anxiety/depression and referrals to a mental health specialist should also be considered for every patient with MCAS.

- There's typically a need for a periodic loop-back to testing on drugs of tolerance, as it's common for patients to experience several months to years of medication trial and error before finding a good combination.

- Anaphylaxis is a true medical emergency and it's important to have a written emergency plan, readily available auto-injectors of epinephrine (as appropriate), and a medical identification bracelet. Patients and family members should be well-versed in the signs of anaphylaxis.

- Survival Overdrive Syndrome (SOS), Kryptopyrroluria (KPU) and Multiple Systemic Infectious Disease Syndrome (MSIDS) offer examples of theoretical explanations for the underlying bigger picture of physiological problems and secondary mast cell activation that can occur.

- Once a patient has the diagnosis of MCAS, it's recommended that they investigate aspects of a "Second-Tier Checklist" by pursuing testing and care under the supervision of a naturopath or functional medicine doctor who is knowledgeable in MCAS or willing to learn about MCAS.

- It may also be useful to consider a series of standard medical tests, a thorough gastrointestinal investigation, tests to address environmental triggers, and other special tests that examine aspects such as genetics and nutritional absorption. Specifically, tests for heavy metals, gluten intolerance, adrenal and reproductive hormones, vector-borne disease such as Lyme Disease and other tick-borne illnesses, and the presence of bacterial infections, viruses, parasites and candida (yeast) may be especially beneficial for the patient who has MCAS.

Chapter Seven
Coexisting Conditions

I f social media is any indicator, it's becoming increasingly apparent that modern medicine is still missing something. The vast majority of patients diagnosed with MCAS don't simply have MCAS. Their Instagram profile is classically something like:

@examplepatient

MCAS / EDS / gastroparesis / rheumatoid arthritis / fibromyalgia / POTS / Hashimoto's / Raynaud's / ME/CFS / bipolar / Lyme / SIBO (etc. etc. etc.!)

This phenomenon is puzzling; it appears that a great number of patients are struggling with many concurrent diagnoses. For the newly diagnosed, this may not be true. But for others, MCAS may be the "gateway" diagnosis that leads to eventual discovery of other issues, and for yet another group of patients, MCAS may be discovered long after other conditions are identified.

Something is making younger generations sicker and sicker. Something is causing widespread immunosuppression (or in some cases, immune overactivity that presents as autoimmunity) and susceptibility to getting more and more burdened with chronic invisible illness.

Is MCAS is to blame for *all* of these comorbidities? Or perhaps *some* of them? Or, as theorized in Chapter 6, is there a bigger-picture systemic issue (like survival overdrive syndrome, multiple systemic infectious disease syndrome, or kryptopyrroluria) serving as the conductor in these patients?

It's evident that MCAS potentially interacts intricately with many of these conditions. This chapter provides an overview of *some* of the more common conditions associated with MCAS. The information is not designed to be all-inclusive information regarding specific diseases.

Rather, the different sections serve as 1) a general overview of information from which one can conduct more individualized investigation and 2) a space for theoretical connections to be brainstormed, based on the literature.

EHLERS-DANLOS SYNDROME (EDS)

EDS is a disease of the body's connective tissue. The prevalence of EDS varies depending on the type, with an average prevalence estimate of one in 5,000 people.[1] The disease is typically diagnosed by a geneticist and most types of EDS have a known genetic etiology. The more common types are classical EDS (cEDS; previously known as type I or II), hypermobile EDS (hEDS, previously known as type III or joint hypermobility syndrome), and vascular EDS (vEDS; previously known as type IV).[1] Other rarer forms also exist.

In 2017 an updated international classification of EDS was published that identified 13 different types of EDS.[2] Twelve of the 13 have specified genetic causation and associated molecular and genetic diagnostic criteria; hEDS is the only type that has not been officially connected to a particular gene.[2] Some experts believe that there are actually 15 types of EDS.[3]

Historically, EDS was coined by two doctors in the 1800s and is characterized by poor healing, skin stretchiness, and joint hypermobility. Initially the disease had a pediatric genetic investigative focus and the hypermobility cases were thought to be "benign." Indeed, it's believed that 2% of the general population exhibit evidence of joint hypermobility, and this trait alone may not be reason for concern.[3] However, the pathological presentation of hEDS involves multiple tissues below the surface that can create a concerning medical condition that ought to be taken seriously.

Many clinicians suspicious of EDS will have genetic testing performed in order to rule out the types with more serious consequences. (And no, home-based DNA testing kits are not sufficient for diagnosis!) Vascular EDS can have a big impact on lifespan because of the risk it poses for blood vessel problems such as an aneurysm (blood vessel that bursts). Classical EDS is more commonly characterized by difficulty with wound healing. All of the types of EDS tend to impact multiple systems. The hypermobile type is most common, followed by the classical type, the vascular type, and the kyphoscoliotic type.[3]

Hypermobile EDS

It appears that hEDS is the most common type of EDS associated with MCAS. Experts affirm that as of 2018, hypermobile EDS research has yet to reveal a genetic mutation of connective tissue protein responsible for the disease. Some theorize that it's possible that hEDS could be the name describing a cluster of symptoms connected to the aberrant mediator release of MCAD, which results in connective tissue abnormalities. Others may associate the etiology of hEDS to theories of genetic mutation (such as the RCCX Theory, discussed in Chapter 4) that connect hEDS to common comorbidities that could all share the same genetic defect.

The hypermobile type of EDS is associated with fragility of connective tissue and joint laxity that can result in hyperextension, subluxation, and dislocation.[2] Some patients with hEDS experience recurrent joint dislocations, while others may experience minor subluxations or inflammation. The joints of the spine may also be impacted.

Due to the nature of the hypermobility, some patients experience severe muscle guarding and myofascial pain, because the muscles are essentially acting as extra stability for the joints which move around too much and lack tight ligamentous support. Tendons, bursae, ribs, and surrounding nervous system structures may also be impacted. Increased ligamentous laxity is often accompanied by reduced proprioception, or a decreased kinesthetic ability to sense where the body or joint is located in space. Decreased proprioception may result in clumsiness or compensatory patterns such as gripping objects forcefully or wearing tight clothing and footwear.

Patients with hEDS often also have system-wide symptoms that reside outside of the orthopedic spectrum. Systemic signs of a generalized connective tissue disorder, such as atrophic scarring, hyperextensibility of the skin, and organ prolapse may be present.[2] Patients with hEDS may experience heart valve problems, and many patients have orthostatic intolerance and dysautonomia, including postural orthostatic tachycardia syndrome (POTS).[2] Chronic pain, anxiety/depression and fatigue are frequently reported.[2] Many patients also experience gastrointestinal problems and sleep disturbances.[2]

While the other types of EDS require testing with a geneticist, as of 2018 one can make a diagnosis of the hypermobility type of EDS by evaluating three sets of criteria. Physical therapists and occupational therapists are potential non-MD clinicians who can help detect this condition. The diagnostic criteria are available on the Ehlers-Danlos Society website (see the link in Appendix 2).

EDS and MCAS

A retrospective study of rheumatology patients conducted in 2017 noted that 45.6% of patients with joint hypermobility, as assessed by the Beighton Scale, also had the diagnosis of MCAS.[4] When evaluating a subgroup of patients who had *MCAS plus other comorbidities* (such as orthostatic hypotension, urticaria, allergic rhinitis, pruritis, tachycardia, aphthous stomatitis, syncope and gastrointestinal complaints), only 0.5% of this subgroup of patients *did not meet the criteria for joint hypermobility*.[4] In other words, the vast majority (99.5%) of patients with MCAS and conditions often associated with it also displayed measurable joint hypermobility that may be consistent with EDS.[4]

Mast cells have been implicated as underlying culprits within connective tissue disorders such as EDS. Mast cells help the body to create connective tissue and collagen in response to stress/strain and the presence of wounds. When mast cells become dysfunctional, it's possible that the results of excess degranulation or elevated concentrations of certain chemical mediators can have a negative impact on the body's normal connective tissue healing process, whether it be in laying down too much scar tissue, or by forming weak bonds with new collagen that result in weak connective tissue. Thus, one theory is that mast cells are responsible for the collagen problems noted in hEDS.

On the other side of the theory spectrum, it's also possible that a genetic mutation causes hEDS (though it hasn't been officially discovered yet) and as a result, connective tissues are innately abnormal. If connective tissues are not healing or laying down new collagen properly, this could also trigger subsequent mast cell activation as the mast cells perceive the abnormality as a threat that triggers a cascade of chronic degranulation.

Complications Associated with EDS

Serious complications can occur with the hEDS patient population. Chiari malformation is one of the most common complications and is theorized to occur with hEDS secondary to ligamentous laxity in the cervical spine (neck) and possible posterior gliding of the condyles.[5] An upright MRI is recommended to detect this condition, where the base of the cerebellum (brain) slips through the opening of the skull. This commonly presents clinically as pain, spasticity in the extremities, difficulty swallowing, paresthesia, chronic headaches, and ataxia.[5] The exact incidence of Chiari malformation in EDS patients in unknown, although it has been noted that the female to male ratio is high (approximately 9:1).[6,7]

Headaches are frequently reported with EDS, and the most common types are migraines, headaches generated by neck muscle tension, and headaches triggered by jaw joint dysfunction. However, some headaches may have more serious causes. A headache that increases with strain such as a cough or a sneeze increases the index of suspicion for Chiari malformation.[5] Spontaneous cerebrospinal fluid leaking is often characterized by a worsening of headache while upright and a reduction in headache symptoms when lying down.[5]

Idiopathic intracranial hypertension (IIH), a condition of elevated fluid levels and elevated pressure inside the brain, can occur in patients with EDS.[5,6] Headache, ringing in the ears, feeling the heartbeat in the ears, visual disturbances, nausea/vomiting, and sensitivity to light may be noted with IIH.[6]

Tethered cord syndrome (TCS) is also associated with hEDS. A 2009 study found that 77% of patients who had symptoms of Chiari malformation also had TCS.[7] Tethered cord involves the conus of the spinal cord being yanked down. This can be especially concerning for patients with Chiari who are already at risk for the upper part of the spinal cord and the brain being compressed.[5] Symptoms may include low back pain, leg weakness and/or sensory loss, and neurogenic bladder symptoms.[5]

Barre-Lieou syndrome can occur when a patient with anterior cervical spine (neck) instability experiences injury to the capsular ligaments. Without these ligaments functioning properly, the cervical spine can translate further forward than it should with movement, which results in the vertebrae pushing on the cervical sympathetic nervous system ganglion. In addition to dysautonomia, patients may also experience tongue numbness, blurred vision, ringing of the ears, dizziness and vertigo, headaches, and neck pain.[5] Patients with EDS who experience a worsening of POTS symptoms in conjunction with neck and head positions may need to consider the diagnostic possibility of Barre-Lieou syndrome.[5]

POSTURAL ORTHOSTATIC TACHYCARDIA SYNDROME (POTS)

Postural orthostatic tachycardia syndrome, also known as "POTS," is a condition where the heart rate increases in response to changes in position (typically, standing up). The word *orthostatic* refers to something caused by upright posture, and *tachycardia* means a fast heart rate. It can also occur when going from laying to sitting, and some patients report intense symptoms with other movements like turning over in bed. This condition is frequently reported in patients who have MCAS and is more common in women between the ages of 15 and 40.[8] POTS is classified as a type of dysautonomia, where the autonomic nervous system is not working properly. There are different types of POTS.

Patients often report an intense heart-pounding sensation in addition to a rapid heart rate. Palpitations and dizziness are also experienced. Some people get light-headed and some people experience fainting in conjunction with episodes. The onset is typically sudden and can sometimes be connected to a trigger such as trauma, emotional stress, infections, viruses, or exposure to toxins.[9] Symptoms in women may be exacerbated around the time prior to their menstrual cycle.[9]

Mast cell disease subject matter expert Lisa Klimas describes life with the condition. "(POTS) can cause very severely disabling symptoms and effects. It can cause a huge array of symptoms, including dizziness; fainting; exhaustion; inability to exercise; nausea; vomiting; major GI disturbances (both diarrhea and constipation); inappropriate sweating; chest pain; coldness, numbness, pain and weakness of extremities; and anxiety. Some patients are unable to stand up at all."[10] Many patients are wheelchair bound due to poor standing tolerance. POTS alone can have a dramatic influence on a patient's quality of life.

Tremors have also been reported in conjunction with episodes.[11] While near-fainting is common, only about 30% of patients will actually pass out, according to one article.[9] One study noted that patients with POTS had greater difficulty with memory and concentration and scored higher on an attention deficit hyperactivity disease (ADHD) rating scale.[12] A 2005 study of 17 patients with POTS noted that tachycardia symptoms were more pronounced in the morning when compared with the evening.[13] Acrocyanosis (discoloration of the legs) and coldness of the skin to the touch is noted in some patients with POTS.[9] Many patients will have low total blood volume on testing.[14]

While the hyperadrenergic type of POTS is not as common in the general population, only comprising about 10% of cases,[9] it appears to be more common in patients with MCAS.[15] Patients with hyperadrenergic POTS tend to present with elevated systolic blood pressure when upright, as opposed to the drop in blood pressure observed in patients with neuropathic symptoms.[15] Increased urine output when upright and increased migraine headaches may be noted with this type of POTS.[11] This type tends to occur in a gradual and progressive manner and may be caused by an excess of adrenaline in the system. Doctors may order supine and upright testing of serum catecholamine levels if the hyperadrenergic type of POTS is suspected. Serum norepinephrine levels are typically >600ng/ml (upright) with these patients.[11] Many believe that there is a strong influence of genetics in the development of hyperadrenergic POTS.

244

Partial dysautonomic POTS (also known as neuropathic POTS) is also sometimes associated with MCAS, and it is believed to be caused by the veins in the legs not working properly, resulting in pooling of blood in the extremities which then tells the brain that the blood pressure is low, which triggers a rise in heart rate to compensate. Patients with neuropathic POTS have been found to have less norepinephrine released (and less sympathetic nervous system activation) in their lower extremities when compared to their upper extremities.[16] This type is considered a mild peripheral autonomic neuropathy and 5:1 cases are female compared to male. Neuropathic POTS development often occurs after surgery, trauma, sepsis, immunizations, pregnancy, or a febrile viral illness.[11] Clinicians may observe an obvious darkening of the color of the legs in the examination room while the patient is seated. There is also a "developmental" partial dysautonomic POTS that typically affects teenagers after they've experienced large growth spurts, which tends to naturally regress over time in 80% of cases.[11]

POTS may be classified as primary or secondary. Patients without any other identified comorbidities may be diagnosed with primary POTS. Patients who have coinfections or other diseases may receive a secondary classification. For example, patients with the vector-borne illness Babesia may have secondary POTS occurring due to the infiltration of parasitic infection.[17] The symptoms may be present for several months and then regress, only to reappear months later. This is *theorized* to occur as the body switches its perception of what viral or bacterial load is the greatest threat at a given time.[17] When the immune system perceives Babesia as the biggest current problem, POTS symptoms may be more likely to occur.[17]

The most common cause of secondary POTS is type II diabetes, a condition that often has inherent peripheral neuropathy.[11] Patients with Parkinson's disease or multiple sclerosis and patients experiencing heavy metal toxicity or undergoing chemotherapy may also experience secondary POTS.[11]

Some experts theorize that median arcuate ligament syndrome (MALS) is connected to dysautonomia and POTS symptoms. This condition, which commonly affects thin women between the ages of 20-40,[18] involves compression of the celiac artery and possibly the celiac ganglia by the median arcuate ligament, resulting in narrowing (stenosis) of the blood vessel that can be noted on ultrasound and CT imaging (on exhale). This compression is believed to cause ischemia downstream to the abdominal tissues, spleen and liver, an audible epigastric bruit sound, vomiting, weight loss, gastroparesis, and other symptoms.[18] MALS has also been connected to dysregulation of the autonomic nervous system due to the increased or continual neural impulses initiated by mechanical pressure on the celiac ganglia.[18]

Some tumors and cancerous conditions may mimic POTS.[11] Conner et al. notes, "Paraneoplastic syndrome associated with adenocarcinoma of the lung, breast, ovary, or pancreas may also present as POTS. These tumors produce auto-antibodies targeting the acetylcholine receptors in the autonomic ganglia in a manner similar to post-viral syndromes."[11]

POTS has also been noted as an adverse effect following the vaccine for human papilloma virus (HPV).[19] In theory this could be from vaccine content or excipient-induced activation of mast cells.[19]

POTS is typically diagnosed in a medical clinic using a standing or tilt table test. A positive test is indicated by the presence of orthostatic intolerance symptoms associated with a sustained heart rate increase of 30 beats per minute (bpm) or absolute rate exceeding 120 bpm in adults within the first 10 minutes of shifting to an upright position.[11] In children, the diagnosis is made if the sustained heart rate increases by 40 beats per minute.[20]

The diagnosis can only be made if the patient has *not* been subjected to prolonged bed rest or medications that interfere with the autonomic nervous system (such as diuretics, vasodilators, anxiolytic agents, and antidepressants). Dehydration, anemia, and hyperthyroidism often cause tachycardia and must also be ruled out.[9]

A "normal" rise in heart rate is about 10 beats per minute from sit to stand. So, a rise of 30 beats per minute is certainly clinically significant in adults. It's important to measure both the heart rate and the blood pressure when testing for POTS. A 2012 study noted that "most patients will have orthostatic symptoms in the *absence of* orthostatic hypotension (a fall in BP >20/10 mmHg)."[11]

POTS and MCAS

It's possible that sympathetic nervous system activation is what triggers subsequent mast cell activation in patients with POTS. A spike in heart rate and/or adrenaline experienced with POTS can actually cause mast cell activation as the body perceives a threat. Patients who have both POTS and MCAS can find themselves in a vicious cycle. The mast cells may release chemicals to try and regulate the heart rate, but this can increase perceived stress and result in a continuous cascade of mast cell activation if the heart rate or adrenaline factor is not resolved properly or continues repeatedly throughout the day, as is common in POTS.

It's also possible that an underlying state of MCAS can be the bigger culprit for a certain subgroup of patients with POTS. Some theorize that reflex sympathetic activation may be caused by circulating chemical mediators that cause vasodilation of the blood vessels (such as those released by mast cells). Many mast cell mediators can trigger a vasodilation or low blood pressure response, including histamine, vasoactive intestinal peptide, heparin, chymase, tryptase, and prostaglandin D2.[21,22] A drop in blood pressure may trigger a compensatory elevation in heart rate. Many patients with POTS describe flushing symptoms that correspond to episodes of orthostatic intolerance.

A 2005 study evaluated 177 patients with long-standing POTS and determined that MCAD should be considered in patients who present with both POTS and flushing.[15] The authors theorized that elevated histamine levels could cause both flushing and vasodilation noted in their patient population. In their study, about 50% of patients with POTS plus flushing reported signs of MCAD.[15]

Research by Zadourian and colleagues noted that in neurogenic cases of POTS, it remains unclear whether the sympathetic nervous system activation leads to mast cell degranulation, or whether the presence of MCAS initiates the release of vasodilators and resultant sympathetic nervous system compensation.[23]

Similarly, POTS researcher Raj summarizes, "It is not clear if mast cell activation (releasing vasoactive mediators) represents the primary event in these patients or if sympathetic activation (through release of norepinephrine, neuropeptide Y and ATP) is the cause of mast cell activation."[9]

This is the golden question, and unfortunately there's not enough evidence out there to make grand conclusions. Whether the cause of POTS is an overactive sympathetic nervous system, underlying mast cell activation, or other complex physiological mechanisms, it appears that the two conditions often go hand in hand.

POTS and Ehlers-Danlos Syndrome (EDS)

Patients who have connective tissue issues, such as those with hypermobile EDS (hEDS), appear to have a higher incidence of POTS compared to the general population. Researchers estimate that up to 70% of patients with joint hypermobility syndrome also have clinical POTS diagnoses.[24]

If the vascular connective tissue has abnormal distention, an orthostatic environment may be facilitated because the patient will experience excess peripheral venous pooling, which tends to have a compensatory heart rate mechanism that can lead to the clinical signs of (neuropathic) POTS.[25] In other words, this theory suggests that the veins get too big, and as a result it's hard for them to return blood upward when standing, so the body perceives the situation as an alarm signal of low blood pressure and makes the heart beat faster to spread the blood more adequately around the body. This is similar to the theory about mast cell mediators causing excess vasodilation of blood vessels, but the implicated mechanism with EDS lies in collagen defects that influence the blood vessels directly and permanently.

Some specialists believe that hEDS patients are prone to similar vascular complications noted in other types of EDS. Critics argue that the influence of collagen on blood vessel diameter may not be the primary mechanism since many patients develop POTS suddenly overnight, whereas patients with EDS would likely have had collagen defects their whole lives.[20] This characteristic of abrupt symptom development supports the possibility of a neurological cause of venous dysfunction in patients with POTS, as opposed to a slow chronic stretching of connective tissue being the sole culprit.

POTS, EDS and MCAS

Many patients with mast cell activation problems will *anecdotally* present with the "terrible triad" or "trifecta" of the three conditions: MCAS, hyperadrenergic POTS and hEDS. Some authors believe that there is one genetic mutation or causal factor that may be responsible for all three conditions, and some assert that the three conditions are actually just three different names for one bigger systemwide diagnosis. However, recent studies evaluating the prevalence of all three conditions in different patient cohorts have differing results.

Researchers Cheung and Vadas conducted a study in 2015 where they evaluated 15 female patients who presented with clinical signs of POTS.[26] In the study, 12/15 (80%) had formal diagnoses of POTS.[26] Nine out of 12 (75%) had both POTS and EDS, and 66% of patients with both diseases also had validated symptoms consistent with MCAS.[26] The authors concluded that collagen disorders, dysautonomia seen with POTS, and mast cell activation appeared to "co-segregate" together.[26] However, this study had a small female-only sample size and the authors concluded that more research is needed.[26]

A separate 2015 study evaluated a larger group of 117 patients with POTS, 74% of which were female.[27] Of these patients, 20% had laboratory evidence of MCAD (specifically, elevated urinary prostaglandins or elevated urinary histamine).[27] The authors did not find a correlation between MCAD and the hyperadrenergic POTS phenotype in this study.[27]

A 2016 study evaluated 41 patients with POTS and found that 63% had a coexisting joint hypermobility syndrome (JHS).[28] When compared with patients with POTS who did not have joint hypermobility, the POTS + JHS group of patients was associated with a longer symptom

248

duration and lower supine norepinephrine levels.[28] Thirty-five percent of patients in the POTS + JHS group had a positive family history for JHS, and 27% of these patients had laboratory evidence of MCAD.[28]

In summary, based on the above studies it appears that POTS and EDS are potentially highly interconnected, MCAS and EDS are potentially interconnected, MCAS and POTS may be interconnected, and thus the three *could* go hand in hand. However, the nature of these studies makes it difficult to create generalizations about the likelihood of shared etiology.

Senior scientist/molecular biologist Lisa Klimas notes, "This is very much a chicken and egg situation where it's not clear exactly what begets what. EDS is a genetic disorder and considered primary. However, that does not necessarily mean POTS or mast cell disease is secondary in this scenario."[29]

Below is a diagram that highlights one theorized potential summary of mechanisms between EDS, MCAS, and POTS.

Table 2. An example of proposed mechanisms between EDS, MCAS, and POTS

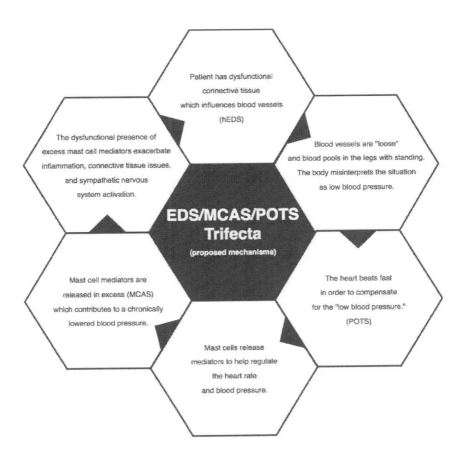

The Driscoll Theory

The Driscoll Theory challenges the concept of a sympathetic nervous system response as the inner source of problems for a *particular subgroup* of patients with POTS. Dr. Diana Driscoll, a therapeutic optometrist and the Clinical Director of POTS Care in Dallas, has devoted much of her research and practice to patients with idiopathic POTS who often have normal autonomic nervous system testing (except for abnormal tilt table results).[30] Driscoll notes that a number of symptoms are characteristic of this subgroup of patients, including fatigue, difficulty breathing, gastroparesis and/or IBS, headaches, depression, and environmental sensitivities, in addition to the classic POTS symptoms.[30]

In her book, "The Driscoll Theory Newly Revised: The Cause of POTS in Ehlers-Danlos Syndrome and How to Reverse the Process," Driscoll describes a subgroup of patients who do not fall into the category of an autoimmune, neurological, endocrine, or metastatic underlying cause for POTS—the *idiopathic* POTS patients—who don't meet the clinical characteristics of neuropathic POTS.[30] She notes that a thorough differential diagnosis process should occur before jumping to the assumption of idiopathic POTS, including evaluation for conditions such as multiple sclerosis, Parkinson's disease, multiple systems atrophy, amyotrophic lateral sclerosis, pheochromocytoma, carcinoid cancer, and others.[30]

The parasympathetic nervous system (PSNS) is responsible for "rest and digest" moments, whereas the sympathetic nervous system (SNS) is known for the "fight or flight" adrenaline response. Many theories point to the SNS being responsible for hyperadrenergic and/or idiopathic POTS, and current POTS testing focuses on the SNS. Indeed, treatments targeting a reduction in sympathetic tone may alleviate POTS symptoms *temporarily*.

Driscoll and her children had experience with chronic mysterious illness and idiopathic POTS, and through her investigation she realized that, in both their cases and in her patients, the role of the parasympathetic nervous system had been missed.[30] No one to date had explored the possibility that perhaps the imbalance in the autonomic nervous system in idiopathic POTS was due to more of *an underactive parasympathetic nervous system*, as opposed to an overactive sympathetic nervous system.[30] Driscoll investigated the role of the vagus nerve (part of the PSNS), intracranial pressure, vascular anomalies, connective tissue problems, inflammation, and immune function in relation to idiopathic POTS.[30] She also began to connect Ehlers-Danlos syndrome and histamine-producing cells to the findings, noting a *secondary* mast cell response in patients.[30]

The Vagus Nerve

As part of the "rest and digest" system, the vagus nerve plays an important role in a plethora of systemwide functions. The vagus nerve and its branches innervate a number of organs and influence the heart, abdominal viscera, larynx, pharynx, bronchi, and more. The nerve influences motor functions, PSNS functions, sensory functions, and even taste.

The main neurotransmitter that affects the vagus nerve is acetylcholine, which attenuates the release of inflammatory cytokines (including TNF and interleukins) from mast cells and other cells.[31] Vagus nerve activation (through an immune system response to inflammation or endotoxins) induces stimulation of the hypothalamic pituitary axis (HPA) and adrenals which modulates inflammation in the body.[31] Stimulation of the vagus nerve has been found to reduce epileptic seizures[32-34] and reduce inflammatory cytokine synthesis and release.[31]

Driscoll postulates that the vagus nerve can be impacted by either elevated intracranial pressure (ICP) in the head or pressure in the blood vessels adjacent to it as it travels through the neck.[30] Theoretically, chronic mechanical pressure to the vagus nerve can result in desensitization and an imbalance between the PSNS and SNS. When the nerve is repeatedly compressed over time, the patient may experience low blood pressure, fainting, difficulty breathing, heart rhythm and rate abnormalities, dizziness and vertigo, low HDL cholesterol, sweating and feeling hot, nausea, ringing of the ears, anxiety, and brain fog or difficulty thinking.[30] Sometimes these patients are labeled with having a panic attack.[30]

Intracranial Pressure and Chiari Malformation

The Driscoll Theory also outlines some interesting potential explanations for the link between EDS and POTS with the symptoms of Chiari malformation.[30] Chiari malformation is traditionally known as a "structural" malformation at the base of the skull that allows the brain to "sink" too low instead of floating above the opening in the skull that permits a passage for the spinal cord. Most mainstream doctors assert that the ligamentous laxity and upper cervical spine instability, commonly noted with hypermobile EDS, are the biggest factors to this slippage of the cerebellum downward through the foramen magnum in this patient population. Thus, many patients are immediately told they have a congenital defect that requires surgery.[30]

However, Driscoll asserts that a lesser known cause of Chiari positioning may be elevated ICP in the head related to the overproduction of cerebrospinal fluid or poor drainage of the fluid around the brain, as is common in patients with EDS. If the pressure is elevated enough on top of the brain, it can cause the same downward displacement of the brain that is noted in

Chiari patients.[30] Driscoll notes that symptoms of elevated ICP include fluid coming out of nose, increased symptoms when straining (such as a cough or bowel movement), dizziness, nausea, headaches radiating to neck, hypersensitivity to stimuli, tremor, pressure in head, ear aches, vertigo, and motion sickness.[30]

Elevated CSF pressure may explain why patients with EDS tend to have poor kinesthetic awareness of where they're at in space (proprioception), something that was previously attributed to ligamentous laxity.[30] The above fluid issues could also explain many symptoms of POTS.[30] Elevated intracranial pressure and a sluggish venous system may also contribute to chronic inflammatory problems, creating a "cytokine storm" and a subsequent dysautonomia vicious cycle while untreated.[30] In addition, Driscoll notes a strong connection between behavioral and emotional conditions and abnormal ICP. "Mildly increased intracranial pressure over long periods of time could also cause hypothalamic dysfunction, exhibited as obsessive-compulsive tendencies, free-floating anxiety and/or the need to over-achieve."[30]

"The Driscoll Theory Newly Revised: The Cause of POTS in Ehlers-Danlos Syndrome and How to Reverse the Process" is an excellent read for patients and providers who are seeking more information regarding the potential physiological mechanisms between POTS, EDS, Chiari malformation, intracranial pressure abnormalities, the vagus nerve, mast cell activation, and much more.[30] Driscoll continues to advocate for these patient populations, is a member of the medical advisory board for EDS Network C.A.R.E.S., and is the president of Genetic Disease Investigators, a corporation devoted to researching POTS, EDS, and their comorbid conditions. Her clinic POTS Care focuses on searching for the underlying causes of POTS and treating it at its source. More information can be found at www.POTScare.com.

COMPLEX REGIONAL PAIN SYNDROME (CRPS)

Complex regional pain syndrome (CRPS) (previously known as reflex sympathetic dystrophy) is a condition that involves pain and inflammation in one predominant body area or limb that is disproportionate in its severity and duration compared to the norm. The pain is typically unrelenting, even at rest. Many patients with this condition go on to develop central sensitization, where the nervous system becomes hypersensitive due to the continual pain message impulses it's receiving. Many patients experience CRPS in the extremities, but it can also occasionally present in the head or trunk.

The cause of CRPS is unknown, though research does indicate that immobilization of a limb (such as casting an extremity following a fracture) may increase the risk of developing the condition. CRPS may be triggered by some type of trauma, such as a sprain or bone fracture, brain injury or prolonged immobilization, a needle stick or surgery, and sometimes there is no known etiological factor.

It's theorized that following a triggering event, the localized area experiences impaired muscle pumping (due to immobility), which can lead to increased edema and over time to the development of adhesions in the connective tissue.[35] These factors increase the strain and reduce the efficiency of the lymphatic drainage system, which can cause decreased oxygen delivery to the tissue, increased acidosis, and increased pain.[35] As this continues, the nervous system is bombarded by (abnormal) afferent pain signals that can lead to central and peripheral sensitization and eventual severe hypersensitivity in the area.[35] This can create an extremely debilitating vicious cycle that can dramatically influence the patient's quality of life.

CRPS nerve-type pain does not follow a specific nerve dermatome (territory). Abnormalities in skin characteristics, such as sweating, redness, and unusual hair growth or the absence of hair often occur, in addition to edema. These symptoms, when combined with increased sensitivity to touch, are hallmark of CRPS. (Often, these patients cannot even tolerate the pressure of a light bedding sheet on the skin.) Patients may also exhibit a movement disorder called dystonia, which is characterized by uncontrollable muscle contractions.

Some assert that the diagnosis of CRPS is very much a clinical diagnosis, as opposed to one based on imaging.[5] And it's very much a true diagnosis, despite some who will accuse these patients of having psychosomatic origins. However, a 2019 review article noted that the diagnosis of CRPS as well as the proposed autoimmune etiology and treatment options are not well supported in the literature, and it appears that it remains a somewhat controversial condition.[36]

Glial cells have been implicated to play a role in CRPS. As part of the immune system protection of the nervous system, the glial cells normally hang around the neurons in case of emergency, and similar to mast cells, the glial cells release cytokines, which go on to cause nerve inflammation.[5]

Mast cells have also been implicated to play at least a partial role in this condition. A 2004 study noted significantly higher levels of mast cell mediators in the limbs of patient with type I CRPS compared to the unaffected limbs.[37] The study also found a significant correlation between pain and tryptase levels in CRPS patients.[37]

Mechanisms between mast cells and the initiation and propagation of long-term changes in pain response are complicated, at best. Research indicates that mast cells reside in close proximity to nerves, which facilitates communication or "cross-talk" between the two cells types.[38-39] This communication is facilitated by substances such as neurotransmitters and cytokines released by mast cells.[38]

A number of mast cell mediators can activate and/or sensitize the neurons involved in the pain experience.[40,41] According to Wirz & Molderings, "When these neurons are stimulated, they send signals to the central nervous system (CNS) and concomitantly release neuromodulators, such as substance P and calcitonin-gene related peptide, the vasoactive intestinal protein, and corticotropin releasing hormone (CRH), which, in turn, can further stimulate mast cell activation creating a bidirectional positive feedback-loop potentially resulting in neurogenic inflammation."[41]

In essence, neurotransmitters can trigger additional mast cell degranulation,[40] leading to a vicious cycle of pain. Bidirectional communication (from the release of cytokines and chemical mediators) between mast cells and the nervous system results.[41] Additional cell recruitment may stir up this process. Theoharides and colleagues note, "Activation of MCs (mast cells) may also contribute indirectly to the development of pain by the recruitment of neutrophils and macrophages, which also release algesic mediators."[40] It appears that the physiological mechanisms connecting mast cells to chronic pain conditions such as CRPS are multifactorial and complex.

GASTROINTESTINAL "MYSTERIES"

Gastrointestinal distress is a very common complaint in patients with MCAS. Unlike the diagnoses of EDS and POTS, however, when it comes to the gut, there does not seem to be one predominant "diagnosis" aside from the labeling of the umbrella term irritable bowel syndrome (IBS).

As noted in the first few chapters of the book, patients with MCAS report everything from IBS and small intestinal bacterial overgrowth to ulcers, diagnoses of Crohn's and ulcerative colitis, GERD and acid reflux issues, gastroparesis, severe distention from abdominal angioedema or third spacing, uncontrolled diarrhea, continual nausea and vomiting, and everything in between.

Dr. Hamilton, a gastroenterologist at Brigham and Women's Hospital, estimated in 2018 that about 50% of his caseload includes patients with MCAD who have gastrointestinal concerns.[42] He asserts that it's very important to look at anything else that could be contributing to symptoms in patients with MCAS who have gastrointestinal problems.[42] He often assesses for inflammatory bowel disease, eosinophilic disorders, bacterial overgrowth, motility disorders, and lactose intolerance in his patients.[42] Hamilton associates some of the

254

gastroparesis and motility issues noted in MCAS patients as potentially connected with a comorbid interplay between Ehlers-Danlos syndrome and dysautonomia influencing the vagus nerve.[42]

In terms of the typical gastrointestinal presentation in a patient with MCAS, Hamilton notes from clinical experience that the majority tend to be chronically on the constipation end of the spectrum but move to loose stools and diarrhea when in a reactive state.[42] He states that the classic gastrointestinal symptoms suggestive of mast cell activation once exposed to a trigger include abdominal distension and bloating, followed by abdominal cramping, followed by diarrhea.[42]

Irritable Bowel Syndrome (IBS)

According to a 2017 publication by researchers Wirz and Molderings, "A majority of MCAD patients complain about abdominal pain and/or cramping usually accompanied by bloating-gassiness of the bowel, diarrhea, constipation, thereby fulfilling the diagnostic criteria for irritable bowel syndrome (IBS). A bulk of results suggest roles of mast cell infiltration and activation in IBS-related pain pathology."[41]

Recent research links small intestinal bacterial overgrowth (SIBO) to the development of IBS.[43] SIBO is the presence of excessive amounts of bacteria in the small intestine (a place that is normally devoid of bacteria, in comparison to the large intestine, which is bacteria-rich). There are two types of SIBO, methane-dominant, which tends to coincide with delayed motility and bloating issues, and hydrogen-dominant, which is associated with diarrhea. While testing is improving for detection of SIBO, it can be a tricky and frustrating condition to eradicate. Some experts believe that small bowel dysfunction in POTS may contribute to the development of SIBO.[43]

SIBO may be an underdeveloped explanation for the breadth of gastrointestinal issues in patients with MCAS. In the alternative medicine world, some assert that SIBO can cause histamine/mast cell issues.[44] While gastrointestinal issues can certainly influence other systems (such as mental health), it may be a stretch to conclude that SIBO alone causes MCAS and the entire breadth of systemic issues associated with it. SIBO could, in theory, be part of the *triggers or confounding variables* for symptoms of secondary mast cell activation. Anecdotally, many patients report that getting better control of their SIBO symptoms and gut health tends to help them with easier management of their MCAS, and vice-versa.

There's an abundance of research that shows increased numbers of mast cells and/or activation in gastrointestinal tissues in certain medical conditions. An increased number of mast cells have been found in both the small and large intestinal mucosa of patients with IBS compared to controls.[45-48] A 2011 study by Frieling and colleagues found that 19 out of 20 patients diagnosed with IBS had signs and symptoms of pathological mast cell activation disease.[49] A 2010 review noted associations between additional diseases such as mastocytic enterocolitis and systemic mastocytosis with an increased number of mast cells in the GI mucosa.[50]

Increased mast cell mediators have been measured in patients suffering from IBS. Elevated tryptase levels have been found in intestinal fluid, blood, and biopsy tissue of patients with IBS.[45-48] Serotonin released by mast cells in the intestinal nervous system has been theorized to be connected to pain in IBS patients.[51-52] A study of IBS patients who exhibited visceral hypersensitivity determined that the mast cell stabilizer ketotifen significantly improved pain and quality of life when compared to placebo.[53]

Gastroesophageal reflux, diarrhea, peptic ulcer disease, malabsorption, and steatorrhea are symptoms that are believed to be caused by mediator release in patients with systemic mastocytosis (SM) and they are possible even in the absence of increased mast cells in mucosal biopsy specimens; similar mechanisms could occur in patients with MCAS.[54]

Mast cells have a number of important roles in the gut. They function as part of the GI tract's immune system and are found in high quantities in the mucosal interface that processes environmental exposures.[50] Substance P and other neuropeptides stimulate mast cells to release inflammatory mediators, which is facilitated by the close proximity of mast cells to nerve terminals in the lamina propria.[50] Histamine and prostaglandin D2 released by mast cells play an important role in the regulation of intestinal motility and chloride and water secretion.[50]

The Vagus Nerve and the Gastrointestinal System

It appears that the physical proximity of mast cells to nerves in the gut creates a two-way communication loop, where nerves influence mast cells and mast cells can also influence nerves.[55] Mast cells regulate gastrointestinal permeability as well as visceral sensitivity and are believed to be involved with the perception of pain in gastrointestinal tissues.[50,56-57] Spinal sensory nerves and major nerves such as the vagus nerve's afferent fibers have receptors for mast cell mediators.[50]

The vagus nerve connects the brain to the gut, which could explain the mast cell–gut–brain pain perception connection. The research shows that motor neurons may react to mast cell

256

degranulation in the manner of excessive propulsion and secretion in the gastrointestinal tract, which could trigger abdominal pain and diarrhea.[58] Nociceptors in the small intestine may become sensitized over time from chronic mast cell degranulation—and, in particular, histamine—resulting in a reduced threshold for pain.[59]

Patients with inflammatory bowel disease may have reduced vagal tone and stimulation of the vagus nerve may be a promising treatment option. According to 2017 research, patients with Crohn's disease (CD) show an inverse relationship between vagus nerve tone and levels of plasma TNF-alpha (a mast cell mediator).[60] The majority of patients with CD responded favorably to vagus nerve stimulation, including over 70% of patients with CD experiencing deep clinical and endoscopic remission at a six-month follow-up.[60]

Handheld vagus nerve stimulator devices applied to the neck have been the subject of recent research and have been shown to effectively activate vagal afferent nerves and reduce migraine headaches.[61] It would be interesting to see what type of an effect vagus nerve stimulation has on (the majority of) patients with MCAS who have gastrointestinal system dysfunction and/or headaches. *Anecdotally,* supplements targeting the boosting of vagus-specific neurotransmitters like acetylcholine have been reported to provide some relief in some patients with MCAS.

The vagus nerve also has a role in the production of stomach acid. Hypochlorhydria, or low stomach acid, has been gaining increased attention in the functional medicine world in recent years. Both gastritis and the use of the proton pump inhibitor omeprazole have been associated with reduced stomach acid and subsequent microbial overgrowth.[62] *In theory*, if a dysfunctional vagus nerve can induce hypochlorhydria, this can contribute to bacterial imbalances in the gut and a heightened immune system response locally in the gastrointestinal tract that could involve overactive mast cells.

Fungal Infections

Candida albicans ("yeast") in the gastrointestinal tract and other areas has been implicated to play a role in chronic gastrointestinal dysfunction. Research dating back to 1974 found that increased histamine was released when rat cells were exposed to a glycoprotein that comes from *candida albicans*.[63] The research indicated that exposure to the fungus elicits a response in mast cells similar to the studied response of mast cells to exposure to bacteria, viruses, and parasites.[63] A more recent study suggested that *candida* colonization in mice may promote sensitization against food antigens via the effects of an array of chemical mediators on gastrointestinal permeability, as mast cells contribute to antifungal host defense.[64]

257

Fungal infection may possibly be part of a "perfect storm" of factors that have been theorized to contribute to IBS problems. The combination of a history of antibiotic use, which decreases the healthy bacteria in the gut, and the presence of certain bacterial strains that can permeate the mucosal barrier may play a role in the symptom etiology.[65] According to Noverr and colleagues, "Antibiotics also lead to overgrowth of the yeast *candida albicans*, which can secrete potent prostaglandin-like immune response modulators."[66] It's possible that a single antibiotic course combined with the presence of *candida albicans* in the gut can result in an immunocompromised state that is more likely to induce subsequent mast cell activation. A study looking at mice found that after five days of antibiotic use and one dose of *candida* infiltration, mice exposed to mold spores had an increased number of mast cells and increased allergic reactions in the lungs.[66]

Bacterial Infections in the Gut

The research regarding intestinal microbiota physiology and interactions with mast cells is still in its infancy in terms of patient populations with normal mast cells.[67] Inflammation from bacterial infections such as streptococcus or staphylococcus may provoke a local immune response inside the gut.[65] Mycoplasma is another common type of bacteria, and it also induces mast cell activation in various organs including the GI tract.[67] The presence of a high number of activated mast cells from a local immune response may trigger an increase in IBS symptoms. Other cell types such as macrophages, B cells, and T cells may also contribute to gut dysbiosis.[65] Furthermore, a poor diet can essentially "feed" bad bacteria, and methane-predominant SIBO can contribute to delayed gastrointestinal transit and further inflammation.[65]

In 2015 Afrin and Khoruts performed a literature review on the interaction between mast cells and microbiota that included 140 different studies.[67] They noted, "Recent environmental factors (e.g., extensive antibiotic use, increased processed food consumption) may underlie decreases in microbiotic diversity and metabolic capacity, in turn altering the function of MCs (mast cells) which, via their proximity to nervous and endocrine system elements, crucially regulate intestinal permeability, visceral sensitivity, and gastrointestinal motility."[67]

Probiotic supplementation has become a popular topic in recent years. Animal research has found that the combination of a high-fat diet and probiotics had an anti-inflammatory response and resulted in reduced numbers of mast cells in the GI tract in mice compared to those who did not receive probiotic supplementation.[68] A high-fat diet (believed to stimulate

258

the vagus nerve) has been associated with inhibition of inflammation and the preservation of gut barrier function in animal studies.[69-72] A detailed discussed on dietary considerations and probiotics is presented in Chapter 10.

Parasitic Infections

Parasitic infections may be underlying (or possibly co-occurring with) some cases of MCAS. For example, infection with the parasite *strongyloidiasis* can provoke systemic symptoms including urticaria, angioedema, anaphylaxis, shortness of breath, coughing, and gastrointestinal issues.[73]

Early research on mast cells focused on their role as pivotal players in the immune system's response against different parasites.[74] In the case of nematodes (roundworms), a mast cell cytokine response was noted in addition to an increased number of mast cells in the gastrointestinal tract, which increased intestinal permeability to assist the body in parasite removal.[74] Furthermore, mice deficient in mast cells have a slower ability to reduce parasites from the body, and in some cases, fail to do so altogether.[75,76] In the case of infection with the parasite *Strongyloides venezuelensis*, mast cells play a role in the primary immunity and removal of eggs.[77] Similar parasite-attacking features of mast cells have been noted in a variety of different types of parasites.[78-81]

The relevance of gastrointestinal permeability to chronic clinical symptoms is still being clarified in the literature. Mice deficient in mast cells had significantly decreased gastrointestinal permeability following parasite exposure when compared to mice with normal levels of mast cells.[82] In additional mice studies, an increased parasitic burden corresponded with increased intestinal permeability, increased numbers of mast cells, elevated levels of histamine in the ileum, and increased systemic circulating histamine levels.[83]

It's possible that the mast cell-associated increase in intestinal permeability can be altered with medications. Research shows that in cases of mastocytic enterocolitis (inflammation with excess mast cells in the lining of the colon), chronic intestinal permeability has been shown to be reversible with use of H1 and H2 receptor antagonists.[84]

Malaria has also been associated with increased numbers of mast cells and ileal histamine levels that resulted in increased intestinal permeability in both mice and non-human primates.[82] The use of antihistamine medications reduced gastrointestinal permeability and yielded more promising results in mice with active malaria infections.[82]

While an increase in mast cells is important for the expulsion of parasites in the intestine, it can also result in a detrimental increase in mast cell mediators, which can cause diarrhea and intestinal malabsorption.[82] Thus, it appears that the role of mast cells in "normal" subjects exposed to parasitic infection can result in a catch-22 scenario in terms of the secondary consequences in the gastrointestinal tract. The intestinal changes are crucial for removal of the parasite to avoid widespread infection, but they also can cause debilitating symptoms, particularly when they are chronic.

When this information is coupled with what is known about the excess levels of mediators present in MCAS, it is easy to imagine that a patient exposed to parasites who also has MCAS could very well experience more gut problems than a "normal" subject. *Theoretically*, if the immune system is already compromised and they are not fully able to remove the parasitic invader, mast cells could elicit a heightened chronic response to the presence of a parasitic infection that could increase gastrointestinal issues further, similar to what can occur systemwide when the body is fighting a chronic viral or bacterial infection.

Inflammatory Bowel Disease

There's still debate about whether mast cells, dendritic cells, or macrophages (or others) are the primary cells responsible for the inflammation associated with inflammatory bowel disease (IBD) (i.e., Crohn's disease and ulcerative colitis).[57] Some experts like Hamilton believe that a secondary mast cell activation is likely occurring in patients who have both MCAS and IBD.[42] Indeed, increased levels of mast cells, mast cell mediators, and mast cell activation have been noted in patients with IBD.[85-90] Increased urinary levels of N-methylhistamine have been found in patients with IBD when compared to controls and patients in remission.[90]

Mast cell abnormalities (such as the presence of c-*KIT* mutations and CD117-positive staining) have been noted in case reports of patients who present with neurofibromatosis and ulcerative colitis.[91,92] The comorbid presence of both systemic mastocytosis and ulcerative colitis has been reported in the literature.[93] There have also been reports of Crohn's disease being misdiagnosed when the patient had underlying mastocytosis.[94,95] While interesting, these associations have not been investigated on a larger-scale manner.

Stress has long been associated with symptomatic flares in this patient population. It's been theorized that stress influences mast cell activation, inflammatory cytokines, and subsequent increased intestinal permeability in patients with IBD, creating another vicious cycle scenario.[96-98]

Some of the major drugs used in patients with Crohn's disease and ulcerative colitis may influence mast cell mediators. For example, TNF-alpha is a mediator that is commonly elevated in mucosal biopsies of patients with IBD, and adalimumab (Humira) targets this regulator of inflammation in patients with IBD.[99,100] However, TNF-alpha is released by a large number of different cells and isolated associations cannot be made.

Additional pharmacological research may shed future light onto associations between IBD and the role of dysfunctional mast cells. Even if mast cells are not the primary generators of pathology in intestinal inflammation associated with IBD, de Winter and colleagues concluded that "mast cell stabilizing drugs or drugs interfering with mast cell mediator activity may be an adjunctive therapeutic possibility in the treatment of IBD."[57]

Operations and Motility

Recent studies have also examined the feasibility of utilizing mast cells medications in the treatment of post-operative ileus. When patients have an intestinal surgery and bowel manipulation, it's common to have problems with delayed gastrointestinal motility that can lead to the development of a post-operative ileus, or reduced propulsion within the intestines that can lead to accumulates of gas and fluid in the bowels. Mast cells may contribute to this scenario by releasing pro-inflammatory mediators that further irritate the tract and increase the intestinal permeability, resulting in an increase in inflammatory infiltrates.[57]

Post-operative gastrointestinal complications including post-operative ileus are an interesting area of debate in terms of the suppression of mast cell activity. Some authors note that delayed wound healing or increased infection risk could result from medications that alter mast cell activity in post-operative patients.[57] However, the authors did not comment specifically on suggestions for post-operative care for patients who have MCAS.

Gastroparesis deserves a chapter of its own in many regards. Gastroparesis is associated with diabetes, the use of certain medications, and surgeries; however, it is often considered "idiopathic." Upper abdominal pain, nausea, vomiting, early satiety, and bloating are common symptoms of gastroparesis. Some patients may exhibit issues with ileocecal valve mechanical function, though it's unclear whether this is the main issue or simply a side effect of something else going on.

Interstitial cells of cajal (ICC) are considered the "pacemakers" for neuromuscular aspects of gastrointestinal motility, and research has noted that mast cells are found in close proximity to these cells.[101] Interestingly, the vagus nerve mediates the relaxation of gastric muscles via the

ICC.[102] While more research is needed, it's plausible that mast cell degranulation and the vagus nerve impact gastrointestinal motility through complex interactions with ICC.

Abdominal Angioedema

Abdominal angioedema has been connected to mast cell activity and is considered a type of *third spacing*.[103,104] Third spacing refers to the movement of interstitial fluid into the tissues where it does not belong. This can occur in the lungs (pulmonary edema), under the skin (angioedema), around the brain (cerebral edema) … technically anywhere in the body.

Many patients with MCAS *anecdotally* report third spacing in their abdominal cavity. This can result in a very painful ascites-like abdominal swelling that can take several hours to days to resolve. Sometimes the pain and swelling are so severe that patients appear to be in the third trimester of pregnancy. Third spacing can cause dangerous complications such as circulatory shock, life-threatening airway swelling, severe dehydration, impaired organ function, and gastrointestinal obstructions from swelling. Third spacing may be triggered by anaphylaxis in some cases,[105] though this is not the case with hereditary angioedema episodes. Abdominal angioedema has been associated with the use of angiotension-converting enzyme inhibitors (ACE inhibitors) used to manage high blood pressure.[106] However, there are numerous other mechanisms that can trigger attacks of third spacing.

While certain mast cell mediators could potentially be responsible for third spacing, in an interview in September 2017, Dr. Afrin stated that he believes that episodes of acute abdominal pain/bloating may be more connected to dysautonomia of the bowel muscles.[107] If GI transit time is delayed and the intestinal contents are left sitting stagnant, this could in theory cause a putrefaction-like process to occur, which could influence levels of certain mast cell mediators and inflammation in the intestinal tissue, further exacerbating pain and swelling and the shift of fluids to other areas. This is one theory that connects abdominal angioedema and MCAD, but clinical research is needed.

SPOTLIGHT ON HEREDITARY ANGIOEDEMA (HAE)

It's important to note that idiopathic cases of angioedema are clinically distinct from the diagnosis of hereditary angioedema (HAE). The presence of a comorbidity such as HAE *may* explain *some* cases of third spacing in patients with MCAD. It's important that physicians consider HAE investigation for patients who present with long-lasting (several-day) attacks of abdominal angioedema (or angioedema in other areas). Experts note that patients presenting with MCAS sometimes experience angioedema, and HAE should be considered on the differential diagnosis list.[22,108] Because HAE is considered a rare disease, it's often overlooked and subsequently misdiagnosed, particularly when it predominantly affects the abdomen.

Most types of HAE are caused by a lack of a protein called C1-esterase inhibitor that regulates the production of bradykinin, a chemical mediator that causes swelling and the movement of fluid outside the tissues. HAE can also be caused by a mutation in the protease factor XII. A subgroup of HAE patients are significantly impacted by estrogen levels.

HAE influences the complement system and can cause extremely painful and debilitating abdominal pain, swelling, and unnecessary surgery, in addition to swelling of the face, airway, groin, brain, extremities, and other areas.[109] Episodes of pain and swelling typically last two to five days at a time. Research notes that the severity of the pain associated with HAE has been indistinguishable from that of labor/delivery and appendicitis and in many cases has been responsible for unnecessary surgery.[110] The swelling of the airway is very distinct from anaphylaxis; with HAE, patients tend to experience a slower and more gradual airway swelling (without the presence of hives) that is longer-lasting than anaphylaxis and does not respond to antihistamines, steroids, or epinephrine.[111] Airway swelling associated with HAE is a life-threatening emergency that can cause death by asphyxiation.

It's estimated that between 1 in 10,000 and 1 in 50,000 people have HAE, classifying it as a rare disease.[109] Though the majority of HAE cases have a family history, approximately 25% of cases occur with no known family history,[112] which is attributed to a spontaneous mutation of the C1-inhibitor gene at conception. There's a 50% chance that children will inherit HAE from an affected parent.[109] Symptoms may be present before age 7, and 66% of patients reported that they became symptomatic with noticeable attacks starting by age 13.[109] The majority of patients will have HAE attacks emerge or worsen by their teenage years or early 20s.[109] It's common for patients to remain undiagnosed, sometimes for decades, and *particularly in the case of abdominal attacks, patients often experience unnecessary surgeries and multiple misdiagnoses.* The mortality rate for HAE was 30% before treatment became available in 2008.[109]

Patients with HAE report a plethora of triggers, from environmental factors and toxins (like exposure to cleaning supplies or a water-damaged building) to drops in barometric pressure, vibrations from car and airplane travel, lack of sleep, certain foods or beverages, exercise, surgery, insect bites or stings, minor trauma, illness such as the flu or a common cold, hormonal fluctuations, dental procedures, and emotional stress (both positive emotions like excitement and negative emotions like anger).[109] Many of the triggers for HAE overlap with reported triggers for MCAS.

A 2016 study found that *patients with HAE were nearly five times more likely to have the comorbid diagnosis of systemic mastocytosis* compared to the general population.[113] This implies that there may be a deeper connection between mast cells and HAE than is currently realized. *Anecdotally*, many patients in support groups report that they have true medical diagnoses of both conditions at once.

It appears that HAE and MCAS can certainly "feed off" each other. Unsurprisingly, epidemiological data on the co-prevalence of MCAS and HAE is lacking. While the medical establishment is currently unable to draw concrete conclusions about whether one may contribute to another, it's plausible that mast cell activation can trigger increased secretion of mediators that increase the severity or duration of HAE attacks.

There are some theoretical connections between HAE and MCAS that relate to mast cell mediators such as bradykinin and heparin. Research has shown that heparin released by mast cells contributes to increased vascular permeability in patients with HAE.[114] Specifically, heparin contributes directly to bradykinin formation via activation of the complement system following IgE-mediated mast cell activation. In animal studies, mice with C1 INH-deficiency had earlier vascular leakage that was longer lasting and increased in quantity following exposure to heparin, when compared to mice without C1 INH-deficiency.[114]

According to Oschatz and colleagues, heparin activates the factor XII contact system pathway which influences bradykinin generation, contributing to mast cell-related inflammation, edema, and low blood pressure.[114] In addition to bradykinin-specific mechanisms, heparin appears to play a more global role in regulating mast cell granule content and function (particularly with proteases, which are fully active enzymes that can contribute to immediate tissue injury during mast cell degranulation), so it's possible that self-regulatory feedback loops could contribute to dysfunctional mechanisms in patients who have both HAE and MCAS.[115,116]

Patients with MCAS often report low blood pressure and drops in blood pressure that are associated with presyncope and syncope during mast cell degranulation. Heparin and the combination of heparin with other substances (such as dextran sulfate in animals, which activates the complement system) have been associated with a drop in blood pressure that can be reversed with icatibant, a medication used to treat HAE attacks.[114] Icatibant (brand name Firazyr) is a selective bradykinin b2 receptor antagonist.

Researchers have also identified allergen-sensitized mast cells as an initiator of pathological edema formation in the mouse model of HAE.[114] Following this discovery, researchers had 38 HAE patients in Switzerland complete a survey identifying attack triggers.[114] Eleven out of 38

264

patients (29%) reported that swelling was associated with allergic reactions to foods.[114] In addition, 8% reported insect toxin-based triggers, and 3% noted that a drug triggered their attacks.[114]

The findings that associate food reactions with HAE attacks support the theory that mast cell-mediated mechanisms *may* be a key component to symptoms in some HAE patients. However, *anecdotally* it appears that most patients with HAE *do not* respond favorably to mast cell-targeting medications. Indeed, an angioedema symptom response to antihistamines and/or steroids is a clinical sign that the patient does *not* have HAE (but could have an "acquired" or "allergic" type of angioedema).[111] Based on this information, while MCAS may not cause HAE attacks, it's plausible that certain mast cell mediators supplement the pathways that are already occurring in HAE patients to trigger an increase in other factors such as the severity or duration of attacks.

Logically, one could imagine how a patient who is already predisposed to elevated levels of bradykinin (genetically) could see an increase in symptoms if their mast cells were hypersensitive or susceptible to increased activation via a number of different triggers. In theory, this could create a *vicious cycle between heparin, the complement system, bradykinin, mast cells, edema, pain, and inflammatory responses.* Furthermore, HAE attacks involve great deals of emotional stress and physical pain, which may very likely exacerbate a repeated pattern of increased mast cell degranulation.

Or perhaps the two conditions share other common variables at the root underlying issue. *Anecdotally*, many HAE patients report intolerance to environmental factors like secondhand cigarette smoke, candles, perfumes, cleaning supplies, laundry detergent, etc. A sluggish liver and high toxin load may contribute to mast cell "attacks" and HAE attacks in the same patient, even though the two types of attacks look very different from each other. Genetic factors may also underlie these two immune system–driven conditions. HAE typically involves low levels of complement C4 and a dysfunctional complement system, and the mutations influencing the complement system have been noted as part of the RCCX Theory (discussed in Chapter 4).

Going a step further, it would be interesting to investigate if certain viral and bacterial loads (such as Lyme disease and Epstein-Barr virus) predispose patients to the development of detoxification issues and subsequent development (or a flare-up in baseline) of HAE or MCAS. Hopefully future research will investigate this area.

In summary, while HAE attacks are distinct from anaphylactic attacks in both mechanism and characteristics, it appears that mast cell mediators and mast cell activation can trigger an increase in factors that may contribute to the intensity or frequency of HAE attacks, and the stress and pain associated with HAE attacks may very well translate to an elevated baseline of inflammation and mast cell activity. This may very well be confounded by the presence of dysautonomia, viruses, bacteria, and other comorbidities or dysfunctional processes that may impair aspects such as gastrointestinal motility or systemwide detoxification. Hopefully the future will bring more concrete research on potential mechanisms between third spacing, HAE and MCAS. Patients with MCAS who experience recurrent episodes of severe third spacing should be strongly encouraged to investigate the possibility of HAE or idiopathic angioedema with their medical team.

FIBROMYALGIA SYNDROME (FMS)

As a physical therapist, fibromyalgia syndrome (FMS) is one of the more frustrating diagnoses to treat, simply because it is poorly characterized by the medical community and tends to describe a cluster of symptoms of mysterious origin that often come with a social hypochondriac stigma. This stigma is inappropriate, and it's more likely that patients with fibromyalgia are suffering with some kind of hidden, chronic and debilitating condition with underlying viral, bacterial, or inflammatory origins.

FMS is characterized by chronic and widespread musculoskeletal pain that is usually accompanied by soft tissue tenderness in trigger point areas, fatigue, cognitive symptoms, bowel and bladder symptoms, and impaired sleep. Patients often report a heightened pain response to light pressure. While the exact cause is undetermined, the condition has been theorized to have connections to a number of conditions such as Lyme disease, chronic fatigue syndrome, post-traumatic stress disorder, irritable bowel syndrome, restless leg syndrome, and others.[117] One review noted that patients with joint hypermobility syndrome are more likely to be diagnosed with fibromyalgia, indicating that there may be a potential connection within hypermobile-type EDS patients.[118]

Li and Ehrlich described fibromyalgia as a wastebasket disease—"defined out of a complex of complaints that could not be attributed to any established diseases diagnosable or treatable by specialists." Essentially, in many cases, fibromyalgia appears to be the label that patients are given when the constraints of the medical system lack ample time for a thorough patient history and testing, or when the doctor doesn't know what to do with the patient.

A 2016 study looking at 105 patients with FMS and 105 controls found that dermatological symptoms such as itching, tingling, burning, and increased sweating were increased in the FMS group.[119] In addition, 92.4% of the FMS group reported cutaneous symptoms and 78.1% of the FMS group had prior diagnosis of at least one dermatological disease.[119] Pruritis was the most common skin symptom reported, with 69.5% of FMS patients reporting skin itching, compared to 24.8% of patients in the control group.[119]

Some theorize that overactive mast cells could be behind the etiology of fibromyalgia. Recent research has begun to focus on mast cell characteristics in fibromyalgia skin biopsies. One study evaluated patients with fibromyalgia compared to patients with rheumatoid arthritis, whiplash injuries, and healthy controls.[120] The authors found that the patients with fibromyalgia had significantly higher signs of degranulated mast cells in the dermis and vessel walls and had a higher reactivity for type III collagen when compared to the other subjects.[120] However, this study had a relatively small sample size.

Mast cells in the skin of patients with FMS were both increased in number and altered in shape (spindle-shaped) in a 2010 study.[121] Researchers evaluated the number of mast cells in the skin of patients with fibromyalgia and controls and found that all patients with fibromyalgia had increased numbers of mast cells, in some cases up to 14 times the quantity of mast cells of the control group.[121]

Musculoskeletal pain is a common concern in patients with MCAS. One study noted that approximately 75% of MCAD patients report musculoskeletal pain, numbness, and tingling that is likely a manifestation of mast cell chemical mediators.[122] A 2017 review by Wirz and Molderings noted that pain is one of the most severe symptoms in patients with MCAD and concluded that a subset of patients with fibromyalgia syndrome may be the clinical manifestation of MCAD.[41] Mast cells may play a role in the actual perception of pain via a number of different mechanisms that revolve around the proximity of mast cells to nerves, the communication pathways, and the chemical mediators that continue to propagate inflammation, as already discussed.

Inflammatory mast cell chemical mediators have been studied in patients with fibromyalgia. In 2016, researchers at Tufts University evaluated 84 patients with FMS and found that serum levels of corticotropin releasing hormone (CRH), substance P, and hemokinin-1 were elevated in the FMS group compared to controls.[117] They also found that certain inflammatory cytokines released by mast cells, including tumor necrosis factor (TNF) and interleukin-6 (IL-6) were elevated, while other cytokines (such as interleukin 31 and interleukin 33) were found at lower levels in the same patient group.[117] Substance P is of particular interest, as it is released by both neurons and mast cells, and it leads to the production of prostaglandins, histamine, leukotrienes, TNF, and IL-6.[38] CRH is also responsible for the release of TNF and IL-6 from mast cells. The authors concluded that the elevated levels of these particular inflammatory mast cell mediators could potentially be connected to the etiology of FMS.[117]

Genetic research has begun to uncover specific genes that are differentially expressed in patients with FMS. While more research is certainly needed, preliminary research with 70 patients with FMS and 70 controls found hundreds of genes that differed significantly between the two groups, and some of these genes may potentially play big roles in allergic reactions and systemic inflammation.[123] For example, the gene CPA3 is a biomarker for mast cell degranulation and was expressed in a different manner between groups in the study. Inflammatory cytokines and FMS diagnosis were strongly correlated in the study.[123]

Research is beginning to investigate the use of mast cell stabilization medications and antihistamines in the treatment of fibromyalgia. A 2016 study evaluated the use of common mast cell stabilizer ketotifen (in maintenance dose levels of 4 mg) as part of a 10-week randomized, double-blind, placebo-controlled trial with 51 patients diagnosed with fibromyalgia.[124] Authors concluded that there were no significant differences in pain sensitivity or overall self-perceived fibromyalgia symptom severity between the patients who received the ketotifen compared to the placebo.[124] However, when compared to the study showing that ketotifen improved IBS symptoms, this study used a significantly lower dosage of the medication, which could explain the lack of significant differences between groups. It's also possible that mast cells do not play a central role in the etiology of fibromyalgia, though nonpharmacological studies beg to differ.

In revisiting the possibility that fibromyalgia is associated with MCAS, definitive conclusions cannot be made yet. It's possible that overactive mast cells release chemical mediators that cause increased hypersensitivity of muscles and tendons, similar to the mechanism observed in the abdominal visceral contents. It's also possible that some other underlying source of inflammation is the main driver of fibromyalgia, and as a result, the condition triggers a secondary surge of mast cell activity in dermal tissue (and elsewhere).

MYALGIC ENCEPHALOMYELITIS/CHRONIC FATIGUE SYNDROME (ME/CFS)

Many patients with MCAS report severe and disabling fatigue, muscular heaviness, and exhaustion triggered by minor everyday activities. Myalgic encephalomyelitis/chronic fatigue syndrome (ME/CFS) appears to be a common diagnostic comorbidity with MCAS. Poor sleep, depression and anxiety, impaired memory and concentration, post-exertional malaise, joint pain, muscle pain, and headaches are symptoms that often accompany disabling fatigue in patients with ME/CFS.[125]

One theory about the origins of ME/CFS focuses on developmental immunotoxicities acquired prenatally. Many patients associate mold and other toxin exposure to periods where the disease becomes more severe. Some associate histamine with the symptoms of the disease. Many studies have focused on the measurement of cytokines, hormones, neurotransmitters, and infectious agents in the etiology of ME/CFS, but no current theory is universally accepted that explains the root cause of the condition.

Mast cells have been theorized to be associated with ME/CFS by Theoharides and colleagues.[126] Specifically, mast cells in the diencephalon area of the brain could be responsible for some of the physiological pathways responsible for ME/CFS symptoms.[126]

Theoharides and colleagues have discussed the effects of different medications in the treatment of ME/CFS. They noted that tricyclic antidepressants have been shown to be effective in patients with ME/CFS and chronic pain and noted that tricyclic antidepressants also have mast cell inhibition properties.[127] Flavonoid compounds that inherently possess mast cell stabilizing properties have also shown successful results in animal studies for ME/CFS.[128,129]

The sparse available research in mast cell connections to ME/CFS is a far cry from anything conclusive. It's possible that ME/CFS could actually be a label for a cluster of symptoms that are derived from MCAS in a subset of patients, or it could be more connected to mold toxins, infectious disease, genetic mutations, or other undetermined factors.

NEUROPSYCHOLOGICAL CONDITIONS: ANXIETY, DEPRESSION AND AUTISM SPECTRUM DISORDERS

Anxiety and Depression

Neuropsychiatric symptoms are common in patients with MCAS, and the prognosis appears positive once underlying mechanisms are addressed. An article by Afrin and colleagues asserted, "Significantly helpful treatment—including for neuropsychiatric issues—usually can be identified once MCAD is accurately diagnosed."[130]

Exactly how much do mast cells play a role in mood? There are some authors who assert that depression is simply an "allergic response to inflammation." Some go as far as to even point to the fact that there are more suicides in the spring when pollen counts are higher. A 2015 systematic review concluded that existing literature indicates that there is a link between allergies and suicide mortality.[131] However, the results for associations between allergies and nonfatal suicidal behaviors were mixed and more research is needed.[131]

Past significant, traumatic events may have both short- and long-term effects on a cellular level. Childhood traumatic experiences are associated with changes in white blood cells and inflammatory processes in adults affected by post-traumatic stress disorder (PTSD).[132] It appears that mast cells play a key role in stress-associated changes and neuroinflammation observed in PTSD, and mast cell activation may influence further development of neurodegenerative and neuroinflammatory diseases, including Alzheimer's disease.[133]

History of physical and sexual abuse are obvious stressors associated with disease, but other types of childhood adversity also appear to significantly increase one's risk of developing depression and cancer as an adult. A 2016 systematic review found that a number of factors including growing up with divorced parents, feeling belittled or humiliated by a parent, neglect, victimization from sibling or peer abuse, family financial difficulties or parental unemployment, or living with a depressed, alcoholic, or incarcerated parent were associated with an increased risk for disease and, in particular, cancer.[134]

There's a good amount of evidence that backs up the connections between mast cell activation and neuropsychiatric conditions. Inflammatory cytokines released by mast cells have been theorized to play a role in depression. Elevated cytokine levels such as interleukin-6 have been found in the brains of suicide victims, and the most violent suicide attempts were associated with the highest levels of inflammatory cytokines.[135] Interleukin 1-beta, Interleukin-6 and tumor necrosis factor (TNF)-alpha were noted in elevated quantities in the prefrontal cortex of teenage suicide victims.[136] A 2013 systematic review noted that the majority of existing evidence associates interleukins, TNF-alpha, and vascular endothelial growth factor (VEGF) with suicidal behavior.[137] They concluded that while an imbalance in immune system function is associated with suicidal ideations and tendencies, this information does not imply the existence of a causal link.[137]

Depression has been associated with high numbers of mast cells in the large intestinal mucosa in patients with IBS.[138] Human studies have also made associations between patients with food allergy and gastrointestinal inflammation and anxiety/depression.[139]

The gastrointestinal tract has been the focus of much research regarding mast cells due to its ease of evaluation using tissue sample stains, but brain mast cell activity has also been evaluated extensively in the literature. According to a 2014 review, an increase in both the number and the activation of peripheral and brain mast cells have been associated with neuroinflammation and chronic pelvic pain.[140] The authors concluded that mast cells may be a viable target for multifactorial management of depression and pain.[140]

Brain mast cells have been shown to be activated by acute stress, which in turn leads to increased permeability of the blood–brain barrier.[141] The blood–brain barrier is a membrane of endothelial cells that normally separates circulating blood from the fluid around the brain. When this barrier is altered, certain molecules such as neurotransmitters are able to pass through and have a more direct impact on the brain, which in theory could trigger more neuropsychiatric symptoms.

As a review of the mechanisms that are responsible for mast cell-associated brain inflammation, in response to physiological and emotional stress, mast cells are activated by a number of different substances that bind to Fc receptors, including cytokines, immunoglobulins other than IgE, neuropeptides, and anaphylatoxins.[141] Corticotropin releasing-hormone (CRH) is one example of a neuropeptide that can activate mast cells, and CRH-linked mast cell activation is believed to be one of the main culprits for the increase in the permeability of the blood–brain barrier.[142] The role of mast cells in controlling what enters the brain area is supported by the observation that mast cell-deficient mice did not exhibit changes to the blood–brain barrier when experiencing stress.[142]

The activation of CRH-1 receptors on mast cells or sensory nuclei leads to the release of vasoactive mediators including histamine, nitrous oxide, interleukin-6, tumor necrosis factor, and vasoactive intestinal peptide, which all contribute to increased permeability of the blood–brain barrier. These substances can cause a *selective* release of chemical mediators from mast cells without a global or "overt" degranulation occurring.[141]

The hypothalamus is the part of the brain that connects the nervous system to the endocrine system and it is considered a key regulatory area that contributes to symptoms of anxiety and depression. One of the major regulators of this brain area is histamine.[143] Histamine is a key player than can specifically trigger the release of CRH in the brain[144] which then increases blood–brain barrier permeability and subsequent brain mast cell activation, which can lead to the release of more histamine. On top of that, research supports that mast cells are not only *affected by* CRH but are also the *source* of CRH synthesis and secretion.[145]

In addition to depression, brain mast cells are believed to modulate anxiety. When levels of CRH rise in a brain area called the central amygdala, there's an increase in stress-induced tonic activity in a zone of neurons called the locus coeruleus, which results in symptoms of acute anxiety and aversion to certain places.[146] This anxiogenic activity is completely reversible with the use of a CRH receptor antagonist, indicating that CRH could be a main trigger in anxiety attacks.[146]

Studies evaluating mice have noted that allergic responses correspond to anxiety-like behavior and activation of the adrenal system.[147,148] Norepinephrine is another neurotransmitter that has been connected to the anxiety response.[146] Histamine has been shown to regulate the release of norepinephrine in the hypothalamus and cardiac tissue of both animal models and humans. [149,150]

Serotonin has been the focus of a specific class of medications used to treat depression in the pharmaceutical industry. Nautiyal and colleagues note, "Selective serotonin reuptake inhibitors increase serotonin signaling and decrease anxiety; therefore, a lack of mast cell derived serotonin may result in an increase in anxiety-like behaviors."[151] However, experts concur that the influences of mast cells on the brain are likely due to a variety of chemical mediators as opposed to one specific culprit.[151]

A 2008 study evaluated blocking peripheral versus central (brain) mast cells in mice via the use of cromolyn sodium (which does not cross the blood–brain barrier).[151] Researchers found no effect on anxiety-like behavior when the cromolyn was injected peripherally but did see a change in anxiety when the cromolyn blockade was applied in the brain, indicating that mast cell induced anxiety is mediated centrally in the brain.[151]

The interplay between mast cells and substances such as histamine, serotonin, CRH, and norepinephrine is complicated. It's likely that the chronic presence of these mediators in combination with an increase in blood–brain barrier permeability can lead to a vicious cycle of anxiety and depression coupled with mediator-induced inflammation, headaches, and neurotoxicity—all of which can have a significant impact on mental health.

Autism Spectrum Disorders (ASD)

While not causal, the research on autism does indicate that associations exist between mast cell activation/degranulation and the development of autism spectrum disorders (ASD). MCAS-specific research is lacking, but studies on patients with mastocytosis do shed some light onto potential connections between mast cells and autism.

Children with mastocytosis have a ten-fold higher prevalence (1 in 10) of autism compared to the general population.[152] With the general prevalence of autism at 1 in 100 and the general prevalence of mastocytosis 1 in 4,000 (as of 2009), this statistic is quite profound.[152] (A more recent study in 2014 noted that 1 in 68 people in the general population have ASD, but that is still approximately 1.5% of the population compared to 10% of patients with mastocytosis.)[153]

There are different theories about the etiology of autism that support a mast cell component. Theoharides and colleagues have connected the increasing cases of ASD with mast cell activation by allergic, infectious, environmental, and neuroimmune triggers that result in an inflammatory chemical disruption of the blood–brain barrier and/or the activation of susceptibility genes.[152] Some theorize that chronic fatigue and fibromyalgia are actually adult-onset autism emerging after an overload of toxins and virus exposure. Known toxins that trigger mast cells, such as heavy metals (beyond mercury) and environmental chemical exposure, both prenatally and in youth, have been (somewhat controversially) associated with the development of autism. The presence of heavy metals, for example, may block the actions of acetylcholine, an important neurotransmitter that impacts vagus nerve function.

The role of heavy metals and environmental factors in the development of autism continues to be disputed, yet less than one-third of cases of autism are considered to have genetic ties.[154] A number of studies note trends between ASD and prenatal exposure to alcohol, cigarettes, cocaine, and pesticides,[155,156] childhood deficiency in elements such as zinc and manganese or excess amounts of copper, lead, mercury, and cadmium,[157-159] premature birth that may result in poor gut and blood–brain barrier protection,[160] use of aluminum cookware, consumption of fish, and exposure to pollution from industrial facilities,[159,161] and the list goes on!

A 2016 literature review concluded, "Environmental causes especially some heavy metal deficiency and some excess of heavy metals are widely discussed with accumulating evidence. However, we are still far away from identifying the central pathogenic mechanism of ASD development thus delaying an effective treatment method."[154]

Direct damage to the vagus nerve may also play a role. Viral infections can influence vigorous immune system activity and viral-associated "cytokine storms" can have a significant influence on the nervous system, the vagus nerve, and the subsequent balance between sympathetic and parasympathetic nervous system tone.[162] Chronic damage to the vagus nerve has been associated with poor digestion, visual-auditory hyperreactivity, performing repetitive motions to calm oneself and induce more parasympathetic nervous system tone, impaired recognition of social cues and others' emotions, and difficulty with detoxification—all hallmark signs of ASD.[163-165]

Theoharides is leading the way with research regarding ASD and such disorders' potential connection to MCAS. According to Theoharides and colleagues, "Perinatal mast cell activation by infectious, stress-related, environmental or allergic triggers can lead to release of pro-inflammatory and neurotoxic molecules, thus contributing to brain inflammation and ASD pathogenesis, at least in a subgroup of ASD patients."[160]

Patients with ASD frequently report allergy-like symptoms, including the presence of urticaria.[160] Allergic problems, including asthma, rhinitis, food allergies, and atopic dermatitis, have been reported at a higher prevalence in patients with autism and Asperger syndrome than in those in the general population.[166-168] Maternal factors during pregnancy, such as the presence of atopic dermatitis, asthma, hay fever, and psoriasis, also appear to increase the risk of development of ASD.[169] However, most of the allergy association research is based on case studies or parental report of symptoms, which limits its interpretation.[160]

In 2010, Angelidou and colleagues evaluated blood samples from 19 children with autism and 16 controls. They discovered the neurotensin was significantly higher in the serum of children who had autism compared to controls.[170] Neurotensin is a mast cell mediator that may have a direct effect on both brain inflammation and ASD. Stress-associated increases in corticotropin releasing-hormone (CRH) may also influence the development of autism prenatally or perinatally.[160] Neurotensin's release by mast cells is triggered by CRH and it may also impact DNA and potential autoimmune-type reactions. Further research by the same group found that neurotensin "induces release of extracellular mitochondrial DNA (mtDNA) that could act as 'autoimmune' triggers"; ASD was associated with anti-mitochondrial antibodies.[171]

In 2014, a Tufts University research group determined that elevated serum neurotensin levels in children with ASD are significantly associated with gastrointestinal symptoms.[153] Interestingly, the same study also evaluated a group of bull terriers (dogs) that exhibited repetitive tail-chasing, similar to behavioral phenotypes associated with autism. When compared to "non–tail-chasing" dogs of the same breed, the tail-chasers (or dogs exhibiting signs similar to ASD) had significantly elevated levels of both CRH and neurotensin.[153]

Kempuraj and colleagues have also looked into the potential links between exposure to low doses of mercury (such as those found in vaccines) and autism. Their research found that mercuric chloride in concentrations as low as 0.1 μM triggered the release of pro-inflammatory vasoactive chemical mediators from mast cells, including vascular endothelial growth factor (VEGF) and interleukin-6.[172] These mediators contribute to inflammation and could also impact the permeability of the blood–brain barrier, as discussed in the depression and anxiety section.

Research into medications for the treatment of ASD may shed additional light on the potential relevance of mast cell activity on symptoms. Cyproheptadine, a serotonin- and histamine-receptor antagonist, provided a significant reduction in symptoms of ASD when compared to haloperidol, an antipsychotic medication.[173] Theoharides and colleagues assert that antioxidant and anti-inflammatory flavonoid supplementation (such as quercetin and luteolin, and their associated products commonly trialed with MCAS) appears to be beneficial with this patient population.[174]

While it was not a blinded randomized controlled trial, in 2012 Theoharides and colleagues did investigate the supplementation of a blend of luteolin, quercetin, and rutin in a liposomal formation utilizing olive kernel oil (known as Neuroprotek) in a group of 37 patients with ASD who had not responded to other forms of treatment.[175] After a four-month treatment time, the authors noted that "GI and allergy symptoms improved in about 75% of children, eye contact and attention in 50%, social interaction in 25% and resumption of speech in about 10%."[175] This supplementation was previously shown to be significantly effective in the stabilization of mast cells[176-179]—more so than cromolyn, according to one study[180]—so these findings implicate that "natural" mast cell stabilization may reduce symptoms of autism, though additional research is certainly needed.

In summary of the available research on autism, Theoharides states that "subjects with ASD susceptibility genes and hypersensitive mast cells may represent a unique subgroup of patients who are more likely to respond to environmental and stress triggers, leading to worsening ASD."[160] It appears that a complex interaction between epigenetics, mast cell triggers, inflammation, and disruption of the gastrointestinal and blood–brain barrier may play a role in the development of autism spectrum disorders.

CHAPTER KEY POINTS

- There are a number of different comorbidities that are commonly reported in patients with MCAS.

- Ehlers-Danlos syndrome (EDS) is a disease of the connective tissue in the body. MCAS appears to be associated with hypermobile EDS, and patients may experience significant joint problems, pain, and dislocations.

- Chiari malformation, intracranial pressure issues, and tethered cord syndrome have occurred in patients with EDS and may need to be considered in a subgroup of patients with MCAS. Vagus nerve impairments may also play a role in altered parasympathetic nervous system tone and digestive issues in these patients.

- Postural orthostatic tachycardia syndrome (POTS) is a condition where the heart rate elevates with changes in body position, and it may be associated with the interplay between mast cell activation, the nervous system, and connective tissue abnormalities that influence blood vessels.

- A wide array of gastrointestinal and abdominal concerns tend to be present in the patient who has MCAS. Fibromyalgia and myalgic encephalomyelitis/chronic fatigue syndrome also appear to be common and potentially associated with mast cell activation.

- Neuropsychological conditions including anxiety, depression, and autism also appear to be highly prevalent in the MCAD population and may be associated with mast cell activation and high levels of inflammatory mast cell mediators.

Chapter Eight

Common Root Issues

CANARIES IN A COAL MINE

Several functional medicine and naturopathic medicine professionals use the analogy of patients with MCAS and other chronic illnesses being "canaries in a coal mine." Back in the day, coal miners would take yellow canaries (birds) into the mines with them while they were working. Yellow canaries are notorious for being extra sensitive to carbon monoxide. When the birds would start passing out, the miners knew that it was time to leave the area to avoid carbon monoxide poisoning.

In medicine, yellow canaries are those extra-special patients who have environmental sensitivities and often present with diagnoses of multiple chemical sensitivity. Yellow canaries are the patients who are most susceptible to environmental triggers, including toxins. If the yellow canary patient can remove predictable triggers from their system's total load, in theory they should have a more stable baseline of health. Logically, this can lead to less strain on the liver, fewer mast cell mediators in the bloodstream and a better overall homeostatic balance.

Patients with MCAS and other yellow canaries ought to prioritize *the elimination of toxic triggers* as opposed to increasing dosages of mast cell medications (while maintaining the same toxin exposure), though a combination of both medications and avoidance may be necessary initially. The effort put in may dictate the outcome, though progress can be slow in this area. Patients who decide that they can't do without processed foods, toxic beauty products, or other sources may not reap the same benefits as patients who commit to a long-term lifestyle change. For some patients, toxin elimination may mean minor changes, such as the addition of a tap water filter and use of an air purifier in the house, the consideration of EMF reduction, and a change in food sources and practices. For others, it may mean making large life changes in living location, particularly if mycotoxins are detected in the home.

While *it's not fair* to be that extra-sensitive person, and it's tempting to get discouraged when comparing oneself to others, it's important to remember that some people can get away with the same toxin exposures with no noticeable effect, *but this does not mean that the toxins are not influencing them negatively under the surface.* For the seemingly immune neighbors, toxin exposure could very well translate to the development of disease down the road. Non-canaries are still at risk, though the process may take longer to experience the same toxic build-up.

TOXIC OVERLOAD

The current industrialized world faces numerous hidden environmental toxins on a daily basis. It's easy for many to dismiss this topic on the basis of appearing like a paranoid conspiracy theorist. However, addressing toxins should be one of the biggest priorities for patients with MCAS and other chronic illnesses. Failing to address this area means that a patient will fail to unlock a dramatic gold mine of healing potential.

Toxicant-induced loss of tolerance (TILT) describes either a series of low-level exposures or a one-time major exposure to toxins that is followed by a loss of tolerance to foods, drugs, and chemicals that previously did not bother the patient.[1] This phenomenon was *not* described to explain the mechanism behind *every* illness, but according to the Hoffman Tilt Foundation, "it's an overlooked process that may occur at the same time as other health problems."[1] TILT is a theory that could explain why many patients with MCAS and other chronic disease, though typically presenting with a long-standing history of chronic ailments, also will report a point in time when they suddenly found themselves unable to tolerate everyday substances and foods.[1]

In 2017, Dr. Pizzorno released a book called "The Toxin Solution: How Hidden Poisons in the Air, Water, Food, and Products We Use Are Destroying Our Health—AND WHAT WE CAN DO TO FIX IT."[2] He noted that not only can toxins contribute to different symptoms and diseases, but they may also serve as a catastrophic catalyst when coupled with the right conditions.[2] "Toxins damage every aspect of our physiological function and play a role in virtually all diseases. They don't act alone. They interact with other factors in our health environment and in many cases *magnify* the disruption caused by other factors."[2]

The human body has mechanisms in place to clear out toxins. *Why then, all of a sudden, does it seem that the younger generations are struggling so greatly to "detoxify?"* Is this growing catchphrase a trend, or is there truth to it?

There appears to be great evidence behind the alarmingly increased toxic burden that humans are exposed to all over the world. Fifty years ago, air quality and soil quality were different, and the body was less burdened with filtering out all of the noise from the

278

environment. However, today the body is faced with a higher toxic load burden, and for most people the amount of exposure exceeds the body's processing ability. When the body is not able to break toxins down, it's forced to sequester them in the bloodstream or tissues somehow until it has an efficient way to remove them.[2] In the cases of certain heavy metals, like lead, the body will store them in the bones until the bones begin to break down (such as during hormonal changes like menopause in women) when they may be released again.

Pizzorno explains, "Many of these hundreds and thousands of chemical toxins simply didn't exist prior to the mid-twentieth century. Our grandparents undoubtedly faced their own unique stressors, but they were nothing like the barrage of chemicals, heavy metals, radiation, electromagnetic frequencies, and pollution that batter people today. Although the human body has an innate capacity to detoxify itself, people are now exposed to a level of consumer, agricultural, and industrial toxins that the human organism never evolved to handle."[2]

In addition to exposure over one's lifetime, humans can be exposed to such toxins prenatally. It appears that each generation is more and more likely to start life as a newborn with a higher toxic burden than their parents' generation, simply from the higher level of toxins that are passed from the mother to the growing fetus.

The Environmental Working Group (EWG) conducted a study in 2005 that examined the umbilical cord blood of 10 newborns.[3] They detected 287 chemicals, of which 208 cause birth defects, 217 are toxic to the brain and nervous system, and 180 are linked to cancer.[3] Flame-retardants, pesticides, gasoline, consumer product ingredients, and waste from burning coal and garbage were some of the sources associated with the measured toxins.[3]

Toxins themselves have been linked to numerous diseases and symptoms, but public knowledge may only encompass a superficial understanding of this. The movie-famous Erin Brockovich, who helped fight for the residents of Hinkley, California, after they were exposed to drinking water contaminated with hexavalent chromium, is an example of one obvious source of toxins.

But the reality is, regular daily effects of hidden toxins are commonly found to be slow, stealthy, and less obvious. Environmental toxins can cause more gradual and silent chronic ailments that go undetected. Over time, neurotoxicity can lead to memory and cognitive decline, headaches, or motor and sensory difficulties associated with brain atrophy, edema, changes in blood flow, alterations to nerve myelin, and influences on receptors and metabolism.[4] Endocrine toxicity can impair metabolic function and is connected to libido and reproductive issues.[5] Immunotoxicity appears connected to everything from asthma and allergies to chronic disease and cancer.[6] Different types of toxins can also act in a detrimentally synergistic manner. For example, aluminum and pesticides create more cell damage when they are both present than when either is alone.[2]

Toxins can also damage DNA, alter gene expression and cause damage on the cellular level.[7] *Could this information apply to the spontaneous, non-heritable mutations that researchers are uncovering in patients with MCAS and other chronic illness?*

Not only do toxins impact the major organs and the body's ability to detoxify, but they may have a direct impact on mast cells. One study found a 72% increase in mast cell degranulation after high-dose, short-term exposure to diesel exhaust fumes.[8] When diesel exhaust particles were combined with exposure to dust mites, histamine levels in nasal wash samples increased threefold![8]

It's been well-established that heavy metal exposure, and in particular mercury, may be associated with autism spectrum disorders. A 2010 study investigated the effects of mercury on human mast cells and found that mercury elicited a degranulation response of histamine, cytokines, vascular endothelial growth factor (VEGF), and interleukin six (IL-6).[9] The authors concluded that this process could influence what crosses the blood–brain barrier and could contribute to the development of autism spectrum disorders.[9]

It seems that much of conventional medicine has been turning a blind eye to the research that confirms the dangers of an increasing toxic burden. In some cases, there appears to be a disconnect between medical provider acknowledgment of the presence of everyday toxins and how these toxins may translate to symptom and pathology development in chronically ill patients. Clinically, one major challenge is the lack of priority given for toxin testing and treatment options. Poor insurance coverage and limited reliability for such tests further complicates matters.

Regulatory agencies are in place to protect consumers, but allowed chemicals vary across different countries. There are some pretty alarming statistics out there about the United States toxin regulations (or lack thereof). According to the Natural Resource Defense Council, there are 80,000 synthetic chemicals out there, most of which have not undergone full testing.[10] Only 11 chemicals are banned in the U.S., compared to over 650 in Canada and over 1,300 in Europe.[10]

In the U.S., the cosmetic industry's panel has only evaluated a small portion (about 11%) of the cosmetic ingredients in the FDA.[10] Perfumes in particular are worrisome, as the word "parfum" is not regulated and could potentially mean a cocktail of harmful chemicals.[10] Perhaps more shocking is the fact there are no laws in place to regulate the words "natural" and "organic" on personal care products.[10]

Common Toxin Sources

Regularly-encountered toxin sources may include poor air quality, chemicals in drinking water and food sources, additional types of heavy metal exposure, and exposure to other environmental possibilities such as mycotoxins that come from water-damaged buildings. Toxins can enter the human bloodstream simply by breathing or by skin contact/absorption. Toxins are present in nail salons and electronic products and are the by-products of living in an increasingly industrialized world. However, there are a number of other toxins that humans are exposed to on a regular basis that need to be examined.

The Agency for Toxic Substances Disease Registry recommends that parents consider the former use of the site, nearby sites/activities, naturally occurring contamination, and the safety of drinking water when seeking a safe location for childcare.[11] There are agricultural and industrial toxins, such as pesticides, hormones, herbicides, pollution, and radiation.[12] Household and workplace toxins may circulate from building materials, rugs, paint, cleaning supplies, and the presence of dangerous materials like asbestos.[12] Toxins are in personal care products, including health and beauty aids, perfumes, and cosmetics.[12] Toxins can impact residents who live near fracking wells, power plants, and sources of coal burning.[12]

Food toxins—including genetically modified organisms (GMOs), food coloring, artificial flavors, preservatives and artificial sweeteners—are becoming increasingly embedded in the food supply.[12] Even organic food sources from grocery stores may not be immune to certain toxins. Short of a home-grown garden, it's difficult to know for certain what exactly the crops have been exposed to. In addition, herbal and other over-the-counter supplements may be toxin-contaminated.[13]

The danger of phthalates are becoming better known in the consumer world, where they can be present in everything from children's toys and makeup to plastic containers.[10] According to the Natural Resources Defense Council, "Phthalates can seep into food through equipment used in processing plants such as tubing, gloves, conveyor belts, lids, adhesives, and plastic wraps."[10] Vinyl items in the home such as blinds, flooring, and shower curtains most likely contain phthalates.[10] Air fresheners contain phthalates, even those labeled as "natural" or "unscented."[10]

Everyday items in the kitchen are hidden toxin sources. Plastic from water bottles, milk jugs, and food storage containers leach into food and beverages.[10] Pizza boxes and popcorn bags aren't safe either! Pizza boxes tend to be treated with perfluorinated alkylated substances (PFAs) which increase water and grease stain resistance.[10] Nonstick cookware, stain resistant fabric/carpet, and Goretex clothing are other common sources of PFAs,[10] and the toxin is associated with liver, pancreas, thyroid and hormone abnormalities.[14]

It's becoming more common knowledge that seafood such as canned tuna, marlin, and sea bass have higher mercury levels. Silver dental amalgams are also high-risk factors for release of mercury in the body. Certain jewelry and household products like broken thermometers, thermostats, and switches may be other sources of mercury exposure. A 2010 review noted that "mercurials may be found in various drugs, in bleaching creams, antiseptics, disinfectants, as preservatives in cosmetics, tooth pastes, lens solutions, vaccines, contraceptives and immunotherapy solutions, fungicides, herbicides and in dental fillings, as well as in fish such as tuna due to water pollution."[9] There's great debate about vaccinations that will be discussed later in this book, but it's important to note that mercury is present in many more everyday products than one may realize.

Additional concerning substances include[15]:

- Arsenic found in rice, non-organic chicken and water

- Benzene found in soda and cigarettes

- Cadmium found in batteries and plastics

- Chloroform (by-product of chlorine) found in water

- Lead found in old paint, antique jewelry, and old plumbing/drinking water

- Vinyl chloride found in dry-cleaning chemicals and cigarettes

- Polychlorinated biphenyls found in non–wild-caught fish ("farmed fish") and certain plastic products

- Polycyclic aromatic hydrocarbons produced from asphalt, burning coal, cigarettes, and charred meats

Tattoos have been associated with chemical toxicity and the masking of cutaneous disease and malignancy.[16,17] Polycyclic aromatic hydrocarbons and phenols are present in black tattoo ink, and it appears that tattoo ink is unregulated and often used for other tasks like printing and painting cars.[18] In addition to the ink-associated risks, tattoo complications can include bacterial and viral infections, localized and generalized inflammatory problems, hepatitis and infectious endocarditis.[19]

The dangers may not be isolated to permanent tattoos. Paraphenylenediamine is a chemical in temporary henna tattoos that has been associated with severe reactions and even fatalities.[20]

Tattoo removal procedures may also pose hazards; a case report noted cardiotoxicity and death in one patient.[21]

There are enough reputable sources on everyday toxins to make one's mind spin! And if one is exposed to these toxins regularly, it's easy to imagine how after a few decades, and certainly by middle age, this could very well trigger a number of symptoms and health conditions, particularly if the body has an inefficient or "clogged" toxin elimination system.

How Does the Body Get Rid of Toxins?

The liver, kidneys, skin, and gastrointestinal tract are some of the body's most important detoxification passageways. Sluggish and dysfunctional livers are more common than one would think. The typical blood tests may only pick up abnormalities with end-stage organ issues, so blood work alone is not ideal for determining if the liver is *thriving* or simply *surviving*. As noted in Chapter 3, an alarming number of patients with MCAS tend to have some type of liver abnormality on testing.

Pizzorno notes that a poorly functioning liver can negatively impact the body's ability to clear certain mast cell mediators.[2] "Liver enzymes break down unwanted chemicals so that they can be harmlessly released, or bound to molecules that render them inactive and easier to excrete. This process renders inactive: inflammatory chemicals, such as histamines and prostaglandins in addition to other chemicals, toxins and drugs."[2]

Logically, if a patient has a sluggish liver, a high toxic burden, and MCAS, it's like a triple whammy. Dietary fiber and gastrointestinal motility also play a role in detoxification, and when the gastrointestinal system is sluggish, the body may *reabsorb toxins* when it cannot eliminate them efficiently.

The ability to remove toxins is influenced by mitochondrial function, exercise, glutathione, nutrients, and thyroid function.[2] When the system has chronic diseases processes occurring on top of a toxic load exposure (which is presumably the case for the majority of people reading this book and a large percentage of people in westernized cultures), the toxins and by-products of other issues can fuel each other.

Symptoms may be specific to the heavy metal that is in excess—though, *anecdotally*, an individual patient with chronic illness often presents with an excess of multiple heavy metals. Elevations in certain heavy metals, like lead, can lead to elevated intracranial pressure and edema.[22] Other heavy metals like cadmium may influence zinc levels and reduce gastrointestinal absorption.[22] These are just *two examples of the 35 metals* that are of largest concern for humans due to the potential for residential or occupational exposure.[22]

It appears that bacteria may "feed off" heavy metals and toxic chemicals present in the body.[23] Thus, it's not a stretch to imagine that toxin exposure on a regular, chronic basis can easily be tied to inflammation "storms" and flare-ups as well as residual, systemwide issues.

Patients with MCAS may be especially susceptible to the effects of toxins. Pizzorno describes the detrimental effects of gut endotoxin metabolites, which are small molecules that result from the presence of the wrong bacteria and toxic chemicals in the gastrointestinal system.[2] These endotoxin metabolites circulate through the system and contribute to histamine levels and hives.[2]

It's very important that a patient addresses their concerns carefully with their healthcare team instead of attempting to detox without medical advice. If a patient does not control or manage their detoxification carefully, and repair the necessary organs (particularly the gut, liver, and kidneys) in a particular sequence, more toxins can be unleashed than the body can safely process.[2] Indeed, a guided stepwise approach is important, and the use of supplements can recirculate toxins if the vital organs are not prepared for the process.

Radiation and EMFs

In addition to the exposure to toxins that are ingested or absorbed through the skin in everyday life, the last few decades of increasing access to technological advancements also put human bodies at more risk for invisible harm. *Anecdotally*, getting off the grid can work wonders for patients with chronic illness.

According to the National Cancer Institute in America, "Electric and magnetic fields are invisible areas of energy (also called radiation) that are produced by electricity, which is the movement of electrons, or current, through a wire."[24] Electric fields occur regardless of whether a device is turned on, whereas magnetic fields occur only when current is flowing.[24]

Electromagnetic field (EMF) radiation exposure is not just a "step away from the microwave" concern. Hair dryers, power lines, shavers, lamps, coffee makers, vacuum cleaners, dishwashers, electric wiring, and electric blankets are examples of common everyday "extremely low frequency EMFs," although some experts claim that this name is misleading because these can cause harmful effects.

The more concerning radiofrequency radiation sources include many of our everyday devices – cell phones, iPads, laptops, smart watches, and e-readers. These are often claimed to be "non-ionizing" sources of radiation, though this is a controversial point. Standing near household electrical motors and digital components in appliances like the refrigerator, using a

284

clock radio, and sleeping near the wall of the house's main power meter may also be EMF sources to consider avoiding.

EMFs have been long associated with problematic health effects *anecdotally*, but it's another area where the medical system seems to turn a blind eye to the growing risks and negative health implications.

The National Cancer Institute (America) maintains that "no consistent evidence for an association between any source of non-ionizing EMF and cancer has been found."[24] They note that while studies have looked for associations between prenatal or preconception exposure via the parents, the results have been inconclusive in this area as well.[24]

Anecdotally, many experts appear to have a healthy dose of skepticism for the National Cancer Institute's stance as well as what they constitute as "non-ionizing radiation." The National Cancer Institute failed to acknowledge studies that, from a research standpoint, provided ample evidence of the harmful effects of EMFs. Furthermore, plenty of evidence exists to show that EMFs are harmful in some physiological way or another (even outside of cancer). This topic is highly controversial and EMF exposure is becoming increasingly difficult to avoid in westernized cultures.

Researchers first noted skin-specific reactions, including skin and mucosa signs of itching and redness, flushing, pain, papules, pustules, and heart and central nervous system symptoms in patients who were exposed to electronic screens and mobile phones in studies conducted back in the 1980s.[25,26] Further research in the early 2000s on electrosensitivity noted headaches in about 85% of cell phone users, and a significant number of subjects also reported fatigue, dizziness, nausea, itching, redness, burning, and cognitive symptoms.[27]

A study in 2004 found that overnight EMF exposure negatively impacted soundness of sleep and well-being in the morning.[28] Interestingly, they also found that patients tended to shift to the side of the bed that was furthest from the source of radiation during the night.[28] A 2007 study in the European Journal of Neuroscience found that mobile phone emissions altered brain waves in adults.[29] In 2009, researchers found that mobile phones operating under the safety cutoff of the International Commission for Non-Ionizing Radiation Protection still altered human lymphocyte function for up to 72 hours after exposure, regardless of whether the person was electrohypersensitive or not.[30]

Multiple scientific review articles assert that using a cell phone for 30 minutes a day over several years or decades increases the risk of developing a brain tumor, in some estimates up to 40%-50%.[31,32] Cell phone radiation has been connected to all sorts of diseases, including childhood leukemia, other types of cancer, neurodegenerative diseases, immune system issues, cardiovascular symptoms, infertility, and allergic and inflammatory responses.[31,32]

In the past decade, electric companies began installing new smart meters (digital gas and electric meters) that track when someone is home. While at first glance they seem like a good idea for energy efficiency and use of resources, some voice concern that the EMF grid radiated from smart meters could cause health problems. Following the mandate for smart meters in Victoria, Australia, a 2014 case series noted that subjects most frequently reported insomnia, headaches, tinnitus, fatigue, cognitive disturbances, dyesthesias (abnormal sensations), and dizziness.[33] While the average radiofrequency emitted by smart meters is no greater than holding a cell phone to the head, it's possible that smart meters emit "brief and very intense radiofrequency pulses" that may have a detrimental effect on health in susceptible individuals.[34-36]

Mast Cells and EMFs

Olle Johannson of Sweden is leading the way with research into the effects of EMFs on mast cell physiology. Johannson describes a phenomenon called electrohypersensitivity where certain patients experience reactions to the full-body penetration of electric and magnetic fields in their environment.[37] Specifically, patient labeling of "environmental illness" or "multiple chemical sensitivity" are the strongest predictors of electrohypersensitivity to EMFs.[37] The World Health Organization acknowledges the condition of electrohypersensitivity and suggests that reduction of EMFs may help people who suffer with chronic fatigue and central nervous system/autonomic nervous system issues.[37]

The unnatural environmental trigger of EMFs can cause systemwide symptoms and alterations in immune system function. Specifically, Johannson noted that "EMFs disturb immune function through stimulation of various allergic and inflammatory responses, as well as effects on tissue repair processes."[37] Johannson describes "hypersensitivity reaction" events and theorizes that they are caused by three different types of antigens: (a) infectious agents, (b) environmental disturbances, and (c) self-antigens.[37] EMFs are most certainly considered environmental disturbances.

Cardiac changes, including heart palpitations and heart attack symptoms, have been found in patients with electrohypersensitivity after being exposed to EMFs, and Johannson theorizes that this could be connected to mast cells present in the cardiovascular system.[37] Brain mast cells may also experience chronic degranulation and subsequent tissue inflammation when

286

under the influence of EMF exposure.[37,38] It seems that no area of the body is immune to the potential EMF effects that can trigger mast cell reactions.

Johannson and colleagues have published several papers that discuss theories for how mast cells and EMFs may interact. Johannson notes that EMFs appear to increase both the size and quantity of mast cells, the migration/infiltration of mast cells, and the rate of degranulation of mast cells in electrohypersensitivity patients.[37]

More specifically, electrohypersensitivity patients have a number of unusual patterns noted in the skin following EMF exposure[37]:

- The normally empty zone between the dermo-epidermal junction and mid-to-upper dermis is filled with a high infiltration of mast cells.
- More degranulated mast cells are present in the dermal reticular layer.
- A larger size of infiltrating mast cells is noted.
- A migration of mast cells toward the epidermis occurs and many of the mast cells release their contents into the dermal papillary layer.

Patients with electrohypersensitivity are more likely to have a dramatic increase in the number of mast cells in facial skin samples compared to norms.[37] Johansson notes, "Alterations have been observed in cell populations of the skin of EHS (electrohypersensitive) persons similar to those observed in the skin damaged due to UV light or ionizing radiation."[37]

The research supports that EMF exposure triggers a classic mast cell degranulation response in the skin and other tissues, which can trigger a cascade of inflammatory events in the body as mast cells degranulate their plethora of chemical mediators.[37,39,40] Johannson's research noted that mast cell mediators like chymase, tryptase and histamine were found to be elevated following exposure to EMFs.[41] Johannson concluded in his summary paper, "From the results of the cited studies, it is clear that electromagnetic fields affect the mast cell and the dendritic cell population, and may degranulate these cells."[37]

It's possible that patients who were labeled electrohypersensitive in the early 2000s are in essence patients who would now be clinically diagnosed with MCAS. This research indicates that such patients are more susceptible to the harmful effects of EMFs, and it's possible that the increased number and/or reactivity of mast cells is to blame for increased symptoms following exposure.

Perhaps this phenomenon is similar to the synergistic effect of different heavy metals on the body. Theoretically, EMFs could be considered another form of toxin that human bodies are exposed to that triggers the release of mast cell mediators. When combined with other types of toxins or chemicals, the result could be a larger and more detrimental immune and mast cell response in patients who are already more susceptible to invisible triggers in their environments.

Mold Illness

Biotoxins are toxins that come from living organisms, and mycotoxins are a type of biotoxin that is the by-product of fungi (mold). Humans can react to certain species of mold allergenically or also more globally in the case of toxic/black mold. Even in the 1980s, it was estimated that up to 50% of illness results from exposure to indoor air pollution,[42] with exposure to water-damaged indoor environments likely being a significant contributor to this.[43] When particles such as mycotoxins are inhaled through the nose, it appears that the olfactory nerve is triggered and the particles make a direct and immediate connection with the brain.[44]

According to a 2013 review on mold illness authored by Hope, "Although respiratory symptoms are common from exposure to water-damaged indoor environments, it is important to note that a typical patient presents with multiple symptoms which are often debilitating, including fatigue, neurocognitive symptoms, myalgia, arthralgia, headache, insomnia, dizziness, anxiety, depression, irritability, gastrointestinal problems, tremors, balance disturbance, palpitations, vasculitis, angioedema, and autonomic nervous system dysfunction. The development of new onset chemical sensitivity is also commonly seen after exposure and can have a severe impact on a person's life."[43,45,46]

In addition to chemical sensitivity, food allergies have been associated with mold exposure.[47] A 2014 review by three prominent biotoxin specialists stated that mold can induce POTS and can also impact adrenal and thyroid function.[47] Mold is also associated with chronic fatigue syndrome, fibromyalgia, diabetes, heart problems, joint problems, various cancers, inflammatory bowel disease and other autoimmune disease, neurological conditions including multiple sclerosis, kidney stones, and Raynaud's disease.[47]

Dr. Ritchie Shoemaker, founder of SurvivingMold.com, has devoted 22 years to providing resources for patients who present with chronic inflammatory response syndrome (CIRS), a condition that results from exposure to different types of biotoxins.[48] According to Shoemaker's website, CIRS is "an acute and chronic, systemic inflammatory response syndrome acquired following exposure to the interior environment of a water-damaged building with resident toxigenic organisms, including, but not limited to fungi, bacteria, actinomycetes and mycobacteria as well as inflammagens such as endotoxins, beta glucans, hemolysins, proteinases, mannans and possibly spirocyclic drimanes; as well as volatile organic compounds."[48]

Shoemaker explains that a vicious cycle occurs in a portion of the population where the body recognizes foreign substances (antigens) but is unable to effectively clear them, so the immune system remains in a constant state of activation, which leads to inflammation and chronic illness.[48] Shoemaker describes a complex biotoxin pathway that affects numerous regulators of cellular function in patients who have an inability to remove biotoxins.[48] Specifically, the pathway influences cytokines, leptin, melatonin, endorphins, melanocyte stimulating hormone, cortisol, sex hormones, and other important regulators of cellular signaling, metabolism, sleep cycles, energy, inflammation, and much more.[48]

It's important to highlight that *only certain people respond in this way* to environmental triggers (most notably, the yellow canaries in the coal mine!). When mold is present in the workplace or home, one's boss or coworkers or family members may be seemingly immune.

How is it possible that some people are severely impacted by biotoxins including toxins from mold, while others can live for decades in contaminated environments without symptoms? Genetics may play a role in individual susceptibility to detrimental effects of mold exposure. Non-susceptible individuals have an immune system that recognizes the offending biotoxins, creates antibodies to them, and removes them through the gastrointestinal tract.[48] In contrast, individuals who are genetically susceptible are unable to remove the biotoxins, so they remain in the body indefinitely, causing cell and immune system damage which leads to systemic inflammation.[48]

In a 2013 summary paper on mold illness, physician Janette Hope explains that there are a number of factors that drive whether an individual will respond to exposure, such as underlying health and nutritional status, genetic factors, and the duration and severity of the exposure.[43] In particular the genetic make-up of the gene "HLA-DR" has been linked to mold toxicity risk and is estimated to be present in about 25% of the general population.[48] This likely explains why some people are more prone to reactions than others.

Some patients may have a "double allele defect" where both HLA-DR patterns are susceptible to mold, which can predispose them to greater mold colonization in the body. According to the 2014 review by Forsgren, Nathan, and Anderson, patients with the double allele defect may have been those who experienced more health problems in youth, such as asthma, ear infections, and sinus infections.[47] They may also be more prone to irritable bowel syndrome, yeast infections, and interstitial cystitis.[47]

Systemic inflammation, infection, allergies, irritant effects, and toxicity are all possible by-products of exposure to indoor air pollution.[43] It's not surprising that people who struggle with mast cell activation are more likely to be mold sensitive or reactive, given the fact that their mast cells are already on heightened alert and susceptible to an elevated baseline activity level from other triggers.

Most people associate obvious discoloration on the ceiling with mold, but mold can present inconspicuously and can even be found in dust particles. In addition to mold, mold spores and mycotoxins, bacterial endotoxins and cell wall components, insects and dust mites, protozoa (amoeba), and rodents can all contribute to building-related toxic exposure.[43] Off-gassing of fumes like formaldehyde also occurs as building materials deteriorate.[43]

Thousands of mycotoxins have been identified. Aflatoxins are some of the most widely recognized of the mycotoxins, which are found growing in certain foods (such as peanuts) as well as in environmental areas. Aflatoxins have been linked to liver cancer and are considered one of the most abundant, potent and dangerous of the mycotoxins.[49] Stachybotrys ("black mold") is another pathogenic mold that is not typically airborne but can be identified through dust sample testing.[47]

In her book "Through the Shadowlands: A Science Writer's Odyssey into an Illness Science Doesn't Understand," math and science writer Julie Rehmeyer described the political controversy around mold (surprisingly similar to what's occurred with Lyme disease) in what she deemed the "mold wars."[50] Rehmeyer ended up needing to go out to a desert with borrowed belongings for several weeks in order to determine that mold was a factor in her debilitating (often neurological and paralytic) symptoms.[50] When one is exposed to mycotoxins on a regular basis, sometimes it can be tricky to put two and two together in terms of the relation to chronic symptoms. Rehmeyer's combined story and scientific journalism is an excellent resource for patients who suspect they may have mold issues.

Basically, even a small amount of water damage in a building (mere inches) can provide the environment of a cellular war zone for someone suffering with MCAD. No matter how clean or renovated the surface may look, older buildings inevitably pose a host of hidden "land mines," and not just in humid and wet climates. Building and insulation materials vary by state, and some drier states may still have increased susceptibility, particularly where swamp coolers or air conditioning units are used.

The objects in the environment are not immune to the contamination. Even with the use of HEPA-type filters and washing with vinegar or other solutions, certain types of materials continue to elicit mycotoxins. Clothing, bedding, and even paper materials can still contain the toxins even after relocating homes. Coming into contact with these products can induce exposure via air particles as well as absorption via skin contact. HEPA air purifiers that have moved locations can also be a source of recontamination.

Food- and Beverage-Borne Mold Sources

Food-borne aflatoxins are present in tree nuts, rice, maize, peanuts and spices and are considered genotoxic and carcinogenic substances[51] that could potentially trigger mast cell activation. A 2014 review noted that a variety of additional foods including coffee, corn, barley, rye, wheat, sorghum, cereal, oats, dried food, peas, bread, some cheese, alcohol, cottonseed, and sugar can be contaminated by mold.[47] Dairy and meat may be cross-contaminated through feed sources for animals (unless grass-fed, since grass does not usually contain mycotoxins).[47]

A 2015 study found that 97% of peanut butter was contaminated with aflatoxins, and this may be due to the tendency for defective/deformed peanuts to be preferentially selected to be made into peanut butter.[52] Raw peanuts appear to pose a lesser risk, with 10-14% of samples testing positive for aflatoxins in recent studies.[52-53]

Coffee beans are another form of ingested mold that go under the radar.[47] Coffee is often contaminated with mold in the way that it is processed, regardless of whether it's organic. Ochratoxin A, a type of mycotoxin, has been measured in higher concentrations in decaf coffee when compared to coffee containing caffeine, though it appears that the risk is less if decaffeination occurs prior to roasting of the beans.[54] A 2015 review confirmed that drying, storage, and transportation practices significantly influence the growth of ochratoxin A on coffee beans.[55] After the coffee cherries are harvested, they are often laid out in water for several days to make the pulp softer, which creates a breeding ground for fermentation and mold. Ochratoxin A appears to be the most common contaminant of coffee, but estimates imply that due to climate change and a tendency for more spores to impact the crop with higher temperatures, aflatoxins may exceed ochratoxins on coffee crops in the next 50 years.[56]

A 2015 study in Spain determined that the estimated daily intake of mycotoxins from coffee produced by a number of different methods (coffee maker, electrical machine, and Turkish process) revealed 99th percentile exposure to mycotoxins among consumers but determined that this was not at levels harmful to the average consumer.[57] Additional research indicates that the (highly prevalent) levels of mycotoxins in coffee tend to be below legal limits.[58,59]

However, a study in Europe found that some commercial samples tested higher than the maximum limit established by the European Commission.[57] Research studies have reported 52%-91% mold toxin contamination rates in coffee beans.[59-61] Regardless of where the bar is set for the suggested legal limits, it's clear that these types of toxins are commonly present in coffee. Supplements that contain green coffee bean extracts also appear to have multiple types of mycotoxins.[62]

The concept of mycotoxins in coffee has been the source of some controversy and debate, especially in light of the suggested antioxidant effects of coffee, and it may be less relevant for people who are in good health and don't have sensitivities. However, patients who are hypersensitive to foods and beverages as well as environmental mycotoxins may want to factor this information into their healing plan.

Lyme Disease and Mold Illness

Lyme disease and mold exposure often go hand-in-hand in chronically ill patients. For many, it's difficult to pinpoint which came first. According to Dr. Wayne Anderson, mold exposure can make a person more susceptible to Lyme disease, and vice-versa.[47] Regardless of what came first, the presence of both issues at once can make treatment more challenging.

It's important that Lyme disease treatment doesn't steal the show. According to Forsgren, Nathan and Anderson, "One of the downsides of 'chronic Lyme disease' is that Lyme often becomes the focus of treatment, when in fact it may not be the dominant stressor that the body is burdened by."[47] Symptoms sometimes gives clues to the immune system perception of what is the biggest threat at a given time when patients are experiencing more than one type of toxic burden.

Many patients experience a "seasonal variance" to their type and intensity of symptoms. Some doctors believe that this is due to increased exposure to mold in winter months which shifts the immune system to re prioritize fungal issues when the weather is damp and cold.[47] This clinically noted tendency may need to be factored in to optimize holistic treatment success. Lyme disease will be discussed at length later in this chapter.

Chronic Fatigue Syndrome and Mold Illness

For the last two decades, increasing links have been made between myalgic encephalomyelitis/chronic fatigue syndrome (ME/CFS) and mycotoxins.[63] Cluster outbreaks of patients in the same geographical areas support that mycotoxins could play a role, though some theories point to an infectious disease origin.[64] Mold does not yet appear to be the universally accepted root of CFS etiology in the most recent literature.

A 2013 study revealed some astonishing results. In it, 112 patients previously diagnosed with ME/CFS had urine tested for three mycotoxins: aflatoxins, ochratoxin A, and macrocyclic trichothecenes.[63] Of those tested, 93% were positive for at least one mycotoxin, and nearly one-third of patients had more than one mycotoxin present in their urine.[63] Ochratoxin A was the most common strain detected (83%).[63] Out of these patients, 90% reported a history of exposure to water-damaged buildings.[63] In comparison, a control group of 55 healthy patients all tested negative utilizing the same urine testing.[63]

However, Osterman (2016) refuted the research conclusions, noting that a methodological limitation to the study was that the control group did not report history to mold exposure.[65] The original authors defended the key point that the entire general population does not harbor elevated levels of mycotoxins, and re-emphasized that the study shows an association but is certainly not causal.[66]

The ability to state one's history of exposure to mold is tricky in itself because it's subjective, and in many cases patients (and controls) have been exposed unknowingly. Whether mold exposure could be one factor or the entire story behind the etiology of ME/CFS, an abundance of additional recent research supports that the two are closely connected.[64,67-72]

Testing for Mold

One approach is to determine whether any existing environments are contaminated with biotoxins from mold. According to the experts, "Testing that can be useful in some situations includes environmental testing for bacteria and endotoxins, mycotoxins, VOCs and polymerase-chain-reaction (PCR) based mold testing such as ERMI to identify species of mold."[43] The Environmental Relative Moldiness Index (ERMI) is an objective test that takes dust samples for analysis of 36 different species. The results are broken down into percentages, which determine one's relative mold burden in the home or workplace. Mycometrics.com is a top company that performs the ERMI, in addition to other useful biotoxin tests. For score interpretation, experts advise that an ERMI score below 2 is desired for patients who have a mold-susceptible HLA-DR type.[47] The drawback is certainly the cost.

According to Hope, mold testing methods are typically expensive and not extremely accurate, particularly if they involve air samples.[43] "Air spore counts are frequently done and, unfortunately, have significant limitations as they typically collect over a short (5 minute) period and can easily result in false negative results."[43]

Additional sources concur that air samples, which represent a snapshot in time, are not especially accurate when compared to the ERMI test.[47] Experts note, "99% of the toxic substances in a water-damaged building are carried by mold fragments too small to be detected by air testing or mold plates."[47]

A 2017 review by Valtonen noted that there are no universal criteria for diagnosing a patient with dampness and mold hypersensitivity syndrome (DMHS). Five criteria were recommended to assist in making the clinical diagnosis:[70]

- The history of mold exposure in water-damaged buildings
- Increased morbidity due to infections
- Sick building syndrome
- Multiple chemical sensitivity
- Enhanced scent sensitivity

The author recommended that all five criteria indicate a probable case of DMHS.[70]

As far as laboratory and clinic-based patient tests go, there's no silver bullet test that can lock in the diagnosis of CIRS. The Visual Contrast Sensitivity (VCS) test is a useful *screening tool* that determines a personal baseline of possible biotoxin-associated illness and can also be used as a follow-up test to determine if a particular treatment has been effective. However, the test alone is not validated as a diagnostic tool for mold illness.

Antibody testing for different types of mold can be performed, and Alletess Medical Laboratory performs IgG testing to various molds, but positive tests could either be the result of fungal colonization or an allergy response to environmental exposures.[47] The ALCAT mold panel is a blood test that's also available to assess intolerances/sensitivities.[47] RealTime Laboratories now offers a urine panel that evaluates for three types of mycotoxins, which may be a useful clinical option.[47] Some clinicians factor in positive genetic testing for HLA when consider the possibility of mold-related illness.[73]

There are several lab tests that Shoemaker recommends to help rule in suspicion of CIRS. His website is extremely informative and offers physician resources for downloading an updated listing of lab tests along with recommendations for specimen storage, diagnosis and

CPT codes, and recommended lab sources. Appendix 2 contains a link to Shoemaker's informative web resources.

C4a (a split product of the complement C4 protein) is one inflammatory marker considered in the evaluation of CIRS. Shoemaker notes that, in his clinical experience, MCAD is *overdiagnosed* in the face of elevated C4a.[74] It's possible that some patients with signs of MCAD may be suffering from an underlying case of CIRS and a secondary mast cell response. *Anecdotally,* many patients with MCAS are certain that they have been exposed to mold, and some report that the mold exposure corresponded to a time frame where their MCAS symptoms increased dramatically. Addressing the possibility of biotoxin illness from water damaged buildings is extremely important in this patient population. Specific treatment guidelines exist that may guide a trained clinician in addressing the presence of CIRS and/or mold illness.

BACTERIAL INFECTIONS: LYME DISEASE/VECTOR-BORNE ILLNESS

Lyme disease has become an infectious disease problem of epidemic proportions. Estimates in 2013 by the CDC showed that the U.S. alone has over 300,000 new cases each year (and that's just the cases that get reported/confirmed).[75] The last decade has seen a big surge of cases of Lyme disease outside of the geographical areas known to harbor ticks with the disease, even as far north as Alaska and Canada. Research confirms that ticks are not the only vector that can carry the disease; fleas, mosquitoes, and other biting insects can carry Lyme disease, and it can be transmitted from mother to infant.[76] Some experts also question whether saliva, cows' milk and sexual activity are possible vehicles for the transmission of Lyme disease, though research does not yet support these claims.

Lyme disease is arguably one of the more controversial comorbidities with MCAS. Its history is controversial, its transmission is not universally agreed upon, and its laboratory detection is muddy at best. On top of that, there are conflicts of interest with members of different governing boards, vaccine conspiracies are debated, "Lyme Literate MD" licenses are attacked in court, and there's no universal treatment that appears effective.

Cases of neurological symptoms, meningitis, encephalitis, and other symptoms began to be connected to tick bites in the early 1900s. However, it wasn't until the 1970s the term Lyme disease was coined (in Lyme, Connecticut) and the U.S. saw its first "official" case.

Much of the mainstream approach to Lyme disease diagnosis and treatment revolves around the belief that ticks are the primary method of Lyme bacteria transmission. Websites traditionally state that the risk of infection is low if the tick is removed within 24-48 hours, but it's believed that human cases may have acute infection transmission even after short (several-hour to several-minute) exposures to ticks in the skin. The transmission time may depend on the exact species. A 2015 review noted that transmission can occur in less than 16 hours, and the salivary glands of the tick have the presence of spirochetes, which could indicate a very rapid potential transmission when feeding.[77]

Some believe that the method of tick removal can also impact the degree to which the insect "dumps" its toxins. If it's pulled right out of the skin or accosted with chemicals or fire, some believe that the barbs get embedded and more toxins are released. The recommended removal method is to scoop the tick from underneath and rotate it 90-180 degrees to remove it from the skin.

The CDC currently defines acute Lyme disease as an active bacterial infection of *borrelia burgdorferi* as the result of a tick bite with the "classic" presentation of the bull's eye rash (concentric circular rings), headache, fever, numbness and tingling, and joint pain.[75] Treatment is typically a 21-day course of antibiotics, commonly doxycycline or amoxicillin, and some experts claim that it can be effective at eradicating acute Lyme disease. Some patients (up to 80% in some estimates) never end up presenting with the rash and assume they have some sort of virus instead.[78]

Acute Lyme has been split into three phases: early localized infection, early disseminated infection, and late disseminated infection. The first phase is localized to the skin where the insect bite occurred. The spirochete, a spirally twisted type of bacterium, is believed to remain in the skin for several days after the tick feeding. The second phase involves spreading of the bacteria into the bloodstream.

If the infection goes untreated for several months, the third phase of late disseminated infection can occur. The third phase is typically where more chronic neurologic symptoms can occur, such as polyneuropathy or Lyme encephalopathy (approximately 5% of patients).[79] Symptoms of chronic Lyme disease are widespread and overlap with many other conditions, including MCAS. Rashes, neck pain and stiffness, headaches, chronic fever, brain fog, gastrointestinal ailments, joint problems, and facial nerve palsy are common. Slow gastrointestinal motility, particularly in the small intestine, is frequently reported.

Some patients may have more of a flu-like state with joint involvement as opposed to neurological symptoms, and this may be associated with the specific geographical area where they were exposed. For example, patients in Europe typically have different symptoms than patients in the United States.

For patients who don't respond to treatment, or who are never originally diagnosed correctly, the development of the chronic form of Lyme is coined *post-Lyme syndrome,* and some experts believe that it has the capacity to trigger autoimmune-like problems in the body.[80] Once the case becomes chronic, patients often do not get better with treating the original bacterial infection and require a more comprehensive approach to assisting the immune system in order for the body to heal.[80]

The Controversy

Post-Lyme syndrome has been coined "the great mimic" due to its symptoms being vague, chronic, and often misdiagnosed as fibromyalgia, chronic fatigue, and a plethora of other common conditions. Additionally, Lyme has the ability to stay dormant in the body, and it's a very slow-replicating disease. Some experts believe that nearly everyone is exposed to Lyme bacteria at some point in life, but it's the ones who experience great stress or trauma or perhaps the perfect storm of genetics and a faulty environment who may actually go on to develop symptoms. Some argue that exposure via ticks is only a small minority of those who go on to develop Lyme symptoms. Some experts assert that the symptoms are not a direct manifestation of the bacteria itself, but rather the effect of the immune system lodging an assault on the invader. Some patients may experience cyclical symptoms if their immune system is responding to different types of bacteria at different times based on the current level of perceived threat from each organism.

It can be difficult to catch the proper moment in time when the antibody levels will test high on traditional testing. Some experts claim that in the case of chronic disease, the body becomes so immunosuppressed that the antibodies will look low as a consequence. This may also explain why some patients need longer treatments and attention to their overall immune system in order to assist in healing.

There are some who believe that Lyme disease may more accurately describe the body responding to a virus, rather than a bacterial infection. Epstein-Barr virus and cytomegalovirus infections were associated with false positive IgM tests for Lyme disease in one study,[81] but there's a scarcity of research in this area.

Many patients and practitioners alike are frustrated that chronic cases of Post-Lyme syndrome seem to get ignored in mainstream medicine and are not prioritized on the federal public health level. Many believe it's a controversial topic because these patients may not test highly positive on the traditional Lyme tests. Some estimate that 1 in 100 people who are symptomatic with a clinical diagnosis of Lyme disease are actually "CDC positive." It's possible that patients can experience immune system or systemic dysfunction from the history of exposure to an organism despite currently appearing "infection-free" in the bloodstream, which is a topic of great debate.

There is great scrutiny in regards to the clinical treatment guidelines that drive physician practice as well as insurance reimbursement. According to the documentary "Under Our Skin," 9 of the 14 panelists who wrote the Infectious Disease Society of America (IDSA) Lyme treatment guidelines had clear conflicts of interest with insurance companies, patents, and vaccines.[82]

The International Lyme and Associated Diseases Society (ILADS) is an advocacy organization for chronic Lyme disease. They specifically aim to increase public awareness and improve physician knowledge about Lyme disease. IDSA and ILADS often clash on their clinical criteria for diagnosis of chronic cases of Lyme disease. According to "Under Our Skin," the IDSA has led to the closure of labs and research ventures and has waged war with many "Lyme Literate MDs" in lawsuits.[82] From one perspective, it's devastating to watch compassionate, caring professionals help thousands of patients get their lives back and then end up losing their licenses due to the "industry" of healthcare. On the other hand, some experts are criticized by colleagues for over-diagnosing Lyme disease without concrete clinical findings. The controversy of many aspects of the diagnosis and treatment of Lyme disease continues to grow.

The standards for testing for Lyme disease involve a two-tiered method. It's important to note that no current lab test can definitively diagnose Lyme disease; the test merely looks at whether a person has been *exposed* to the bacteria and has detectable levels of antibodies. The CDC definition for diagnosis is contingent upon the positive test plus the clinical presentation of symptoms. The first test is known as the Lyme Screen Test, which is a blood test looking for antibody levels of IgG and IgM. If this is positive, the second test performed is the Lyme Western Blot test, which examines a larger series of antibodies that the body can make once it's been exposed to Lyme.

A 2014 study found that only 10%-18% of Western Blot testing comes back positive in patients with suspected Lyme disease.[83] Symptoms of Lyme disease certainly overlap with those experienced in other chronic conditions, but there is also valid concern about the testing methods themselves.

Research in 2017 found that using the conventional two-tiered protocol, the Western Blot test exhibited a very poor sensitivity (25%) in patients in the early stage of Lyme disease with acute erythema migrans rashes.[84] (Tests in medicine are considered "good" if their sensitivity is 95% or higher.) A systematic review and meta-analysis of data in Europe found no clear benefit to the two-tiered approach over single test approaches.[85] Similarly, a meta-analysis conducted in 2016 in United States laboratories recorded a very poor (53.7%) sensitivity when the two-tier methodology was used.[77]

Functional medicine doctors who are testing for Lyme disease may also look at indicators of the overall quality of the immune system. Additional tests can include a standard panel of immune markers, T and B cells, genetic testing and immunoglobulin levels. They may also look at inflammatory markers for a baseline and to determine how someone is responding to treatment. Tick bites are also associated with alpha-gal allergies which can trigger MCAD and/or allergic disorders, so alpha-gal antibody testing may also be warranted, particularly in patients who experience delayed allergic reactions to meat.[86]

Many experts include consideration of the presence of coinfections in patients with symptoms of Lyme disease. Bartonella, babesiosis, anaplasmosis, ehrlichiosis, mycoplasma, and Powassan virus are all examples of diseases carried on insects and may be considered, since their symptoms are similar to those experienced with Lyme disease. It's not uncommon for testing to reveal more than one vector-borne illness.

Lyme and MCAS

Lyme has been called a "do-it-yourself" disease. Many patients find themselves having to be their own advocates until they find the right physician willing to order the right tests and consider a clinical diagnosis—even if the tests don't reflect the disease perfectly on paper. (Sound familiar?!)

Most treatments and specialists are not covered by insurance and can run upwards of $100,000 per year for two years or longer at Lyme "specialty" centers. *Anecdotally*, once diagnosed, some patients self-treat with herbal combinations found online, some pursue expensive blood ozone and intravenous therapy treatments, some rig up home devices for ionic footbaths and infrared technology. Some patients end up having to take matters into their own hands in order to move forward and stay afloat.

There are many similarities in what patients go through with Lyme compared to MCAS. Both groups of patients are often told that they have chronic pain, fibromyalgia, or chronic fatigue, often with some hints of "it's all in your head" thrown in. There are many medical professionals out there who are undereducated about both diseases and how to diagnose and treat them. Lyme is definitely better-known than MCAS, but both diseases do carry many similarities. MCAS is certainly a "do-it-yourself" disease, too!

Whether Lyme disease is tick-borne or not, whether its origin is bacterial or viral (or some other undiscovered factor), one thing is certain: Patients with MCAS are more likely to have heightened reactions to foreign "invaders," and it's probable that Lyme disease triggers mast cell activation. One of the more well-known studies in this area evaluated the effect of *borrelia burgdorferi* spirochetes on rodent mast cells in vitro.[87] The researchers found that the spirochetes induced the synthesis and secretion of inflammatory cytokines (such as TNF-alpha) from mast cells.[87] Mast cells certainly play an active role in the immune response to environmental toxins, insect bites, and "invaders," so this connection comes as no surprise.

While Lyme bacteria likely induce a secondary mast cell activation, it's also probable that patients who already have MCAS are more likely to experience a more reactive state if they are to acquire Lyme disease later in life due to their propensity for overactive mast cells.

Afrin believes that some patients asserted to have Lyme disease (despite relatively little laboratory evidence of such) might actually be cases of MCAS; he suspects that true cases of Lyme disease sometimes trigger additional mast cell activation in patients where (in most cases) MCAS predated the Lyme disease.[88]

It's also possible that chronic MCAS may make one more susceptible to developing Lyme disease. Additional research shows that a protein called histamine-releasing factor (HRF) is secreted in the saliva of *borrelia burgdorferi*-containing ticks, and it appears to be crucial for the transmission of Lyme disease.[89] HRF stimulates a number of cells, including mast cells and basophils, and researchers believe that the cascade that results from the presence of this protein increases vascular permeability to facilitate easier tick engorgement into the skin and thus greater likelihood of Lyme disease transmission (via ticks).[89] Researchers found that blocking the effects of HRF in mice reduced the efficiency of tick feeding and likewise reduced the total burden of *borrelia burgdorferi*.[89] While this provides interesting preliminary data for potential vaccine-based preventive measures against Lyme, one could also theorize that heightened circulating levels of chemical mediators released by mast cells, such as histamine, may make one more susceptible to acquiring Lyme disease from tick exposure. Of course, this idea is *purely extrapolation* at this point.

Ticks have also been shown to contain and secrete prostaglandins when in contact with a host, and elevated prostaglandin levels have been found in the synovial (joint) fluid of patients with Lyme disease.[90,91] While a separate study asserted that the immunosuppression induced by ticks was not prostaglandin-related, prostaglandins and other chemical mediator elevations may play an influential role in patients with Lyme disease (and, in particular, patients with both MCAS and Lyme disease).[92]

The scarcity of research on mast cells, their chemical mediators, and *borrelia burgdorferi* is somewhat surprising, and the conclusion that "more information is needed" prevails. While Lyme bacteria exposure is not the root of all (or possibly any) MCAS-related problems, it certainly can contribute to the "perfect storm" of viral, bacterial, and toxin-based problems that can clog the system and increase one's baseline of mast cell activity.

Lyme disease, like MCAS, may possibly be part of a much bigger picture of chronic immune system issues. For some patients, focusing solely on Lyme disease as the "bad guy to be eradicated" appears to be a problematic approach, as opposed to supporting the immune system more naturally so that it can better do its job in light of multiple confounding variables. However, it's important that patients with MCAS are aware of this common comorbidity and are prepared to address all bacterial and viral influences that may impact their healing potential.

Lyme Disease Plus MCAS, SIBO, POTS, CIRS and Mold Exposure

It has been observed clinically that Lyme disease seems to co-occur with other conditions, especially MCAS, SIBO, POTS, CIRS, and mold illness.[93] Across these conditions, some of the same triggers are noted that exacerbate symptoms: excess stress, exposure to water-damaged buildings, excess sugar consumption, lack of sleep, and alcohol use.[93] All of these conditions may involve immunosuppression and similar chronic inflammatory symptoms.

What do Lyme disease specialists think about the presence of these comorbidities? Some specialists theorize that the assault on the gastrointestinal system's microbiome (bacterial balance) and the increase in autoimmune conditions and susceptibility to immune system coinfection over the last 50 years has led to an increased the number of patients struggling with these conditions.[93]

Researchers have looked at whether certain Lyme-transmitting bugs live in mold-infested areas, but that theory has been inconclusive.[93] Another "left field" possibility is that patients with certain genetic backgrounds or certain body odors emitted by an unbalanced microbiome may attract insects more readily. It's also been theorized that ticks are responsible for the minority of Lyme disease transmission, and that the bacteria is getting passed on in other manners and could "take hold" in a body that is already immunosuppressed.

It's possible that Lyme disease and/or mold exposure are the root cause of a secondary MCAS and gastrointestinal microbiome disruption. Cytokines and other chemical mediators released by mast cells in response to bacterial invasion can certainly have a negative impact on both the immune system and the gastrointestinal system. Cytokines appear to be linked to a dysfunctional microbiome and/or the presence of "leaky gut," both of which are associated with SIBO.

So, the logical mechanism could be:

Mold exposure and/or exposure to Lyme/vector-borne illness → secondary mast cell activation → release of chemicals that create an environment for leaky gut and SIBO, plus increased future susceptibility to inflammation and environmental toxins including mold

Many patients with Lyme experience a "Herxheimer Reaction" or "die-off" reaction cyclically, which is a detoxification process thought to be related to the life cycle of the bacteria. This can create flu-like symptoms and an overall flare-up and may be associated with mast cell degranulation. The same type of reaction can occur with patients who are being treated with medications or herbal products following mold exposure.

But what about all of the patients who have had clinical signs and symptoms of MCAD since they were young/decades prior to the suspected vector-borne illness exposure? And what about the patients who have clinical evidence of mast cell clonality? Perhaps the underlying presence of MCAD involves a mechanism that "turns on" the Lyme infection more readily or chronically.

So, maybe it's more likely that:

A person is born with primary MCAD → which in itself predisposes them to GI issues, leaky gut, SIBO → they are genetically more susceptible to environmental toxins and bacterial infections, or their mast cell activation plays a role in this immune system state and susceptibility → they happen to be exposed to Lyme, another vector-borne illness, and/or mold

Mold toxicity and Lyme disease are both biotoxin-associated illnesses that involve an immune response that's modulated by mast cells. Some experts theorize that either 1) Lyme disease is much more common than realized and is the root for much of these other coinfections (which is only amplified in a MCAD host) or 2) since mold illness and Lyme disease are biotoxin-related, perhaps the recipients are the unlucky population who have a genetically influenced poor detoxification system in the first place and happen to be hit with both diseases independently. Experts recommend evaluation and treatment of both Lyme disease and mold illness when one or the other is first identified, as outcomes tend to be better when both are addressed.[73]

Perhaps genetic factors load the stone in the slingshot, but a patient's lifestyle is what pulls it back and aims. Many functional medicine doctors attribute a genetic–environment combination in the etiology of chronic illness. This may explain why one family member may be especially sick despite all members being exposed to the same area with ticks or mold. Perhaps a stressful life event, vector-born exposure, or dietary practice is the tipping point for that one family member. While there are several theoretical explanations but no clear answers as to the exact mechanisms between these comorbidities associated with Lyme disease, an approach that factors in the whole picture (beyond simply Lyme or simply MCAS), *in theory*, will reap the most rewards. Adequate attention to potential underlying bacterial infections is crucial for patients who have MCAS.

VIRAL INFECTIONS: EPSTEIN-BARR VIRUS (EBV)

Cytomegalovirus, varicella-zoster virus and Epstein-Barr virus (EBV) are examples of common viruses that could be responsible for secondary mast cell activation. EBV has gained more attention in recent years as a possible underlying factor tied to chronic immune system issues. EBV is transmitted through saliva, and once a person has been exposed, it may remain dormant in one's body indefinitely.[94] It's believed that EBV can also be transmitted in utero, and recent research in the United Kingdom found that 25%-50% of children who were age two and younger tested positive for EBV.[95] Literature supports that patients are often initially asymptomatic when affected during infancy or childhood.[96] The lifetime prevalence of EBV has been estimated to be at least 90%.[97,98]

EBV may become symptomatic from dormancy following stressful life events. EBV is the virus that causes mononucleosis or "mono," and when it's acute it can also cause enlargement of organs like the spleen and the liver and can even be life-threatening.[99] The chronic form of EBV can be a stealthy infection that can wreak havoc systemwide. Chronic EBV often presents as fatigue, aching muscles and joints, depression, swollen lymph nodes, thrombocytopenia, and other flu-like symptoms.[100] Patients with chronic EBV often also exhibit rashes, hypersensitivity to mosquito bites and anemia.[98]

Patients with immunodeficiencies appear to handle EBV infection poorly, and there are also indicators that healthy subjects are susceptible to EBV-associated malignancies.[99] EBV has been studied in regards to its interplay with cancers such as lymphoma,[101] leukocyte migration in airway allergic reactions,[102] and cross-reactions with the influenza virus,[103] to name a few. Thyroid conditions like Hashimoto's thyroiditis and Graves' disease have been associated with the positive expression of EBV in laboratory testing.[104]

Research continues to investigate the potential role of EBV in a plethora of different health conditions. However, there's little research on potential interactions between EBV and mast cell activation. One study found that children with Hodgkin's lymphoma were more likely to have positive tests for EBV and they noted the presence of higher infiltrations of mast cells with more advanced stages of the virus.[105]

Many of the symptoms of EBV overlap with the symptoms of MCAS. Is it possible that this virus (and potentially others) could be causing a physiological state of secondary mast cell activation? It's certainly plausible that EBV infection (and/or the presence of other viral infections) is one of the missing pieces of the bigger picture for many patients who suffer with MCAS.

CHAPTER KEY POINTS

- A number of environmental factors such as toxins (including mold) and EMF exposure appear to negatively influence patients with MCAS.

- Bacterial infections appear to trigger an increase in mast cell activation. *Anecdotally,* Lyme disease is a commonly reported condition in patients with MCAS.

- Viral infections appear to trigger an increase in mast cell activation. *Anecdotally,* Epstein-Barr virus is a commonly reported condition in patients with MCAS.

- A holistic plan that addresses potential environmental, bacterial and viral factors (as opposed to just focusing on mast cells) will best optimize quality of life considerations for patients with MCAS.

Chapter Nine

Conventional Treatment Approaches

The following information is not intended to be medical advice, and it is not all-inclusive. A patient should always consult with their medical team for individualized advice, diagnosis, and treatment tools.

MCAS TREATMENT STRATEGY

I t's tempting to focus on medication-based management of MCAS; after all, modern culture seeks a quick fix in a fast-paced world. Patients with MCAS have (likely) been suffering for decades and tend to be burning the candle on both ends while struggling to make ends meet financially. However, patients should be encouraged to consider healing a multifaceted process and should be prepared for a number of potentially difficult lifestyle changes to foster a realistic path to long-terms goals, particularly if they are avoiding the "Band-Aid" approach to symptoms as an end goal.

Patients should be encouraged to dig deeper than simply seeking the right combination of antihistamines, mast cell stabilizers and other mast cell-targeting medications. Afrin emphasizes a "lock and key" approach, where the patient ought to try different over-the-counter and prescription medications until they find those which seem to satisfactorily control their particular variant of MCAS.[1]

This aspect is *step one*, the achievement of a stable "symptomatic baseline," and though it should not be the only approach, it is *very* important. Many patients are so unstable that they repeatedly experience anaphylaxis or other severe symptoms, so the primary priority is to help facilitate a more *stable individualized baseline* in every patient. Pain management and low bone mineral density treatment should also be included in the pharmacological considerations as part of a holistic baseline treatment plan.

However, once a stable baseline has been achieved, *step two* includes delving into the root cause of the disease. For decades to come, the research will likely focus on genetic mutations linked to MCAS. While genetic factors do appear to play a role in tipping the scales to influence which patients are more susceptible to mast cell issues, holistic care for MCAS must zoom out even further.

Blaming everything on genetics can create a pattern of learned helplessness in patients who are diagnosed with a chronic disease. Even if a patient was born with the disease, the mental weight of "I was born this way, and nothing I can do will change it—I guess this is just my lot in life" is an unhealthy approach. Some degree of overall acceptance is important, but the more difficult (and more fruitful) approach is to consider genetics as one small piece of the puzzle and to focus on what is in one's power to change. This applies to patients who have monoclonal MCAS as well; even though they may have a larger influence (on paper) from aspects outside of their control, *anecdotally* some patients with Primary MCAD are able to achieve meaningful goals for a reduced symptomatic baseline and, in some cases, complete remission of certain symptoms or all symptoms.

In reality, the management of MCAS is not as simple as a two-step process. Patients tend to experience flare-ups and may jump back and forth between trying to find symptom stability and exploring underlying root mechanisms. Medication testing can be a lengthy trial-and-error process.

A Simple Analogy: Tree Orchard

The big-picture, long-term approach can be hard to grasp on day one. In order to envision the importance of the two-step approach, imagine two trees in an orchard, planted side-by-side. One tree develops large deep roots when it is planted, but its neighbor has smaller more fragile roots.

Over time, both trees are subjected to the same environmental conditions (wind, sunlight, rain, etc.). However, the one with small roots has less ability to tolerate many environmental stressors. Following a windstorm, it starts to lean. When a bird builds a nest on it, it tips even further. When it's sprayed with pesticides, the roots shrivel even more. And suddenly, another small trigger releases those roots from the soil and it topples completely. The original problem (weak roots) didn't cause the tree to topple right away, but when coupled with the right stressors and toxins to its system, it was much more likely to struggle compared to its deep-rooted neighbor.

In this analogy, patients with MCAS obviously can't control the *original roots* that caused the disease but can certainly aim to reduce exposure to new factors, remove the environmental triggers that have been keeping the body out of harmony, and influence the body's ability to grow new roots. And the good news is, with the right tools, not only can the tree thrive upright again, but it can foster the growth of brand new deeper and stronger roots that will make it better able to withstand unpredictable forces in the future.

However, this process does not happen overnight, just as it tends to become clear, upon deeper examination, that the original issue did not crop up overnight. Healing the roots usually takes years, and this anticipated time frame is an important reality to share with patients newly diagnosed with MCAS. The other important reality is that an approach that *only* focuses on mast cell medications may serve as external supports that make the tree appear stable from afar but likely won't correct the original issue or prevent it from worsening in a big storm.

INITIAL CONSIDERATIONS FOLLOWING MCAS DIAGNOSIS

Identifying All Allergens and Triggers

Upon diagnosis, patients should review potential triggers of mast cell activation with their medical team and consider what triggers seem unique to them in particular. Some of the less-obvious triggers that may surprise patients and trigger acute attacks include fevers, muscle relaxants, opioids, contrast media used in diagnostic imaging, and nonsteroidal anti-inflammatory drugs.[2] Some patients may already know this, but it's important that all patients are educated initially about these (and other) trigger sources. Identification of true allergies is also important in initial stages, if it has not yet been performed. Hymenoptera venom allergy testing may be of particular importance for a subgroup of patients with MCAD and a history of adverse reactions to insect stings.

Tips for the Newly Diagnosed

Starting on day one, adequate attention should be given to the following:

- Prepare for acute episodes.
- Obtain a medical alert ID bracelet or necklace.
- Carry emergency medications at all times and stash them in car, gym bag, etc.
- Carry a card or paper that summarizes medical instructions for the event of an ER visit. Include past medical history, emergency contacts, conditions, and the patient's medication list.

- Consider purchasing a mask to wear if needed for contact with smokers, perfumes, cleaning supplies, etc.

- Communicate with family members and come up with an emergency plan with specific roles identified. Go over potential scenarios that could arise and have everyone practice with the EpiPen training injector if applicable.

- Complete a thorough assessment of any and all potential triggers.
  - Environmental
  - Dietary
  - Medication-based
  - Physical

- Consider a temporary symptom log as the patient is adjusting foods and medications.

- Assess the environment for stealthy hidden contaminants (e.g., mold in the walls of a building, chemicals in skin products and cleaning supplies).

- Evaluate one's lifestyle/schedule and reduce as many daily stressors as possible.

- Ensure adequate sleep, clean drinking water, organic food, and HEPA-filtered air for maximal success.

- Consider ways to assist the body in detoxification. Epsom salt baths, sweating, and colonics may be useful, though not all MCAS patients can tolerate these approaches.

- Focusing on certain foods and supplements with the help of a natural medicine provider may help this process.

- Focus on a positive mindset and make sure to address any unresolved emotional trauma. Talk therapy, EMDR techniques, Tension and Trauma Releasing Exercises (TRE), sound healing, meditation, prayer, yoga, affirmations, reading, and podcasts can all be helpful. (More suggestions are shared in Chapter 12.)

MAINSTREAM MEDICATIONS FOR MCAS TREATMENT

Medication Options

Once diagnosed with MCAS (and typically in the period leading up to diagnosis), the patient should work with their medical team to identify medications that may help stabilize their symptoms.

A patient may be prescribed a combination of the following types of medications:[3,4]

- Emergency medications for use in anaphylactic type reactions
  - Auto-injectable epinephrine, inhaled medications for airway, and diphenhydramine (Benadryl)
- Preventive medications that <u>block the action</u> of released mast cell mediators
  - Antihistamines (H1 and H2 blockers, diphenhydramine), leukotriene antagonists, TNF antagonists, IL-1 antagonists
- Preventive medications that <u>inhibit the release</u> of mast cell mediators
  - Oral or inhaled disodium cromoglycate (cromolyn), tyrosine kinase inhibitors, omalizumab, benzodiazepines, cannabidiol, ketotifen
- Preventive medications that <u>inhibit the production</u> of mast cell mediators
  - NSAIDS and aspirin (with caution), steroids, vitamin C
- Preventive medications to address osteoporosis/osteopenia, if present
- Cellular therapy and allogeneic stem cell transplants are very rarely used, and then only in the case of aggressive MCAD (typically, systemic mastocytosis and mast cell leukemia)
- Hydroxyurea is sometimes considered for MCAS patients; other drugs such as alkylators, taxanes, fludarabine, cladribine, cytarabine, alemtuzumab, and daclizumab are considered for some cases of mastocytosis, though there are other treatment options available for mastocytosis.[5]

*Note: There is some discrepancy in the literature about certain medications and their mechanism of action (i.e., whether they inhibit the *release* or *production* of mast cell mediators). Some medications also appear to work by more than one mechanism of prevention.

While there are many options for mast cell-targeting drugs out there, there is a scarcity of pharmacological research that is specific to MCAS itself. According to a 2016 review, only three medications have been studied specifically in patients with MCAS: omalizumab (Xolair), continuous IV infusions of diphenhydramine (Benadryl), and hydroxyurea.[4] Since then, an additional case report was published on the use of IV infusions of diphenhydramine and subsequent use of imatinib for a patient with MCAS; further research on omalizumab with patients who have MCAS and monoclonal MCAS were also located.[6-8] These studies and others will be presented in this chapter.

First-Line through Sixth-Line Medication Options

A 2016 review by Molderings and colleagues suggested the following sequence of medication considerations:[4]

- o First-line therapy: If H1 and H2 antihistamines, disodium cromoglycate (also known as cromolyn), vitamin C, and ketotifen are not sufficiently effective even at maximal doses, add:
- o Second-line therapy: immunosuppressive drugs
- o Third-line therapy: omalizumab
- o Fourth-line therapy: inhibitors of tyrosine kinase and other kinases
- o Fifth-line therapy: investigational drugs
- o Sixth-line therapy: cytoreductive drugs, polychemotherapy

A subsequent article by Wirz and Molderings supported the same sequence, noting, "With no predictors of response yet available, a cost-based approach to sequencing therapeutic trials in a given patient seems reasonable."[9] The authors noted that it remains unclear whether it's effective to take the mediator that tested high (like histamine, or prostaglandin D2) and to pair it with a medication that targets the same mediator. There simply is not enough research available yet to help guide these types of specific clinical decisions. A personalized, patient-specific approach that starts with the most affordable options is advised.[9]

Therefore, the above sequence may mirror the flow chart that the physician follows in terms of trialing new medications if first-line therapy is not successful. *Keep in mind, however, that many patients do very well with first-line therapy for the management of MCAS.*

Another factor to remember is that sometimes less is more (in terms of the number of medications utilized), and that more-expensive treatment options do not mean better care. Many patients respond well to the over-the-counter options; the less widely used medications (like fourth- to sixth-line treatments) tend to be reserved for patients who generally have more severe cases of MCAS and do not respond to other options first.

The following discussion of medications is organized by *theorized mechanism of symptom reduction* and does not reflect the above-recommended chronological order for first- through sixth-line therapy.

Medication Trial Considerations

The trial and error process can take months or even years to find the right combination, dosage, and brand of medication. Patience and attention to detail are crucial in this process. It's important to make ONE change at a time—this applies not just to *types or brands* of medications, but also to the *dosage* and *frequency* per day. According to the experts, for most medications a one-month trial will generally be sufficient to determine if the current medication/dosage will be of significant benefit.[10,11] This time frame is dependent on the particular medication, however. (For example, ketotifen and cromolyn trials generally take longer—up to several months—to determine efficacy. When in doubt, check with the prescribing doctor.)

For each medication, patients ought to be educated to expect a several-week time frame from starting a new medication to noting any symptom relief.[12] Dosages will also likely vary. For example, with antihistamines, Seneviratne and colleagues note, "Most patients (with MCAS) need a higher dose (between two to four times) the dose used for treatment of mild hay fever symptoms. Many patients find a 2-3 times daily dosing to be more helpful than a once daily dosing regimen."[12]

It's important to consider each new medication trial a step-by-step process. Medications that are questionably helpful should *not* be continued after a trial period; absolute certainty that a medication is helpful is recommended. It should be fairly obvious whether a new medication is a "keeper."[11] If less than optimal treatments are continued while other new meds are added, unmanageable polypharmacy can develop; this should be avoided.[12] A quality—rather than quantity—approach is ideal.

According to Afrin, "If at any point it is thought that a given medication is no longer providing significant benefit, it should be stopped or weaned (as appropriate for that medication) to see what happens. No patient with any disease should be taking one more milligram of one more medication if it is not clearly providing significant benefit."[11]

Keep in mind that many patients react to fillers/dyes/additives and may need to trial many versions of the same active ingredient before ruling it in or out. For example, a patient may tolerate the generic H1 blocker cetirizine but react to the brand name Zyrtec medication. That same patient may do better with the brand name Allegra and react more to the generic versions of the same active ingredient. Patients may even react to the capsule itself. It may be beneficial to try compounding pharmacies that have more hypoallergenic filler options. Certain supplements and medications (including aspirin and quercetin) may contain plant-based substances called salicylates, which can also be the source of intolerances in some individuals.

Many supplements and medications also contain grains like gluten and corn, even though these ingredients may not be obvious from reading the label. Some companies have been found to falsely advertise ingredients and the true quantity of an active ingredient, so caution is warranted with online purchases. Reputable companies will be more expensive but may be better options for patients with sensitivities to ensure that the appropriate ingredients and dosage are being obtained. The source of the supplement may also be vaguely explained on the label; patients with allergies to shellfish and nuts should be especially careful, as some supplements may be derived from or cross-contaminated with such ingredients. For example, the cheapest sources of quercetin are derived from peanut shells and fava beans, and when they are in a "proprietary blend" with questionable purity, they could trigger reactions in patients with g6pd deficiency or peanut allergies.[13]

Many patients will experience side effects from medications, some of which have been reported to disappear over time, while others may persist. In general, some medications actually cause a flare-up of mast cell activity in patients with MCAS in the first days or weeks of use, which may then be followed by significant relief. It's important to do some research and be aware of these types of patterns for each medication that is trialed. It's also important to be clear on what types of reactions can be "tolerated" and what types necessitate immediate cessation of a particular medication. It's very important to discuss all of the above with one's individual medical team.

Of course, there's also the possibility that a patient may not realize that a medication is significantly effective until they cease using it. Generally, the desired response to a given medication should be fairly profound in terms of symptoms, but some patients find that cessation of the medication is the ultimate telltale indicator of efficacy.

It's important to be aware of longer-term sudden reaction possibilities. Patients may experience times where they suddenly react to a medication they have been taking for a long time without issues. In this case, it can be helpful to assume detective-mode as it's possible that the pharmacy may have changed brands or excipients in the medication without notifying the patient. However, if no explanation can be found, ultimately any medication that is ineffective or harmful should be immediately stopped.[10]

It's also possible that new, sudden reactions to previously "safe" medications could be in the nature of MCAS over time. According to Afrin, "Or perhaps—if an initial beneficial effect wears off within a few days to a few weeks—the patient's mast cell activation disease has 'learned' to react to one or more of the excipients in the particular formulation of the drug being taken, such that intentionally switching to a different formulation with different

314

excipients might suddenly improve the drug's tolerability. It's always possible, too, that the patient's mast cell disease has changed/evolved (even further mutated) and is simply no longer responsive to one or more of the drugs to which it was previously responsive."[11]

There are many other considerations that may streamline the process of trial and error in this area. Vitamins and supplements should always be examined as they are potential sources of additives and ingredients that could trigger reactions. Some experts recommend temporary abstention from gluten, yeast, and dairy product consumption while trialing new mast cell medications for best results.[9]

Patients receiving medications intravenously may have additional considerations. According to Afrin, "MCAS patients who react to seemingly every IV treatment they're given may be reacting to microparticulate material being shed by the plastics in IV bags and/or tubing. For example, many IV bags and tubing contain a plastic molecule whose chemical name is abbreviated as DEHP, and an occasional MCAS patient reacts to exposure to DEHP. Such a patient would want to seek DEHP-free bags and tubing for his/her IV treatments."[5] Multi-dose medication vials are more likely to have preservatives when compared to single-dose containers, another factor to consider with certain medications.[14]

The temperature of the medication or the water taken with it can even, in some cases, play a role in reactions. According to Afrin and Khoruts, "Some 'allergies' (e.g., to iodine or even water!) may seem psychosomatic until the recognition of excipient (e.g., povidone in iodine/povidone solution) or physical (e.g., temperature) triggers."[15]

There's no perfect formula for the right number of medications and the right dosing per day. Many patients report that a steady/continual dosing of medications (more than once per day) may be better for stability. However, some patients with milder cases of MCAS find once-a-day dosing sufficient. Some medications may cause drowsiness and therefore may be better tolerated at bedtime. Others can have the opposite effect and need to be taken in the morning. Some may need to be taken on an empty stomach, while others should be taken on a full stomach. Dosing may be higher or lower than what appears as a "standard dose" on over-the-counter medication bottles, depending on the patient.

It's important to investigate whether any of the medications interact with each other (or alcohol) and to come up with a way to organize and streamline the medication process. Pill organizers can be useful to make sure the patient doesn't forget to take medications. Symptom logs are also important in the initial phase of trial and error until the regimen is determined to be effective.

When thinking of the big picture, it's helpful to think of a sliding scale in terms of finding a stable baseline via medications. As an example, patients may require multiple H1 and H2 blockers, prescriptions such as ketotifen or cromolyn or leukotriene antagonists, plus more "natural" substances such as vitamin C and quercetin to achieve a stable baseline initially.

Over time, patients may find that their baseline status shifts, necessitating an increase or decrease in the dose or number of medications they need to stay stable. An episode of acute anaphylaxis may shift the patient baseline to increased reactivity and they may be prescribed a short-term steroid in the weeks to follow. The addition of factors such as stress reduction techniques, mold remediation, or supplements that reduce mast cell mediator activity/assist in detoxification may help the patient slide to a level of greater stability and taper off certain prescribed medications over time (with the help of their medical team).

What's of the utmost importance in this process is that the patient 1) achieves a stable baseline to move from and 2) feels supported in the process, while also being educated that patience and meticulous trial and error must be part of the process. Upon initial diagnosis, it's natural to want to dive into trying everything at once, but this will make it very difficult to determine what medications are effective and need to be a regular priority. Patience, patience, and more patience are mandatory!

There's also the question of whether newly diagnosed MCAS patients should continue medications that they had been taking for prior diagnoses or symptomatic management. The short answer to this is: yes, *if they are helpful*. At an educational conference directed at healthcare providers in September 2017, Dr. Afrin suggested only *eliminating* drugs for previously diagnosed conditions if they're *not* of a clear benefit to the patient.[14]

Research supports that the majority of patients with MCAS will eventually find some degree of relief of symptoms from pharmacological treatment. Molderings and colleagues noted in a 2011 review that "especially in non-aggressive disease (comprising the great majority of patients), at least partial improvement is usually attainable with one regimen or another, and thus the practitioner is obligated to persist with therapeutic trials until no options remain."[10]

One of the most important factors is putting in the extra effort to get to know one's local pharmacist(s). According to Dr. Afrin, "The number one most valuable asset a patient must acquire on the path toward achieving therapeutic success with MCAS is finding a local doctor who is willing to learn, and willing to try. The number two asset is finding a local pharmacist who is willing to learn, and willing to try."[14] Strong communication with pharmacy staff can help ensure that the MCAS patient is fully aware of ingredients (including fillers and dyes) in prescriptions, the change of brands that can occur without notice, potential side effects, and other important considerations that may otherwise go under the radar.

Flare-Up Medication Considerations

When experiencing anaphylaxis, the immediate response should be to administer epinephrine that's been prescribed for the patient, unless otherwise directed by one's doctor. Patients with MCAS and a history of anaphylaxis *or* monoclonal disease with no history of anaphylaxis should have access to at least two auto-injectors of epinephrine at all times and should not assume that they will have time to report to the emergency room (without self-administration) if reactions escalate.[16] (The most likely exception to this is in the rare case that a patient with MCAS is also taking a beta blocker, a drug which may impact the effectiveness of epinephrine. In this case, glucagon may be the medication of choice. This special scenario should be discussed very carefully with one's doctor.)

Patients may be initially unsure whether to use epinephrine, even when they know they are experiencing an acute reaction. Some may be concerned about the cost of the drug and may want to be sure that they are experiencing anaphylaxis so that they don't waste the medicine. Others may not be completely convinced that they are experiencing anaphylaxis or may think that it is wise to wait until they *absolutely need it*. Some patients may not be sure what triggered them and may second-guess their symptoms initially. Still others may be concerned that epinephrine could be harmful to the body. There are also cases where medical personnel are uneducated on anaphylaxis and give improper advice because the patient may not be experiencing visible signs of anaphylaxis like hives or swelling (which are not always present in true anaphylaxis).

To these concerns, it's important to emphasize that 1) epinephrine is safe when used properly, and 2) it can be VERY dangerous to wait and *not* administer epinephrine when one needs it. Acute attacks can escalate very quickly (in a number of seconds sometimes), and it is never a good idea to postpone life-saving medication. The pros of using the medication outweigh the cons, and there is low risk in using it, presuming the patient has been cleared by their doctor to do so.

A 2008 committee statement by the World Allergy Organization noted that "epinephrine is currently underused and often dosed sub-optimally to treat anaphylaxis, is under-prescribed for potential future self-administration, that most of the reasons proposed to withhold its clinical use are flawed, and that the therapeutic benefits of epinephrine exceed the risk when given in appropriate intramuscular doses."[17] The authors described anaphylaxis as something that occurs on a continuum and noted that it can be very dangerous to wait until the patient presents with multi-organ symptoms, as delayed administration is often associated with poor outcomes.

Some patients end up being hospitalized for their MCAS-related reactions and may need additional care beyond epinephrine. In 2015, Afrin published an abstract reporting a series of cases in which continuous intravenous infusion of diphenhydramine (Benadryl) was used to treat patients with severe MCAS. Afrin noted that patients with severe MCAS experienced a seesaw-type effect where the patient would experience another flare as the medication levels dropped to subtherapeutic levels repeatedly throughout the day when the drug was *not* continuously infused. According to Afrin, "Most patients who come to need continuous diphenhydramine infusions have already been taking the drug in 25-50mg doses ten times a day or more to maintain merely marginal control over their anaphylactoid symptoms, and by switching to continuous diphenhydramine infusions, these patients can gain substantially better control while simultaneously reducing their total daily dosage of diphenhydramine."[5] Afrin advocates for the careful consideration of continuous IV diphenhydramine for patients who experience life-threatening MCAS that is difficult to stabilize.[18]

Afrin's patient cases included 10 females with MCAS who all had been hospitalized for continuous MCAS-associated anaphylaxis and/or dysautonomia with pseudo-epileptic or hypotensive-type complications.[18] Dr. Afrin noted that nine out of the 10 patients stopped flaring once they achieved continuous IV doses of 10-12 mg/hr, ceased flaring 12-24 hours after the start of the IV, and were discharged from the hospital 18-48 hours later.[18] These nine patients were sent home with indwelling lines and portable pumps with capacity for additional demand dosing as still needed to control flares of symptoms from time to time.[18] Thus, it appears that *for severe MCAS cases*, the use of continuous diphenhydramine infusions is supported in this patient population with special guidelines for inpatient management as well as post-discharge care.[18]

A second case report was published in 2017 on the use of continuous IV diphenhydramine for an 18-year-old patient with MCAS who was experiencing serious continual anaphylactic episodes including one that induced cardiac arrest.[6] The patient presented with elevated episodic tryptase and prostaglandins on testing, but her bone marrow biopsy was inconclusive with no evidence of mastocytosis or the *KIT* mutation.[6] The patient had been symptomatic for a number of years and had previously trialed a great number of H1 and H2 receptor antagonist medications and steroids.[6] She had also trialed one dose of omalizumab, which triggered anaphylaxis.[6]

318

When she was admitted to the University of Minnesota intensive care unit, she was administered a continuous infusion of diphenhydramine (starting at 5 mg/hour, increased by 2 mg/hour until she reached the target of 15 mg/hour) and continued the medication from there, which resulted in a dramatic reduction to one to two anaphylactic episodes per month.[6] She eventually also began treatment with imatinib (starting at 100 mg/day and titrating up to 400 mg/day), which resulted in even greater reductions in attacks to one every two to three months.[6]

This case highlights the importance of individualized care that is catered to the patient based on the severity of their MCAS. For patients who present with severe, uncontrolled MCAS, a more intensive medication regimen and dosing plan may be essential to achieve stability and improve quality of life, regardless of potential side effects or long-term concerns. What started out as emergency care in this case carried over into a long-term plan that was very justified.[6]

The authors noted that one to two anaphylactic episodes per month "felt like a miracle to the patient."[6] Continuous anaphylaxis and other severe presentations of MCAS can be incredibly challenging for the patient and their family, and it's crucial that each care team individualizes their treatment plan with adequate attention to quality of life factors.

This case study serves as a reminder that it's crucial that all patients are taken seriously and treated with respect, regardless of whether they meet the inclusion criteria for systemic mastocytosis or not. Some hospitals like the University of Minnesota have historically been more exposed to MCAS-specific treatment measures such as continuous diphenhydramine thanks to the physical presence of Dr. Afrin, but keep in mind that many other hospitals may not be as open to considering this option.

It may be helpful and sometimes necessary for MCAS patients to come armed with a slew of resources to show emergency room physicians. Physical printouts of case studies like the ones mentioned above may be useful. *Anecdotally,* patients report that they often have poor experiences with emergency room staff in the event of anaphylaxis and MCAS flares, and many patients have been accused of "faking it." Patients and their families may find themselves in the position where they need to be gentle educators—or even vocal advocates—for treatment options when facing doubting providers.

While the case reports identify a subgroup of patients who may truly need continuous Benadryl or other potent medications, this appears to be a minority of MCAS patients. On the other end of the spectrum, many patients with MCAS experience much smaller flares that are not considered anaphylactic-type reactions but may require some supplemental medication in addition to their typical daily prophylactic medication routine for symptom management. Oral diphenhydramine, antihistamines, glucocorticoids, and benzodiazepines may be useful for managing *minor* flares.[11]

There are some "fast-acting" forms of medications on the market that could be helpful during minor flares. For example, liquid forms of Benadryl may be faster acting than the tablet and capsule forms. Some antihistamine brands offer faster-acting versions of the same drug. Epinephrine sprays for anaphylaxis appear to be in development, though it currently appears that intramuscular formulations are the fastest-acting option.[17]

PREVENTIVE MEDICATIONS THAT <u>BLOCK THE ACTION</u> OF RELEASED MAST CELL MEDIATORS[3]

- H1- and H2-receptor antagonists
- Leukotriene inhibitors
- TNF antagonists
- Interleukin antagonists

Antihistamines: H1 and H2 Receptor Antagonists

Antihistamines have been available for treating allergies since the 1940s.[19] Antihistamines are most often associated with medications that block H1 receptors, but there are also H2-receptor antagonists on the market that are useful in the treatment of MCAS. H1-receptor antagonists and H2-receptor antagonists are sometimes also referred to as "H1 blockers" and "H2 blockers," respectively.

H1-Receptor Antagonists

According to The Mastocytosis Society, this class of medications helps with "itching, abdominal pain, flushing, headaches, and brain fog."[20]

First-generation antihistamines were initially effective but have heavy sedating properties and side effects because they cross the blood–brain barrier, which inspired the development of second-generation antihistamines in the 1980s.[21] These second-line drugs have more selectivity for H1 receptors, a longer bio-availability, and less interference with cognitive function.[19] Second-generation antihistamines also have stronger anti-inflammatory actions, fewer anti-cholinergic effects, and less risk for adverse cardiovascular reactions when compared to first-generation versions.[19] However, a few second-generation drugs (terfenadine and astemizole) exhibited serious cardiac complications and were removed from the U.S. market[21] and, from there, a new third generation class of medications became available to replace them that were free of cardiac toxicity. Second- and third-generation antihistamines have a carboxylic acid group substituted molecularly and are therefore considered *non-sedating carboxyl group* medications.[19]

Below are some generic medication names accompanied by one example of a name brand of medications in each class (noted in parentheses). This is *not* an all-inclusive list.

Examples of first-generation ("sedating") antihistamines:[22]

chlorpheniramine (Chlor-Trimeton), diphenhydramine (Benadryl), promethazine (Phenergan), hydroxyzine hydrochloride (Atarax), meclizine (Bonine), clemastine (Tavist), doxepin hydrochloride (Sinequan)

Examples of second-generation ("non-sedating carboxyl group") antihistamines:[22]

loratadine (Claritin), cetirizine (Zyrtec), levocetirizine (Xyzal), desloratidine (Clarinex), ketotifen (Zaditor/Zaditen in Europe)

Example of third-generation ("non-sedating carboxyl group") antihistamine:[22]

fexofenadine (Allegra). *Additional third generation medications were in formulation but had not been released to the market at the time this book was written.*

The second- and third-generation medications tend to cause less drowsiness than first-generation antihistamines, but some of them still do cause some degree of fatigue or tiredness.

There is great concern about whether all generations of antihistamines are safe. A 2017 review article by Yanai and colleagues helps clarify the differences between different types of antihistamines.[19] First of all, first-generation antihistamines are more likely to have both short-term and long-term cognitive impacts.[19] For example, the cerebral half-life of sedating antihistamines such as diphenhydramine (Benadryl) is longer than the plasma half-life at 30 hours, which explains why many patients who take it at bedtime still feel drowsy the following day.[19] For some patients, first-generation antihistamines provide relief of anxiety.

Secondly, the affinity of the medication to bind directly to H1 receptors varies among different medications and thereby impacts potency.[19] However, potency does *not* equal clinical efficacy. The authors clarify, "More than a hundredfold difference exists in binding affinity (potency) among various antihistamines. Based on potency, non-sedating antihistamines can be classified into low- (loratadine, fexofenadine) and high-potency groups (bepotastine, olopatadine, cetirizine, epinastine, levocetirizine). However, though potency varies greatly among antihistamines, clinical efficacy as represented by maximum responsiveness is the same if administered in sufficient dosages."[19]

Thirdly, antihistamines ought to be considered in terms of whether they possess anticholinergic activity.[19] Anticholinergics are medications that inhibit the actions of acetylcholine, a neurotransmitter that triggers the release of histamine. Anticholinergic drugs have been under recent scrutiny due to their association with the development of dementia. A 2009 review found that 25 out of 27 eligible studies associated anticholinergic medications with dementia, delirium, and cognitive impairment.[23] In addition to potential cognitive consequences, anticholinergic drugs may influence other areas of the body, such as the muscles that control the initiation of urine or gastrointestinal motility.[13] Antihistamine medications that are considered in the anticholinergic class include: diphenhydramine (Benadryl), hydroxyzine (Atarax), cyproheptadine (Periactin), and chlorpheniramine (Chlor-Trimeton).[19,24] Second- and third-generation antihistamines are generally considered to have low anticholinergic activity.[24] Of course, this also means that the non-sedating antihistamines don't get into the brain like the anticholinergic medications and may not have the same short-term anti-anxiety effects.

A 2014 review on urticaria published guidelines that state that the dosage of non-sedating antihistamines may be increased two to four times the typical dose when the typical dose is insufficient to manage symptoms.[25] These dose-increase guidelines only apply for *non-sedating carboxyl group* antihistamines that *do not have anticholinergic action*.[25] In other words, additional dosing (within reason) of second- and third-generation antihistamines is permitted as needed to manage mast cell-related skin symptoms according to these guidelines.[25]

A 2015 study of over 3,400 patients evaluated medications that have anticholinergic effects, including antihistamines, and found that higher use of such medications was associated with an increased risk of dementia.[26] However, this study classified other types of drugs such as incontinence medications and antidepressants as anticholinergics, so the study was not directly specific to the sole use of antihistamines.[26]

A study in 2016 further investigated the use of anticholinergic medications including antihistamines on executive function test scores and brain scans and found increased brain atrophy and reduced brain glucose metabolism accompanied a clinical decline in cognitive function in patients using anticholinergic medications.[27] This study, which considered a

322

number of different drugs as anticholinergic, failed to separate patients based on which exact medication they were taking.[27]

On the other hand, while a lot of the research has focused on the potential negative long-term consequences of antihistamine use, one recent study found that clemastine fumarate (brand name Tavist) appeared to improve optic nerve function and possibly contribute to re-myelination of nerves in patients with multiple sclerosis.[28] Subjects reported fatigue, but no adverse events were reported.[28] Medication use was 10-72 mg per day in twice-daily doses.[28] The group that received the drug for three months followed by a two-month period without it had beneficial carry-over effects into the months when they were not taking it.[28] Dosing was not standardized and long-term effects were not determined in the study; future research will likely aim to further investigate these areas and replicate findings.

In summary, it appears that the anticholinergic and sedating potentials (i.e., first-generation classification) of certain antihistamines are what are currently believed to pose the greatest threat for long-term side effects. The 2017 review on antihistamines concluded that in terms of suppressing allergic activity, "from this perspective, long-term use of non-sedating antihistamines in monthly regimens is desirable as adverse reactions are uncommon. *Carboxyl group-containing non-sedating antihistamines* are particularly suitable for long-term use due to their reduced anticholinergic activity."[19]

The bottom line is that every patient is different, and the pros and cons need to be weighed, keeping in mind that there's a sort of ebb and flow to MCAS treatment and that some medication regimens may be temporarily necessary for certain time frames. If the patient is stable enough to have the choice, based on the research it appears that avoidance of first-generation antihistamines may possibly reduce the risk of dementia development.

Not all patients with MCAS use H1-blocking antihistamines, but they are recommended to be trialed as first-line treatment for MCAS by all. A 2015 review notes that second-generation non-sedating H1 antihistamines given twice a day is a proper initial treatment trial for prophylactic therapy in MCAS.[16] Experts in MCAD concur with the recommendations from the urticaria research that "doses to 4 times what is considered normal may be needed if urticaria is present."[16]

Flare-ups and breakthrough symptoms may be managed by first-generation (sedating) medications such as diphenhydramine and hydroxyzine.[16] Other patients with severe MCAS may necessitate anti-cholinergic drugs on a chronic basis (particularly Benadryl), and in those patients, the benefits and impact on quality of life *likely* strongly outweigh the potential risks, as highlighted in the above description of the case studies utilizing a continuous IV drip of diphenhydramine.

A third sub-group of patients with MCAS may find that once they have symptoms better under control, they can successfully transition from regular antihistamines to more natural compounds that have antihistaminic effects on the body and may opt for antihistamines during flares only. And lastly, there are patients who may not respond to antihistamines at all and may opt for other types of medications.

If a patient with MCAS is concerned about long-term consequences of H1-receptor blocking antihistamine use, according to the research, they should talk to their doctor about second-generation carboxyl group-containing non-sedating antihistamines or look into different, more natural treatment options with their medical team. All medications and supplements have the potential for side effects and interactions with other drugs and should be under the same scrutiny as the H1-receptor antagonists. Unfortunately, when compared to the H1 blockers, there's not nearly as much research out there for some of the other medications used to treat MCAS (and their specific applicability for this diagnosis).

H2-Receptor Antagonists

According to The Mastocytosis Society, this class of medications helps with "gastrointestinal symptoms and overall mast cell stability (all mast cell activation symptoms)."[20]

While H1-receptor antagonists suppress generalized histamine-mediated effects in the body, H2-receptor antagonists are more specific to the parietal cells and the suppression of gastric acid secretion by blocking histamine receptors in the stomach. They are commonly used for the treatment of gastroesophageal reflux disease (GERD), but can also be effective for both chronic management of MCAS and during acute flare-ups. H2 blockers are *different* than proton-pump inhibitors, which act by a separate mechanism.

It's important to note that some patients use H1-/H2-receptor antagonists for MCAS and add a proton pump inhibitor to control GERD as well. According to the Mastocytosis Society webpage on medications to treat mast cell disorders, "The H1 and H2 antihistamines are necessary to stabilize receptors on the mast cell. Therefore, if additional medication is required for control of gastroesophageal reflux (GERD), a proton pump inhibitor may be added to this protocol, but it cannot replace the H2 antihistamine."[20]

H2-receptor antagonists are typically recommended in twice-daily dosing for patients with MCAS, particularly those who present with abdominal symptoms.[16]

Examples of H2 blockers include:

famotidine (Pepcid), ranitidine (Zantac), cimetidine (Tagamet), nizatidine (Axid)

Combining H1 and H2 blockers for the treatment of conditions like urticaria has been investigated dating back to the 1970s.[29,30] Both medications have been shown to cause a dose-dependent reduction in inflammatory cytokines released by mast cells.[31] Improved patient outcomes have been cited in the literature in regards to acute cutaneous reactions with the use of H1 and H2 blockers.[32] Difficult cases of chronic urticaria also appear to be better managed with the combined treatment of H1- and H2-receptor antagonists plus montelukast sodium.[29,33] However, a recent systematic review determined that the existing evidence is not of sufficient quality to make conclusions about the *sole efficacy* of H2-blocking medications for the urticaria patient population.[34]

H2-receptor antagonists are frequently part of acute attack/anaphylaxis management recommendations by allergists. Surprisingly, based on a 2014 meta-analysis, it's unclear whether H2-receptor antagonists are effective in these scenarios.[35] The majority of research with H2-receptor antagonists focuses more on associations with the gastrointestinal system and stress ulcers. More research is certainly needed in the area of the role of H2 blockers in the management of allergic conditions and anaphylaxis.

There are concerns about the impact of regular use of H2-receptor antagonists on vitamin B12 deficiency. A 2013 study confirmed an association and noted that the risk increases as the length of time on the medication increases.[36] Many other studies support this finding,[37-40] and it may be extra problematic for patients who are also taking metformin for diabetes.[41-42] This may warrant a conversation with one's medical team about the pros and cons of H2 blockers, as well as the potential implications for vitamin supplementation.

While there is great concern about the development of dementia with H1-receptor antagonists, H2-receptor antagonists may not pose the same risk. A 2002 study in the journal *Neurology* found no associations between H2 blocker use and the development of Alzheimer's Disease.[43] However, a 2007 study of an African-American population found that continuous H2-receptor antagonist use was associated with greater risk of cognitive impairment, even after controlling for a number of factors including additional anticholinergic medication use.[44] When compared to the research on the use of an H1-receptor antagonist, there is a scarcity of peer-reviewed evidence in the area of H2-receptor antagonist use and its association with dementia and utility in patients presenting with symptoms of MCAD.

Leukotriene Inhibitors

According to The Mastocytosis Society, leukotriene-receptor antagonists and leukotriene inhibitors help with "respiratory symptoms and overall mast cell stability (all mast cell activation symptoms)."[20]

Examples of leukotriene inhibitors include:

montelukast (Singulair), zileuton (Zyflo), zafirlukast (Accolate)

In addition to those afflicted with respiratory inflammation, patients with elevated prostaglandins in particular may see symptomatic relief with the use of montelukast.[16] Leukotrienes appear to have a role regulating mast cells in the bone marrow as well as in the recruitment of mast cells into the tissues before maturation.[45] Thus, inhibition of their binding pathways could directly impact a number of symptom-generating factors. Some of these medications (like zileuton) block the production of leukotrienes by inhibiting an enzyme involved in their synthesis, while others (like montelukast) are leukotriene-receptor antagonists that prevent leukotrienes from binding to their receptor sites on smooth muscle cells.

According to Seneviratne and colleagues, leukotriene-receptor blockers are widely used for chronic urticaria and asthma patients and are generally well tolerated.[12] Some patients with MCAS do better taking the medication twice daily.[12]

A 2010 review of montelukast noted that in addition to targeting mast cells, it appears that the drug also has potent anti-inflammatory properties impacting other cells like eosinophils, monocytes, and neutrophils (which have a poor response to corticosteroids).[46] In studies with mice, three months of treatment with montelukast not only reduced the clinical severity of collagen-induced arthritis, but it also reduced the levels of TNF-alpha (a mast cell mediator) and the number of mast cells in their arthritic paws.[47]

According to a review by Riccioni et al., leukotriene-targeting medications have been investigated in clinical studies, case reports, and reviews for a number of diseases outside of asthma/respiratory symptoms.[48] While research has not evaluated their efficacy with MCAS patients, they do show promising potential for the treatment of sinus issues, migraine headaches, systemic mastocytosis, irritable bowel syndrome, urinary issues like interstitial cystitis, chronic urticaria, and atopic dermatitis, to name a few.[48]

A 2004 case report described the use of a leukotriene-receptor inhibitor for the treatment of systemic mastocytosis in a young child and reported that when it was added to his regimen of antihistamines it significantly improved his wheezing and skin vesicles.[49] Likewise, when it was removed, he had flare-ups of those symptoms.[49] A more recent (2012) case report of child with systemic mastocytosis reported that refractory abdominal and urinary symptoms were successfully treated by adding montelukast to the medication regimen.[50]

These case studies indicate that leukotriene-targeting medications may be useful adjuncts for patients with MCAD, but it's clear that more research is needed in this patient population.

TNF Antagonists

Tumor necrosis factor (TNF) is an inflammatory cytokine released by mast cells (and a number of other cells). TNF antagonists are immunosuppressive drugs that are often prescribed for patients with autoimmune disease but may also be useful for patients with MCAS experiencing chronic inflammation who aren't achieving optimal symptom relief with other options. These medications are prescription drugs and may have greater side effects and risks than over-the-counter mast cell medications.

Examples of TNF antagonists include:

etanercept (Enbrel), adalimumab (Humira), infliximab (Remicade)

TNF blockers are commonly prescribed for patient with psoriasis. A 2014 study noted that patients who are less likely to respond to TNF blockers to manage psoriasis are patients who smoke or are overweight or obese and patients who had higher baseline severity scores.[51]

TNF blockers are also commonly prescribed for patients with rheumatoid arthritis, inflammatory bowel disease (such as Crohn's disease and ulcerative colitis), and ankylosing spondylitis. The majority of the research focuses on these conditions. While MCAD-specific research is lacking, *in theory* medications targeting a blockage for the effects of TNF should have a positive impact on certain patients with MCAD who have TNF-driven symptoms.

There has been some concern about the development of cancer and, in particular, lymphomas in patients who have used TNF blockers. A 2010 review evaluated 48 cases in children and concluded that treatment with TNF blockers may increase the risk of malignancy, but the use of immunosuppressants and comorbidities may play a role in these cases.[52] A 2011 meta-analysis of 74 randomized controlled studies indicated less than 1% short-term risk of malignancy for patients using TNF blockers; the authors concluded that based on the evidence they were unable to refute or verify whether their use truly raised the short-term risk of developing cancer.[53]

On the other hand, research supports that the use of TNF blockers may offer protective benefits for the cardiovascular system in patients with rheumatoid arthritis.[54] The overall inflammation inhibition created by TNF antagonists may be beneficial for certain patients.

Interleukin Antagonists

Interleukins are another type of inflammatory cytokine released by mast cells (and other cells), and they are increasingly being targeted pharmacologically in inflammatory conditions.

Examples of interleukin antagonists include:

IL-1 antagonists – anakinra (Kineret)

IL-1β antagonists – canakinumab (Ilaris)

Patients (particularly those who have arthritic symptoms) may find great relief with interleukin antagonists. Research has evaluated the role of certain interleukins in autoimmune diseases and has determined that their blockage may improve inflammation-mediated effects, including loss of hearing and vision and poor organ function.[55] Interleukin antagonists appear to be beneficial in reducing symptoms in asthmatic patients.[56] They are being increasingly utilized in patients with MCAS.

Keep in mind that many TNF antagonists and interleukin antagonists should not be used in combination simultaneously because of risk of serious complications relating to immunosuppression. Generally, for MCAS, one or the other is deemed to be effective and is the focus.

In Development

New medications are being developed that may block the release of mast cell mediators. H3-receptor blocking medications and drugs that inhibit tryptase and chymase are currently in development.[3] As of 2017, the development of H4-receptor antagonists for clinical use also appears to have growing interest.[57]

PREVENTIVE MEDICATIONS THAT INHIBIT THE RELEASE OF MAST CELL MEDIATORS[3]

- Cromoglicic acid (cromolyn sodium)

- Omalizumab (Xolair)

- Benzodiazepines

- Tyrosine kinase inhibitors and mTOR inhibitors

- Immunosuppressors (azathioprine and others)

- Cannabinoids

While H1 and H2 blockers prevent the binding of substances to receptors on the mast cell, this class of medications prevents mediators from being released into the circulation.

Cromoglicic Acid (Cromolyn Sodium)

Cromoglicic acid ("cromolyn sodium" or "cromolyn") is one of the more well-known medications that inhibits the release of mast cell mediators. Cromolyn is effective via the modulation of the chloride current and G-protein coupled receptor 35, a common target in asthma and inflammatory conditions.[4] The drug is available in a number of different formulations, including oral liquid form, inhaled form, and eye drops. It appears that a systemic (IV) form of sodium cromoglicate is in development.[12]

Early research supported the use of cromolyn in rodent peritoneal mast cells for histamine inhibition,[58] but there was no effect seen in mucosal mast cells even at high concentrations of the drug.[59,60] In human studies, very high doses of cromolyn were required in order to see inhibition from human tonsillar and lung mast cells.[61] A 2011 study found that a cromolyn substance (delivered by iontophoresis into the skin) was able to prevent itching following injections of intradermal histamine, but instead of exerting antihistaminic effects on skin mast cells, the authors determined that the itching was alleviated through actions of the cromolyn on sensory C-fiber nerve endings.[62] And interestingly, more than one study reported that patients developed contact dermatitis from eyedrops that contained cromolyn.[63,64]

The oral liquid form is most commonly prescribed for patients with MCAS. The medication comes in small plastic tubes that are to be added to a full glass of water 30 minutes before each meal. Most patients are instructed to use the medication three to four times per day in doses up to 800 mg/day,[12,16] slowly titrating the dose up over the series of several weeks or months to tolerance to the prescribed amount.

For patients with food sensitivities and persistent gastrointestinal symptoms, cromolyn can be very helpful. However, there is very poor absorption of cromolyn in the body (less than 2%) and it's essentially limited to the gastrointestinal tract (outside of potential interactions with the nerves in the gut), negating any potential systemwide effects.[13,16]

High cost, slow response time (weeks to months), and tedious dosing are some reasons why patients may not use cromolyn, even if they tolerate it well. Other patients with MCAS may be deterred by side effects or find that they become sensitized to the medication and need to take higher dosages over time. *Anecdotally*, some patients swear by cromolyn for their day-to-day survival, while others claim that certain side effects and a worsening baseline of symptoms resulted from their trial of cromolyn.

Oral cromolyn is a drug that's certainly worth a try if the patient is not responding to other types of first-line therapy for MCAS. The inhaled and eye drop versions may also be considered for certain patients with MCAS. *Anecdotally*, the liquid formulation may also be useful topically to assist in MCAS-related dermatological issues.

Omalizumab (Xolair)

Omalizumab is another commonly utilized treatment option for patients with MCAS and is considered third-line treatment. Originally designed for patients with asthma and chronic urticaria, omalizumab is a monoclonal antibody that binds to free human IgE that is not already occupied at cell receptor sites, thus preventing the allergic inflammation cascade from occurring.

Omalizumab is administered as an injection, and its downsides are the high cost and requirement to return for subsequent regular injections. However, copayment assistance plans exist, and it's definitely worth looking into if the patient's medical team is offering the drug as an option. The main reported adverse effect is anaphylaxis, but it's reported to be extremely rare (0.001 to 0.002% of patients).[65,66]

Omalizumab has well-documented benefits for patients who suffer from chronic urticaria, allergic angioedema, asthma, and drug allergies,[67] so it's not a stretch to infer that patients with MCAD may also benefit from its use.

Fortunately, there are multiple MCAD-specific studies to report. In 2011, Molderings and colleagues published a report on four patients with therapy-resistant MCAD who were treated with omalizumab.[67] Two of the patients in the report had systemic mastocytosis and two of the patients had monoclonal MCAS.[67] Overall, "two patients achieved an impressive persistent clinical response to treatment with omalizumab."[67] Symptoms gradually improved in the third patient, and the fourth patient had one injection of omalizumab after which the drug was discontinued due to a flare-up in symptoms.[67] Thus, three out of the four patients were responders to the drug.[67]

The patient with the poor response was one of the patients with monoclonal MCAS; however, the other patient with monoclonal MCAS had a significantly positive response to the injections of 300 mg every four weeks.[67] Around the six-month mark, the patient who responded well to omalizumab experienced a significant cessation in symptoms such as hives and flushing and noted less fatigue.[67] She was able to reduce her number and dosages of other mast cell medications and expand her dietary options.[67] In addition, her urine N-methylhistamine levels normalized.[67] The authors concluded that omalizumab can lessen the intensity of the symptoms of systemic MCAD.[67]

A 2011 review on MCAS management noted that "Recently, anti-IgE treatment with the humanized murine monoclonal antibody omalizumab has alleviated high intensity symptoms of MCAD. Since treatment with omalizumab has an acceptable risk-benefit profile, it should be considered in cases of MCAD resistant to evidence-based therapy."[10]

In 2012, Bell and Jackson published a case report on an 11-year-old boy who met the diagnostic criteria for MCAS and had monoclonal MCAS and mastocytosis ruled out.[8] The patient reported chronic systemic symptoms as well as anaphylaxis triggered by food several times per month initially.[8] While symptoms improved somewhat on antihistamines and a prolonged course of corticosteroids, he was still unstable, at which point he began omalizumab injections (150 mg) every four weeks.[8] He had a rapid response to the omalizumab therapy and reported only one episode of urticaria in the 10 months that followed the initiation of his treatment.[8] The authors concluded that omalizumab may be an appropriate addition to traditional antihistamine therapy in certain MCAS patient cases.[8]

Omalizumab has support for improving—and in some cases, inducing remission of—recurrent cases of anaphylaxis[2,68] and also shows efficacy in reducing anaphylactic reactions with Hymenoptera venom immunotherapy in patients with monoclonal MCAS.[7] Omalizumab also has a variety of evidence supporting its efficacy in patients with systemic mastocytosis.[10,69,70] Recent reviews and case reports continue to support its effectiveness in patients with MCAD.[2,68,71-73]

Benzodiazepines

Additional medications that inhibit mast cell mediator release include benzodiazepines, a class of medications that are commonly prescribed for anxiety. Many patients with MCAS experience anxiety which *anecdotally* can often be alleviated or completely resolved when mast cell mediator release is prevented. Lorazepam, clonazepam, and alprazolam are examples of benzodiazepines utilized with some MCAS patients.

In mice, benzodiazepines (diazepam and midazolam) were effective in reducing mast cell proliferation and the release of mediators such as TNF-alpha and nitrites.[74] Early research also noted that benzodiazepines were effective in the inhibition of serotonin released by mast cells.[75]

It's also plausible that there is an indirect loop that downregulates mast cell activity based on other properties of benzodiazepines, such as the enhanced GABA (neurotransmitter) activity in the brain, or immunomodulation effects with the binding of certain drugs to translocator proteins.[76] If the overall level of stress and anxiety is reduced in the brain, it could be theorized that mast cells will be subsequently less reactive. A 2015 review of systemic mastocytosis noted that "even anxiety may trigger mast cell degranulation, for which benzodiazepines may be considered."[77]

Tyrosine Kinase Inhibitors

Tyrosine kinases are types of enzymes that are responsible for activating proteins by adding phosphate groups to the proteins. Thus, tyrosine kinase *inhibitors* prevent this protein-phosphate binding step from occurring, which halts the cellular cascade and could prevent mast cells from proliferating. In theory, tyrosine kinase inhibitors block mutated c-*KIT* activity and could be a useful type of medication for patients with MCAD.[78]

Based on the mechanism by which these medications act, *in theory* patients with monoclonal MCAS or clonal disease (who are more likely to have evidence of a c-*KIT* mutation and/or an increased proliferation of mast cells) would be on the end of the spectrum more likely to benefit from this class of drugs. However, that does not mean that they are not necessarily beneficial as an option for MCAS patients who don't present with such findings. They are considered a fourth-line treatment option for patients with MCAS and should only be considered in patients who don't respond to first-, second- or third-line treatment options.[4]

The decision to begin tyrosine kinase inhibitor use is not one to be taken lightly. Tyrosine kinase inhibitors are used as chemotherapy agents with the intent to induce mast cell death in patients with mast cell leukemia. There are different types of tyrosine kinase inhibitors. Imatinib mesylate, dasatinib, and midostaurin (also known as PKC412 in the literature) are some of the more commonly researched tyrosine kinase inhibitors. Imatinib (Gleevac) is a well-known chemotherapy medication. Careful monitoring of kidney and lung function is required for patients who are on these types of medications, as they carry a higher risk of infection. They also pose a list of potential significant side effects to be aware of.

The research for tyrosine kinase inhibitor use with MCAD appears to be all over the map. Most of the research focuses on patients who have systemic mastocytosis or mast cell leukemia, with a range of zero response to significant benefit being reported but no consistent overall trend. A 2010 review from the Mayo Clinic of 342 patients with SM and the literature to date recommended cladribibine and interferon alpha and noted limited treatment success with imatinib mesylate and other anti-*KIT* D816V inhibitors.[79] Some studies noted that specific tyrosine kinase inhibitors do not show any preferential ability to kill human mast cells in patients with systemic mastocytosis and mast cell leukemia.[78,80] Other research has noted a change in mast cell burden, improvements in liver function and spleen size, a decrease in skin symptoms, or a reduction in measurements of circulating chemical mediator levels including histamine and tryptase.[81]

As a whole, it appears that based on the high-quality evidence, the impact of tyrosine kinase inhibitors is, at best, partial resolution of symptoms in patients with systemic mastocytosis.[4] However, many case reports offer more positive support for their use.[4] In a 2016 review article on the pharmacological management of MCAS, Molderings et al. noted, "As with all drugs used in therapy of MCAD, their therapeutic success seems to be strongly dependent on the individual patient, again underscoring the observed mutational heterogeneity of the disease."[4]

More recent studies provide additional theoretical and clinical support for the use of imatinib and midostaurin in patients with MCAS. Authors of a 2017 study called midostaurin "a magic bullet that blocks mast cell expansion and activation."[82] They discussed the results of a multicenter phase II trial that found an overall response rate of 60% for midostaurin in patients with advanced SM.[82] In their conclusion, they offered hope for this drug in the reduction of mediator-related symptoms in the MCAS population as well, though midostaurin has yet to be studied outside of the SM population.[82]

In the 2017 case report, one patient with severe MCAS who did not meet the diagnostic criteria for systemic mastocytosis was treated with 400 mg/day doses of imatinib (once her continuous anaphylaxis was under improved control with IV diphenhydramine), which led to further intervals between anaphylactic episodes and an improved quality of life.[6] The authors noted that "imatinib provides benefits in *KIT* D816V-negative mast cell disorders due to other unknown mutations."[6] Thus, tyrosine kinase inhibitors may prove to be useful for a certain subgroup of MCAS patients in the future, and research appears to be heading in this direction.

A similar class of drugs called mTOR inhibitors has been investigated for its anti-cancer effects. These drugs inhibit the target of rapamycin, a specific protein kinase. mTOR inhibitors may be under consideration for use of MCAS in the future.

Bruton's tyrosine kinase (BTK) is an enzyme that is involved in the activation of mast cells and basophils when allergens bind to IgE that's attached to high-affinity IgE receptors. Food, medications, and insect venom trigger anaphylactic responses via this pathway.

According to a 2017 review, some BTK inhibitors were on the market and others were in development that looked promising as treatments for patients with MCAD.[83] The authors concluded that in addition to episodic use for anaphylaxis to food and other substances, "Given their excellent safety and tolerability profiles, it may also be possible to utilize BTK inhibitors on a more chronic basis for the treatment of other mast cell disorders where reactions are more frequent or unpredictable, such as idiopathic anaphylaxis, mast cell activation syndrome, and mastocytosis, if these disorders prove to be mediated by FcεRI or other BTK-dependent pathways."[83] BTK inhibitors may be another future clinical direction for patients with MCAS, but more research is needed to evaluate whether this theory could translate into efficacious clinical results.

Immunomodulators

Immunomodulators such as azathioprine, methotrexate, cyclosporine, and prednisone are also sometimes used for patients with MCAS to inhibit the release of mast cell mediators via a general state of immunosuppression. Azathioprine (Azasan) is typically used in patients with rheumatoid arthritis or who are at risk for organ transplant rejection. Methotrexate (Trexall) is typically used in patients with psoriasis, rheumatoid arthritis, and cancer. Cyclosporine (Neoral) also tends to be prescribed for patients with psoriasis or rheumatoid arthritis or who face the risk of organ rejection after transplant.

Interestingly, a 2016 review noted an association between systemic mastocytosis and rheumatoid arthritis (RA) and reported a case study where antihistamines were effective in a patient with RA.[84] It's possible that a specific subgroup of MCAD patients may also benefit from RA-targeting immunosuppressive drugs (and vice-versa), though more research is needed.[84]

Prednisone (Deltasone) is probably the most well-known immune-modulating glucocorticoid drug that covers a wide range of inflammatory, autoimmune, and malignant conditions and is also used to assist in short- and long-term care for allergic reactions. Several authors support the use of systemic steroids in patients who experience frequent anaphylaxis that is unresponsive to other anti-mediator medications.[2] Prednisone is commonly used in the acute, one- to two-week phase after an anaphylactic reaction. Prednisone is sometimes used on a longer-term basis for prevention of idiopathic anaphylactic attacks (sometimes for up to 9-12 months at a time) and in these cases, it appears that about 20% of patients with frequent cases of idiopathic anaphylaxis end up *unable* to wean off the drug.[85] Ketotifen appears to be a helpful addition for anaphylaxis-prone patients who are having difficulty weaning off prednisone.[85]

Seneviratne and colleagues note, "Oral steroids may be prescribed for acute episodes of MCAS symptoms that involve airway issues, but they should not be taken on a long-term basis. Low-dose inhaled steroids may assist patients with MCAS who have high airway hyper-reactivity."[12] Risk of side effects, infections, and long-term complications are some of the reasons that pharmacologic immunomodulators are not first-line choices for the treatment of chronic systemic MCAS symptoms.

Allergy desensitization therapy is considered a form of immunomodulation that is sometimes used with MCAS. Allergen desensitization is sometimes performed in the clinic sublingually or with injections and should be closely monitored by one's medical team.

Stem-cell transplantation has been recently investigated in patients with systemic mastocytosis (SM). A 2014 study retrospectively evaluated the use of allogeneic hematopoietic stem-cell transplantation treatment in a patient population with *advanced SM*.[86] The treatment was associated with long-term survival and the majority of patients (70%) had some type of positive response, although it appeared less effective in patients with mast cell leukemia.[86]

An updated (2017) review concluded that allogeneic stem-cell transplantation is a realistic option for patients with advanced SM in drug-refractory disease who are young and fit and have a suitable donor.[87] While initial research looks promising for patients with severe MCAD, this type of treatment is generally not considered with the MCAS patient population.

Cannabinoids

Endocannabinoids are naturally-occurring substances found within the body. Endocannabinoids are found in breast milk and have also been linked as the source of the "runners high" one can get with exercise. Endocannabinoids are part of a neurotransmitter system that promotes relaxation and regulates other body functions like sleep, hunger, memory, and even aspects of the immune system. They have been touted as big players in the maintenance of homeostasis in the body.

Phytocannabinoids are very similar to endocannabinoids and come from plants. One of the more common and potent sources on the market comes from the hemp plant. Cannabidiol (known as "CBD") is the non-psychoactive component of the cannabis plant that stimulates cannabinoid activity. Due to the stigma associated with the psychoactive tetrahydrocannabinol (THC) ingredient in marijuana, CBD oil has unjustly received a bad rap based on association by those who are not aware that the two compounds operate distinctly.

A 2015 peer-reviewed review article in *Neurotherapeutics* noted that THC can be addictive, while "cannabidiol (CBD), in contrast, appears to have low reinforcing properties with limited abuse potential" and that it appears to inhibit drug-seeking behavior.[88] However, it may take a while for American mainstream medicine to jump on board fully with the use of CBD, in-part due to its stigma but also due to the limited research studies conducted in the U.S. (thus far).

That being said, more and more peer-reviewed research articles on CBD use in other countries are coming back with some astonishing results. According to the 2015 review, "Human studies on CBD corroborate preclinical findings on its therapeutic effects on nausea, inflammation, and cerebral ischemia."[88] Epilepsy, anxiety and depression, cardiovascular disease, endometrial inflammation, neurological conditions, and atopic dermatitis are a small example of the conditions that show promising results in CBD research.[88-91] CBD has promising initial research into potential use for patients with addictions and opioid abuse.[88] Its use has also been associated with a reduction in allergy symptoms, and cannabis appears to have a bronchodilating effect in the asthmatic population.[90,91] CBD appears to decrease autonomic nervous system activation[88] and it would be interesting to study its effects in a population of patients who present with MCAS and hyperadrenergic POTS.

It appears that to date there is no high-quality research evaluating CBD use in patients with MCAS or mastocytosis. A 2005 study evaluated the role of cannabinoid receptors (CB1 and CB2) in human cutaneous mast cells including one patient with mastocytosis.[92] Ständer and colleagues concluded, "The abundant distribution of cannabinoid receptors on skin nerve fibers and mast cells provides implications for an anti-inflammatory, anti-nociceptive action of cannabinoid receptor agonists and suggests their putatively broad therapeutic potential."[92]

Additional sources support that CBD appears to have a therapeutic impact on mast cell activation. CBD use reduces the production of cytokines (such as interleukins released by mast cells) in human subjects.[93] An Italian research team conducted a review of studies examining

CBD and mast cell activation in 2008.[90] They noted evidence of in vitro animal and human prevention of mast cell activation via different pathways following cannabinol exposure.[90] The authors concluded that "cannabinomimetic compounds, including PEA and its congeners, act to control MC (mast cell) activation and degranulation early during the inflammatory response, thus leading to a swift resolution and preventing the development of chronic inflammatory disease."[90]

Furthermore, a 2017 review of pain management in the MCAS patient by Wirz and Molderings concluded that CBD offers a promising future for analgesic therapeutic options for patients with MCAD.[9] While the research is somewhat preliminary, it appears that CBD has tremendous neuroprotective, anti-inflammatory, antimicrobial, and antioxidant effects on the human body and offers a promising potential for patients with mast cell overactivation and allergic disease. CBD oil does not contain THC and has been approved in all 50 U.S. states.[94]

Anecdotally in the online MCAS community, both CBD and THC have been reported to be helpful for some patients, particular those with high pain levels, inflammation, and insomnia. CBD may have potential side effects, depending on the dosage. Patients have reported GI issues, tiredness, lightheadedness, and low blood pressure.[88] Patients with MCAS may need to factor these possibilities into their decision to use CBD, as they are often already prone to these symptoms. Many patients find that using CBD oil at bedtime is most optimal to prevent side effects and assist with symptoms of insomnia. However, studies have noted both sleep-inducing and wakefulness characteristics with CBD use, so it's not certain that it assists with insomnia.[88]

Initial caution may be needed as CBD oil, like any new medication or supplement, could in theory cause reactivity in patients with MCAS. Long-term effects are currently unknown, and CBD is metabolized in the liver and could in theory interact with other drugs metabolized in the same area, such as pain medications and steroids.[88] CBD oil can also interact with certain medications such as tricyclic antidepressants and anti-anxiety meds, so it's another topic to discuss with one's medical team.[88]

PREVENTIVE MEDICATIONS THAT INHIBIT THE PRODUCTION OF MAST CELL MEDIATORS[3]

- Steroids
- Nonsteroidal anti-inflammatory drugs (NSAIDs)
- Hydroxyurea

- Vitamin C
- Ketotifen

Steroids

According to a 2011 review on MCAS management, "If symptoms are resistant to therapy, as a next therapeutic step toward reducing mast cell activity and thereby decreasing mediator release, treatment with prednisone, ciclosporine (cyclosporine A), low-dose methotrexate or azathioprine can be considered."[10] These drugs are also considered to inhibit the release of mast cell mediators (in addition to inhibiting their production)[3] and have already been discussed in the above section titled "Immunomodulators."

Nonsteroidal Anti-Inflammatory Drugs (NSAIDs)

NSAIDs comprise a medication group that includes many well-known over-the-counter anti-inflammatory drugs. Ibuprofen (Advil, Motrin), naproxen (Aleve), and aspirin (Bayer) are examples of NSAIDs.

Aspirin appears to be the NSAID most commonly recommended for a therapeutic trial in patients with MCAS. Specifically, aspirin has been cited to be potentially helpful for patients with MCAS who have elevated prostaglandin levels.[4,16] However, it's very important to note that in some patients, aspirin can actually trigger a worsening of mast cell activation and symptoms. Patients with a known salicylate intolerance should avoid aspirin. Patients who wish to consider a trial should begin with very low doses (81 mg or less, titrated up to a potential maximum of 325 mg twice per day) under doctor supervision.[16] Other NSAIDs possess the potential to trigger reactions with MCAS so patients should proceed with caution.

Hydroxyurea

Hydroxyurea is a cytotoxic agent that works to reduce the number of blood cells in the bone marrow. Specifically, it inhibits an enzyme called ribonucleotide reductase that decreases the production of single units of DNA.

Hydroxyurea (Hydrea) is commonly used in the treatment of sickle cell anemia, chronic myeloproliferative leukemia, and head and neck cancers. It's also used in patients with systemic mastocytosis and polycythemia vera and is considered second-line treatment for psoriasis. In patients with sickle cell anemia, its use is predominantly to reduce the need for blood transfusions and to reduce the frequency of painful episodes. Hydroxyurea sometimes improves mast cell activation symptoms in patients with systemic mastocytosis, and it's plausible that it could be utilized for MCAS as well.[95]

There are mixed reviews about the efficacy of hydroxyurea in the systemic mastocytosis (SM) population. A 2008 study evaluated 43 patients with MCAD (SM/SM-ANHMD/MCL) who utilized hydroxyurea as a primary treatment and noted that partial or moderate response was noted in about nine patients (about 21%) and no complete response in any patient.[96] This was low when compared to the other treatment options in the study including the cytoreductive agents interferon alpha (with or without prednisone) and chlorodeoxyadenosine, which had nearly double (41%-46%) the response rates.[96]

A case report by Sheikh et al. described two patients with systemic mastocytosis (SM-ANHMD) who responded favorably to the addition of hydroxyurea.[97] Both patients had a reduction in tryptase levels within two months of beginning the medication.[97] Changes were noted on the follow-up bone marrow biopsy of one patient, with a reduction in bone marrow mast cell infiltration and a conversion from positive to negative CD25 and other aberrant markers in a significant proportion of mast cells.[97] The second patient also noted improvement in ascites and skin lesions.[97]

"Idiopathic" soft tissue and bone pain, or diffuse aching, is common in MCAS and often nonresponsive to traditional pharmacological pain management options. Afrin published a case series in 2013 that described five patients with MCAS who responded well to the use of hydroxyurea.[95] In all five cases, the addition of hydroxyurea to the medication regimen promptly and dramatically reduced diffuse aching in the legs and other areas noted by the patients.[95] Several patients had significant declines in their pain level (such as from 8 out of 10 to 3 out of 10 on the numeric pain rating scale).[95] There are a number of brands for this drug, and three of the five patients had to try different formulations of the drug until they found a tolerable version (likely due to reactions by their dysfunctional mast cells to certain excipients in various formulations of the drug).[95] One patient had to stop the medication due to the development of a low red blood cell count.[95]

Afrin discussed the similarities in diffuse aching pain experienced by patients with both sickle cell anemia and MCAS and posed the possibility that, based on his case findings, 1) MCAS may be an unrecognized comorbidity in some patients with sickle cell anemia, and 2) the efficacy of hydroxyurea in patients with sickle cell anemia could be connected to inadvertent treatment of MCAS.[95] He concluded that his cases show support of relatively low-dose hydroxyurea in treatment of bone and soft tissue pain for MCAS patients, and that further research is needed to identify optimal dosing and the patient subpopulation characteristics likely to benefit from the drug.[95]

Vitamin C

Vitamin C is a well-known antioxidant that functions as a scavenger of free radicals and is an important component involved in the synthesis of neurotransmitters and hormones. Vitamin C boosts the function of the immune system and has antimicrobial properties. Vitamin C *deficiency* is not only associated with scurvy but is also correlated with elevated histamine levels.[98] Vitamin C has the ability to both increase the breakdown of histamine and decrease the rate of histamine formation.[4]

There are other pathways in which vitamin C (also known as ascorbic acid) may be beneficial for patients with MCAD. Vitamin C interacts in a beneficial way with glutathione, and it appears that prevention or reduction of glutathione deficiency can occur with adequate ascorbic acid.[99] Glutathione is an important part of the body's detoxification system, which may already be impaired in the patient with MCAS. In theory, the more efficient the detoxification process in the body, the more quickly the body will remove potential mast cell triggers. Research has found that vitamin C supplementation even at lower levels (500 mg/day, an amount attainable with diet alone) results in a significant rise in red blood cell levels of glutathione.[100]

A 2007 study evaluated eight patients with asthma who took vitamin C supplements in the form of 1500 mg ascorbic acid per day for two weeks.[101] The subjects had a number of factors measured pre- and post-supplementation with vitamin C or placebo following an exercise test.[101] In addition to improvements in pulmonary function scores, urinary leukotriene and prostaglandin levels were significantly lower in the group receiving the ascorbic acid when compared to the placebo.[101]

Nausea and motion sickness have been associated with histamine, and one study found that 2 g of vitamin C supplementation helped reduce boat-associated motion sickness in younger subjects (under age 27).[102] However, this study did not specifically evaluate patients with MCAS.[102]

There are other formulations of vitamin C, such as gel-like mixtures of liposomal vitamin C that have reportedly better bioavailability in the bloodstream. A 2008 study compared 1 g of an oral ascorbic acid to a liposomal ascorbic acid formulation and found almost double the plasma levels available from the liposomal version compared to the traditional oral supplement.[103]

340

Ascorbic acid may also be useful when used in IVs as opposed to oral supplementation. A 2013 study evaluated 89 patients with either allergic or infectious disease.[104] Following IV infusion of 7.5 g ascorbic acid, there was a significant decline in serum histamine levels.[104]

There is some debate in the MCAS community about the optimal dosage of vitamin C, as some rumors exist that excessively high levels can actually induce mast cell activation. Thus, its benefits for this patient population may very well be dose-dependent and (as always) individual-dependent. While the body flushes out vitamin C that it cannot utilize fairly quickly, large quantities may trigger diarrhea or other symptoms.

A 2017 review noted that dietary intake of vitamin C of 100-200 mg/day (enough to provide adequate saturating levels) was sufficient for prophylactic prevention of infection in healthy subjects.[105] However, the authors noted that "treatment of established infections requires significantly higher (gram) doses of the vitamin to compensate for the increase inflammatory response and metabolic demand."[105] Nonetheless, based on the lack of existing evidence for the supplementation of ascorbic acid in the MCAD population, there is not sufficient proof for a research-based dosage recommendation to be made for the treatment of MCAS. This question may be best posed to one's medical team.

Ketotifen

Ketotifen is considered by some to be both anti-histaminic and mast cell-stabilizing via different mechanisms.[12] It's available in the U.S. from compounding pharmacies as an oral medication; ketotifen fumarate (Zaditor) eye drops also exist for allergy sufferers. While the drug seems to be a relatively novel option for the treatment of allergic disease, it's actually been around for quite a while (since the 1970s). It's generally well-tolerated, although some patients report severe drowsiness, dizziness, lightheadedness, an increase in appetite, and weight gain when using it.[12]

The issue for many patients has been access to the medication, as only certain compounding pharmacies make it. Oral ketotifen can be more expensive in the United States when compared to other countries.[12] Outside of the U.S., it is more readily available under the brand name Zaditen. Recently it appears that ketotifen has been easier to locate online, although it's important to be aware that non-compounded versions of the medication are more likely to have fillers and other ingredients added. Extra caution is warranted against pharmacies selling ketotifen overseas that don't require prescriptions.

Some patients have better results when taking ketotifen in doses spread out throughout the day.[12] Capsules are typically available in 0.5 mg-2 g dosages. Soderberg notes in a 2015 review that dosing at 1-2 mg twice a day may be beneficial for gastrointestinal symptoms in patients with MCAS.[16]

Ketotifen has been studied in a number of different populations. It has shown to be beneficial for patients with irritable bowel syndrome.[106] Many studies also support its use for chronic urticaria,[107-110] and one study found it effective for urticaria pigmentosa associated with cutaneous mastocytosis, although the study was small and performed with questionable methodology.[111,112]

Patients with systemic mastocytosis appear to respond favorably to ketotifen.[113] Bone, gastrointestinal, skin, and neuropsychiatric manifestations of SM have shown improvements with the utilization of ketotifen.[114-116]

"Mast Cell Stabilizer" Controversy

In the literature, both cromolyn and ketotifen are sometimes considered to inhibit the release of mast cell mediators. They are sometimes referred to as "mast cell stabilizers" in studies. There's some controversy in labeling certain medications as mast cell stabilizers, particularly if they only selectively prevent degranulation of certain mediators and not others. Theoharides asserts that while cromolyn and ketotifen (weakly) inhibit histamine and prostaglandin release, neither medication blocks inflammatory cytokine release, and neither medication should be considered a true mast cell stabilizer in humans.[117]

PREVENTIVE MEDICATIONS TO ADDRESS BONE MINERAL DENSITY ISSUES

Osteoporosis is a highly documented comorbidity in patients who have systemic mastocytosis (SM). Some sources claim a slightly increased risk, while others report the prevalence to be over 40% of patients with SM.[118,119] High numbers of mast cells are associated with accelerated bone turnover and loss.[120] Specifically, patients with SM have decreased trabecular bone mass and an increase in osteoblasts and osteoclasts, which are bone-remodeling cells.[121] This finding has been noted regardless of whether the patient has cutaneous manifestations of mastocytosis.[121] Higher levels of urinary N-methylhistamine have also been associated with increased osteoporotic findings in patients with systemic mastocytosis.[122] Vitamin D deficiency, a significant risk factor for the development of osteoporosis, may also be responsible for the decreased bone mineral density noted in patients with SM.

A 2016 review by Austin and Akin recommends that patients who have clonal mast cell disease (monoclonal MCAS and SM) maintain good calcium and vitamin D supplementation to reduce potential complications associated with osteoporosis and consider bisphosphonates and denosumab as options.[2]

Molderings and colleagues note that bisphosphonates should be the first treatment option for patients who have bone pain, osteolysis, osteopenia, and osteoporosis.[4] They consider vitamin D and calcium second-line options due to "limited reports of success and an increased risk for developing kidney and ureter stones."[4] They also cited consideration of calcitonin.[4] Teriparatide may be used with caution as liver failure has been known to occur.[4] Anti-RANKL drugs like denosumab are also recommended, but with caution due to the reports of severe osteonecrosis of the jaw (in patients with poor dental health or recent invasive dental work).[4] Intravenous zoledronate has also been reported in the literature for a patient with SM who could not tolerate the gastrointestinal side effects of calcium, vitamin D, and bisphosphonates.[123]

Despite research indicating that patients with systemic mastocytosis ought to consider supplementation to prevent osteoporosis, physiological mechanisms related to osteoporotic risk factors are just beginning to be researched in the MCAS population. Patients with MCAS *may* also be at higher risk for bone mineral density problems, but it may be due to a mechanism other than vitamin D deficiency.

In 2017, researchers in Germany theorized that patients with MCAS would be more likely to be deficient in vitamin D, which has mast cell stabilization properties.[124] Germany is a northern country with less annual sunshine, so researchers theorized that the lack of vitamin D could explain the high prevalence of MCAS in Germany.[124] The researchers compared 100 patients with MCAS to patients in the general German population.[124] However, they ended up finding a pattern contradictory to their theory.[124] Thirty-four percent of patients with MCAS were deficient in Vitamin D, compared to 75% in the general German population.[124] Vitamin D levels were in the "sufficient" range for 53% of patients with MCAS, compared to 8% in the general German population.[124] Thus, patients with MCAS who are concerned about bone mineral density should not assume that they are automatically at risk, and should have testing done with their medical team to assist in supplementation and osteoporosis prevention decisions.

PAIN MANAGEMENT AND HOSPITAL MEDICATION CONSIDERATIONS FOR MCAS

According to a 2017 review by Wirz and Molderings on pain management for the MCAS patient, there are a number of considerations for medication choices that aim to reduce subsequent mast cell activation.[9] Opioid receptor agonists (such as morphine, oxycodone, methadone, tramadol, meperidine, and fentanyl) may be *more* likely to induce mast cell activation.[9] The authors noted that etoricoxib and celecoxib medications are *less* likely to activate mast cells when compared to nonsteroidal anti-inflammatory drugs (NSAIDS) like ibuprofen and acetylsalicylic acid.[9]

Anecdotally, some patients note that fentanyl and tramadol are better tolerated than the other opioid receptor agonists, and Zofran may also be utilized for nausea. The narcotic Dilaudid may also be tolerated, depending on the patient.

In the cases of acute pain management (typically in the hospital during acute attacks and very high pain levels), the 2017 review recommends consideration of the following:[9]

- o Remifentanil, alfentanil, fentanyl, oxycodone when individual tolerance is known
- o Piritramide
- o Ketamine
- o Dipyrone
- o Acetaminophen up to 1 g/day (caution for liver toxicity!)
- o Flupirtine
- o Etoricoxib, celecoxib
- o Ibuprofen or acetylsalicylic acid when individual tolerance is known (used with caution—may induce mast cell activation)
- o Peridural anesthesia with lidocaine (used with caution—may induce mast cell activation)

In preparation for surgical procedures, the appropriateness of anesthesia should be discussed. Patients who have a history of anaphylaxis to anesthesia and those who have systemic mastocytosis should be considered high risk.[9] Patients should keep clear records of exactly what types of anesthesia have been used in past procedures (both successfully and those that triggered reactions) to help assist in the process.[9] Premedication with sedatives such as benzodiazepines should be considered in cases where surgical anxiety may trigger mast cell degranulation.[9] The surgical team should be aware of any potential physical trigger factors for the MCAS population, including friction, infusion of cold solutions, sudden temperature changes in the operating room, and widespread tissue trauma.[9] Procedures that involve radiocontrast media should be considered with high caution.[9]

In terms of general operative considerations (surgeries and endoscopies), Wirz and Molderings recommend intravenous premedication that includes a glucocorticoid, ranitidine, and dimetindenmaleate about 30 minutes prior to the procedure.[9] Exact recommendations depend on disease intensity and body weight.[9] The authors also note that ethanol-based solutions should be avoided in patients with MCAD.[9] A link to the original article that contains additional specifics can be located in Appendix 2.

When it comes to postoperative pain management, Wirz and Molderings recommended consideration of remifentanil, alfentanil, fentanyl, oxycodone, and piritramide.[9] Out of those options, piritramide is the only *opioid analgesic* that has support for inhibition of mast cell activity.[9] Seneviratne and colleagues noted that "narcotics, too, commonly are triggers; fentanyl, tramadol, and hydromorphone tend to be better tolerated than other narcotics in MCAD patients."[12]

It's important to keep in mind that opioid analgesics like morphine, codeine, and pethidine are more likely to induce mast cell mediator release and should be avoided.[9] Ketamine is another type of pain medication that has potential mast cell inhibitory effects, but it tends to have side effects.[9] For lower-level postoperative pain, acetaminophen and dipyrone may be useful in the MCAD patient population.[9]

Chronic pain management holds some additional considerations. A 2015 review noted that chronic pain management utilizing mast cell stabilizers, cannabinoids, the cannabinoid-like compound N-palmitoyl-ethanolamine (PEA), and nociceptin agonists, in addition to conventional analgesics, may offer improvements in symptoms.[125]

Wirz and Molderings noted that the therapeutic efficacy of pain-targeting medications can vary between patients and may be poor.[9] "The absence of any response of the pain to or even its aggravation under classical pain therapy must not be misconstrued as a somatoform disorder. In MCAD, the different pain sensations have to be treated specifically, if possible deduced from their putative mast cell mediator-related causes."[9]

This brings up an excellent point. Patient response to pain medications is unpredictable in all scenarios and may be especially so in patients with MCAD. Patience and trial and error may be initially necessary in this area of acute management, just as it is necessary when attempting to determine chronic triggers and come up with a comprehensive long-term medication plan for the patient with MCAS.

MEDICATIONS TO BE AVOIDED

A 2016 review article examined the available literature and came up with following medications that have a higher risk of mast cell mediator release. [4]

Table 1. Medications that may trigger reactions for patients with MCAD[4]

TYPE OF MEDICATION	DRUGS THAT HAVE PROVEN OR THEORETICAL RISK
antibiotics	cefuroxime, gyrase inhibitors, vancomycin
anticonvulsive agents	carbamazepine, topiramate
cardiovascular drugs	ACE inhibitors, ß-Adrenoceptor antagonists
intravenous narcotics	methohexital, phenobarbital, thiopental
local anesthetics	amide-type: lidocaine, articaine; ester-type: tetracaine, procaine
opioid analgesics	meperidine, morphine, codeine
peripheral-acting analgesics	acidic NSAIDS such as ibuprofen
peptidergic drugs	icatibant, cetrorelix, sermorelin, octreotide, leuprolide
plasma substitutes	hydroxyethyl starch, gelatin
muscle relaxants	atracurium, mivacurium, rocuronium
selective dopamine and norepinephrine reuptake inhibitors	bupropion
selective serotonin reuptake inhibitors	all
x-ray contrast material	iodinated contrast medium, gadolinium chelate

Based on the literature, it may be wise to avoid the above-mentioned medications or to speak with one's medical team if concerned. The original 2016 review by Molderings and colleagues suggests therapeutic alternatives to the medications in Table 1 and serves as an excellent resource for an in-depth understanding of the variety of pharmacological options for this patient population.[4] This chapter is not all-inclusive and patients and clinicians should access the full text recommendations available in Appendix 2.

MANAGEMENT OF OTHER SYMPTOMS/COMORBIDITIES

Most patients with MCAS have some sort of gastrointestinal (GI) ailment present. The 2016 Molderings review recommended a number of medications to help manage GI symptoms.[4] For patients experiencing diarrhea, the authors recommended the use of nystatin, cholestyramine, montelukast, or 5-HT3 receptor inhibitors such as ondansetron.[4] Acetylsalicylic acid (aspirin) may be trialed incrementally in doses of 50-350 mg/day for patients who have diarrhea; extreme caution is recommended for the use of aspirin products as they can potentially cause mast cell degranulation.[4] The authors recommended a five-day trial of a particular drug in order to determine whether it will be effective in reducing diarrhea.[4]

On the other end of the spectrum, abdominal distention pain from gas can be treated with metamizole or butylscopolamine.[4] For patients with MCAS who experience nausea, dimenhydrinate, lorazepam, 5-HT3 receptors, and NK1 antagonists such as aprepitant are recommended.[4] The treatment of colitis is typically best tolerated with the use of budesonide or prednisone (20 mg/day).[4] Protein pump inhibitors may also assist with GERD/gastric concerns.[4] For patients who experience angioedema during reactions, tranexamic acid or icatibant may help manage symptoms,[4] but both do have the potential for serious side effects.

Anemia has some special considerations unique to patients with MCAS. Iron supplementation (in both oral and parenteral forms) for a patient with iron-deficiency anemia has a risk of inducing "potentially intense mast cell activation" and should be given cautiously.[4] Red blood cell transfusion may be considered as an alternative for anemic patients.[4]

Chronic joint symptoms ("rheumatoid symptoms") are sometimes treated with COX2 inhibitors (etoricoxib or celecoxib) or acetaminophen.[4] Triazolam may be tolerated well for insomnia.[4] Zolpidem (Ambien) is another medication for insomnia that works in part by actions on histaminergic neurons and may be appropriate for some patients with MCAS who suffer from insomnia.[126]

As mentioned in Chapter 5, bladder issues and symptoms of urinary tract infections (often with no evidence of infection) appear to be fairly common in this patient population. Pentosan polysulfate sodium (Elmiron) or amphetamines are typically used for patients with MCAS who suffer with interstitial cystitis, or pain and pressure around the bladder.[4] Pentosan polysulfate sodium is also considered a medication that inhibits the release of mast cell mediators.[3,4]

For skin itching, the authors recommend either palmitoylethanolamine-containing care products or a cromolyn-containing ointment.[4] Cases of eye inflammation (conjunctivitis in particular) in the MCAS patient are best treated with eye drops that are preservative-free versions of H1 antihistamines.[4] Cromolyn, ketotifen, and glucocorticoids (brief courses) may also be used for eye inflammation.[4] However, it's important to determine the underlying cause and make sure a secondary disease is not responsible for any new eye concerns.[4]

For patients who experience obstructive/mucus-based respiratory symptoms with compulsive throat clearing, leukotriene receptor blockers are recommended.[4] In certain countries, leukotriene synthesis inhibitors (like zileuton) are also available and useful for respiratory issues[4].

High cholesterol is a common finding, and it appears to be independent of diet and may be due to the inhibition of transport into the cells in patients with MCAS.[4] The drug atorvastatin may be trialed for hypercholesterolemia in this patient population.[4]

CHAPTER KEY POINTS

- Achieving a stable baseline with medication assistance should be the first priority for patients with MCAS, *step one*. Over time, patients may find that addressing underlying factors that impact the immune system (such as viruses, bacteria, and toxins) may assist in reducing the usage or reliance on medications, *step two*.

- There's no shortage of medication options to address MCAS. Most patients are initially prescribed a combination of H1- and H2-receptor antagonists and should follow a stepwise approach to trialing other pharmaceutical drugs with the assistance of their medical team.

- Medication trials should be meticulously isolated to one drug at a time. In general, one month is usually sufficient to determine the efficacy of a single medication on symptoms.

- There are a number of over-the-counter, prescription and inpatient-administered substances and medications that should be avoided for patients with MCAS due to their likelihood of inducing mast cell degranulation.

Chapter Ten

Natural Treatment Options and Special Considerations

A TEAM APPROACH

Holistic Specialist Care

Holistic care aims to address the root cause(s) and trigger(s) of mast cell activation and also strives to foster lifestyle modifications for long-term management. It's important to create a care team that incorporates multiple areas for healing success (e.g., a doctor who focuses on MCAS, physical therapist, allergist, acupuncturist, mental health specialist, naturopath).

It is strongly recommended to pursue care *right away* with a functional medicine doctor or naturopath who can help evaluate additional underlying causes contributing to or flaring the symptoms. (This should *not*, however, replace medical advice from the professional who diagnosed the patient with MCAS. This should be considered a crucial supplemental piece of the team.) An example of a holistic team approach to MCAS is shown in Figure 1.

Anecdotally, many patients exhaust all mainstream medicine options before considering the more alternative/natural routes of care. Some patients put off the advice for a naturopathic approach for years and then may regret not instigating such care sooner in their healing journey. Thus, in the early stages, *once one has a stable baseline of health achieved after the diagnosis of MCAS,* it's recommended that the patient investigates and addresses a number of underlying factors that could impact the degree of mast cell activation they are experiencing. Addressing other comorbidities may not "cure" the patient of MCAS but will likely have a positive impact on their quality of life, level of symptoms, and amount of medications necessary to control it.

Figure 1. Example of a Multidisciplinary Team Approach for Management of MCAS

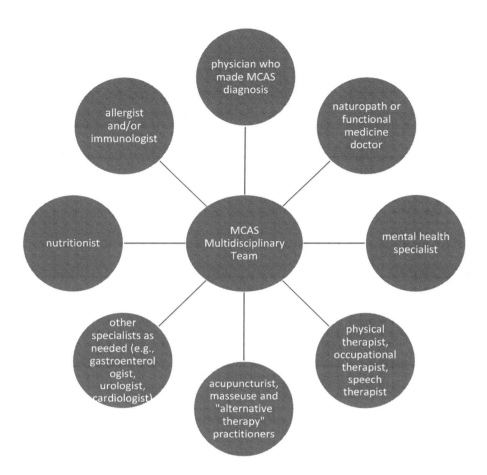

Breaking the Vicious Intergenerational Cycle

In the patient world, the perfect storm of forces encountered in utero (exposure to viruses, bacteria, heavy metals, etc.) plus continual toxins encountered on a daily basis (pesticides, cleaning products, unclean air and water, mold- and water-damaged environments, skin products, etc.) can all contribute to dysfunction. This dysfunction may be related to the by-product of westernized diets that are lacking the tools the body needs to fight invaders and heal. It may be increased by the presence of one particularly toxic event (such as the removal of mercury amalgam fillings, for example). It's possibly impacted by an increase in technology, including the near-constant presence of wi-fi and other frequencies. It is likely triggered by underlying emotional trauma and stressful life events, both big and small.

According to this theory, over time, as the immune system is weakened, the body picks up various insults such as parasites, Lyme disease, mycoplasma pneumonia, Bartonella, Epstein-

Barr virus, shingles, mold toxins, and heavy metal toxins. As these types of insults reduce efficiency and add inflammation to the system, additional problems may manifest like eczema, insomnia, GERD, endometriosis, SIBO, gluten intolerance, polycystic ovarian syndrome, thyroid issues, migraines, arthritis, fatigue, and so much more. The cumulative effects "clog" the bloodstream, render the lymphatic system sluggishly slow, and put extra stress on vital organs including the liver.

From a functional medicine perspective, as the body runs out of effective ways to "detox" from the continual daily input of environmental toxins (particularly in certain patients who appear to have genetic predispositions to reduced detoxification efficiency), the body begins to revolt in certain ways. Food reactions and sensitivities may suddenly develop.

Many people with MCAS note that their allergic reactions can be variable. For example, a patient may say, "I've been eating avocados every day, and all of a sudden, I had anaphylaxis to one today." One theory is that this is not likely a true *IgE-mediated* allergy, but more of the body's way of signaling that it's unable to process the backlog of "junk" clogging things up. Similar to the histamine bucket theory where the body reaches a spillover effect, it appears that the body's mast cells will both chronically react to triggers and also sporadically react when the overall system is overloaded and has no way to process and detoxify new inputs.

Just as patients with MCAS often react to fillers and dyes in medications, there's a good chance that they are also reacting to chemicals contaminating the food and water supply, household environments, beauty products, etc. These are likely things that they've been exposed to their whole lives but, at some point, reached a tipping point in terms of their baseline mast cell activation and subsequent sensitivity. In terms of food sources, extra mast cell degranulation may occur if an item was contaminated in the chain of handling before it was ingested.

Pesticides have both direct and indirect effects on the immune system.[1] Research dating back to the 1980s determined that pesticides trigger the release of histamine and other chemical mediators.[2] It's not surprising to find that pesticide-induced mast cell activation occurs and may be dose-dependent,[3] seeing as how mast cells can react to every other "unnatural" trigger out there as part of the body's innate self-protection mode. Similarly, a variety of types of heavy metal exposure also appear to be triggers for mast cell activation.[4-6] Addressing the toxic load is one giant piece of the puzzle.

Why do younger generations seem to be more plagued by these problems? One theory is that younger generations are experiencing these types of symptoms earlier and earlier in life due to an exponentially higher rate of exposure to toxins coupled with decreased efficiency in the body's ability to process them. The baby boomer generation began to show symptoms around the age of retirement and menopause. The current 20- and 30-somethings are now alarmingly symptomatic, and their kids are often severely symptomatic starting at infancy. In addition to increased exposure throughout life, it appears that each generation is passing more and more toxins like heavy metals, bacteria, and viruses from the mother to the fetus, which only compounds the issue of individuals arriving into this world predisposed to a greater toxic buildup.

Mainstream medicine is important and has its role and time and place; there's no denying that. *Step one*—achieving a more stable symptomatic baseline to get the body to a more parasympathetic-dominant nervous system state with less continual inflammation and anaphylactoid-type reactions—is an essential aspect of MCAS patient care. However, the addition of a naturopathic or functional medicine type approach as part of *step two* will, over time, (hopefully) be the game-changer to help patients achieve long-term goals and reduce the overall assault on the immune system.

This chapter contains information about options for nonpharmacological supplement treatment that are sometimes recommended for patients with MCAS, as well as a deeper look into special topics including considerations for vaccinations, venom immunotherapy and the management of MCAS in pregnancy and in the pediatric population.

ALTERNATIVES AND/OR SUPPLEMENTS TO MEDICATION REGIMEN

Flavonoids

Flavonoids are "polyphenolic compounds found in fruits, vegetables, nuts, seeds, herbs, spices, tea, olive oil and red wine with antioxidant properties. Flavonoids have potent anti-oxidant, anti-inflammatory, and mast cell blocking activities."[7,8] Quercetin is one of the better-known naturally occurring flavonoids that has been associated with beneficial effects on mast cells. Luteolin, which is structurally similar, has also been the subject of research regarding its impact on mast cells.

Flavonoids like quercetin, apigenin, and kaempferol work to reduce mast cell degranulation via the inhibition of certain pathways such as spleen tyrosine kinase. Luteolin impacts mast cells though another pathway and is an API transcription factor inhibitor.[9] Luteolin, in addition to reducing inflammation and inhibiting microglia and mast cell reactivity, appears to be a weak metal chelator, offering some utility for patients with cognitive issues like brain fog and higher toxic burdens.[10]

Numerous studies support the use of quercetin and luteolin for patients with autism, as presented earlier in this book.[11-15] Quercetin may also assist in the body's ability to detoxify harmful substances, as evidenced by its ability to reverse sleep deprivation/stress-induced reductions in brain glutathione levels in mice.[16,17] Brain inflammation and detoxification issues are commonly experienced in patients with MCAS, and quercetin appears to be one of the more popular "natural" treatments of MCAS.

Quercetin and other flavonoids have also been the subject of mast cell research. Animal (mouse and rat) studies have shown that the release of mast cell mediators including interleukins, tumor necrosis factor (TNF), and histamine can be inhibited by flavonoids.[18-21] Quercetin and luteolin have shown inhibitory effects of leukotrienes, histamine, and prostaglandin D2 from human cultured mast cells, and they also reduced secretion of serotonin by platelets.[20,22] Quercetin alone also inhibits TNF, tryptase, cytokines, and histamine release from human mast cells.[23-25]

Theoharides is one of the research leaders in the area of natural polyphenolic flavonoids. His team is investigating the most optimal formulations for absorption, the determination of dosage guidelines, and additional potential anti-allergic, anti-inflammatory and anti-cancer mechanisms of action for certain flavonoids like quercetin and luteolin.[26]

Quercetin vs. Cromolyn

Research dating back to the 1980s had already begun to investigate what natural substances could inhibit histamine secretion from mast cells.[27] One early study noted that quercetin inhibited histamine from rat peritoneal mast cells by 75% at a low dose of 10 uM, while very high doses of cromolyn (1000 uM) were necessary for similar (but reduced) results (65% inhibition).[8,27]

Weng and colleagues conducted an extensive study in 2012 comparing quercetin and 100 uM cromolyn on human cultured mast cells.[8] Two formulations of quercetin were used: an equimolar formulation of quercetin ("Q") and 100 uM water-soluble quercetin ("WSQ").[8] Authors noted that Q is half as active as WSQ, and 100 uM of WSQ is approximately equivalent to the 1 g/day dosing of quercetin commonly used in human studies.[8] In contrast, the study used concentrations of cromolyn that were approximately *10 times* the typical concentration of oral cromolyn evenly distributed throughout the day in an 80 kg (about 176 pounds) human.[8]

The authors initially determined that cromolyn was ineffective when administered prior to the trigger, so it was used at the same time as the trigger, while quercetin was administered 30 minutes prior to the trigger in all parts of the study.[8]

In the first part of the study, human cord blood–derived cultured mast cells were stimulated with IgE/anti-IgE, which resulted in the release of mast cell mediators including histamine, prostaglandin D2 (PGD2), and leukotrienes.[8] Cells that were pretreated with quercetin saw an 82%-87% (Q-WSQ) inhibition in histamine secreted, compared to a 67% inhibition in cells treated with cromolyn.[8] Prostaglandins were 77%-81% (Q-WSQ) inhibited with quercetin pretreatment compared to 75% with cromolyn, and leukotrienes were inhibited 99% with both formulations of quercetin and 88% inhibited with cromolyn.[8]

Substance P is a mast cell mediator that has been associated with contact dermatitis and other inflammatory skin conditions. It has also been shown to induce further mast cell activation. In the second part of the study, the mast cells were treated with substance P instead of the IgE/anti-IgE sequence (plus preincubated with either Q or WSQ or treated at the time of exposure with cromolyn).[8] Two hours following this trigger, histamine was reduced by 78% with WSQ (which was actually lower than the control!), 51% with quercetin, and 71% with cromolyn.[8] Twenty-four hours after substance P was administered, interleukin-8 levels were reduced by 33%-74% (Q-WSQ), and only reduced by 17% with cromolyn.[8] Tumor necrosis factor (TNF) levels were reduced 77%-85% (Q-WSQ) compared to a 15% reduction with cromolyn one day following the trigger.[8] The release of IL-6 following stimulation with substance P and pretreatment with quercetin was found to be dose-dependent.[8] IL-6 was reduced by 71% (10 uM dose quercetin) and 87% (100 uM dose quercetin) which were both lower than the control value, compared to a 37% reduction with cromolyn.[8]

In the third part of the study, researchers found that quercetin inhibited intracellular calcium levels following substance P administration as a trigger, while cromolyn had no effect.[8] (Intracellular calcium release is believed to be a crucial step prior to the release of mast cell mediators.) They also found that WSQ more effectively inhibited NF-kB nuclear translocation (a step necessary for the production of cytokines) when compared to Q and cromolyn.[8]

What does all of this mean? There are a few take-home messages. Both quercetin and cromolyn effectively inhibit histamine, leukotrienes, and PGD2 in human mast cells. However, quercetin is much more effective in the reduction of inflammatory cytokines released from human mast cells. The more active water-soluble version of quercetin was superior to regular quercetin and cromolyn in all tests. Interleukin-6 had a significant dose-dependent effect in terms of quercetin efficacy. With the exception of the comparison of histamine levels with regular quercetin compared to cromolyn (which was still less effective than the water-soluble quercetin solution), all other formulations of quercetin were superior to cromolyn for all remaining mediators and conditions tested. Furthermore, cromolyn had to be added at the exact same time of the trigger to have any effect at all, whereas quercetin was effective as a prophylactic treatment.[8] Both formulations of quercetin showed better results in terms of the carryover effects into the next day when compared to cromolyn. [8]

This study was highlighted and explained more thoroughly in this chapter because it's one of the groundbreaking studies that support the use of a more natural substance to reduce human mast cell activation with direct comparison to a pharmacologic drug. The implications are powerful in terms of cost-effectiveness, as cromolyn tends to be much more expensive than quercetin (depending on insurance coverage, of course). This study was important because although rodent models have previously shown that cromolyn reduces histamine levels, it appears to be less effective in human mast cells.[8] The study was also powerful because despite significant differences in dosing (10 times the typical daily dose of cromolyn compared to half to full daily dose of quercetin), the quercetin still exceeded the effects of the cromolyn dramatically.

Skin Conditions and Quercetin

The 2012 study by Weng and colleagues also included a separate clinical portion of their research.[8] They had human subjects wear nickel patches while receiving regular pre-administration of WSQ.[8] Patients treated with WSQ showed significant reduction in contact dermatitis (over 50%-100%), skin itching, and the irritant dose necessary to achieve skin redness.[8] The authors concluded, "Here we report for the first time to our knowledge that quercetin can be beneficial in contact dermatitis and photosensitivity in humans, conditions that are typically difficult to treat."[8] Prior research supports that these conditions do not tend to respond significantly to antihistamines and cromolyn.[28,29] This may have implications for future investigation into the flavonoid treatment of skin conditions like eczema, atopic dermatitis, and psoriasis, as well as mast cell-activation disease-associated dermatological issues.

Flavonoid Supplementation

One limitation to the supplementation of both cromolyn and quercetin in water soluble formulations is their poor oral absorption. WSQ, while very effective in test tubes, is likely less useful in the gastric environment in human subjects due to stomach acidity. However, Weng and colleagues noted in 2012 that "a liposomal or enteric coated formulation may offer advantage for increased bioavailability. A phytoquercetin is now under development and appears to have much higher oral absorption."[8]

Six years after the study was published, there appears to be more bioavailable formulations of quercetin on the market. NeuroProtek is an over-the-counter formulation of quercetin, luteolin, and rutin created by Algonot that's mixed in olive and sunflower extracts to increase absorption and promote the anti-inflammatory effects with less metabolism prior to reaching the brain. A lower-concentration version is also available that is lower in phenols. (Some adults and children may be sensitive to phenols so might need to start with this version.)

Some formulations (such as ProstraProtek) also include olive kernel extract and chondroitin sulfate as active ingredients which serve to correct GI mucosal damage and improve absorption. Chondroitin sulfate may also exhibit antihistaminic effects.[30] However, it's important to note that ProstaProtek does contain shellfish, which is a common allergen and could in theory cause reactivity in the patient with MCAS, so caution is needed when trying this particular version.

Thorne now has a product called Quercetin Phytosome that binds the quercetin to phosphatidylcholine (derived from sunflower), which enables it to cross the gut barrier more easily before being broken down. Thus, it appears that multiple companies have begun to include formulations that in theory should enhance the oral absorption of flavonoids. According to the manufacturers, it may take from one to six months to see the full benefits of flavonoid supplementation.

It also appears that flavonoid skin products and nasal sprays are in development and could potentially offer a more direct route for flavonoids to access the brain.[10] While flavonoids are available without a prescription, the downside is that there are few companies producing these supplements. Plus, if patients use the supplements according to dosing instructions, they can be costly.

It's important to weigh out all factors. MCAS prescription and over-the-counter medications can also be costly, and it's entirely possible that a flavonoid supplement could be as effective as or more effective than a regimen of mainstream prescription medications—and could come at a reduced price in the long run.

Low-Dose Naltrexone

Low-dose naltrexone (LDN) is being increasingly prescribed in the autoimmune and chronic illness community. LDN works to block opioid receptors and enhance immune system function by upregulating the production of the body's natural opioids. A 2018 case report found that a patient suffering with severe POTS, small intestinal bacterial overgrowth and MCAS responded well to the use of LDN in conjunction with other treatments.[31] LDN is inexpensive and may reduce inflammation in a certain subgroup of patients, though more research is needed.

Nonprescription Supplements

There are a number of other treatment options that do not require a prescription that should be discussed with one's medical team. It's important to remember that supplements and herbal remedies still have the potential to have contaminants and/or excipients. Patients should use extra caution when ordering supplements online, as overseas websites or even Amazon sometimes contain products that may be misleading. In many cases "natural" supplements may be processed through the same detoxification pathways in the liver as traditional pharmaceutical drugs. A meticulous and lengthy trial is advised for supplements in patients with MCAS, just like prescription medications.

Some MCAS specialists include trials of substances including DAO, n-acetyl-cysteine, and alpha-lipoic acid in their arsenal of treatment options. Sources of omega-3 fatty acids and methylfolate have also been discussed as part of treatment for this patient population, in addition to products that aim to improve vagus nerve function and overall nerve function. Natural bowel motility agents, antiemetics, bronchodilators, pancreatic enzyme supplements, and antidepressants may also be considered with help from one's medical team.[32]

Vitamins and Minerals

Some patients may be deficient in certain vitamins and minerals and may need specific supplements. The supplementation of vitamin C has already been discussed. *Anecdotally* magnesium and vitamin D deficiency are especially common in the MCAS community.

Vitamin D is known for its role in bone health and in assisting in calcium absorption, but it's also important for brain function and development, as well as skin health. Vitamin D synthesized in the skin is taken up by mast cells and stored inside their granules.[7] Vitamin D3 is associated with the protective benefits of interleukin-10 in cutaneous mast cells, and topical vitamin D medications are sometimes used for the treatment of psoriasis and other skin conditions.[7]

Vitamin D's effects are far-reaching, as it's known to regulate over 900 genes and contribute to multiple influential roles in the equilibrium of systemwide health. Vitamin D deficiency has been implicated in conditions like diabetes, cardiovascular disease, cancer, autoimmune conditions, and neurological disease.[33-35]

Research indicates that vitamin D deficiency is associated with respiratory issues including asthma. A 2011 European study evaluated vitamin D levels in children and found that the children who had low serum levels tended to be asthmatic with poor respiratory function testing following an exercise challenge.[36] Additional research supports the correlation between low serum vitamin D levels and severe therapy-resistant asthma in children.[37]

It's possible that vitamin D *deficiency* puts one at higher risk for issues with mast cell activation. Low bone mineral density and high osteoporosis risk (associated with low vitamin D levels) are noted in studies of mastocytosis patients, so one could infer that a similar phenomenon could be playing a factor in patients with MCAS.[38-40] On the other hand, as previously discussed in the osteoporosis section, a German study in 2017 noted that patients with systemic MCAD actually had *lower* rates of vitamin D deficiency (34%) than the general population (75%).[41]

Vitamin D appears to decrease mast cell activation. Specifically, it appears that when vitamin D3 binds to its receptor, it inhibits the release of vasoactive compounds in mast cells.[42] Mast cell-mediated suppression of skin inflammation and pathology was achieved following dosage of vitamin D in mice that were subjected to chronic UVB radiation.[43] A 2014 study found that vitamin D3 metabolites suppressed the production of mast cell mediators through vitamin D receptor mechanisms in a laboratory setting.[44] Further evaluation using mice found that vitamin D3 metabolites were able to reduce skin swelling during IgE-mediated allergic reactions.[44] Vitamin D3 supplementation is sometimes included in a treatment plan for MCAS, particularly when the patient's levels test low.

Magnesium is crucial for many bodily functions, including everything from major organ function and heart health to blood sugar regulation, metabolism, muscle function, bone health, nervous system function, and gastrointestinal motility, to name a few. Magnesium regulates the calcium inside cells; increases in magnesium outside the cells is theorized to be part of its mechanism in reducing inflammation in the body. In animal studies, magnesium deficiency is associated with an increase in mast cells in the small intestine, kidney, bone marrow, and liver.[45] Another study found that magnesium deficiency resulted in elevated urinary histamine and reduced DAO levels in rats, which was reversible with supplementation.[46] Further research has confirmed that rats deficient in magnesium exhibited excess inflammatory free radical and cytokine production and an exaggerated response in immune stress.[47]

In one human case study of a female patient with mastocytosis, researchers noted that low baseline magnesium levels appeared to promote degranulation of mast cells.[48] However, a retrospective review in the 1990s of 21 patients with systemic mastocytosis at Brigham and Women's Hospital only noted one patient, out of the entire cohort, who had reduced magnesium levels on testing.[49] Hopefully future research will delve more into the role of magnesium in the MCAD patient population.

There are different forms of both nutrients, and they are also available as injections (vitamin D) and in IV form (magnesium), so all options should be evaluated if supplementation is indicated. Magnesium is available in many different oral formulations, some of which may cross the blood–brain barrier and have greater impacts on anxiety (magnesium threonate) or have bigger implications for alleviating constipation (magnesium citrate), so it's important to keep in mind that not all supplements are alike.

Vitamin E is also an important regulator of immune function. In addition to antioxidant functions, vitamin E analogues are involved in mast cell and protein kinase pathways that in effect modulate mast cell migration, proliferation, life cycle, and degranulation.[7] Vitamin E is also important for cardiovascular health and vision. Vitamin E contributes to the reduction of oxidation of low-density lipoprotein (LDL) cholesterol which, according to researchers, may also reduce mast cell activation.[7] Some experts assert that true vitamin E deficiency is rare, while others attest that it's more common than once believed. Seeds, nuts, avocado, broccoli, mango, and spinach are some examples of foods containing vitamin E. Supplementing this vitamin can be tricky, and toxicity can occur. Plus, many supplements have soy added or are synthetic versions instead of natural vitamin E.

Deficiencies in B vitamins also appear common in MCAS patients, *anecdotally*. There are eight different types of B vitamins, all with unique purposes in the body. Some are utilized in metabolism and energy regulation, some play crucial roles in fetus development in pregnancy, some help regulate the good type of cholesterol, and others fight inflammatory free radicals. In addition, one study found that vitamin B6 supplementation during pregnancy increased levels of DAO, the enzyme that breaks down histamine.[50]

The advent of easy-access personal genetic information at one's fingertips has stirred up quite the discussion on the role of the B vitamins. Some patients appear to have a genetic predisposition to difficulty with methylation and poor processing and utilization of the B vitamins. Without getting too much into the topic of methylation, it's important to know that inadequate bioavailability of B vitamins can have a negative impact on the body's ability to detoxify everything from daily exposures to the chronic buildup of heavy metals and other toxins in the system that may have been present for decades. In theory, the more junk that clogs the system with poor exit routes, the greater the presence of potential mast cell triggers, and the more overflowing the mast cell mediator bucket will be.

Thus, the B vitamins are another important group to test for and address properly with a medical team. B vitamin supplements often cause nausea but there are some different options out there (such as powder to put in smoothies) that may be better tolerated or absorbed.

It's possible that many of the recommended daily vitamins (or lack thereof) can influence mast cells, so the best advice is to have all major vitamins and minerals measured to get a "baseline" and rule out any deficiencies present, and to get supplement recommendations from one's medical team to ensure the best possible absorption and combination with other medications.

It's important to note that while many patients may appear to have normal circulating levels on tests, it's possible that they could still be malnourished if the body is not utilizing the vitamins properly. Plus, traditional testing only provides one snapshot in time relative to a recent meal and other daily factors. More recent testing advances (such as those offered by Spectracell Laboratories) provide a comprehensive nutritional panel that has the ability to show vitamin and mineral levels as an average value for estimates of the past six months, plus overall immune function ratings, and may be more accurate for patients with chronic conditions such as MCAS.

Alpha-Lipoic Acid

Outside of quercetin and luteolin (already discussed above), alpha-lipoic acid (ALA) is one of the more common supplements recommended by MCAS specialists, particularly for patients who experience nerve-related pain and numbness/tingling.[51] ALA is synthesized in plants and animals, but it has a low production rate in humans.[52]

Research supports ALA supplementation for a number of diseases, including sepsis, cancer, diabetes, neurodegenerative disorders, tissue regeneration, and aging.[52] In addition, a meta-analysis of 10 randomized controlled trials found that ALA supplementation had a statistically significant association with weight loss in humans.[53] In animal models, ALA also reduced intra-abdominal adhesions and may be of assistance to prevent post-operative complications.[54]

ALA has good support for the reduction of neuropathic pain and dysfunction related to diabetes, and when used in combination with omega-3 supplements it appears to reduce cognitive and functional decline with activities of daily living in patients with Alzheimer's.[55,56]

ALA also possesses qualities that assist with detoxification. As a potent antioxidant and chelator of heavy metals, ALA appears to reduce the cognitive impairments associated with heavy metal toxicity (aluminum) in mice.[57]

Research also supports its use for bladder-related problems. ALA appears to be neuroprotective for the urinary bladder in patients who have spinal cord injuries.[58] It also appears to reduce symptoms of painful bladder syndrome and vulvodynia when combined with omega-3 fatty acids.[59]

Burning mouth syndrome is believed to a neurological condition and it's been theorized that mast cells may play a role in its etiology. A 2015 study evaluated patients with burning mouth syndrome and found that ALA supplementation of 600 mg/day for two months reduced symptoms in over 60% of patients, and none of the patients taking it experienced a worsening of symptoms.[60] Several subsequent additional studies showed the reduction of symptoms of burning mouth syndrome with use of ALA.[61-63]

However, there have also been a few studies in patients with burning mouth syndrome that found no difference when compared to placebo,[64,65] and one study that noted nearly a 90% improvement rate, which was nonetheless not different from the placebo.[66] A 2015 review concluded that based on the existing studies, alpha-lipoic acid shows good results for burning mouth syndrome but the long-term effects and potential for complete remission are unclear.[67]

Bromelain

The enzyme bromelain has been shown to inhibit prostaglandin synthesis. Bromelain is a proteolytic enzyme mixture that comes from the fruit, stem, leaves, and peel of the pineapple plant. A review of several studies found that bromelain supplementation (combined with rutoside and trypsin) resulted in equivalent pain reduction for those patients taking it compared to those who were taking diclofenac, an NSAID (nonsteroidal anti-inflammatory drug) for active osteoarthritis.[68] Bromelain and quercetin are often combined for a natural anti-inflammatory and antihistaminic oral supplementation in patients who have histamine intolerance or MCAD.

Glutathione: Cysteine, Glycine, and Glutamate

Glutathione is an important fundamental building block for detoxification and optimal liver function. In addition, Lyme disease specialist Dr. Horowitz notes that some of his patients who have oral or IV glutathione treatments have reduced levels of pain.[69] He adds, "Glutathione may be acting to metabolize toxins in the short term, and may have an effect on cytokines, prostaglandins, interleukins, oxidative stress, and immune modulation in the long term. We have found detoxification to be crucial in helping patients deal with their chronic resistant pain."[69]

Glutathione is composed of three amino acids: cysteine, glycine, and glutamate. Supplements have been developed to provide the body with these important fuel sources for detoxification. Forms of glutathione supplementation have been studied both in the context of chronic illness and acute (critically ill) patients. Enteral glutathione use has been associated with a reduction in hospital stay length, as well as in reduced mortality in patients suffering from burn injuries.[70]

Glutathione is available as an intravenous infusion, though this formulation can be cost-prohibitive for many patients. The biosynthesized form of glutathione is not available as a supplement, but supplementation with its building blocks is a mainstay of treatment for patients looking to improve detoxification.

N-acetyl cysteine (NAC) is one of the three building blocks that facilitates systemwide detoxification. NAC, the precursor of l-cysteine, contributes to liver-mediated detoxification. NAC has been studied extensively and appears beneficial for the treatment of a variety of conditions such as cancer, Epstein-Barr virus, liver conditions, polycystic ovarian syndrome, inflammatory bowel disease, asthma, and neurological conditions.[71,72] NAC is a potent antioxidant that is not found in natural sources, though it is sometimes added to foods and supplements.

Glycine, the second building block of glutathione, is more readily available in the diet in foods such as spinach, kale, cauliflower, kiwi, beans, cabbage, pumpkin, banana, and animal proteins. The combination of both cysteine and glycine supplementation appears to promote sufficient restoration of glutathione in adults.[73] *Anecdotally* some patients with MCAS and gastrointestinal issues report difficulty with l-glutamine supplementation (the third precursor to glutathione). Patients who don't tolerate l-glutamine well may want to consider the other building block (NAC and glycine) options. Patients with MCAS *may* also find better results when multiple glutathione building blocks are trialed separately and eventually combined into their plan.

364

In theory, enhancement of the body's natural detoxification system should benefit patients who have overactive mast cells that are easily influenced by toxins, viruses, and other degranulation triggers. Patients with MCAS may need to carefully trial and slowly titrate up the doses of these supplements. Some precursors of glutathione are available in powder form for easy dosage adjustment, as well as oral pill-based formulations, some of which contain added substances to assist in better absorption and bioavailability.

When increasing substances that help remove toxins from the body, it's always important to ensure that other systemic methods of detoxification (such as gastrointestinal motility) are functioning well to avoid a detrimental buildup of waste products with no route of elimination. It's important to work with one's medical team in order to ensure that the supplementation and detoxification processes are being managed appropriately.

Curcumin (Turmeric)

Curcumin is another popular supplement in the MCAS and chronic illness communities for its anti-inflammatory and antioxidant powers. Curcumin is the active compound in turmeric, an ancient Indian spice. On the physiological level, curcumin regulates pathways of inflammatory cytokines, protein kinases, and growth factors, all of which are controlled at least in part by mast cells.[74]

In animal research, curcumin suppressed the degranulation and secretion of mast cell mediators including TNF-alpha, histamine, and interleukin-4.[75,76] Curcumin interferes with the Syk kinase pathway that activates mast cells and inflammatory cytokines.[75] Curcumin has been show to inhibit prostaglandin E2 production in several studies.[77,78] Multiple animal studies have shown that curcumin can inhibit passive cutaneous mast cell-mediated anaphylactoid reactions.[75,76,79]

In the literature, the efficacy and safety of curcumin are supported with osteoarthritis, inflammatory diseases, cancer, and complications of diabetes.[74] Similar to other compounds, its use as a supplement offers relatively low bioavailability, but its absorption can be improved with phytosomal formulations (such as curcumin combined with phosphatidylcholine).

Mangosteen

Mangosteen comes from a tropical tree of Southeast Asia that produces fruit rich in xanthones. The active constituents in mangosteen are considered to have mast cell stabilizing properties. Specifically, mangosteen suppresses certain pathways (such as spleen tyrosine kinase) by decreasing the levels of certain phosphokinases and may also reduce calcium influx on the cellular level.[80] A 2012 study found that the active substances in mangosteen inhibited bone marrow–derived mast cell chemical mediators including interleukin-6, leukotrienes, prostaglandins, and histamine.[81] Additional research supports the antihistaminic and anti-prostaglandin effects of mangosteen.[82]

As a supplement, mangosteen has a diverse range of activity. According to a 2017 review, mangosteen has numerous antibacterial, antimalarial, anticarcinogenic, antiatherogenic, and antifungal properties and is protective against heart conditions, neurodegenerative conditions like Alzheimer's disease, and much more.[83] The research supports that the substance can work simultaneously toward multiple comorbidities or targets that may be present.[83] Mangosteen also appears promising in initial investigation of the treatment of asthma and atopic dermatitis in mice.[84,85] Despite the support, there have been few clinical pharmacodynamic studies to date, "which seriously impedes their promotion from empirical studies to an evidence-based, clinically applicable pharmacotherapy."[83] Nonetheless, mangosteen offers a promising natural potential option and hopefully future research will investigate its utility in the MCAS population.

Khellin

The Ammi species plant-derived khellin has long been cited as a natural mast cell stabilizer, and its early research data was part of the original inspiration behind the drug disodium cromoglicate.[86] A 2013 review noted that the plant has many antibacterial and antifungal properties in addition to promoting relaxation of vascular smooth muscle.[87] Khellin has literature support of over a dozen studies for the treatment of skin conditions such as psoriasis, vitiligo, and hypopigmentation tinea versicolor in humans.[87] Khellin is readily available in tincture forms.

Resveratrol

Resveratrol is considered a phenol that is found predominantly in the skin of red grapes, berries, and peanuts. It's difficult to achieve high levels of resveratrol dietarily, and oral supplements are available.

Resveratrol has been shown to have protective effects against cancer, aging, inflammation, bacterial infections, and cardiovascular disease.[88,89] Resveratrol appears to possess regulatory influences of mast cell-mediated inflammation in laboratory research. Specifically, it regulates calcium inside the cell and suppresses interleukin-6, interleukin-8, and TNF-alpha expression in human mast cells.[90] At low concentrations, resveratrol has also been shown to inhibit prostaglandin biosynthesis.[91]

In a 2017 animal study, mast cells pretreated with resveratrol reversed the experimental intestinal ischemia that otherwise leads to acute lung injury.[92] Thus, the compound may also potentially impact the gastrointestinal and respiratory systems, although it remains to be researched in humans.

A 2018 study found that chronic prostatitis in mice was alleviated via resveratrol supplementation.[93] Authors theorize that chronic prostatitis is induced by mast cell infiltration, and thus the addition of resveratrol was able to improve fibrosis and urinary function by suppressing mast cell activation and chemical mediator pathways.[93]

Silibinin

Silibinin, also known as milk thistle extract, is a flowering plant native to Mediterranean Europe. The efficacy of silibinin as a supplemental adjunct for different types of cancer has been well-investigated.[94-97] It also has antiviral, cholesterol-lowering, and immunomodulating potential. Recent research in animal models also indicates that it is protective against osteoarthritis.[98]

It's also the source of health benefits for a variety of liver conditions, such as hepatitis, cirrhosis, and liver poisoning. Silibinin has protective effects on glutathione stores and is instrumental in the body's detoxification process. It's used in Europe parenterally in cases of acute liver toxicity from mushroom poisoning. Milk thistle is generally well tolerated in the gastrointestinal tract, although it can occasionally have a laxative effect.[99]

It appears that silibinin has the ability to selectivity increase and decrease certain interleukins, and as a whole it appears to suppress TNF activity.[99] Silibinin inhibits the production of prostaglandins and leukotrienes in the liver.[99] It appears to have a protective effect against histamine-modulated allergic reactions, asthma, and anaphylaxis.[99] Silibinin has potent antioxidant and anti-inflammatory properties and may also benefit the nervous system.[99]

Melatonin

Melatonin is a hormone produced by the pineal gland that helps regulate sleep and waking cycles. Melatonin is available orally, sublingually, and in transdermal patches. It has been touted for decades as a solution to insomnia and has recently gained attention for potential utility in cancer, neurological conditions, and gastroparesis (among many other conditions).[100]

A 2018 umbrella review evaluated 195 studies on melatonin and determined that out of the pool of studies, 31 were of high quality methodology, and out of those, seven studies had statistically significant p levels of <0.001.[100] These seven studies supported the use of melatonin for improving sleep quality in insomnia, decreasing preoperative anxiety, reducing the risk of breast cancer, and preventing agitation.[100] The common overall consensus was that melatonin exhibits beneficial antioxidant, anti-inflammatory, and immunomodulatory properties.[100] While there were hundreds of suggested mechanisms for melatonin's protective properties, reduction of cytokines appeared to be a common finding across multiple systems.[100]

In a 2017 article on the neuroendocrine properties of mast cells, Theoharides commented on additional theoretical support for the ability of melatonin to modulate mast cell secretion.[101] Specifically, he noted the findings of a 2014 study where melatonin appeared to inhibit mast cell proliferation[102] and a study of frogs where melatonin inhibited the expected increase in the number of mast cells following a trigger.[103] Additionally, in the rat thyroid gland, mast cells are observed to fluctuate in numbers and reactivity as part of a daily rhythm;[104] this "clock" observed with mast cells follows the traditional circadian rhythm controlled by the pineal gland.[105] Theoharides concluded, "recent evidence indicates that mast cell reactivity exhibits diurnal variations, and it is interesting that melatonin appears to regulate mast cell secretion."[101]

Chinese Herbal Formulations

A number of herbs are commonly used by Chinese medicine practitioners to address allergies and mast cell activity. One example of this is Shuang-Huang-Lian (SHL), a three-herb formula has been studied in China for its mast cell stabilizing properties. SHL has been found to stabilize mast cells and reduce allergic activity by activating the mitochondrial calcium importer, which reduces cytosolic calcium levels.[106] This formulation combines the Chinese herbs lonicera, forsythia, and scute together and is available in oral formulations. While it's claimed that these herbs have been used successfully for centuries in Asian medicine, the majority of support in the literature is based off test-tube and animal studies, though there are limitations in western medicine's interpretation due to language differences.

Additional Sources

There are a number of additional supplements and food sources (herbs, spices, fruits, and vegetables) listed in Chapter 11 that *may* exhibit a beneficial effect on mast cells. For example, pomegranate seed oil appears to prevent prostaglandin synthesis.[107] Berberine is a common natural supplement that exhibits COX-2 inhibitor activity in studied doses and could also be of some benefit in reducing prostaglandin synthesis.[108] Some specialists include garlic, clove, berberine, perrilla, albizzia, and other supplements in their treatment plan for MCAS when SIBO or other root issues are identified. Some herbs may work synergistically together, particularly in patients with multiple bacterial and viral infections or parasites.

Many recommended fruits, vegetables, and herbs are readily available in one's everyday supermarket or health food store. Some of the supplements are also available as tinctures or teas (such as green tea, chamomile tea, nettle tea, and holy basil tea) that may influence mast cell activation. For example, green tea has been shown to stabilize mast cells in patients with inflammatory bowel disease.[109] Some are also available in powder form. Adaptogens such as chaga mushroom may have mast cell stabilizing properties.[110]

Reminder: Even though many supplements, vitamins, and minerals are available online or over the counter and are advertised as "natural," that does not mean that they are all safe or created alike. They may contain additives, pesticides, or other chemicals. Toxicities, drug interactions, and overdoses can occur. It is crucial to work with one's medical team to come up with the right individualized combination.

Toxin Binders

As part of a program to help the body detoxify from mold exposure or other toxins, some patients may have a brief (several-week to several-month) trial of toxin binders. Examples of toxin binders include cholestyramine, activated charcoal, bentonite clays, chlorella, zeolite, apple pectin, diatomaceous earth, cilantro, and others. Over time these may help reduce the presence of heavy metals and other potential mast cell triggers, which can result in a reduction in symptoms. In some cases, the use of certain toxin binders is also advised for longer time periods.

Toxin binders are tricky in that they must be carefully spaced away from other medications and supplements and sometimes even foods. And just like anything else, they do have the potential to trigger anaphylactoid reactions in patients with MCAD. Working closely with a specialist is crucial when utilizing these compounds; if the body's detoxification pathways are not working efficiently or the patient is not having regular bowel movements, these products can rerelease toxins back into the tissues and can cause major problems. They may also pose a risk of malnutrition if they are not timed and spaced appropriately. However, when included as part of a comprehensive plan, *anecdotally* toxin binders may be helpful to reduce secondary triggers of mast cell activation.

Probiotics

How exactly does the gut microbiota interact with the immune system? Some believe that microbiotic diversity is something that is partially determined at birth and during early childhood years. It's been theorized that microbiotic diversity has the ability to regulate immune reactions to environmental allergens. The microbiome also appears to play an important role locally in terms of influencing gastrointestinal motility, as well as in the interaction with vitamins that dictate our everyday energy production and absorption.[111]

However, not all is lost if a person missed out on "good gut bacteria" in those early years or if they took a lot of antibiotics in their lifetime. Probiotic supplementation options offer the chance to boost the system if a patient is missing the mark dietarily (and/or historically). There are many factors that influence the gastrointestinal bacterial balance. Chronic alcohol consumption has a negative impact on gut microbiota, as do antibiotics and many medications.[112] The role of oral probiotics is a repopulation of the gut with a more balanced "healthy" bacteria level that can boost the immune system. But there is some debate on public forums about whether the patient with MCAS should take probiotics.

The short answer to the question appears to be "yes," according to leading MCAS experts. It's important to keep in mind that probiotics offer a lot outside of simple gut health. Based on a review article on MCAS and microbiotic reactions by Afrin and Khoruts, human and mouse studies indicate that probiotics inhibit mast cell degranulation.[112] According to the 2015 review, based on a number of studies, "There are increasing suggestions, too, that microbiotic manipulations may be able to prevent colorectal cancer, an effect possibly dependent on microbiotic interactions with MCs (mast cells) and perhaps unsurprising given not only long-recognized associations between MC (mast cell) activation and initiation and progression of cancer but also an ability to improve outcomes of human malignancies on recognition and treatment of comorbid SM or MCAS."[112] And there are certainly other microbiota biomes outside of the gastrointestinal system that are also important for health, such as the mouth, lungs, skin, and sinuses.[112] The role of mast cells in these other areas are still being defined, according to researchers.[112]

The more difficult answer to "what type of probiotics?" remains less clear at this time. The answer may depend on the patient and the context. A 2015 study noted that in rodent models with inflammatory bowel disease, the probiotic *lactobacillus reuteri (hdc+)* suppressed colonic inflammation via the reduction of cytokines and special signaling pathways.[113] However, these pathways may theoretically result in the conversion of histadine to histamine and it's unclear how that would impact patients with MCAS. Further, Afrin and Khoruts note that "little is known about how dysfunctional MCs (mast cells) interact with microbiota. Given that microbiotic manipulations can reduce normal MC (mast cell) activation, perhaps some abnormal MCs might be similarly quiesced."[112]

A 2013 study evaluated the effects of two different probiotics on inflammatory markers in mice that were on a high-fat diet. The mice that were on *lactobacillus rhamnosus* GG and *propionibacterium freudenreichii* spp. *shermanii* both had fewer intestinal mast cells following treatment when compared to the control group.[114] In addition, both probiotics resulted in a decrease in proinflammatory markers (both locally in the gut and systemically) which, given the high-fat diet, were originally expected to increase over time.[114]

Dr. Hamilton, a gastroenterologist at Brigham and Women's Hospital, believes that intestinal dysbiosis may be a root issue that contributes to the reactive immune system in patients with MCAS.[115] Fecal transplants are a new treatment to correct intestinal dysbiosis but are currently only FDA-approved for the treatment of C. Difficile infections.[115] As an alternative, Hamilton recommends that MCAS patients supplement with probiotics (specifically, VSL#3 which has the most number of strains and the highest amounts of bacterial to help re-populate the gut).[115]

Nutritionist Rebecca Snow recommends certain probiotics for the MCAS population, including *bacillus spp., lactobacillus rhamnosus GG, bifidobacterium longum* BB536, and *bifidobacterium bifidum* BGN4, which are believed to be histamine-degrading probiotics.[116] Snow also recommends *saccharomyces boulardi* which is histamine neutral, and notes that different strains of the same probiotic species may have different effects.[116] Functional medicine doctor Jill Carnahan recommends *lactobacillus rhamnosus* and *bifidobacterium spp.* probiotics for her MCAS patient population experiencing mold illness.[117]

Nutritionist Heidi Turner notes that she tends to see really good tolerance to the strain *bifidus infantis* in isolation, which reduces hypersensitivity in the digestive tract and reduces the histamine response.[118] Align probiotic, while derived from dairy and containing additives, seems to be tolerated fairly well with patients who have MCAS.[118] Turner recommends starting with 1 billion units of one single strain until the body can work up to multiple strains and higher dosages, as opposed to starting with something like VSL.[118] While *bifidus* sometimes is better tolerated than the *lactobacillus* strains, she finds that some patients with MCAS may tolerate Culturelle, which contains *lactobacillus rhamnosus GG-inulin*.[118] For patients who have zero tolerance to probiotics, Turner recommends aiming to get a prebiotic, such as acacia fiber, into the diet.[118]

Topical probiotics are under investigation. A 2010 study evaluated the use of *bifidobacterium longum* (a nonreplicating bacteria) in lysate form as a whole-body lotion skin product (or placebo) to 66 female volunteers with reactive skin.[119] After approximately one month of use, subjects who received the probiotic lotion reported less skin fragility, less sensitivity, and minimal dryness when compared to the placebo group.[119] Due to the general poor tolerance of skin products in the MCAS population, topical products may not always be an ideal option.

It's clear that various specialists have differing clinical opinions on which probiotics are best tolerated in this patient population. The bottom line is that, just like other medications and supplements, the probiotic process should be customized and built up over time to a regimen that is tolerated well by the individual.

Infusion of IV Fluids

Senior scientist and molecular biologist Lisa Klimas has written a number of resources for patients with MCAS considering the use of regular intravenous infusion of fluids for the management of chronic symptoms.[120] (This is separate from the topic of continuous infusion of IV diphenhydramine for acute management, previously discussed.) Klimas notes, "There has been no organized study for the use of intravenous fluids to manage symptoms from mast cell disease. Despite this fact, use of intravenous fluids in mast cell disease is increasing in popularity, largely because it works, and word of effective treatment travels fast in a rare disease community. While there is no firm answer for why it helps, there is a reasonable explanation: it treats both deconditioning and POTS and many mast cell patients have one or both."[120]

Another potential explanation that Klimas offers is that mast cell activation can result in third spacing, the shift of fluids from the blood vessels to the tissues where it is unusable, which can result in dehydration.[120] IV fluids can help restore homeostasis in the body and prevent the physiological effects of dehydration.[120]

IV use poses the risk of infection and blood clots and can also be costly (with poor likelihood of insurance reimbursement for some patients) and is not a decision to be taken lightly. Since patients with MCAS tend to be hyperreactive to many things in their environment, not all of them tolerate IV fluids well. Some may also react to the materials of the bag or line itself, the tape used, and the preservatives present in the solutions. In a "mixed bag" full of a dozen different vitamins and minerals, it can be difficult to determine what may be causing reactivity and whether it is dosage-dependent. Some naturopathic offices offer more "hypoallergenic," preservative-free fluids that may be better-suited for the MCAS population.

That being said, *anecdotally* many patients with MCAS tolerate basic electrolyte solutions well. Some may also find that IV treatments such as blood ozone and glutathione help assist with detoxification and reduction of viruses and bacteria in the bloodstream, which in theory could reduce overall mast cell activation. High-dose vitamin C with other vitamins and minerals, hydrogen peroxide, and other IV solutions exist that are also purported to reduce the load of toxins, bacteria, and viruses that may be triggering mast cell hypersensitivity reactions on a chronic basis. For now, these statements lack literature investigation for this patient population, but it's anticipated that future studies will investigate these potential treatments for MCAS.

Some patients with MCAS and other chronic conditions may utilize a port catheter ("port") or peripherally inserted central catheter ("PICC line"). A port is a device that is placed in a large main vein, generally in the upper chest area, that serves as an alternative to an IV that may be placed in the arm or the hand. Generally, these patients require regular blood draws or infusion of medications, nutrition, and fluids, and some ports may be necessitated by poor vein access peripherally. PICC lines are a form of long-term venous access that extend from a peripheral site to the central area of veins in the body. Patients with gastroparesis may also have a jejunal feeding tube in place for short- or long-term time frames.

Hormones

Estrogen is probably the most widely discussed sex hormone in terms of its potential to influence symptoms in chronic illness. *Anecdotally* some MCAS patients find that their symptoms are altered depending on whether they are taking estrogen-containing medications or consuming estrogen-high foods and beverages. Mast cells have a high-affinity estrogen receptor and the potential to be influenced by estrogen,[121,122] which may be a trigger for mast cell degranulation.

Dr. Benoit Tano, a Minnesota-based allergist/immunologist and author of "The Layman's Guide to Integrative Immunity," notes that many of his MCAS patients find relief when they eliminate xenoestrogen, phytoestrogen, and other chemical sources.[123] He notes that treatment of MCAS involves a thorough evaluation of the patient to uncover the mast cell and basophil activators, lifestyle changes, and a complete hormonal evaluation including thyroid hormones.[123] Tano adds, "In most cases, estrogen overload (progesterone deficiency), many environmental toxins, household chemicals, and chemicals found in cosmetics and cosmeceuticals are the major mast cell and basophil activators."[123] Clinically, Tano has noted that balancing the hormones can reverse or halt some reactions.[123] Patients may also benefit from discontinuing traditional birth control that is estrogen only, progesterone only, or estrogen/progesterone-containing, as well as intrauterine devices that contain progesterone such as Mirena and others.[123]

NONPHARMACOLOGICAL PAIN MANAGEMENT

Outside of pharmacological management, there are a number of treatments that may be of benefit for the patient with MCAS who also experiences musculoskeletal or neuropathic pain. Working with a physical therapist (PT) may be a helpful starting place as stand-alone treatment or in conjunction with other approaches for pain management. A PT who specializes in chronic pain and includes hands-on "manual therapy" and dry needling in their arsenal of certifications may be especially beneficial. Craniosacral therapy may be a useful approach with this patient population. Visceral manipulation could also be especially helpful for the patient suffering from abdominal cavity pain and delayed GI motility.

There are PTs who specialize in conditions like EDS and joint hypermobility issues, so it's important to do case-specific research to find the best match. PTs can also assist in developing an appropriate exercise plan and progression for patients who experience dysautonomia or POTS. Some PTs focus predominantly on certain areas such as TMJ pain or women's health and can offer very specific essential tools for isolated concerns. Ergonomic assessments can be very useful for patients who have spine pain and spend a lot of time seated at a computer.

Acupuncture *may be* a useful treatment for patients experiencing pain. Mast cells appear to be present in higher densities at acupuncture points compared to "sham points," and acupuncture in animal models resulted in an increase in degranulation in the surrounding skin and muscles.[124] Therefore, acupuncture should be approached cautiously in the MCAS population in order to determine the systemic effects and potential mast cell degranulation response. *Anecdotally*, it can be very helpful for some patients.

Occupational therapy, speech therapy, massage therapy and cognitive-behavioral therapy may also be useful resources for pain and symptom management. Establishing rapport with these types of professionals can be of great help for preventing chronic symptoms and managing acute flare-ups. Somatoemotional release may be an important consideration; more information on these types of therapies is presented in Chapter 12.

MCAS AND VACCINATION DECISIONS

For decades there's been debate about vaccines and mercury content, resulting in the removal of thimerosal (a mercury-based preservative) from all childhood vaccines starting in 2001.[125] According to the Centers for Disease Control and Prevention (CDC), ethylmercury (found in thimerosal) is distinct from methylmercury (found in fish).[125] Ethylmercury is cleared more quickly from the body and helps to prevent bacterial and fungal growth when added in small doses to vaccines. Methylmercury is more difficult for the body to process and has been connected to conditions like autism. The CDC maintains that thimerosal is safe in the doses present in vaccines and the typical side effects are limited to redness around the injection site.[125] However, most vaccines are now available in mercury-free forms for those who remain concerned.

The CDC publishes an up-to-date chart of all ingredients found in every approved vaccine.[125] Virtually all vaccines contain the weakened or killed disease antigens, plus preservatives (to prevent contamination), adjuvants (to help stimulate an immune response), and stabilizers (that help keep the vaccine viable while it is being transported). Antibiotics, inactivating ingredients, and cell culture materials are also added in the manufacturing process.

For example, according to the CDC, in 2017 the Afluria brand Influenza (flu) vaccine contained[125]:

sodium chloride, monobasic sodium phosphate, dibasic sodium phosphate, monobasic potassium phosphate, potassium chloride, calcium chloride, sodium taurodeoxycholate, ovalbumin, sucrose, neomycin sulfate, polymyxin B, beta-propiolactone, thimerosal (multi-dose vials)

Different brands of the same vaccine can include different "fillers" and active ingredients, similar to medications. The Afluria brand was one of the nine brands offering the flu vaccine (as of June 2017) and all nine options contained different blends of ingredients.[125] All discussions about mercury aside, it's obvious that there are many ingredients in the list that could potentially affect mast cells (just like *any* medication that is trialed). This does NOT mean that a person with overactive mast cells should automatically avoid vaccines. The whole goal of a vaccine is for the body to build up antibodies to a particular pathogenic foreign invader. The preservatives (like thimerosal) prevent microbial growth, and microbial growth can also trigger mast cell reactions.

It's very difficult to attribute the origin of potential side effects of vaccines in patients with MCAD when there are multiple ingredients in each vaccine and multiple external factors that can influence one's mast cells on a particular day. In theory, patients with MCAD could react to something as simple as vaccine "fillers," just like those found in oral antihistamines, and vaccine side effects are not necessarily tied to the main/active ingredients. And, some patients with MCAD experience no side effects at all.

Injections of other antibody-promoting substances or triggers that require desensitization (such as Xolair or Hymenoptera venom) are actually encouraged and indicated for certain patients with MCAD. Followers of the "hygiene theory" will argue that a childhood lack of exposure to vaccines, probiotics, viruses, etc. can lead to immune system suppression and susceptibility to allergic diseases.

When the specific ingredients commonly found in vaccinations are researched, there's no denying that certain substances have the potential to trigger mast cell degranulation and chemical mediator release. Multiple studies have found that mercury can induce histamine release and mast cell degranulation.[126,127] Formaldehyde, a common inactivating ingredient used to kill toxins, has also been shown to trigger mast cell reactions.[128] Many vaccines contain heavy metals beyond mercury, like aluminum, which has been shown to increase the risk of autoimmune conditions, long-term brain inflammation, and associated neurological complications.[129] Citric acid, soy, MSG, and egg albumin are other common food source and vaccine ingredients that are linked to mast cell degranulation.[130-132]

It's overwhelming to research this area, because there are a lot of nonprofessional commentary sources (on both sides of the argument) to weed through that are not based on a clear understanding of the high-quality evidence. There's a subgroup of individuals who may be advised to steer clear of vaccinations, such as those with organ transplants or severe immunodeficiencies. For everyone else (MCAD patients included), many experts agree that the risk of death from avoiding a vaccination outweighs the risk of potential side effects. The human influenza virus is one example where serious consequences can happen when a person goes unvaccinated, particularly in vulnerable populations. However, there's certainly great debate about whether each years' flu vaccine truly protects against the most common strains.

According to mast cell disease subject matter expert Lisa Klimas, "Mast cell patients are recommended to receive all vaccines per CDC (or relevant governmental body) guidelines.

376

Pre-medicating with antihistamines is practiced by many mast cell patients prior to receiving vaccines. (Please note that steroids can interfere with vaccine action, and as such should be avoided if possible.) Simply having mast cell disease is not a contraindication to vaccination."[133]

However, a 2017 review on pharmacological management of MCAD noted that "when MCAD is suspected, therapies that strongly activate the immune system (e.g., vaccinations with live vaccines or autohemotherapy) must be given with caution (especially if similar therapies were previously already poorly tolerated), as such interventions sometimes dramatically worsen MCAD acutely and/or chronically."[134] Thus, the type of vaccine and the individual patient history with vaccines may help the patient and medical team in the vaccination decision-making process.

The decision of whether or not to vaccinate as an adult is obviously up to that individual. It's possible that patients with MCAD are inherently more likely to experience side effects from vaccines, so each individual ought to weight out the pros and cons and always consider taking extra mast cell mediator medications prior to and following a vaccination (as per doctor advice). Individuals who experience regular anaphylaxis clearly have more justified concern over vaccinations than, say, a person who suspects a low-level histamine intolerance issue; these patients need to address the topic of vaccines closely with their medical team. It may also be useful to reference charts of vaccination ingredients and different vaccine brands when making a decision.

In addition to the short-term concerns, it's important that the patient with MCAS is fully aware that vaccines can trigger longer-term flare-ups in baseline symptoms, particularly in patients whose detoxification systems are already compromised. It may come down to weighing the (potential) costs vs. (potential) benefits. This decision should be very individualized to the patient and their history and should always involve a thorough discussion with the patient's medical team.

VENOM IMMUNOTHERAPY (VIT)

As previously noted, there's a high incidence of anaphylactic reactions to Hymenoptera venom in patients who have MCAD. Hymenoptera is a species of insects that comprises bees, wasps, ants, and sawflies. The Hymenoptera venom allergy patient is typically reactive to honeybees, wasps, yellow jackets and hornets. (Anaphylactic reactions and tips to manage them are located in Chapter 6.)

It's widely accepted that patients in the general population who have had severe reactions to insect stings are at high risk of experiencing future reactions if they are re-stung. For this reason, venom immunotherapy (VIT) is a recommended treatment plan for patients with Hymenoptera venom allergies. VIT has some drawbacks, mainly being that it is costly and time-consuming. There is also some *(anecdotal)* concern that VIT can negatively influence the symptom baseline of mast cell activation in patients with MCAD.

Once the specific venoms are identified, patients are injected with gradually increasing concentrations of the venom, until they reach a "maintenance" dosage level. Patients are monitored closely for systemic reactions during this period. Once they reach the maintenance dosage, the patient returns to the clinic on a predetermined schedule, which is often weekly, eventually progressing to monthly.

It may seem logical that VIT would be avoided in patients who have MCAD due to their already-heightened level of mast cell activation. However, the opposite is actually recommended by doctors. (It appears to come down to the fact that the risk of death by insect sting outweighs the negative side effects.)

A 2017 study in Italy looked at the length of VIT in patients who had experienced systemic reactions to Hymenoptera venom.[135] They noted that VIT treatment of 3-5 years appears to be sufficient for protecting *most patients* from severe subsequent reactions after discontinuation of the allergy shots.[135]

The high-risk category did well in terms of being protected *during* the five-year duration of VIT in the same study.[135] However, in the high-risk group, the protective benefits did not extend beyond the VIT treatment period, compared to subsequent continued protection in the patient population who did not present with severe reactions or signs of MCAD.[135] The study's authors determined that high-risk patients ought to consider lifelong venom injections.[135]

Most patients who lost the protective benefits of VIT at treatment cessation were ones who had mastocytosis.[135] Interestingly, in this particular study, 6 out of 24 patients (25%) who had mastocytosis and severe Hymenoptera venom anaphylaxis histories had *normal tryptase levels*.[135] The authors concluded that patients who present with severe reactions to Hymenoptera venom should only cease VIT treatment once mastocytosis has been ruled out as a possibility.[135]

Other authors agree that patients who have both mastocytosis and Hymenoptera allergies are recommended to continue allergy shots indefinitely, since multiple systemic reactions to future stings have been reported in the literature after stopping VIT.[136] Furthermore, experts recommend that patients who develop severe allergic reactions to insect venom after they've completed venom immunotherapy ought to consider the diagnosis of mastocytosis.[137]

The overall recommendations are that VIT is effective and should be considered a lifelong treatment in patients with severe Hymenoptera reactions, such as those who present with monoclonal MCAS or mastocytosis.[135,136] *Anecdotally*, VIT appears to be well-tolerated by some patients and very poorly tolerated by other patients with MCAD. In a 2017 interview, Dr. Afrin noted that in regards to cases of severe anaphylaxis to Hymenoptera venom, the decision to initiate and continue VIT may not be black and white; patients need to weigh personal risk factors into the decision.[138]

CONSIDERATIONS FOR CONCEPTION AND PREGNANCY

Pregnancy is a special topic in MCAS that has probably been one of the most difficult areas to research, due to the scarcity of existing quality information thus far in this relatively new diagnosis. Hopefully the second edition of this book will reflect more research findings and resources for MCAS considerations in this patient population.

Conception

In terms of male factors in conception, a 2010 review noted that "In males, MCs (mast cells) are present in the testes and are increased in oligo- and azoospermia, with MC (mast cell) mediators directly suppressing sperm motility in a potentially reversible manner."[122] Specifically, tryptase and histamine have been shown to impair sperm motility, but this phenomenon appears reversible with the use of anti-tryptase antibody and ketotifen.[139-141] Infertility in men has been associated with an increase in testicular mast cells.[142-144] While interesting, no causative conclusions can be made with certainty.

Hormonal and Chemical Mediator Influences

Hormones have a crucial regulatory role during labor. Progesterone plays a role in the maintenance of pregnancy, cervical integrity prior to labor initiation, and the migration of mast cells in response to chemokines.[122] Estrogen plays a role in the birthing process as well, particularly in the regulation of contractions.[122]

Mast cell degranulation has been associated with uterine contractility during pregnancy.[145] Specifically, histamine is connected to the production of prostaglandins during pregnancy, which is responsible for initiation of labor.[146] Some authors believe that elevated histamine and

379

mast cell activity may contribute to preterm labor.[146] Premature labor and premature rupture of membranes has been associated with low DAO levels.[147]

Additional mediators are believed to influence labor and delivery. Prostaglandins appear to contribute to cervical ripening and fetal membrane rupture.[148,149] Overproduction of chymase and tryptase have been associated with severe preeclampsia and spontaneous miscarriages, respectively.[150,151] Serotonin appears to influence myometrial contraction in a dose-dependent manner.[152,153] In the postpartum phase, tryptase may contribute to the fibrinogenolysis that occurs with uterus tissue remodeling,[154-156] though it's not clear if this is associated with an increased risk of postpartum hemorrhage.

Anaphylaxis and Pregnancy

Multiple studies have evaluated the effects of chemical-induced activation of mast cells on myometrial contraction.[157,158] In guinea pigs, the length of pregnancy was approximately 4-5 days shorter in animals that had anaphylaxis induced via intraperitoneal exposure to ovalbumin; early labor was prevented when the animals were administered ketotifen, a mast cell medication.[158] Interestingly, *anecdotally* many non-pregnant patients with severe allergies report uterine-like contractions during attacks.

There's growing research on anaphylactoid-type reactions during pregnancy. One study noted that anaphylactic-type mast cell activation from a shellfish allergy induced preterm labor, which was halted with the use of steroids and antihistamines and went on to full term.[159] A 2017 case report described a food-induced anaphylaxis at 25 weeks' gestation that was treated with typical protocols (two intramuscular injections of epinephrine, saline, nebulizer treatment, H1 antihistamine, and methylprednisolone).[160] The mother went on to deliver at full term without any complications for her or her child.[160] The authors concluded that "management of anaphylaxis in pregnant patients is basically the same of that in non-pregnant ones. Treatment should commence immediately to prevent further development of the anaphylaxis reaction and fetal neurological deficiency."[160] However, it's important to remember that the treatment of anaphylaxis with medications like epinephrine and steroids is controversial during pregnancy, and this was only one patient case report. For obvious reasons, this is a difficult area to research in humans.

Most cases of anaphylaxis during pregnancy are caused by antibiotics or medications administered during labor.[161] There are less common triggers of anaphylaxis in pregnancy noted in the literature, such as ant bites, food reactions, latex, exposure to biological agents, and consumption of an Asian milk formula that contains prebiotic galacto-oligosaccharides.[161,162]

A 2016 study in the UK determined the prevalence of anaphylaxis in pregnancy to be 1.6 per 100,000 maternities.[163] Out of the 37 cases of anaphylaxis that were reported over three years, approximately 1/3 of cases were caused by reactions to prophylactic use of antibiotics prior to cesarean section.[163] Nineteen percent of the cases of anaphylaxis had severe maternal morbidities (such as cardiac arrest or hemorrhagic events).[163] All of the babies survived, but 41% of babies whose mothers had anaphylaxis prior to delivery ended up in the neonatal intensive care unit.[163]

One complication of anaphylaxis is hyperfibrinolysis triggered by elevated tryptase levels, which is becoming better diagnosed with the availability of certain tests.[164] In cases of anaphylaxis that trigger airway obstruction, bronchospasm and cardiac complications, emergency cesarean section is typically performed.[164]

Should women who have been receiving allergy immunotherapy prior to pregnancy continue the therapy during pregnancy? Multiple recent reviews determined that continuation of allergy immunotherapy appears safe during pregnancy, but that allergy immunotherapy should not be *initiated* during pregnancy.[165,166] This topic should be thoroughly discussed with one's medical team, particularly in light of the special considerations that may be relevant for the MCAD patient.

DAO and Histamine During Pregnancy

Diamine oxidase (DAO) and histamine levels may influence complications in pregnant women who have MCAS. A 2008 review concluded that "the balance between histamine and DAO seems to be crucial for an uncomplicated course of pregnancy. Reduced DAO activities have been found in multiple heterogeneous complications of pregnancy such as diabetes, threatened and missed abortion and trophoblastic disorders."[147] Mast cells are present in the placenta,[167] and it appears that DAO may act as a barrier in the placenta to prevent excess histamine from entering fetal circulation.[147]

Maintz and colleagues concluded that, based on a number of studies, "It has long been observed that maternal plasma DAO activity levels rise exponentially during the first 20 weeks of gestation to levels which are about 1,000 times higher than before pregnancy, leading to a decline of circulating maternal histamine levels."[147] Histamine levels tend to be naturally higher during the first trimester of pregnancy but do not differ significantly from "normal non-pregnancy levels" in a healthy patient population.[147] Rises in placental histamine levels and mast cell numbers are correlated with an increased severity of preeclampsia and increased prevalence of hyperemesis gravidarum.[147,168]

Potential Positive Effects of MCs in Pregnancy

It appears that there's conflicting evidence about the implications of mast cells and their mediators in terms of having a healthy pregnancy. A 2011 review entitled "The role of mast cells and their mediators in reproduction, pregnancy and labor" reveals further clarification based on evaluation of 30 years' worth of research (hundreds of studies) in this area.[122] They concluded that "with respect to pregnancy, MCs (mast cells) are redundant during blastocyst implantation and although their mediators can induce myometrial contractility, there is no epidemiological link of preterm birth with allergy, suggesting a non-essential role or robust regulation."[122]

Furthermore, it's important to note that the presence of certain levels of mast cell activity and histamine *are important* during pregnancy. For example, inhibition of a histamine-producing enzyme called HDC is associated with delayed implantation of the fetus in animal models, implying that histamine plays an important role in the initial aspects of conception.[169] Histamine also plays a role in regulating fetal circulation, which may be beneficial in cases of hypoxia.[147]

Maintz and colleagues add that low histamine levels and decreased mast cell numbers could pose potential risks for fetal underdevelopment.[147] "Conversely, a decreased number of mast cells and histamine concentration has been observed in placentae of intrauterine growth retarded pregnancies compared with placentae obtained from gestationally matched preterm controls."[147]

The beneficial effects expand beyond histamine. According to Woidacki and colleagues, "MCs (mast cells) have been shown to exhibit beneficial function in pregnancy by contributing to implantation, placentation and fetal growth through their release of the glycan-binding protein galectin-1 and, thus, are critically implied in the fetomaternal interface. In addition, MCs influence pregnancy by modulating non-immunological responses by contributing to tissue remodeling, angiogenesis, and spiral artery modifications."[146]

Just like in adults, one could theorize that mast cells likely play a protective role in terms of transmission of viruses and bacteria to the fetus. It appears that a "happy medium" level of mast cells and histamine are ideal for pregnancy, just as they are for many other important physiological processes.

Research evaluating patients with "milder allergic conditions" (such as food allergies, urticaria, eczema, and allergic rhinitis) was not indicative of adverse pregnancy outcomes,[122] and no data currently exists to confirm or deny an increased risk of such complications in the MCAS population. A 2011 review concluded that "there is little evidence to suggest any adverse pregnancy outcomes in women with these milder allergic conditions, suggesting that myometrial MCs (mast cells) are sufficiently regulated to prevent adverse outcomes."[122]

Flare-Ups During Pregnancy

Women with MCAS may be concerned with how pregnancy could affect the baseline level of MCAS symptoms. *Anecdotally*, some patients experience a remission of MCAS-type symptoms during pregnancy, while others are extra-flared. Some patients find a significant change (for better or worse) in symptoms during the postpartum period as well.

It's evident that hormones play a complex role in this phenomenon. Research by Vasiadi and colleagues shows that progesterone inhibits the secretion of histamine from mast cells, which could explain why some patients with a history of inflammatory conditions have relief during pregnancy.[170]

Woidacki and colleagues published a review in 2014 entitled "Mast cell-mediated and associated disorders in pregnancy: a risky game with uncertain outcome?"[146] In the review, they focused on psoriasis, atopic dermatitis, urticaria, asthma, mastocytosis, and pruritic urticarial papules and plaques.[146] The authors noted conflicting improvement vs. worsening statuses across the majority of the conditions. For example, chronic spontaneous urticaria tends to be alleviated for some patients during pregnancy but may be aggravated in others.[146] For many conditions, flare-ups in symptoms coincided more with certain trimesters as opposed to others.[146]

Physiologically, the differences in symptom statuses between trimesters could be hormone and/or mast cell mediator-modulated. During pregnancy, several immunological shifts occur: the beginning phase of pregnancy is more Th1-response dominant, which is influenced by mast cell mediators[171] including cytokines. Th1 cells are the body's first defense line and are typically involved in preventing viral and bacterial infection from occurring, via "cell-mediated" immunity. This corresponds with a higher inflammatory response in the first trimester and start of the second trimester that is important for clearance of cellular debris and uterine tissue remodeling.[172-174]

Mid-pregnancy, the body shifts toward a Th2-response that is important for maintaining the pregnancy and is influenced by estrogen, progesterone, and cortisol levels.[175] Th2 immunity tends to target toxins, allergens, and bacteria via the production of antibodies. It's possible that the hormonal stimulation of mast cells contributes to the Th1 to Th2 switch that occurs in pregnancy.[146]

A specific cytokine called interleukin-33 (IL-33) has properties that assist in the survival, adhesion, and maturation of mast cells.[122] Th2-immunity and subsequent inflammation are also controlled by IL-33,[122] supporting the role of mast cells in both the Th1 and Th2 phases of pregnancy.

The rise in these hormones during pregnancy has the potential to influence mast cells in either a proinflammatory or anti-inflammatory manner,[146] further complicating predictions of disease status during pregnancy.

In general, different diseases tend to be more associated with either Th1 or Th2 pathways. For example, asthma is traditionally more Th-2 driven, and one study found that 35% of women had a worsening of asthma in the third trimester.[176] Th-1 driven conditions appear to worsen more during the first and third trimesters,[172-174] and one study found that patients with mastocytosis did worse in the first and third trimesters.[146,177]

According to Woidacki and colleagues, "…disorders that are mediated by MCs (mast cells) or in which MCs are involved may turn into an unfavorable direction. It is however also possible that the symptoms ameliorate due to the hormone-modulated behavior of MCs."[146] Based on this consensus, it appears that patient symptoms could truly go either way during pregnancy.

There's limited research available on the topic of mastocytosis and pregnancy.[146] Three studies concluded that 20%-33% of patients with mastocytosis experienced an overall worsening of symptoms with pregnancy.[177-179] This worsening may be attributable to the tendency to decrease medication doses during pregnancy.[146] Another study noted that undiagnosed or inappropriately managed mastocytosis can be associated with severe pregnancy complications, such as fetal demise.[180] This highlights the importance of proper control of MCAD, if possible, prior to pregnancy.

Medications During Pregnancy, Labor, and the Postpartum Period

Another common question in pregnancy is whether one can continue taking certain medications to manage MCAS. *This is an important question to address with one's medical team.* Fetal exposure to a number of over-the-counter medications (such as H2 blockers, acid-suppressive medications, and proton pump inhibitors) has been associated with the development of asthma and allergies in offspring.[181,182] It appears that long-term oral steroid use increases the risk of gestational diabetes and preterm labor during pregnancy.[183]

Premedication is often recommended for the MCAS patient when labor begins, but many medications may need to be avoided for the majority (or entirety) of pregnancy. It appears that MCAS-specific patient recommendations for considerations during pregnancy have not been published in scientific studies, but in some cases, patients may be advised to followed the guidelines recommended for patients with other types of MCAD, such as mastocytosis.

For mastocytosis, one review noted that some patients were required to continue certain medications (such as antihistamines) during pregnancy, but it appears that the doses were typically decreased due to fetal safety concerns.[178] During labor and early postpartum, it's advised that women with mastocytosis avoid the use of epinephrine, antihistamines, and glucocorticoids, if possible.[184] Epinephrine can cause uterine contractions, and patients who need regular use of epinephrine should also discuss this with their specialist team.[184] C-section deliveries are especially complicated in this patient population due to the potential for anaphylactoid reactions from anesthesia.[146]

There's a huge plethora of studies and statements available for the majority of drugs on the market, and each drug, whether over-the-counter or prescription, should be examined one by one. The FDA has guidelines and a "class" rating system based on available evidence on pregnancy risk for each individual medication.

Clinical Considerations During Pregnancy

Dr. Castells at the Mastocytosis Center for Excellence at Brigham and Women's Hospital notes that about 60% of women with a history of asthma or allergic disorders tend to get better during pregnancy as many mechanisms are in an inhibitory state.[185] She attributes some of this to the fact that progesterone, oxytocin, and other placental hormones and receptors may have an impact in reducing immune system hyperactivity.[185]

Castells suggests the following tips for patients with MCAD during pregnancy:[185]

- Minimal use of medications is highly recommended.
- Patients should stick to safe foods and avoid triggers as much as possible.
- Three to four meals per day are advised.
- Getting enough sleep (at least eight hours) per night is really important.
- Stress-reducing techniques should be encouraged.

According to Dr. Afrin, women with MCAS who are considering pregnancy should go into it with awareness of several considerations. Some women feel better or go into remission during pregnancy, but the majority of the MCAS patient population seen by Dr. Afrin (biased toward those with more severe illness) seem to experience:[138]

- flares in MCAS symptoms during the pregnancy, and/or

- complications with the pregnancy and delivery, and/or

- persistent escalations in baseline mast cell misbehavior following the pregnancy.

This may be in part attributable to the efforts to decrease medication usage during pregnancy, though this likely is not a principal explanation in most of the women observed to be having these problems.[138] According to Afrin, the symptom level does not always return to its prior baseline once the patient is postpartum, so women may need to mentally prepare themselves for the possibility of experiencing a new heightened baseline level of disease after delivery.[138]

Offspring with one or both parents with MCAS may manifest the disease earlier than their parents and may suffer from a more severe form of MCAS than their parents.[138] Afrin explains that this is a phenomenon called "anticipation," which is seen in many diseases rooted in epigenetic mutations.[186] While it has not been proven that MCAS is rooted in epigenetic mutations, some researchers in the field suspect that this could be happening, but little research data has been gathered thus far.[186]

Preeclampsia and early miscarriage appear to be common problems among pregnant women with MCAS. MCAS is certainly not a reason to avoid pregnancy, but it's important that families are aware of potential complications during pregnancy, as well as potential risks to the child.[138]

Summary on Pregnancy

In summary, research indicates that mast cells and their chemical mediators play a role in many factors of labor and delivery, and their excess could theoretically be linked with certain inflammatory complications (such as preterm labor, preeclampsia, or spontaneous miscarriages). That being said, review authors note that "the importance of MCs and their mediators during implantation, menstruation and pregnancy, and their contribution to the initiation and progress of labor, is not yet fully understood."[122] More research is certainly needed in this area.

Clinical experts have noted that some patients with MCAS experience a reduction in symptoms during pregnancy, while others may have flare-ups. A 2014 review concluded that "pre-existing MC (mast cell) mediated and associated disorders may affect disease progression and the disease itself may influence pregnancy outcome... In general, there is no contraindication to pregnancy when MC (mast cell)-related pathologies are under appropriate medical control. Women who were diagnosed with MC mediated or associated disorders and especially those whose disease is active, should be carefully advised by medical specialists to avoid severe pregnancy complications and to monitor disease progression."[146]

A NOTE ON PEDIATRICS

Pediatric guidelines for MCAS are hard to find since this disease is so newly coined and research is still in its infancy (pun intended). Unfortunately, there are only a handful of studies that address this topic. A pediatric specialty team is crucial to the successful management of MCAS in young children.

A 2018 article noted that symptoms outside of the skin, including anaphylaxis, are less common in pediatric cases of MCAD; when they are present, they tend to be found in children with extensive skin involvement, bullous lesions, and a high mast cell burden.[187] Friction, heat, fever, and insect stings appear to be triggers that frequently exacerbate symptoms in children with MCAD.[187]

To date, only one study has evaluated considerations for *MCAS diagnosis* in the pediatric setting. A 2018 study retrospectively evaluated the charts of 104 children who were evaluated for MCAS.[188] Serum tryptase and urinary prostaglandins, histamine and leukotrienes were routinely tested.[188] Utilizing adult reference values for norms, 32 patients had at least one elevated mast cell mediator test.[188] Six patients (6%) had the subsequent diagnosis of MCAS, four patients were diagnosed with cutaneous mastocytosis, and one patient was diagnosed with systemic mastocytosis.[188] The authors noted that some patients with normal lab values on the first round of testing had elevated mast cell mediator values on the second round of testing when they were symptomatic.[188]

The authors noted that the average age at diagnosis was nine years (plus or minus five years).[188] Urinary prostaglandins were more likely to be elevated than serum tryptase in the children.[188] Symptoms of flushing, diarrhea, and abdominal pain were more associated with elevated prostaglandins when compared to tryptase.[188] Patients with pruritis and urticaria were more likely to have elevated tryptase than prostaglandins.[188] The authors concluded that it appears that prostaglandins are the mast cell mediator that is most frequently elevated in pediatric cases of MCAS.[188] They recommended that all mediators be tested when evaluating children for mast cell activation disease.[188]

For young children, mediator testing can pose an additional challenge. A specially designed diaper exists for urine collection, but with the MCAS-specific tests, this method would theoretically be unable to maintain the refrigerated temperature requirements necessary for the urine tests.[10] Theoretically, catching the first urine in the morning may provide an ample sample for mediator testing, though further research is needed to compare this to 24-hour urine specimens.[10]

In a 2018 interview, Dr. Castells noted that children with MCAS seem especially influenced by stress, emotion, heat, and other triggers.[185] Castells recommends that all children presenting with signs of MCAS be evaluated for food and environmental allergies and have an evaluation for mastocytosis if skin rashes or lesions are present.[185] She recommends the aid of a dietician who can help families with meal planning, and notes that it can be helpful to avoid spicy foods, chocolate, fast food, and foods that are high in artificial sugar.[185] Castells notes that a low histamine diet is *not* a recommendation for children, and that the diet should be more personalized to include a lot of fresh fruits and vegetables plus a protein source.[185] When it comes to diet, she notes that there are no fast and hard rules because—like adults—every kid is different.[185]

In terms of medication management, Castells notes that clinically, it appears that H1 and H2 blockers are great choices for kids initially, although it's important to utilize the minimally necessary medications, as it's a long-term proposition to start a kid on mast cell medications.[185] Castells notes that the medication cromolyn, utilized either topically for mastocytosis lesions or orally, has been shown to be effective in reducing skin flares and gastrointestinal symptoms in kids.[185] Quercetin and luteolin are also sometimes trialed with children.[185]

CHAPTER KEY POINTS

- Natural supplements may be useful for the patient with MCAS and should be discussed with one's medical team. Flavonoids such as quercetin and luteolin are some of the most-studied natural approaches to management of mast cell activity, and there are many other options that are supported in the literature.

- Vaccination decisions for the MCAS patient should be made carefully with one's medical team; preplanning that factors in vaccine ingredients, individual anaphylaxis potential, and potential premedication may be advised.

- Patients who have monoclonal MCAS or mastocytosis and Hymenoptera venom allergies are candidates for venom immunotherapy. Based on the literature, this population may need to consider the treatment indefinitely.

- MCAS patients have special considerations during pregnancy, labor, and delivery that should be discussed with one's medical team.

- In children with suspected MCAS, all chemical mediators typically tested in adulthood should be evaluated. A comprehensive and holistic approach should be utilized in the management of MCAS in children.

Chapter Eleven

Dietary Considerations for MCAS

OVERALL DIETARY CONSIDERATIONS

E ating and the avoidance of food reactions can be a very frustrating aspect of life for many patients with MCAS. Most patients, by the time they're reached their diagnosis, have tried at least a handful of different eating plans in attempts to alleviate symptoms. Patients sometimes experiment with eliminating combinations of the following:

- Salicylates (found in plants, preservatives, and medications)
- Nightshades (present in potatoes, peppers, tomatoes, eggplant)
- Candida (sources include malt, vinegar, simple sugars, carbs, yeast, fermented foods)
- Histamine (higher in aged cheese, alcohol, fermented/smoked foods, and more)
- Galactose-alpha-1,3-galactose or "alpha gal" (found in beef, pork, lamb, venison; may be present in dairy, gelatin and some medications)
- Oxalates (found in foods that may increase risk of kidney stones)

Salicylate intolerance is a topic that is growing in interest in the literature. Salicylates in their natural (plant-based) form offer beneficial health effects and anti-aging, antioxidant, and anticancer properties.[1] A variety of fruits, vegetables, teas, herbs, and spices contain natural salicylates. Synthetic versions are also present in fragrances, cosmetics, and medications.[1] The most notorious salicylate-containing medication is aspirin. Symptoms of salicylate intolerance include wheezing, urticaria, rhinitis, headaches, palpitations, irritable bowel symptoms, joint pain, and potential neuropsychological symptoms including anxiety, depression, panic attacks, restlessness, inattention, and irritability,[1] making it difficult to distinguish from "classic" MCAS symptoms at times.

Like any diet that eliminates nutritious food options, it's important that dietary decisions are guided with the help of one's medical team. Experts affirm that "because a salicylate exclusion diet restricts many fruits and vegetables, it is important patients do not continue the diet as a long-term measure."[2] While some patients opt for strict avoidance once they are certain that they are salicylate intolerant, research has shown that—with the help of one's medical team and in a hospital setting—patients may be able to desensitize to salicylates including aspirin, though more research is needed in this area.[1]

Long-term dietary approaches that are "anti-candida" are also somewhat controversial, since they typically revolve around elimination of a number of healthy foods including fruits. *Candida albicans* is the most common human fungal pathogen, and while it's a normal part of the gut flora, when in excess or in immunocompromised patients, candida can cause problems.[3] It appears that other approaches (such as the use of phenolic agents or coconut oil to reduce candida colonization in the gut) may offer alternative options (alone or as an adjunct to dietary changes) compared to antibiotics, although this area certainly needs further research.[3,4]

Patients with MCAS have also reported alpha-gal allergies. Alpha-gal sugar is most commonly found in red meat, and patients with an alpha-gal allergy may have delayed allergic reactions (often anaphylactic) two to six hours after consumption of the offending food.[5] Research also shows that alpha-gal is also present in intravenous cetuximab (a form of chemotherapy) and may trigger immediate anaphylaxis in exposed patients.[5] Patients with alpha-gal allergies often have a history of a lone star tick bite; the tick is believed to have alpha-gal sugar in its gastrointestinal system, which is then passed to the host when bitten.[5] When the antibody cross-reacts during future meat ingestion, a delayed allergic reaction is triggered.[5]

Additional Dietary Approaches with MCAS

Diet is possibly one of the more controversial topics when it comes to managing MCAS. Some patients who have MCAS and gastrointestinal issues or irritable bowel syndrome (IBS) stick to a low-FODMAP diet. A 2015 review by Afrin and Khoruts noted, "Dietary management is important in IBS. The most successful diet (FODMAP [fermentable oligosaccharides, disaccharides, monosaccharides and polyols]) decreases colonic gas and SCFA (short chain fatty acids) production."[6] SCFA are the end products of fermentation of dietary fibers and the breakdown process is controlled in part by the intestinal microbiota. Specifically, a *low*-FODMAP diet is advocated for patients with IBS, and in theory it may be useful for patients with MCAS who suffer from poor digestion, delayed colonic transit, and bloating/distention.[7]

Examples of some of the more "notorious" foods that are higher in FODMAPs include garlic, cauliflower, onion, and asparagus. A number of other vegetables and fruits are also considered high FODMAP foods. The low-FODMAP diet is not intended to be followed for long-term time frames but can reduce inflammation and gastrointestinal discomfort. A *very short-term diet* that eliminates certain types of foods will make it more likely that the patient can resume dietary variety, ensure nutritional adequacy, and minimize impact on the gastrointestinal microbiota when compared to longer-term restrictive diets.[8]

Afrin and Khoruts noted that alcohol use and the consumption of processed foods may increase immunosuppression and have a negative impact on the role of mast cells in patients with IBS.[6] It appears that patients with MCAS are more likely to have an increase in mast cell activation with alcohol use, in part due to the additives (such as sulfites) and by-products. Chronic alcohol use also alters the human gastrointestinal microbiome and can lead to immune system hyperactivation.[6]

There are a number of other current dietary trends, such as Paleo eating or a Ketogenic diet. Some patients pay attention to additional factors relevant to their eating plan, such as a focus on cooking and pureeing vegetables (or the opposite—only consuming raw fruits and vegetables), juicing or smoothies, rotating foods, or intermittent fasting. *Anecdotally* these have mixed reviews in the chronic illness communities. Regardless of the approach that best suits the individual, patients with MCAS should focus on maximizing healing nutrients and reducing inflammation and exposure to toxins. Many patients find that paying close attention to hidden sources of gluten and eliminating all or some grains (such as corn, wheat, barley, quinoa and rice), refined sugar, canola oil, caffeine, dairy, processed foods, and so on may be helpful for reducing inflammation.

In addition to trialing a reduction in certain classes of foods or beverages, patients may need to follow particular standards in terms of their dietary *source selection*. Some patients find that, for whatever reason, certain foods or beverages just don't mesh well with their system. It's easy to get frustrated when certain brands are more problematic than others, or when there is a day-to-day difference in tolerability. This could be explained by hidden factors underlying food or beverage processing, or it could be more associated with the general mast cell activation baseline that may vary from day to day.

Discrepancies in coffee products are one example of this phenomenon. As explained in Chapter 8, coffee can be contaminated with mold-related toxins in the way that it is processed, stored and transported.[9] The bean roasting process may kill the mold, but does not appear to remove the actual Ochratoxin from commercial coffee.[10,11] Thus, patients with MCAS may find that they tolerate certain coffee sources better than others, and this could be connected to the bean harvesting location, practices, altitude, climate and other factors. Patients may also exhibit different sensitivity levels to caffeine itself.

Patients may also find relief with avoiding processed foods that are laden with preservatives. Lyme disease specialist Dr. Horowitz notes a connection between preservatives, artificial food dyes/flavorings and food intolerance.[12] Food additives can cross the blood–brain barrier more easily in children, who may be at higher risk.[12] The Feingold diet eliminates petroleum-based preservatives and other artificial additives that may trigger symptoms in sensitive individuals.[12]

If a patient with MCAS is debating a change in diet but doesn't know where to start, they could start with elimination of preservatives, food dyes, and flavorings. In the United States, there are over 3,000 FDA-approved preservatives.[13] They are added to prevent the spoilage of food in transit. Essentially, the only "safe" foods are those grown in a home garden, or perhaps those organic sources found in a local farmers market. Reading labels can seem like a daunting task, and many words are coded in a "healthy" way to disguise that they are preservatives: "natural flavoring," "citric acid," "sodium nitrite," "sulfur dioxide," "potassium sorbate," and "benzoic acid" are some examples.[13]

The easier option is to buy organic-only foods and avoid shopping in the packaged grocery aisles, instead sticking to the fresh produce sections. Use fresh herbs instead of purchasing "seasoning" type spices, which often contain hidden ingredients. Make olive oil salad dressing, homemade juice, and loose-leaf tea. Utilize coconut oil or avocado oil instead of canola and corn oil. If a product contains a label, make sure to read it to avoid additives. Even frozen berries and pre-chopped salad greens often contain preservatives.

As part of a comprehensive treatment plan, Dr. Hamilton, gastroenterologist at Brigham and Women's Hospital, advises a diet of whole foods that avoids processed foods and preservatives.[14] "Eating intentionally" by avoiding processed foods can seem daunting at first in a fast-paced culture, but it can make a dramatic difference on one's health. And when processed foods are *replaced* with organic natural choices, many people find that the grocery bill actually goes down instead of up, contrary to popular belief. For those feeding larger families, it can help to start with small steps, such as prioritization of purchasing the "dirty dozen" foods in the organic section.

Spontaneous Food Reactions

The fact that a certain food can trigger symptoms one day and be totally fine the next can be puzzling for this patient community. The use of a control spot in allergy testing aims to reduce testing errors, but *anecdotally*, false positives sometimes occur on IgE testing when a patient has overreactive mast cells in the skin, adding further confusion to dietary choices. When the offending culprits are healthy food choices, it can put up roadblocks to patient healing. There are a few theories as to why the body may "spontaneously" react without consistency to different inputs.

It's possible that mast cells react to certain healthy foods sporadically because:

1. the body is reacting to toxins or "additives" in the foods (like pesticides on an apple) and not the food itself; or

2. components of the healthy food may be contributing to the attack of an invader (virus, bacteria, etc.) and this may trigger a mast cell response and symptoms, even though what's occurring on the cellular level is helpful in the long run; or

3. the body is overloaded with toxins from the environment and is struggling to remove them, so mast cells are overreactive when they shouldn't be because the overall inflammatory or mast cell-triggering load is too high.

All three theories could explain why some days are better than others in terms of individual food tolerance. It's also quite possible that all three things are occurring at once. *It's important to carefully delineate between mild food reactions and a true anaphylactic emergency and to move forward with food decisions accordingly depending on the spectrum of mast cell activation that's occurring.*

ELIMINATION DIETS

An elimination diet can be useful for a span of a month or two for the patient with MCAS. Elimination diets are best done with the supervision of a specialist or with nutritionist guidance. This is essentially starting with one "safe" food and gradually adding in one food at a time to determine reactions. The goal is to keep careful track of symptoms in order to determine what food(s) may be triggering a response. According to a 2017 review article by Seneviratne et al., "As with medication trials, diet trials typically need to last only 1-2 months to determine if they are going to be significantly beneficial. The implementation of more than one change around the same time (e.g., a dietary change around the same time as a medication change) can be greatly confounding and should be avoided."[15]

The patient should avoid using spices, oils, and other additions to foods during an elimination diet—the aim is to piece-by-piece determine one specific item at a time. It's crucial that while doing an elimination diet, only organic foods without additives are utilized. The most accurate results will be reflected if the patient avoids processed foods and items that could be cross-contaminated. Experts also recommend the bare minimum in terms of vitamins, supplements, and medications (within reason) in order to figure out what is causing flares during an elimination diet. Most experts recommend waiting at least three days before adding in something new; it should be a slow and methodical process. Elimination diets are not designed to be performed for long-term periods as they can result in malnutrition and possibly an increase in food sensitivities.

It's important to remember in conducting a short elimination diet that not all food reactions occur immediately. Delayed reactions due to IgG antibodies can occur one to two days following exposure to a trigger and may not be recognized as the causative factor. Thus, it's important to go slowly, keep a meticulous food/symptom log, and consider the possibility of delayed reactions during the elimination diet trial period.

Both food and chemical sensitivities can trigger similar symptoms in some patients. With different triggers eliciting the same response, it can be tricky to determine what a patient is reacting to. Once a patient finds a "baseline" diet, it may be useful to expand the concept of the elimination diet to include one-by-one introduction of non-dietary sources of chemicals, such as products used regularly (like toothpaste, shampoo, skin care, and makeup) in order to best isolate the findings and address as many potential triggers as possible.

If the patient opts for an elimination trial, the ultimate eventual goal is re-diversification of healthy dietary components. Creating a healthy lifestyle plan isn't necessarily all about taking things away—it's about adding healthy practices to enhance healing potential, with proper attention to avoidance of toxins (in the diet and environment) that may serve as barriers.

HISTAMINE CONSIDERATIONS WITH MCAS

Histamine has been in the limelight for a number of years now and is one of the best-known mast cell mediators due to its role in allergic reactions and the numerous pharmaceutical antihistamine medications that are available over-the-counter. As discussed in Chapter 2, histamine is one of the chemical mediators that contributes to the "soup" of triggers for inflammation that occur with MCAD. Histamine is released by mast cells and basophils as part of the body's immune response to "invaders," and it can be present in food sources and can grow in quantity on foods after they've been cooked and are not immediately ingested (i.e., leftovers).

Genetically, some people are more likely to struggle with histamine than others. There are two enzymes that help the body break down histamine: diamine oxidase (DAO) and histamine n-methyl transferase (HNMT). People who have MCAD *may* show genetic susceptibility to lacking the right amount of these enzymes. DAO is believed to be the main enzyme responsible for the metabolism of histamine that is acquired dietarily.[16] DAO scavenges the histamine outside the cells, while HNMT primarily acts on histamine inside the cells.[16] Though deficiency in either of these enzymes is not causative to developing MCAD, it can certainly exacerbate the effects that histamine has on the body.

Many sources refer to a bucket theory when it comes to histamine. According to this analogy, if one is ingesting a lot of histamine-rich foods and beverages, AND experiencing stressors or injury, bodily histamine levels will be higher (like water being added to a bucket), until eventually over time there's spillover from the bucket and the patient experiences symptoms. The bucket baseline water level may be higher in patients who have MCAS and naturally have higher circulating levels of mast cell mediators. The baseline water level may also be influenced by genetic factors, the presence of a buildup of toxins, viruses, bacteria, mold, or other environmental triggers that increase mast cell activation, and the predisposition to a difficulty in breaking down and eliminating histamine from the body. The offending food may not be the biggest factor, but it could very well be the *tipping point* in terms of whether symptoms occur with eating or not. If the body's detoxification pathways (like the liver, kidneys, and gastrointestinal tract) are clogged, the bucket's baseline water level may hover very close to the top and make it more susceptible to frequent spillovers with minor triggers.

Histamine from food sources is considered a biogenic amine. There is great attention on websites and social media to the low-histamine diet trend. Indeed, many food and beverage sources increase plasma levels of histamine after consumption. Histamine levels increase on foods and drinks that are fermented, are highly processed, and contain added preservatives. A 2016 review article evaluated 14 studies of the best evidence in this area and determined the following foods to have the highest histamine levels: dried anchovies, fish sauce, fermented vegetables, cheese, fish and fish productions, and fermented sausages.[17]

Alcoholic beverages are liquid culprits associated with triggering histamine reactions. Histamine is believed to be one of the reasons why some people tend to get red or flushed when drinking alcohol. Researchers joke about whether a "red wine test" could help identify people with histamine intolerance. However, other aspects of wine (including compounds such as sulfites and tyramine or conditions such as a grape allergy) could also be playing a role in these symptoms.

An increase in histamine is more likely to occur in foods that have been overcooked or overripened, or that have spent a lot of time on the counter or in the fridge after being cooked. Reheating food more than once should be avoided, and many patients use small separate containers to freeze leftovers. In addition to food selection, meal composition and intervals between meals may also affect histamine-related symptoms.[18]

Foods that are generally accepted to be naturally high in histamine, or that trigger release of histamine, include:

- o Aged cheese
- o All alcoholic beverages
- o Canned foods
- o Chocolate
- o Energy drinks, soda, and soy milk
- o Fermented or bacterially ripened products (kefir, kombucha, yeast, sauerkraut, vinegar)
- o Gluten-containing foods (breads, cereals, etc.)
- o Nuts, legumes
- o Preserved meat (dried, marinated, or smoked) i.e., bacon, cold cuts, dry-cured ham
- o Shellfish and other fish
- o Specific fruits: strawberries, raspberries, citrus fruit, pineapple, banana, etc.
- o Specific vegetables: spinach, tomato, eggplant, avocado, etc.

Specific Levels of Histamine: A Food List Example

Interpreting histamine numbers in food sources can get a little confusing. There are dozens upon dozens of different web resources, books, and studies that cite histamine numbers for different foods. It seems that there's quite a bit of variability in these numbers.

To illustrate this point, three different published sources that specify histamine levels for different types of foods and beverages were selected at random. Georgia Ede published a review in 2017 on dietary histamine and why "freshness" matters.[19] Adriana Duelo, a nutritionist in Spain, helped provide resources in 2017 for the Spanish Diamine Oxidase

Society.[20,21] Mariska de Wild-Scholten published a book in 2013, "Understanding Histamine Intolerance & Mast Cell Activation" (3rd edition).[22]

Table 1. Food Histamine Content Levels According to Three Different Sources

FOOD OR BEVERAGE	EDE 2017[19]	DUELO 2017[20,21]	DE WILD-SCHOLTEN 2013[22]
Conventional dark chocolate	10 to 20 mg/kg	ND to 0.5 mg/kg	Less than detectable limit
Fresh fish	(not studied)	ND to 19.75 mg/kg	1 to 136 mg/kg
Spinach	30 to 60 mg/kg	20 to 30 mg/kg	26 to 62 mg/kg
Avocado	23 mg/kg	23 mg/kg	0 mg/kg
Ripened cheeses	2.21 to 2500 mg/kg	ND to 2000 mg/kg	2 to 1710 mg/kg
Dry aged sausages	up to 357.7 mg/kg	ND to 350 mg/kg	0 to 314.3 mg/kg
Frozen fish	(not studied)	ND to 894 mg/kg	(not studied)
Red wine	up to 24 mg/L	ND to 13 mg/L	0.5 to 26.9 mg/L
Champagne	670 mg/L	67 mg/L	(not studied)

ND = not detectable

Using this comparison, it's obvious that there are no universally agreed upon values for histamine in different foods. The different sources cited some of the foods, such as spinach, in a similar value range. Others, such as fresh fish, red wine, and chocolate, had more variability. Perhaps most interesting was the difference between champagne according to Duelo and Ede. Ede cited exactly ten times the level of histamine in champagne compared to Duelo;[19,20,21] perhaps there was a typo/error in her article.

Nonetheless, it's clear that the numbers are not uniform and that a multitude of factors can impact measured histamine content in food. Testing parameters and conditions, phase in ripeness, handling conditions and temperatures for storage, geographical location, and many other factors could certainly cause variability between published numbers.

Another factor to consider with these numbers is the difficulty in comparing quantities, since the numbers are not cited based on serving sizes. As an example, one kilogram of spinach certainly looks different than one kilogram of dark chocolate.

One commonality, however, is that one type of food can have a wide range of published histamine levels within the same food category. Cheese is a great example of this. According to de Wild-Scholten (2013), Brie cheese has 2-87 mg/kg histamine, whereas cheddar cheese has 1710 mg/kg.[21] Cottage cheese and young edam cheese have less than 5 mg/kg histamine,[21] whereas the more aged cheeses will most certainly, by nature, have higher histamine levels. Swiss cheese has 500 mg/kg histamine, but when it's been ripened for 24 weeks it has 750-1290 mg/kg histamine.[22]

According to the comparison of fresh vs. frozen fish histamine levels cited by Duelo (2017), fresh fish has significantly less histamine content.[20] This observation appears to be supported in the literature.[23] However, histamine levels rise on fresh fish very quickly with improper handling and storage due to the increase in histamine-producing bacteria,[23] so fish that is fresh may not always be ideal, depending on a number of specific details surrounding its timeline and protocols for the time from ocean to table. Fish that is flash-frozen or fileted immediately after it's been caught while on the neighbor's fishing boat in Alaska is going to be safer than fish that had delays between these steps. In some cases, fresh fish that was *immediately frozen* may be safer than the unfrozen form at the supermarket, but the numbers show that, in general, frozen fish is at higher risk. It is completely case-dependent, making it very difficult to make decisions unless one is getting the food directly from the source.

Organic vs. nonorganic food sources may also make a difference. When comparing regular dark chocolate to organic dark chocolate, there was a significant difference in histamine content cited by Ede (2017): 2-4 mg/kg for organic, and 10-20 mg/kg for conventional dark chocolate. As a whole, notable discrepancies in histamine values are reported between a large number of studies, books, and websites.[19-22,24-26]

Histamine-Reducing Practices

It's recommended that histamine-sensitive individuals 1) provide an environment for the least amount of cross-contamination and "pollution" (using clean kitchen practices, eating organic high-quality grass-fed and pasture-raised sources, freezing leftovers etc.), 2) strictly avoid the actual allergens and major high-histamine culprits, such as processed meats and alcohol, and 3) supplement their diet with natural histamine-lowering foods and consider herbal supplements (with their medical team's help).

The late Yasmina Ykelenstam, also known as the "low-histamine chef" and creator of healinghistamine.com, suffered from MCAD and advocated for a number of tactics to reduce the overall histamine load. She recommended minimizing triggers by avoiding certain foods that are especially high in histamine, avoiding certain beauty products that may trigger reactions, adapting lifestyle factors to reduce stress, and filling the diet with healthy antihistaminic nutrient sources.[27] Her web-based resources offer more specific tips plus wonderful recipes and recommendations for food sources that naturally lower inflammation and may potentially reduce mast cell reactivity.

There are many foods that have natural antihistaminic or mast cell-stabilizing properties. This chapter contains several comprehensive charts of herbs, fruits, and vegetables that have been cited in the literature to have antihistaminic and mast cell stabilizing properties (Table 2, Table 3).

The DAO enzyme has been shown to be effective as a supplement with the "histamine intolerant" population in one study.[28] DAO supplements are typically made from porcine (pig) kidneys or peas and act locally in the GI tract without systemic absorption. There are other products on the market that a patient can trial for use before eating, like quercetin and bromelain, which may also help to reduce the impact of mealtime mast cell mediators. Some patients report symptom relief with supplementation of the enzyme DAO in the pill form 30 minutes before meals to help break down histamine, though *anecdotally* there are mixed reviews in those who suffer with very high histamine levels or mast cell hyperreactivity, such as someone who has MCAS.

Low-Histamine Controversy

The low-histamine diet has been challenged by the literature and clinicians alike, particularly when it is performed for a long-term time frame or when it is followed blindly without attention to individual-specific intolerances. In these instances, it's common to observe patients who experience the frustration of getting down to a small handful of "safe" foods. Many patients initially follow website lists and may radically eliminate all foods on the lists, including nutritious fruits and vegetables.

Ykelenstam summarized her stance on low-histamine diets in a 2013 publication. "Once you understand that histamine is just one of many inflammatory mediators leaked into our bodies by unstable mast cells, you begin to reach the root of the issue. I no longer see the point in solely focusing on low histamine or diamine oxidase: I choose to address the more general problem of mast cell instability and inflammation that creates a fertile environment for mast cell degranulation and the subsequent release of pro-inflammatory agents like histamine, prostaglandin D2, heparin, tryptase, serotonin and others."[29]

A 2016 review noted some practical challenges in reducing the intake of histamine and other amines for patients with histamine and/or mast cell issues.[17] The authors noted that following a low-histamine diet is difficult in terms of detecting ingredients when eating away from home and knowing the exact histamine content of a particular food. They also noted more general application limitations due to the lack of standardization in the research methodology and clinical tools that are available thus far in this area.[17]

A 2017 review article by German researchers supported the standpoint that current research is inconclusive about the utility of a low-histamine diet for *histamine intolerance*.[18] "The scientific evidence to support the postulated link between ingestion of histamine and adverse reactions is limited, and a reliable laboratory test for objective diagnosis is lacking."[18]

Indeed, some authors question the recommendation for a low-histamine diet based on the confounding research on the diagnosis of histamine intolerance itself, with a lack of universally validated testing criteria. Oral provocation tests with 75 mg liquid histamine are often used, but a randomized double-blind study "failed to reproduce histamine-associated single symptoms in many patients. One may suggest that histamine-intolerant subjects reacted with different organs on different occasions."[28] Another study found that about 50% of "asymptomatic" control subjects reacted to the dose of 75 mg of histamine, posing additional question to its appropriateness as a diagnostic test.[30]

An article entitled "Histamine intolerance: overestimated or underestimated?" noted that "further evidence is necessary both for histamine being the responsible agent and for a compromised enzymatic barrier function. Therefore, diagnosis of histamine intolerance should provide evidence that symptoms are unequivocally associated with histamine present in food and not other causes."[31]

Furthermore, the German review article challenged the utility of a low-histamine diet as a form of treatment for histamine intolerance.[18] The authors noted that, based on the literature, diagnosis based on DAO levels in the blood is not conclusive, and other studies were not up to par with standards for *histamine intolerance* diagnosis.[18] They also drew attention to a study that found that about half of patients with suspected histamine intolerance responded to dietary changes, but only one of the patients was proven to have the *diagnosis of histamine intolerance*.[18,32]

Outside of the obvious controversy around making a clear clinical diagnosis of histamine intolerance prior to utilizing a low-histamine diet as treatment, there are also some concerns voiced about whether a histamine-free approach is appropriate for patients. A 2016 review article noted some concerns with the diet as a form of therapy.[17] Martin and colleagues discussed the importance of establishing a proper histamine baseline level (as opposed to a completely histamine-devoid diet) and working to improve dietary options and thresholds or

402

tolerance levels over time.[17] This approach supports maintaining some degree of histamine-containing foods in the diet, as opposed to the traditional approach that essentially eliminates all potential sources of histamine, regardless of individual tolerance.

The 2017 review article also admonishes restrictive diets for patients who have symptoms of histamine intolerance.[18] "A diagnostic work-up, combined with individualized nutritional therapy that focuses primarily on nutrient optimization and helps patients reliably to differentiate symptoms, is to be preferred over generalized, restrictive diets."[18]

According to Reese et al., "Some of the dietary recommendations that are currently circulating are not supported by scientific evidence. For example, numerous low-histamine diets prohibit foods that do not contain histamine (e.g., yeast), or encourage the avoidance of so-called 'histamine liberators' (pharmacologically active substances that have a histamine-releasing effect), despite there being no reliable evidence of their existence in foods or of their clinical relevance in the onset of adverse food reactions. The inconsistent data on biogenic amines in foods make it difficult to issue safe recommendations on diagnosis and define treatment measures."[18]

Instead of a restrictive low-histamine diet, the 2017 review article recommends a three-phase plan to regain health and dietary options.[18] Phase one, the "avoidance" phase, aims to reduce symptoms as much as possible.[18] It's recommended to last 10-14 days, with a focus on nutrient optimization, a mixed diet with emphasis on vegetables and reduced histamine/biogenic amine intake, changes in meal composition, and principles of a balanced diet.[18] Phase two, the "test" phase, lasts for up to six weeks and focuses on expanding the food choices while taking individual risk factors (such as stress, medication use, and menstruation) into account.[18] Phase two involves determination of individual histamine tolerance baseline levels.[18] Phase three, the long-term diet, focuses on a high quality of life and a continuous, balanced supply of nutrients.[18] This phase should remain individualized and guided by patient-specific food tolerances but should be a nutrient-dense, diversified diet.[18]

It's important to note the suggested time frames for each dietary phase. Too much time spent in phase one could, in theory, make food reintegration difficult, particularly for the MCAS patient. Food intolerance experts note that "exclusion of potential dietary triggers should be for as short a period as necessary to achieve symptom improvement, followed by gradual food reintroduction to individual tolerance."[8]

Reese and colleagues concluded in 2017, "The treatment approach should be largely guided by the individual tolerance of affected individuals. Generalized restrictions on food selection are only relevant for diagnostic purposes and do not help affected patients in the long term.

More research is needed to establish the relevance of measuring biomarkers, risk factors in intestinal function and barrier, as well as the histamine dose that elicits the pharmacological effects of histamine. Until then, expert nutritional counseling can help patients to avoid diets that result in an unnecessary reduction in their quality of life."[18]

What do MCAS experts think about the low-histamine diet? In 2017, Dr. Afrin stated that "there is no one 'low-histamine diet' that works for everyone—every patient is different."[33] He added that diet, just like medications, is a big trial-and-error process, and that most patients will figure out in one month's time whether any particular diet being tried is significantly helpful (and thus should be retained in the regimen) or not (and thus should be stopped).[33] As noted in Chapter 10, Dr. Castells stated in a 2018 interview that the low-histamine diet is not an appropriate choice for children who have MCAS, and that the focus should be on a well-balanced diet that includes fruit, vegetables and protein sources and avoidance of triggering or allergic foods.[34]

WHAT IS OPTIMAL FOR HEALING?

After evaluating both sides of the perspective, it appears that some believe that a long-term low-histamine diet is not appropriate for healing, while others support its use. As is the case with so many topics, the hope is that MCAS-specific research will be conducted in this area soon.

However, regardless of whether research shows that symptoms can be alleviated in the short-term with the diet, many question its long-term appropriateness. Is the low-histamine diet simply "putting a Band-Aid" on symptoms, while the underlying MCAS cause continues to go on undeterred? And further, does long-term avoidance of important nutrients set one up for more health problems down the road?

Foods that are considered high in histamine or that facilitate the release of histamine also include healthy options like spinach, avocado, and ripe bananas. While these foods have relatively low histamine when compared to the consensus on aged cheese and meats, for example, many patients following the diet will eliminate all potential sources on the list, regardless of whether the resultant diet is full of healing (fruit- and vegetable-based) nutrients and regardless of whether they actually have sensitivities to the food that they are eliminating. This is not the case with all patients but appears to be more common than one would think, particularly in newly-diagnosed patients who may look to low-histamine diet advice on websites or social media platforms.

Further, too much of a focus on the numbers can be unhealthy. It's easy to drive oneself crazy analyzing the histamine charts, and some assert that it's inappropriate to come up with a strict list of "no" foods based solely on histamine levels (although eliminating some of the utmost highest culprits that are unhealthy, such as alcohol, can be useful). For someone who has MCAS, the combined list of the foods that one is truly allergic to, the ones that seem to trigger other mast cell symptoms, and the ones that are high in histamine, salicylates, etc., can eliminate a great deal of food options, leaving the diet devoid of nutrients that are important for healing.

While foods may serve as the immediate trigger to a reaction, it's wise to consider the other factors that may have caused the bucket to fill up and overflow. When envisioning a pie chart, histamine is just one small slice of the whole picture, and focusing solely on histamine may keep a patient in a vicious cycle of reactions and eliminations and a false sense of control that becomes a slippery slope into more dietary restrictions.

Figure 1 shows an example of the number of different factors that *may* influence mast cell activation with *nonfactual sample ratios* shown in pie graph form. Histamine ingested in the diet may appear to be one of the more obvious triggers, but when one looks under the surface, it's possible that other factors play a bigger role in systemwide predisposition toward mast cell activation. Histamine, represented as the smallest sliver on the pie graph, could be more of the "straw that broke the camel's back" in this scenario.

Figure 1. Factors That *May* Influence Mast Cell Activation, as an Example Pie Chart

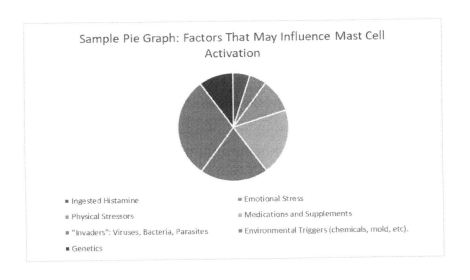

405

The take-home message is this: Short-term elimination diets can be helpful initially, but a long-term dietary plan ought to be as diverse as the individual can tolerate and focused on natural, non-processed, organic healing nutrients. It may be useful to avoid the biggest "high-histamine" culprits, such as aged cheese, cured meats, and alcohol (which in addition to being high in histamine may also be pro-inflammatory and hormone- or additive-laden). A "low-toxin diet" should trump a singular focus on histamine in patients with MCAD and may be a more appropriate response. Dietary changes should be individualized and guided with the help of one's medical team. The end goal should be a well-balanced diet full of antioxidant and anti-inflammatory fruits and vegetables, regardless of their histamine content numbers.

Factors that influence gastrointestinal digestion and absorption may need to be considered. Some patients do better with produce that is cooked compared to raw. Some patients do better with at-home juicer machines, smoothies, or pureed foods compared to whole foods. Again, trial and error are important to find an optimal way to maintain individualized healing nutrients in the diet.

Fatty Acid Considerations

It's theorized that diet can influence other mast cell mediators beyond histamine, including prostaglandins. Fatty acids are precursors to prostaglandins. A good balance of increased healthy omega 3 fatty acids with fewer omega 6 fatty acids *may, in theory,* equate to lower levels of plasma prostaglandins. The ideal ratio for omega 6 to omega 3 fatty acids has been reported to range from 5:1 (reducing asthma symptoms) to 2-3:1 (inflammation suppression), but the typical Westernized diet often looks more like 15:1 to 16.7:1![35]

Fatty acids are termed "essential" because the body does not create them and they need to be obtained dietarily. Alpha-linolenic acid is a plant-based fatty acid that is found in foods such as flaxseed, chia seed, linseed, walnuts, hemp seed, soybeans, kale, chard, some algae, and cold-water fish (tuna, wild salmon, herring, halibut). Evening primrose oil and a high-quality B vitamin are believed to assist with the production of this "good" type of fatty acid. The body converts a percentage of alpha-linolenic acid (omega 3 source) into DHA (docosahexaenoic acid) and EPA (eicosapentaenoic acid), which play a role in anti-inflammatory protective properties against heart disease and other conditions.[35] Linoleic acid, on the other hand, is termed the "bad" fatty acid that's found in products like corn oil, safflower oil, canola oil, sunflower oil, fried food, and processed food.

HEALING THROUGH DIET

For the patient with MCAS, going directly to the food source (as opposed to purchasing supplements that may trigger reactions due to their fillers and preservatives) may be a beneficial approach for certain foods. For example, some patients may tolerate citrus fruit well but have a poor tolerance to ascorbic acid supplements that contain additives. In other patient cases, the opposite may be true, where certain supplements may be better tolerated than the original food source. In some instances, the studied recommended dose of the fruit/extract is more than is traditionally obtained dietarily, which can pose an additional challenge.

Below is a chart based off multiple scientific sources listing natural fruits, vegetables, and grains that *may be* beneficial for someone who suffers from food allergies, food sensitivities, hives, anaphylaxis, inflammation, etc. Keep in mind that much of the available research is test-tube and animal-based and does not necessarily reflect a human patient symptomatic response. *The chart, below, reflects a literature investigation for each listed food with theoretical benefits but is not considered all-inclusive.*

A number of foods—including apple, beet, black rice bran, citrus fruit, cucumber, garlic, mangosteen, onion, peach, pomegranate, and watercress—consistently have literature support implicating careful consideration of their *potential utility* for patients who experience symptoms consistent with MCAS. However, some of these foods may fall into certain classes (such as the birch family) that sensitive individuals may react to; *as always, an individualized approach is advised.*

A do-it-yourself garden approach helps ensure that the end product on the table is clean and chemical free. Farmers markets can also make the process of adding more fruits and vegetables fun, while supporting the local economy. For patients who live in cold climates, indoor "stackable" gardens can be set up with a trip to the hardware store and may be a good option for winter months.

Table 2. Fruits, Vegetables, and Other Foods That *May Be* Helpful for the MCAS Patient

HEALING FOOD	PROPOSED BENEFITS	SOURCE(S)
Amaranth	inhibits anaphylaxis, IgE production, and cytokines	Hibi et al. (2003);[36] Patil et al. (2012)[37]
Apple	antihistaminic, suppresses mast cell activation, antiviral	Shealy (2017);[38] Tokura et al. (2005);[39] Kanda et al. (1998)[40]
Apricot	anti-allergy, anti-inflammatory, antiviral	Shealy (2017)[38]
Artichoke	source of rutin/luteolin (mast cell stabilizing), anti-inflammatory, antiviral	Fratianni et al. (2014)[41]
Avocado	aids skin rashes, antibacterial, antiviral	Shealy (2017)[38]
Beet (root and leaves)	reduces bradykinin-mediated swelling, anti-inflammatory, reduces cytokines	Jain et al. (2011),[42] Nagase et al. (1975),[43] Martinez et al. (2015)[44]
Black rice bran	suppresses mast cell mediators, reduces edema	Choi et al. (2010)[45]
Broccoli	anti-allergy, anti-inflammatory, antiviral	Shealy (2017)[38]
Buckwheat	inhibits histamine and cytokine release	Kim et al. (2003)[46]
Butternut squash	suppresses IgE antibody production	Imaoka et al. (1994)[47]
Cabbage	reduces airway inflammation	Shealy (2017)[38]
Capers	antihistaminic, inhibits mast cell mediator release	Trombetta et al. (2005)[48]
Carrot	reduces inflammation, boosts the immune system, assists with skin and wound issues	Shealy (2017)[38]
Cherry	anti-allergy, anti-inflammatory, antiviral	Shealy (2017)[38]
Chicory	anti-allergy, anti-inflammatory	Das et al. (2016)[49]
Cilantro	reduces food allergies, boosts the immune system, aids detoxification	Verma (2014)[50]
Cucumber	reduces prostaglandin/histamine/serotonin/bradykinin	Kumar et al. (2012);[51] Agatemor et al. (2015);[52]

	/proteases, antioxidant, analgesic, aids skin conditions, reduces respiratory ailments	Shealy (2017)[38]
Fig	soothes respiratory ailments, reduces inflammation	Shealy (2017)[38]
Garlic (fresh)	anti-allergic, immune boosting, reduces airway inflammation, reduces IgE-mediated swelling	Shealy (2017);[38] Kyo et al. (2001);[53] Kim et al. (2012)[54]
Grapefruit	assists respiratory problems	Shealy (2017)[38]
Green Pepper	anti-allergy, anti-inflammatory, antiviral	Shealy (2017)[38]
Lemon	reduces airway inflammation, anti-allergy, source of flavonoids	Shealy (2017);[38] Hwang et al. (2012)[55]
Lime	reduces chest and throat inflammation, immune-boosting	Shealy (2017)[38]
Mangosteen	antihistaminic, inhibits mast cell degranulation, reduces prostaglandins, leukotrienes, interleukins	Nakatani et al. (2002);[56] Chae et al. (2012)[57]
Oats	antihistaminic, antioxidant, boosts the immune system	Chatuevedi et al. (2011)[58]
Onion	reduces food allergies, antihistaminic, stabilizes mast cells, reduces airway inflammation	Aggarwal & Yost (2011);[59] Shealy (2017)[38]
Orange	reduces airway inflammation, anti-allergy, source of flavonoids	Shealy (2017);[38] Cardile et al. (2010)[60]
Parsley	antihistaminic, anti-inflammatory, analgesic	Al-khazraji (2015)[61]
Pea sprouts	source of flavonoids, antioxidant	Liu et al. (2016)[62]
Peach	anti-allergy, antihistaminic, reduces cytokines	Kim et al. (2013);[63] Shin et al. (2010)[64]
Pomegranate	antihistaminic, reduces prostaglandins, inhibits mast cell-derived cytokines, anti-inflammatory	Miguel et al. (2010);[65] Barwal et al. (2009);[66] Lee et al. (2010)[67]
Sweet potato	antihistaminic, anti-inflammatory, analgesic	Meira et al. (2012)[68]
Tangerine	anti-allergy, anti-inflammatory, antiviral	Shealy (2017)[38]
Watercress	antihistaminic, immune-boosting, anti-	Shealy (2017);[38] Sadeghi et al.

409

	inflammatory	(2014)[69]
Zucchini	anti-inflammatory, analgesic, antihistaminic	Karpagam et al. (2011)[70]

There are also many plants and herbs that are purported to have similar benefits, as depicted below in Table 3. Black cumin seed, chamomile, coriander, echinacea, elderflower, ginger, goldenrod, holy basil, lotus root, marshmallow, nettle, peppermint, red ginger (galangal), saffron, thyme, and turmeric are supported by multiple literature sources as *theoretically beneficial* for patients with symptoms of MCAS. Many of these are available in organic tea form as well as in powdered spice form for use with cooking.

There has been some recent concern about the potential for turmeric to reduce DAO levels. A 2016 study noted a reduction in DAO levels when rats with acute enteritis had seven days of the supplement.[71] However, the same subjects showed a reduction in TNF-alpha and certain interleukins, indicating a reduction in overall inflammation.[71]

The concern over turmeric and DAO levels is an example highlighting the importance that though these are "natural" supplements, much of their physiological effects and interactions with mast cells are still being determined, so a general level of caution is warranted. Patients with MCAS are far from uniform in terms of tolerance to difference foods and supplements, so these charts should serve as a starting point from which to evaluate on a case-by-case basis.

Table 3 reflects a literature investigation for each listed plant/herb with theoretical benefits but is not considered all-inclusive. Herbs, plants, and spices can interact with other medications and can be toxic in certain levels, so experimentation in this area should be closely guided by one's medical team.

Table 3. Plants, Herbs, and Other Sources That *May Be* Helpful for the MCAS Patient

HEALING PLANT/HERB	PROPOSED BENEFITS	SOURCE(S)
Agrimony	reduces long-term food allergies	Shealy (2017)[38]
Ajowan	reduces food allergies	Aggarwal & Yost (2011)[59]
Aloe vera	aids skin rashes	Shealy (2017)[38]
Annato	antihistaminic, reduces vascular permeability	Yong et al. (2013)[72]
Ashwagandha	reduces mediator release/vascular permeability	Lee et al (2012)[73]
Astralagus	assists with multiple allergies	Shealy (2017)[38]
Baikal skullcap	reduces allergic rhinitis and hay fever	Chevallier (2016)[74]
Basil	boosts the immune system, reduces sinus and chest inflammation	Shealy (2017)[38]
Berberine	reduces prostaglandin synthesis	Dharmananda (2017)[75]
Black cumin seed	reduces food allergies, antihistaminic, suppresses prostaglandins and leukotrienes	Aggarwal & Yost (2011);[59] Gholamnezhad et al. (2015);[76] Tembhurne et al. (2014)[77]
Boneset	reduces allergic rhinitis and hay fever	Chevallier (2016)[74]
Burdock root	aids skin rashes	Shealy (2017)[38]
Butterbur	reduces seasonal allergies	Low Dog et al. (2012)[78]
Cardamom	aids respiratory problems	Shealy (2017)[38]
Caraway seeds	antihistaminic	Sachan et al (2016)[79]
Catnip	reduces seasonal allergies	Low Dog et al. (2012)[78]
Chamomile	antihistaminic, reduces allergies and rashes	Hussein et al. (2017);[80] Shealy (2017)[38]
Cinnamon	reduces airway inflammation	Shealy (2017)[38]
Clove	reduces airway inflammation	Shealy (2017)[38]
Common plantain	relieves allergic rhinitis and hay fever	Chevallier (2016)[74]
Coriander	stabilizes mast cells, inhibitory for MC mediators, assists respiratory problems, hay fever, and allergies	Bhat et al. (2014);[81] Shealy (2017)[38]

Cumin	boosts the immune system, reduces severe allergies	Shealy (2017)[38]
Devil's claw	reduces seasonal allergies	Low Dog et al. (2012)[78]
Echinacea	reduces allergic rhinitis and hay fever, immune-boosting, reduces throat inflammation	Chevallier (2016);[74] Shealy (2017)[38]
Elderflower	relieves allergic rhinitis and hay fever, sinusitis	Chevallier (2016);[74] Low Dog et al. (2012);[78] Shealy (2017)[38]
Evening primrose	reduces seasonal allergies	Low Dog et al. (2012)[78]
Eyebright	relieves allergic rhinitis and hay fever	Chevallier (2016)[74]
Fenugreek	reduces skin rashes, airway and sinus inflammation	Shealy (2017)[38]
Flaxseed oil	aids skin inflammation, antihistaminic	Park et al. (2011)[82]
Galangal (red ginger)	reduces food allergies, suppresses mast cell degranulation, prevents anaphylaxis, lowers prostaglandin E2	Aggarwal & Yost (2011);[59] Zaidi et al. (2014);[83] Ravindran et al. (2012)[84]
Ginger	inhibits leukotrienes and prostaglandins, soothes throat inflammation	Shealy (2017);[38] Kiuchi et al. (1992)[85]
Ginkgo	reduces airway inflammation	Shealy (2017)[38]
Goldenrod	reduces allergic rhinitis, hay fever, and respiratory inflammation	Chevallier (2016);[74] Pursell (2015)[86]
Holy basil	antihistaminic, anti-anaphylactic, stabilizes mast cells	Singh et al (2007);[87] Choudhary (2010);[88] Rahman et al. (2011)[89]
Honey	reduces allergic rhinitis, throat inflammation, and respiratory issues	Shealy (2017),[38] Asha'ari et al. (2013)[90]
Lemon balm	reduces allergies, aids respiratory issues, antihistaminic	Shealy (2017);[38] Birdane et al. (2007)[91]
Lemongrass	boosts the immune system, antioxidant	Shealy (2017);[38] Cheel et al. (2005)[92]
Licorice root	anti-allergy, reduces airway inflammation, aids rashes	Shealy (2017);[38] Shin et al. (2007)[93]
Lotus root	stabilizes mast cells, anti-inflammatory	Mukherjee et al. (2010);[94]

		Sharma et al. (2017)[95]
Marshmallow	reduces allergic rhinitis, hay fever, throat and skin irritation	Chevallier (2016);[74] Shealy (2017)[38]
Milk thistle	reduces food allergies and inflammation, stabilizes mast cells	Shealy (2017);[38] Lecomte (1975)[96]
Mint	reduces food allergies	Aggarwal & Yost (2011)[59]
Moringa	inhibits mast cell degranulation, antihistaminic	Thakur et al. (2013)[97]
Neem	antihistaminic, anti-inflammatory, antioxidant	Atawodi et al. (2009);[98] Sonika et al. (2010)[99]
Nettle leaf	reduces food allergies, rashes, allergic rhinitis, hay fever and seasonal allergies, anti-histaminic, stabilizes mast cells	Chevallier (2016);[74] Low Dog et al. (2012);[78] Pursell (2015);[86] Shealy (2017)[38]
Olive (fruit/leaf/oil)	stabilizes mast cells, antihistaminic	Chandak et al. (2009);[100] Persia et al. (2014)[101]
Oregano	antihistaminic, may inhibit prostaglandin release, anti-inflammatory	Silva et al. (2012);[102] Baser (2002)[103]
Peppermint	antihistaminic, reduces sinus and lung inflammation	Shealy (2017);[38] Grigoleit (2005);[104] Inoue (2001)[105]
Plantain leaf	reduces allergies and aids rashes	Shealy (2017)[38]
Pycnogenol	inhibits histamine release	Sharma et al. (2003)[106]
Red clover	anti-allergy, reduces skin reactions	Shealy (2017)[38]
Rosemary	aids skin issues, antibacterial and antifungal	Shealy (2017)[38]
Saffron	antihistaminic, reduces throat and airway inflammation	Shealy (2017);[38] Boskabady et al. (2010)[107]
Sage	aids recurrent coughs and allergies	Shealy (2017)[38]
Schisandra	inhibits mast cell cytokine release, antioxidant	Kang (2006),[108] Wilson (2007)[109]
Slippery elm	reduces food allergies	Shealy (2017)[38]
Spirulina	antihistaminic, anti-inflammatory, reduces allergic rhinitis, inhibits	Kim et al. (1998);[110] Yang et al. (1997)[111]

	anaphylaxis	
St. John's wort	aids skin rashes	Shealy (2017)[38]
Tarragon	anti-inflammatory, analgesic, may inhibit mast cell mediators	Eidi et al. (2016);[112] Maham et al. (2014)[113]
Thyme	reduces food allergies, rashes, itching, allergic rhinitis and hay fever, stabilizes mast cells, inhibits anaphylaxis, boosts the immune system	Chevallier (2016);[74] Shealy (2017);[38] Boskabady (2012)[107]
Turmeric (curcumin)	reduces food allergies, antihistaminic, inhibits mast cell reactions and anaphylaxis, reduces airway inflammation	Aggarwal & Yost (2011);[59] Shealy (2017)[38]
Yarrow	aids sinusitis, hay fever, and allergies	Shealy (2017)[38]

THE IMPORTANCE OF A WELL-TRAINED NUTRITIONIST

One of the most overwhelming aspects of daily life for patients with MCAS lies in dietary decisions, particularly when the gastrointestinal system is inflamed or dysfunctional. A patient survey published in 2018 noted that only 10.7% of patients with MCAD reported being referred to a dietician, highlighting the dire need for more clinical attention in this area.[114]

As apparent in a quick glance at the above charts, navigating the nutritional world with MCAS—particularly when patients with MCAS can be seriously reactive to different foods—is extremely tricky. Nutritionists can be a knowledgeable resource for the initial and ongoing management of MCAS. Just like any discipline, it's useful to call ahead and verify that a practitioner is knowledgeable in one's medical condition(s).

In addition to addressing food types and nutrient needs, dieticians and nutritionists can help the patient navigate other diet-related decisions, such as how much fiber to consume. Recent research suggests that dietary fiber (especially polysaccharides and oligosaccharides) and its metabolites (short chain fatty acids) may inhibit mast cell activation and degranulation.[115]

Rebecca Snow, MS, CNS, a licensed nutritionist and herbalist in Maryland, has a multifaceted approach to management of patients with MCAS. She advocates for a comprehensive plan that includes reducing overall histamine load, stabilizing mast cells, replenishing deficient nutrients, focusing on detoxification and reducing overall toxin load, healing the gut, and reducing overall inflammation—all through the use of dietary changes and supplements.[116]

There are a number of resources that help the body clear histamine more efficiently. According to Snow, based on the research, these include cofactors copper, vitamin B6, vitamin C, protein, oleic acid, SAM-e, methylfolate, and methylcobalamin.[16,116] Snow also considers other substances to assist patients with MCAS: cannabinoids, flavonoids (quercetin, luteolin, and rutin, among others), and herbs with potential to stabilize mast cells (schisandra and Baikal skullcap).[116] Emodin from rhubarb/yellow dock and substances that help balance the TH1/TH2 immunity (n-acetylcysteine, curcumin, reishi, alpha lipoic acid) may also be useful in certain patients.[116] Vitamin D3 and iron supplementation may be important for patients with MCAS, but Snow notes that they can also be "overdone" in some cases.[116] According to Snow, non-histamine-promoting probiotics, l-glutamine, omega 3 fatty acids, quercetin, slippery elm or marshmallow powder, molybdenum, and deglycyrrhized licorice may be products to consider for assisting with gut healing.[116]

Snow addresses various sources of daily toxins with her patients, including those that are dietary (GMO, pesticides, sugar), environmental xenobiotics (pthalates, parabens), medical inputs (chemotherapy, radiation), lifestyle and home environment (EMF, mold, drinking water), occupation (sick building), and psychosocial inputs.[116] She recommends hydrotherapy or sweating therapy (which may be challenging for MCAS clients due to their sensitivity to heat and fluctuating temperatures), fiber (such as chia and flax), hydration, and liver-supporting supplements like milk thistle, n-acetyl cysteine and other amino acids, and liposomal glutathione for patients with MCAS who need extra detox support.[116]

Heidi Turner, MS, RDN, is an integrative registered dietitian and nutritionist who works with patients with MCAS and other chronic conditions at her practice Food Logic in Seattle, Washington. She is passionate about increasing education and awareness for the MCAS patient population and is a wonderful resource with an abundance of clinical expertise in this area.

In a 2018 interview, Turner shared some insight into nutritional strategies that may assist this patient population. Ultimately, there's no cookie-cutter approach to navigating the tricky world of diet with patients who have MCAS.[117] *It's crucial that the approach is individualized and guided with the help of a licensed professional.* However, she notes that the tendency is for patients to jump on the internet and start experimenting with things, an approach that can certainly lead to trouble.[117]

It's quite difficult to give generalized dietary advice due to the spectrum of characteristics possible with patients who have MCAS. And by the time patients end up in Turner's office, they are typically extremely restricted in what they can do dietarily.[117] As a general approach, Turner tends to start by reviewing the basics: Has the patient already looked at the usual food suspects like gluten and dairy? Are they being exposed to processing, chemicals, or pesticides in their diet?[117]

Once these areas are addressed and the obvious factors (like true allergies) are considered, Turner tends to start thinking through the lens of histamine.[117] She notes that while some patients do fine, for others, foods with high histamine content may be adding to "the bucket."[117] In these patients, it's most likely that their DAO and HNMT (histamine breakdown) systems are overtaxed, so removing that constellation of foods can temporarily calm the system down.[117]

The next consideration is typically investigating whether the patient is being influenced by high FODMAP foods.[117] Turner notes that, particularly in patients who have small intestinal bacterial overgrowth (SIBO) or are in a dysbiotic state, fermentation can be adding to the overall histamine load.[117] In 2017, researchers McIntosh and colleagues found that a three-week low FODMAP diet reduced circulating histamine levels by eight-fold.[118]

If the above doesn't work, Turner may then resort to investigating other factors like salicylate, oxalate, and sulfur intolerances with her patients who have MCAS.[117] However, she notes that these areas tend to be the "bottom of the pyramid" in terms of priority, as they involve great difficulty to implement and are generally utilized only for the more severe cases.[117]

For some patients, there's no discernible pattern. Turner notes that, in a subgroup of patients with MCAS, the issue is not necessarily a class or type of food, but that the digestive process is so taxed that anything entering it is reactive.[117] She clarifies, "The digestive tract is a large immune system and sometimes becomes overly hypersensitive, leading to reactivity to the digestive process itself."[117]

At the end of the day, Turner's approach tends to be more focused on the big picture in terms of helping calm down the system and get the gastrointestinal system moving optimally and with more options for increased "input" over time.[117] She notes that you have to be careful, because if you take too much out, the body adapts.[117] Turner adds, "We're dealing with a petulant child of an immune system that doesn't want to be messed with."[117] Removal of non-trigger foods on the premise of containing a particular substance can sometimes backfire and cause more sensitivities.[117] This is one of the many reasons why it's so important to work together with a professional throughout this process.

Turner explains that she doesn't tend to see a lot of true allergies in patients with MCAS, but more often she notes reactivities.[117] Reactivities to a food one day that was previously tolerated prior to that point is more of an indicator that the body's pathways are struggling; the pathway is in disorder, which can create a bigger buildup of histamine.[117] A number of daily factors (like environment, stress, and time of day) can influence chemical mediator levels and create day-to-day variations in the bucket spillover effect.[117] Turner notes, "It's not that the patient has allergies to these foods… it's that the body does not want to digest them."[117]

Aside from dietary modifications, Turner also works with patients to optimize gastrointestinal bacterial balance, facilitate optimal levels of stomach acid and digestive enzymes, assist the body in removal of toxins with binders, and upregulate the parasympathetic nervous system (PNS).[117] Just as there is no single approach to medications or dietary strategies, Turner notes that probiotic supplementation advice is individualized.[117] While many patients with MCAS don't tolerate any probiotic very well, she recommends starting small and going with single strain options.[117]

Stomach acid is a common concern for patients who have MCAS. Turner notes that hypochlorhydria (low stomach acid) seems more common in this patient population, particularly in patients with chronic constipation and delayed gastrointestinal transit issues.[117] For these patients, she tends to see positive results with digestive bitters sprayed on the tongue before a meal.[117] She recommends Better Bitters by Herb Pharm, which may help stimulate the gut and the vagus nerve to let the body know that food is on the way.[117] Many patients with MCAS may end up on a high protein diet following food eliminations, and Turner explains that the more we can help the body process proteins, the better, since high protein combined with low stomach acid may go hand in hand with a poorly functioning vagus nerve and gastroparesis.[117] For patients who present on the diarrhea end of the spectrum, hyperchlorhydria (high stomach acid) may be a bigger reality and these patients may need to work more in the medication realm to get things calmed down.[117]

Turner's focus is less on adding specific foods to influence motility and more on calming everything down in order to open the door and get more food and nutrient options in.[117] She finds that magnesium and vitamin C supplements may be tolerated by this population (though high-dose vitamin C appears to exacerbate some patients, particularly those who have interstitial cystitis).[117] Epsom salt baths are a great option for gaining magnesium and assisting the body's detoxification systems.[117] Going as organic as possible is also important, and she suggests that patients prioritize shopping organic for the Environmental Working Group's dirty dozen at a minimum.[117]

Turner also notes that she is seeing a positive trend for the use of toxin binders (such as activated charcoal, Great Plains liquid bentonite clay, and GI detox products) in patients with MCAS.[117] Specifically, she is getting about 80% positive feedback in tolerance to once-daily binder use from patients who are severely compromised.[117] Of course, as mentioned in Chapter 10, caution and assistance are warranted with binders, as they can also compromise nutrients and medication absorption when not used properly.

Lastly, Turner emphasizes the importance of addressing the parasympathetic nervous system, which is often poorly functioning in patients with MCAS. She recommends utilizing exercises for the vagus nerve, exercises for breathing patterns, acupuncture (or acupressure if needles are not tolerated), visceral manipulation, and craniosacral therapies as useful adjuncts to nutritional approaches.[117]

Snow and Turner are great examples of specialized nutrition and herbal experts with extensive knowledge regarding MCAS. At the end of the day, when it comes to nutrition considerations for the MCAS patient, the bottom line parallels other aspects of patient care: advice must be individualized and guided by a well-qualified professional. The importance of working with a nutrition expert who is familiar with MCAS, POTS, EDS, and other comorbidities cannot be underestimated. Patience and discipline are essential aspects of the gut healing process, but the rewards can be plentiful when the patient has a comprehensive and holistic medical team in place to help them navigate the proper path.

CHAPTER KEY POINTS

- Many patients focus on websites that state histamine levels for different food sources. The numbers are not perfect, and there are so many variables that can influence the level of measured histamine in foods. There is not one "gold standard" chart of numbers to follow.

- Focusing on histamine numbers can be dangerous because it may cause one to eliminate healthy, nutrient-dense foods that otherwise could be well tolerated and beneficial for healing. However, some patients find it helpful to eliminate the biggest culprits on the list (like cheese, alcohol, and certain fish) from their diet to minimize histamine bucket spill-over.

- Focusing solely on histamine may be suboptimal management for a patient with MCAS. Many other mediators influence physical symptoms. It's likely that ingested histamine is only a small percentage of the total everyday triggers that stimulate mast cells.

- When patients are diagnosed with MCAS, they are often already limited in the number of foods they can tolerate. Working with a specialized nutritionist can help ensure adequate nutrients and calories.

- A low-histamine diet can be very restrictive in addition to food allergies and sensitivities. Instead, an elimination diet may be helpful in the first weeks or month to determine exact individual triggers. It's helpful to differentiate what foods trigger anaphylactic-type reactions (those to be strictly avoided) as opposed to foods that may cause mild and sporadic symptoms that could eventually be reintroduced down the road.

- It's important to also consider factors in the chain of handling that could impact the food. Additives and preservatives, cross-contamination, and poor hygiene practices or improper temperature regulations could all trigger increased symptoms in patients with MCAS. A preservative- or additive-free eating plan may be a good starting point for the patient with MCAS.

- Eliminating processed foods, nonorganic produce, gluten and other grains, caffeine, refined sugar, and dairy may also be beneficial for overall health and inflammation reduction. Though this type of approach is difficult and requires discipline, when done correctly over time it may foster an increased healing potential.

- Patients may find that eliminating other types of non-dietary environmental triggers (such as exposure to fragrances, toxic mold and cleaning chemicals) may have a more profound impact on food reactions than a strict and lengthy low-histamine diet. This is because elimination of these other big "slices of the MCAS pie" essentially reduces the overall mast cell mediator load in the bucket, which could lead to reintroduction of certain foods and a more varied diet that was not possible in the presence of the offending products or toxins.

- Supplementing the diet with certain herbs, plants, and healing foods may assist in helping the body reduce levels or effects of mast cell mediators. It's important to always consult one's medical team when considering changes in the form of dietary supplements.

Chapter Twelve
Holistic Healing

WHAT IS HOLISTIC CARE?

A holistic approach to illness typically involves attention to *physical, intellectual, emotional, and spiritual* factors that influence healing. In addition to the dietary considerations and recommendations for a two-tier diagnostic approach and a two-part treatment plan presented in prior chapters, there are a number of other practices that may be valuable for the patient with MCAS.

There's an incredible outpouring of emotions that typically happens in this patient population when newly diagnosed. Patients with chronic invisible illness typically experience initial phases of emotions that can include euphoria/joy at finally having a name for their suffering, cynicism toward the medical community, deep depression at the realization that what they are experiencing is lifelong and without "cure," exhaustion/feeling overwhelmed at the prospect of continuing to fight what they are up against, and much more. Outside of the obvious physical treatment needs, there are several actions that should be taken following diagnosis to assist in navigating the emotional impact of MCAS.

A holistic approach to MCAS can be very empowering because, over time, it may reduce stress-related flares or triggers and shift one's focus away from reliance on doctor visits and prescriptions to place more tools in the patient's own back pockets. Consider it a bunch of extra (crucial and potentially cost-effective) supplemental tools to add to an existing medication, supplement, and dietary plan of care.

EXPECTATIONS FOR LIFE WITH MCAS

Setting realistic expectations for oneself and others is an important aspect of the initial phase of emotional healing. Certain expectations may need to be adjusted in some circumstances, both in short-term and long-term disease-management considerations.

Expect bumps along the road. Try not to take the "bad" days too personally. It's easy to get discouraged each time anaphylaxis, severe gastrointestinal symptoms, seizures, or other types of flares in symptoms occur, but don't let the discouragement derail hope or reduce a positive mental attitude. Expect that healing is not linear and that there will be lots of ups and downs along the journey.

Expect to encounter skeptical medical providers. By the time the patient is diagnosed, they will likely already have experience in this area. Expect that certain professionals may continue to negate symptoms or insinuate psychosomatics despite diagnostic clarity. Expect that certain providers may challenge the patient, and others may incompetently manage flares or emergency room scenarios. Expect that the majority of providers will probably never have heard of MCAS; expect to be an ambassador in terms of sharing resources and information with open-minded medical providers.

Expect the journey to be difficult in unimaginable ways. This disease has the ability to affect one's interpersonal relationships tremendously. Not only is it difficult on a daily basis in terms of the physical and mental challenges, but it's a great challenge to friendships and relationships with coworkers, one's family and significant other. Patience is key on both sides. And eventually as things improve—and they generally improve or become more stable as long as the patient keeps fighting—as cliché as it sounds, one will realize that the trials and tribulations on relationships have truly made those relationships stronger. Just as toxic physical triggers should be removed, toxic relationships may need to be let go of in the healing process.

Expect to "find out who your friends are" in a rather blunt way. (For those who have experienced chronic pain or illness for a long time, this has probably already happened.) Embrace those friends who have been there and continue to provide support, and make sure that they are well-supported, too. Instead of dwelling on past hurts and losses, patients should surround themselves with people who have similar values, enhance their outlook on life, and radiate a positive attitude.

Expect that almost nobody will fully "get it" or understand. Life becomes easier if the patient can let go of the desire for people to fully understand or empathize with the daily challenges. Support groups with people in similar scenarios can definitely help the patient feel less alone. Journaling can assist in releasing some of the emotional turmoil, and professional counseling services are also strongly encouraged.

When explaining the diagnosis to friends and family, *expect some engaged curiosity and some polite courtesy—and possibly some negativity.* When people ask a general "How are you?" they usually expect a one-line positive answer, particularly when they are acquaintances. Have a

422

prefabricated summary on the tip of the tongue to summarize the condition, and also be prepared to field questions with people who are genuinely interested in learning more.

Some friends may have hours of questions, where others really just want to know the bottom line: "Are you surviving? Good, let's change the subject." Both responses will come and go. A quick summary could be as simple as, "I was recently diagnosed with a disease that affects certain cells in my immune system. It causes a lot of invisible symptoms, but I'm learning to manage it." That leaves it open for people to ask more questions or change the subject.

Certain friends or family members may come from a particular background, opinion, or personality that questions the diagnosis or the validity of the symptoms or belittles some (or all) aspects of treatment and flare prevention. For example, many patients report experiencing animosity from family members and friends when the patient requires dietary and/or odor accommodations.

Expect to feel like you're letting people down at first (regardless of whether they truly agree). It's common to compare today's level of function to a prior season, which can sometimes promote feelings of guilt, discouragement, and even self-loathing, particularly when the patient is suddenly restricted in terms of the ability to leave the home or work.

Healing must start from within. Acceptance of one's current limitations and a strong sense of self-love are fundamental keys to unlocking healing. Setting boundaries with others and oneself and respecting the time needed for adequate self-care are so important in this process.

Expect tunnel vision and embrace distractions and shifts in attention from time to time. It's important to find a balance between thinking about the condition/symptoms and healing plan and setting one's attention elsewhere. The balance between internal vs. external focus often seems quite skewed at first and can vary greatly from person to person. But as a whole, some amount of distraction is important for mental health, in order to avoid constructing an identity that is completely wrapped up in MCAS. Focusing on a healthy dose of advocacy and awareness is one thing, but *personal identity* should be fostered with care and caution in terms of chronic illness.

This could mean watching a funny movie, creating art, or reading a nonmedical book in one's spare time. It could mean taking a day off from social media or the cell phone. It could mean a getaway to a cabin for a few days or perhaps setting up walking dates with a friend. It could mean committing to tasks that one can work on from home to help with the kids' school, church, or a nonprofit organization.

Believe it or not, there are plenty of hobbies that are MCAS friendly! Even if the patient is not able to be mobile outside of the house yet, it's important to take a mental breather from it all. Even when the symptoms are so "in-your-face" that it's impossible to not think about them, make a point to devote a particular, set-aside time each week to focusing on other things that bring intrinsic joy. It's incredible how much healing can occur when the perspective is shifted externally.

Expect journeys to vary. Avoid comparing one's situation with others who have similar diagnoses, which can add stress and frustration. What works for so-and-so is not always the solution for everyone. Swim the race in your own lane and keep in mind that invisible factors may give the neighboring athlete a short sprint compared to the longer distance event necessary for others.

Expect it to take time. Be patient, more patient, and then even more patient. The symptoms probably did not arrive overnight, so it's important to be realistic about expectations for the time frame to see improvements. Dial the pressure down and work on baby steps in the direction of one's goals. Respect limitations and let go of people who aren't willing to do the same. Surround oneself with people who are life-giving and, over time, when coupled with a holistic plan of care, change will emerge.

Letting Go

Releasing frustration over years of mistreatment within the medical community can be one of the more challenging aspects for the newly diagnosed patient. When a breakdown in patient-provider confidence and respect occurs multiple times over the years, this can lead to a patient's family members and friends labeling the patient as a hypochondriac, which only worsens the depths of anxiety and depression that can occur with regular chemical mediator "explosions." The patient will either get angry and continue to persevere and seek more answers for what they sincerely know to be real and true, or they may start to believe that medical provider and, over time, may sink lower and lower into self-loathing or helplessness. Suicidal thoughts are not uncommon.

"Great news! Your labs are normal!" is one of the more despised forms of commentary from doctors for patients with MCAS. It seems backward to hope that a doctor finds evidence of a big medical condition. But when the patient has been suffering with mysterious and debilitating ailments that are worsening over decades, they may really start to hope for something terrible to be the root problem.

It remains a mystery why some physicians cannot simply say, "I don't know what's wrong with you, but I believe that your symptoms are real." Or even rarer, "I don't know the cause, but I will work with you until we uncover it."

As a patient, it's easy to become bitter at the mainstream medical system and much harder to reach inner peace and acceptance of prior mislabeling once a patient has finally reached the verified answer of MCAS. However, it's *especially important* as part of the healing process to let go of any animosity toward past injustices experienced as a patient, as difficult as it may be.

It's important to remember that, by design, the (American) medical system is not set up to allow for thorough care for the majority of patients who are medically complex. It's important to recall that doctors are, in most cases, simply doing their job the way they've been trained. It's important to not take it personally.

CULTIVATE CALMNESS THROUGH PREVENTION AND PREPARATION

Flare-ups can create panic and anxiety. Anxiety can trigger a reaction or heighten an already-occurring flare. While it's impossible to be prepared for any and every scenario that could occur with MCAS, there are some preventive steps that may help streamline the process.

MCAS-specific everyday factors to consider in advance:

- Order medical alert identification with the patient name, conditions, allergies, emergency contact, and other important information. Consider push-button emergency alert devices or other emergency scenario options if frequent anaphylaxis results in the inability to speak.
- Carry a mask for unexpected environmental triggers.
- Stash mast cell calming medications in various areas—next to the bed, in a purse or day bag, in the car (while keeping in mind that certain meds can't be exposed to extreme temperatures).
- Educate family and friends on what to do in the event of an emergency. Have them *actually practice* with an EpiPen simulator.
- Type out a *medical summary page* and make copies of it to keep with all locations of medications and to travel along with the patient in the event of an emergency.

- Include diagnoses, current medications, allergies, drugs to avoid, typical protocol for handling reactions, a list of labs that may need to be ordered during acute reactions, emergency contacts, and MCAS doctor information.

- With the help of one's medical team, construct *scenario-specific guidelines* as part of an emergency action plan for the following scenarios. Attach it to the medical summary page and make sure it addresses:
  - acute emergencies (emergency room visits)
  - surgical considerations
  - inpatient (hospital) stays

- If frequent emergency room visits occur, designate a specific backpack that is pre-supplied with basic personal belongings to grab on the way out the door.

- Carry a large first aid kit in vehicles and a small one in a day pack or purse for outings or hikes.

- Stash "safe" foods in various places. Throw a cooler in the car with premade meals for longer days.

- Draft up what a comprehensive medical "dream team" looks like. Prioritize specialties and begin to compile a list of practitioners. Establishing care with a naturopath or functional medicine doctor (in addition to other specialists) can potentially identify underlying factors triggering mast cell activation, which may ease overall anxiety and the feeling of helplessness.

Travel Preparedness

In 2017, the World Allergy Organization Journal published an article on allergic reactions that occur during air travel. Patients with medical conditions may be more likely to experience symptoms during air travel, in part due to air pressure changes that impact oxygenation, the dry cabin atmosphere that impacts the mucosal membranes of the mouth and respiratory tract, dehydration risk, and uncontrolled exposures to allergens such as peanuts onboard.[1] The Federal Aviation Administration requires epinephrine to be part of the plane's emergency kit, which also typically contains inhaled bronchodilators and oxygen, steroids, and antihistamines.[1]

However, the best approach is one of prevention. The article included a number of recommendations, including avoidance of airline pillows and blankets, wiping down tray tables, and not consuming the airline-provided food.[1] Some airlines offer "buffer zones" for passengers with fragrance sensitivity or pet allergies.[1] Passengers can also request special

426

accommodations so that peanut/tree nut snacks are not distributed or that announcements are made instructing other passengers to avoid consuming nuts.[1]

Wearing a respiratory mask in-flight, plugging into music right away, wearing blue-light blocking glasses, utilizing antihistamines (or other medications) of choice, and being equipped with ample emergency medications may also reduce the likelihood of escalating reactions during air travel. Medical preboarding and having a wheelchair arranged in advance may also assist in a smoother travel experience. *Anecdotally*, some patients find that premedicating prior to the flight, during the flight, and/or right before landing may be helpful.

No matter how much one prepares, there are factors related to neighboring passengers (like perfume, cigarette smoke, or food choices) that may inevitably impact patients with MCAS on flights. It's best to develop a friendly rapport immediately with flight attendants and to prepare for the event that one needs to request to switch seats.

WIDESPREAD TRIGGER ELIMINATION

Prevention is key when it comes to the patient's home, work, and vehicle environments. Set aside some time initially (and also periodically) to complete a thorough environmental assessment followed by drastic elimination of all identified triggers. Sometimes it's helpful to go room by room when evaluating one's home for potential MCAS-related triggers.

Suggested checklist for initial environmental assessment:

OVERALL ASSESSMENT

- Is there mold or water damage? If found: relocate* or *carefully* remediate with professional help! (*Relocation is the most optimal option and can have a tremendous impact on MCAS symptoms and quality of life. Remediation is typically dangerous and difficult. Remediation can release more toxins and make the patient sicker.)

- Are pesticides, insecticides, or herbicides used around the exterior of the home? Vacate the premises if this is scheduled, or better yet, reconsider these treatments and investigate more natural options, if possible.

- Is the environment cluttered, dark, or unaesthetically pleasing? Living spaces may influence the human body. When clutter is reduced from the home or work environment and when the space is a place that generates peace, some believe that the body may also be better able to detoxify and heal.

ALL ROOMS: GENERAL ASSESSMENT

- Are candles, air fresheners, or other synthetic scented products present? Are essential oils helping or hurting?

- If the home is new-ish, is off gassing of carpets/flooring and furniture an issue?

- Are natural cleaners present? Consider replacing any chemical-based cleaners with something like lemon juice, probiotic solutions, or distilled white vinegar instead of traditional cleaners. Microfiber cloths and water can also be considered for sensitive patients.

- Seek hypoallergenic latex free gloves and a facial mask for cleaning to minimize contact of irritants with skin pores and the respiratory system.

KITCHEN ENVIRONMENT

- Is the tap water filtered? A reverse osmosis or carbon filter may be advised to reduce exposure to heavy metals, volatile organic compounds, water treatment additives, bacteria/viruses, and other potential water contaminants.

- Is there a designated allergen-friendly space for food preparation? Use color coding for cutting boards, knives, and cooking materials that are specific for the MCAS patient, if needed. Make sure there's a designated separate sponge as well.

- Is there a designated allergen-free section of the fridge/freezer?

- Is there adequate ventilation in the kitchen (fans, windows?)

- Are glass-only food storage and non-plastic eating/drinking vessels being used? Avoid plastic Tupperware, aluminum foil, plastic wrap, etc. and avoid heating plastic kitchen components in the dishwasher or microwave.

- Are there plastic containers (or bags) holding food or beverages in the fridge? Mesh bags are a good alternative to plastic storage of produce, and glass bottles and containers should replace any plastic kitchenware.

- Are groceries organic and free of additives, preservatives, and chemicals?

- Are the bags in the trash can odorless?

BATHROOM

- Is hand soap laden with chemicals? Seek more natural options.

- Does deodorant contain aluminum/other chemicals?

- Are additional shower, makeup, and skin beauty products appropriate? Get out every single product used and do some research, aiming to eliminate and reduce the majority that are synthetic/chemical-based. There are apps that may help with this step.

- Are feminine hygiene products free of chlorine, dyes, pesticides, and other chemicals?

- Is shower water filtered? A filter to remove chlorine and other chemicals may be helpful.

- Are adequate ventilation and cleaning techniques used in the bathroom to prevent mold/mildew growth?

- For the patient with regular constipation, is a toilet footstool ready for action? If gastrointestinal issues are present, elevating the knees above the hips (on a "Squatty Potty" type step) can be a tremendous aid for facilitating easier bowel movements.

BEDROOM

- Are electronics that emit EMFs (including alarm clocks and cell phones) near the bed? Are laptops or TVs used in bed? Create a sanctuary for sleeping in bed and base electronic use elsewhere.

- Is dirty laundry stored in a separate area from the bedroom? This may reduce reactivity.

- Do clothes contain fabrics pretreated with anything? Waterproofing materials (like Goretex) and clothes exposed to bug treatments should be avoided.

- Is bedding hypoallergenic? Also, consider the use of hypoallergenic pillow covers and a hypoallergenic mattress encasement.

- Is anything made out of memory foam? Memory foam and other special bedding/pillow material may possibly emit toxins.

- Is the mattress new? It's likely been treated with a chemical to retard flames and may experience some off-gassing.

- Are pillows hypoallergenic and replaced regularly? Dust mites or contaminants may influence patient tolerance to bedding and subsequent sleep quality.

LAUNDRY ROOM

- Remove dryer sheets and scented detergents from use. Distilled white vinegar is a chemical-less alternative to traditional laundry detergent. Wool balls for the dryer may be considered as an alternative to dryer sheets and fabric softeners.

- Is the dryer filter checked regularly?

LIVING AREAS

- Are pets allowed on furniture (or in bed)? This can increase cross-contamination of triggers.
- Are houseplants present? Certain houseplants are known for their ability to contribute to cleaner air.

VEHICLE

- Is the vehicle new? (Does it have off-gassing issues or seat covers that were chemically treated?)
- Is the vehicle old? (Does it potentially have invisible water damage?)
- Drive with the windows down periodically to reduce exposure to inhaled irritants within the vehicle (presuming that it's not a scenario involving inhaling car exhaust or cigarette smoke).
- Avoid inhaling fumes when pumping gas. Consider delegating the task or using a mask and waiting for gas to pump from inside the vehicle.

WORKPLACE

- Assess lighting and ventilation factors.
- Is the location close to a wireless internet router or other EMF sources?
- Assess postural ergonomic factors.

OTHER TIPS FOR TRIGGER ELIMINATION

- Remove shoes before entering home to reduce "cross contamination."
- Invest in a HEPA-type air purifier with a carbon filter (or several, depending on the room/living area size). Do not relocate these from previously contaminated environments. Replace the filter regularly (don't clean it!).
- Ensure clean water adherence when out of the home. Use glass containers and avoid bottled water/beverages from plastic bottles!
- Avoid exposure to paint, and if the house needs to be painted, ensure that low- or no-VOC paint is used.
- Consider hardwoods floors and rugs as opposed to carpet.

- Change the house furnace filter quarterly.

- Vacuum often and consider delegating this task to other family members. Delegate additional house-cleaning tasks and leave the house when they are done, if possible. Try not to do all of the house cleaning at once and make sure to open windows/increase ventilation with fans.

DETOXIFICATION

Basic Detoxification Strategies

Minimizing exposure to toxins and the process of detoxification have already been touched on in terms of their importance for patients with MCAS, and specific strategies should be *guided with the help of a medical professional.* First and foremost, optimizing gut, liver, lymphatic, and kidney health is key to assisting the body in the removal of toxins.

Chapters 10 and 11 describe supplement and dietary considerations that may assist the body in the detoxification process. Adequate hydration and proper attention to a healing anti-inflammatory, antioxidant-rich diet cannot be emphasized enough. Some patients also finding that juicing and fasting practices can be built into their healing plans to assist with detoxification.

Additional strategies such as colonic (enema) therapy, massage, beverages that promote liver cleansing (such as lemon water), focusing on certain foods, avoidance of certain products and environmental factors, and "gentle" sweating (with special attention to heat flare-up considerations for patients with MCAS) may be appropriate. Some practitioners recommend specific types of therapies such as infrared sauna or ionic footbaths for detoxification. Techniques to enhance lymphatic drainage may also be useful for patients with MCAS.

Detoxification strategies should be performed *carefully and slowly*, and short-term flare-ups in symptoms may be expected for patients with MCAS as well as the general population. Massive detoxification reactions should be avoided. The topic of detoxification is shared multiple times in this book to highlight its importance in the MCAS patient population. A full personalized plan of strategies should be agreed upon with one's medical team.

Massage

There is some debate about the utility of massage in patients with MCAS. Supporters claim that massage offers detoxification support by helping flush out toxins and waste, and it may also promote relaxation, stress reduction, and pain relief. Others highlight concerns for the potential of mechanically induced pressure to trigger mast cell degranulation.

The research supports that mast cell mediators like histamine and TNF-alpha contribute to the pain perception experienced with mechanical pressure to the skin.[2] However, this may be a dose-dependent or intensity-dependent response. Similar to the mechanism in which exercise provides protective effects in patients with MCAS with the proper quantitative characteristics like intensity and duration factored in, massage *may* also offer beneficial physiological responses when it's performed in the right manner.

The best approach *once a patient has reached a stable baseline* is to introduce a short, 10- or 15-minute session of light, relaxing massage, and to build from there gradually over time. Attention to detail may assist in providing for a more healing scenario; scented products and lotions should be avoided. Having patients bring their own MCAS-friendly lotion may help, and patients may also benefit from bringing in their own sheets that have been washed in a patient-friendly manner.

Patients may want to call ahead if scheduling a professional massage in order to ensure that certain aspects of the experience are at minimal risk to induce reactions. Requesting an odor-free environment can help, and mold-sensitive patients may want to investigate the building prior to scheduling. Avoidance of meals or other triggers prior to the session and consideration of potential premedication may be advised on a case-by-case basis. When in doubt, light pressure is a good starting place to assess mast cell response. Frequent breaks may be a useful initial approach during the session, and extra hydration is advised afterward.

Lymphatic Drainage

Lymphatic tissue carries waste from the tissues and cells back to the heart. It's hypothesized that an increasing toxic/bacterial/viral load can reduce the efficiency of the lymphatic system to the point where it becomes sluggish and impaired. There are a number of strategies that appear to assist in fostering helpful lymphatic flow. Hydration, massage and skin brushing are considered key tools. Gentle skin brushing involves using a coarse brush on the skin in movements from the extremities toward the heart, stimulating sweat glands and skin circulation.

Light rhythmic activities like swimming, hula hooping, jumping rope, or jumping on a trampoline/rebounder may assist with lymphatic drainage. Special hula hoops have been designed that are more weighted to assist in abdominal area lymph stimulation. Wearing looser-fitting clothing while performing lymph-targeting rhythmic activities may promote additional lymphatic flow.

Lymphatic drainage specialists offer manual therapies, positional considerations, compression instruction, and/or light therapy machines aimed to reduce the lymphedema that can accumulate. Reflexology lymphatic drainage aims to stimulate lymphatic reflexes in the feet and may be another resource.

Mighty Mitochondria

Mitochondria are the "powerhouse" of the cell. They convert nutrients and oxygen into something called ATP. ATP powers the cell to perform all sorts of functions and is crucial for the body's ability to meet the needs of usual daily activities and athletic demands. There are several reasons why mitochondria can become dysfunctional; stress, toxins, and hormonal and nutritional deficiencies can all impact the body tremendously. Factors in the current modern lifestyle such as Wi-Fi signals and pesticides in the food supply can deplete cellular energy reserves to the point where the body is playing catch-up to try to make extra energy to remove daily toxin accumulation.

Essentially, mitochondria control all of the critical systems in the body, including detoxification, and their efficiency decreases naturally with aging. That decreased efficiency is accelerated with exposure to environmental triggers. Many believe that a thorough detoxification program should include strategies to boost mitochondrial health.

A high-fat diet that induces ketosis has become a recent trend to boost mitochondrial performance. Ketosis occurs when carbohydrates are eliminated from the diet and the body utilizes fat and protein for energy instead. There are mixed reviews in the literature about the efficacy and safety of the ketogenic diet for different health conditions.[3,4] Severe depletion of carbohydrates is not generally suggested as a long-term solution for health and can add stress to the adrenal system. Medium chain triglycerides are sometimes used to trigger ketosis-like effects on the body, but it's unclear whether this is a recommended strategy.[5]

For patients with MCAS, these types of trends should be taken with a grain of salt and on a case-by-case basis; mitochondrial boosting techniques may need to be secondary to other considerations for the entire system as a whole in patients suffering from chronic disease, particularly initially. For additional mitochondrial support, some experts recommend diets that are high in antioxidants and polyphenols, foods that boost neurotransmitters, and tips for the avoidance of toxins already discussed.[6,7] Some strategies, such as cold showers and intermittent fasting, are met with mixed reviews in the literature.[8-12]

Intermittent fasting is where one consumes the majority of daily meals within a six- to eight-hour window. Intermittent fasting appears to boost myelin, the sheath around nerves, and has been shown to reduce cytokine levels in animal research.[13] Intermittent fasting is controversial and not recommended for high-level athletes who have higher caloric intake requirements and multiple workouts per day; it *may* also be unwise in patients who already have limited diets or secondary caloric restrictions or glucose issues as the result of mast cell activation disease. While intermittent fasting may boost certain aspects of cellular function and give the gut extra time for healing, it may not be appropriate for certain types of patients, such as those who suffer from diabetes or adrenal issues.

EXERCISE AND MCAS

Histamine and tryptase levels have been shown to be elevated following exercise in patients with mastocytosis,[14] but it's unconfirmed whether the same phenomenon occurs with MCAS. Regardless, this possibility should not deter patients from considering an exercise routine. According to Afrin, "There is absolutely no question that exercise is helpful in all MCAS patients who can tolerate exercise."[15]

However, certain types of exercise may be a trigger that increases mast cell symptoms or, in severe cases, anaphylaxis for patients with pre-existing MCAD. It's important to factor in the type, quantity, intensity, and duration to find the optimal level of exercise according to each individual, while also being cognizant of the physical environment where the exercise is taking place. *And it's important to tackle this goal once the patient has achieved step one, the "stable baseline" of MCAS management.* Pushing into a new, aggressive fitness routine when anaphylactic reactions are not under control is never a good idea.

Exercise-Induced Anaphylaxis

In the literature, exercise-induced anaphylaxis (EIA) appears to be a rare but serious occurrence in the general population. Wheezing, chest tightness, nausea, diarrhea, angioedema, urticaria, and itching typically appear during or shortly after exercise in these patients, with airway compromise and circulatory collapse as potential consequences.[16] Food-dependent EIA typically occurs when food is consumed from minutes to within two hours before exercise, though cases have occurred up to six hours post-exercise.[17]

It is interesting to consider that there's a potential subgroup of patients with exercise-induced anaphylaxis who (unbeknownst to them) are reacting to something that they consumed, possibly even several hours beforehand. Wheat/gluten is a type of food more commonly associated with EIA.[18] Some research indicates that it's the presence of both factors (exercise and something ingested) that are responsible for cases of EIA, whereas the same isolated food or exercise may be tolerated independently in other scenarios.[19] Thus, careful pre-exercise dietary considerations are important for patients with MCAS; trying new foods or food sources the same day as planned exercise should be discouraged in patients with a history of anaphylactoid-type reactions.

Running, strenuous weight lifting and even a casual stroll have been reported to trigger EIA.[16,20,21] Cases do not appear to be fully repeatable or predictable—in other words, the same type of exercise does not always trigger the same response.[21] Some patients do not find relief with preventive antihistamines, and case reports support the use of medications including omalizumab and hydroxychloroquine for preventive management in patients with EIA, though more research is needed.[16,20] A 2016 review noted that some cases of EIA occur after aspirin and NSAID ingestion, so it's important to keep in mind that certain medications may also be triggers.[22]

It's absolutely crucial that patients with MCAS are clear on what symptoms constitute anaphylaxis and what symptoms necessitate immediate cessation of exercise. Patient management of EIA can be tricky. Avoidance of outdoor exercise when pollen counts are high may be helpful for some patients. Likewise, avoidance of extreme heat, cold, and humidity may be wise for patients who experience EIA[22] or exercise-associated MCAS flares.

A case report of EIA advised the patient (in subsequent sessions) to exercise with companions, carry epinephrine, and be alert for the initial signs of anaphylaxis during exercise (such as fatigue, flushing, and itching), upon which he was instructed to stop exercise immediately and lie flat on the ground in preparation for epinephrine administration.[23] However, patients with MCAS may already experience these types of symptoms at baseline (when compared to the general population) and it can be tricky to know where to draw the line in terms of symptom interpretation. As previously discussed, "riding out the storm" and waiting to administer life-saving medications is dangerous and not recommended. To best determine activity recommendations and to most accurately interpret individual symptoms during exercise, patients should always consult their medical team prior to initiating a new exercise routine.

In the grand picture of things, EIA appears to be much *less common* than other triggers. A 2017 study of 223 patients admitted to the emergency department with signs of anaphylaxis over one year reported that approximately 41% were triggered by drugs, 27% were triggered by venom, and 20% were triggered by foods.[24] A four-year Belgian study noted that approximately 46% of reactions were triggered by drugs, 3% were triggered by Hymenoptera venom, and 51% were triggered by foods.[25] Despite the variability in findings between studies (for example, whether food or drugs were the biggest factor), exercise-induced attacks were not nearly as common and were infrequently mentioned in epidemiological studies.

Exercise Considerations

In light of available information, a 2016 review on MCAS concluded that "In spite of the substantial fatigue and malaise that many MCAD patients experience, they should be strongly encouraged to exercise regularly."[26] Dr. Horowitz noted that in his multiple systemic infectious disease syndrome (MSIDS) patient population, "I have seen patients significantly improve their symptoms and recover their health once they begin to exercise."[27]

Exercise in an important tool for both physical and mental health. Dr. Hamilton notes that in his clinical experience, many patients with MCAS have post-traumatic stress disorder from bad reactions in the past and would benefit from regular exercise, meditation, and yoga.[28]

Anecdotally, some patients with MCAS find that they are intolerant to mild to intense cardiovascular exercise (such as running, cycling, and gym machines like the stair stepper, rower, and elliptical). Swimming poses additional potential challenges due to the presence of chemicals like chlorine or bromine and poor ventilation in indoor settings, although this factor does not influence every patient with MCAS. Beginning with gentler exercise like walking and body weight exercise may be a better initial approach for some patients.

Goal-setting can be especially useful for the MCAS patient. It's important to have several tiers of goals and to avoid jumping into something aggressive overnight. On the flip side, it's important to avoid putting exercise off until "tomorrow" indefinitely, as exercise may unlock tools for healing and further detoxification, improved functional mobility, and improved quality of life in this patient population. There is a difference between being "stable enough" for exercise vs. feeling that one is must reach the optimal end-goal picture of health before initiating exercise, and it's important to figure out where this line is drawn for each patient with the help of one's medical team. *Medical clearance for exercise with consideration of all comorbidities is absolutely necessary prior to initiation of a new exercise routine.*

Patients in higher risk categories (as determined by one's medical team) would benefit from initiating an exercise routine with skilled professionals, such as a cardiac rehabilitation specialist (for patients with heart comorbidities) or a physical therapist who can monitor vitals/reactions, suggest exercise types and parameters based on individual findings, and assist in goal-setting, form, and exercise progression. Patients who have POTS may have special exercise considerations due to instability in vital signs when in the upright position, and these patients should begin a program with specialist assistance and have regular measurements of heart rate and blood pressure while exercising. A heart rate monitor can be useful as the patient progresses to independent exercise. The POTS-specific Levine Protocol is sometimes requested by doctors, which involves a gradual and graded approach to introducing exercise for this patient population.

Patients with EDS and MCAS may be especially good candidates for physical therapy–assisted exercise programs that address unique considerations for joint hypermobility, tissue laxity constraints, and bracing or devices for stability when appropriate. Exercises specific to activation and coordination of the deep stabilizing muscles may be especially helpful. Patients with fibromyalgia and MCAS may benefit from analysis of postural and ergonomic factors when creating an exercise routine. Pursuing a specialist who is well-versed in EDS, MCAS, POTS, and other comorbidities and who has experience in chronic pain or fatigue may enhance the chances that the patient and provider are a good match.

Patients ought to delineate, in advance, what symptoms constitute halting exercise (and administering emergency medications) and what types of flare-ups may be acceptable during and immediately after exercise. The exercise environment (ventilation, cleaning supplies, building water damage) should be considered carefully. Patients should always avoid exercising within two hours of consuming food (or exposure to other potential triggers) to reduce the likelihood of co-reactions occurring.

The type of exercise should be flexible in terms of day-to-day variance and can start out as something very basic. For example, some patients set goals for walking to the mailbox on flare days and once around the block on good days, while others may do 45 minutes of moderate to high intensity cardio on good days, and 20 minutes of light weight-lifting or body weight exercise with less heart rate fluctuations on flare days.

There is a huge variability in fitness level and baseline exercise tolerance in patients with MCAS, and it's best to avoid making comparisons to others. The most optimal goal-setting approach involves setting personal short-term, medium-term, and long-term goals as well as "flare-day goals" that follow the "SMART" acronym: specific, measurable, attainable, realistic, and timely. Flare-day goals could involve something as simple as 10 minutes of meditation and breathing exercises. Goals that focus on *functional mobility* (like getting in and out of the car unassisted or walking two laps around the grocery store) tend to work better than goals that focus on factors like the number of pounds lost or the number of repetitions of a particular exercise.

The short-term goal may be based off something that is already occurring (but perhaps not regularly yet) so that it's not a huge leap but rather more of a confidence booster. Previous recent history with exercise tolerance can help assist in setting optimal goals. For example, if a patient knows they have symptoms at 30 minutes of walking but are fine with shorter time spans, they should adjust activity to below the symptoms threshold. In this example, a short-term goal could be one walk that lasts 20 minutes, or two 15-minute walks per day. Adding in specifics (such as where the exercise occurs, how often per week, how many minutes, light vs. moderate intensity, and the exact time frame) can be helpful.

Writing out goals and posting them somewhere in the house helps provide a nice reminder but should not serve as a source of depression on flare-up days. Patients with MCAS should also write out the flare-day goals and kind reminders for self-care and self-compassion. All goals, including short-term goals, may need to be frequently reassessed and revised.

Long-term goals should aim for the 2018 American Heart Association recommendation, which is 150 minutes of *moderate-intensity* exercise per week (the equivalent of 30 minutes x five days a week), or 75 minutes of *high-intensity* exercise per week (the equivalent of 25 minutes x three days a week) plus moderate-to-high intensity muscle strengthening at least two days per week.[29] Patients who tolerate shorter-duration bouts should be encouraged to split up their sessions in modified forms (such as more than one bout of exercise per day).

It's important to plan out exercise considerations to optimize success. Laps around an area that has benches may be smarter than an out-and-back course. Walking on a trail away from vehicles will reduce inhaled exhaust. Having a friend or family member present is strongly advised in patients who regularly experience anaphylaxis (in addition to carrying emergency medications at all times). Many running-type waist belts fit two epinephrine auto-injectors. A portable blood pressure cuff should also be readily accessible, and patients should wear some type of medical alert identification.

The goal activity should be something that is enjoyable as opposed to being a chore. Some patients like to involve their families, pets, or a buddy in their routine to make it more fun and to enhance accountability, which is a good idea as long as flare-up variability can be respected. Financial constraints or environmental sensitivities can sometimes make exercise tricky. However, there are a number of body-weight exercises that can be done in the home environment for patients who are home-bound, sensitive to pollen or extreme temperatures, or looking to save money.

Yoga/Pilates and MCAS

Yoga is generally a great option for patients with chronic illness, because it is low-impact and incorporates breathing techniques and stress reduction. Person-to-person modifications are encouraged to customize to personal needs as well as day-to-day fluctuations in symptoms. EDS-specific modifications can be made for yoga poses, and physical therapists can assist in helping to create an individualized routine. *Anecdotally*, hot yoga is generally less tolerated than traditional yoga due to the potential for extreme heat to induce mast cell degranulation.

Yoga may be especially beneficial for those suffering from allergies, headaches, and asthma.[30] One study evaluated mast cell mediator long-term response to yoga. A randomized controlled trial conducted in 2009 found that asthmatic patients who performed eight weeks of regular yoga had improvements in pulmonary function, quality of life assessments, and the usage of rescue medications.[31] However, the two-month trial showed no change in urinary prostaglandin levels following the intervention.[31]

Substantial evidence supports the many additional health benefits of yoga, including but not limited to: aiding walking tolerance, improving balance and sleep, increasing strength, lowering blood pressure, and improving cardiovascular health, health-related quality of life, and control of chronic conditions.[32] Yoga has been shown to reduce anxiety and contribute to a more balanced autonomic nervous system.[33] Some theorize that the very nature of yoga fosters more parasympathetic nervous system innervation, compared to more strenuous exercise like a triathlon that may induce an increase in sympathetic nervous system activation.[34]

For patients with irritable bowel syndrome (IBS), the activation of the sympathetic nervous system via exercise has been theorized to contribute to intestinal vasoconstriction and decreased intestinal blood flow, which can cause an increase in abdominal pain.[34] Mast cells have been linked to the pathophysiology of IBS, and mast cell mediators may contribute to abdominal pain perception and colonic hypersensitivity in patients with IBS.[34] Yoga, on the other hand, has been associated with increased intestinal blood flow and may be a more appropriate choice than strenuous exercise for patients who have both IBS and MCAS, or those who experience intestinal discomfort with exercise.[34]

Pilates has also been investigated as an exercise form for certain patient populations, including women who suffer with dysmenorrhea (painful periods). One study evaluated whether eight weeks of Pilates exercise alone or Pilates plus supplementation with caraway would impact pain levels and blood prostaglandin levels in adolescent females.[35] Both measures (pain and prostaglandins) were significantly reduced in both groups at the end of the study, suggesting that Pilates alone may provide physiological benefits.[35]

High-Intensity Interval Training

Endurance training, resistance training, and high-intensity interval training (HIIT) have all been shown to improve function on the cellular level.[36-38] HIIT involves strenuous activity with brief periods of "active rest." HIIT can take the form of different types of exercise. For runners, this could mean a track or hill workout that involves aggressive sprinting. HIIT approaches can also be created with gym exercises and many machines. Ultimately, the goal is to elevate the heart rate to near-maximal levels for certain intervals of time. This type of exercise is *not* meant to be performed every day, and typically no more than three times per week. Like any type of exercise, HIIT should be cleared with one's medical team and may not be appropriate for all patients.

A lot of the literature has focused on the use of HIIT in patients with cardiovascular disease. A 2015 meta-analysis compared moderate intensity continuous training (MICT) with HIIT.[36] The HIIT prescription that is commonly studied involves four intervals of 4 minutes of HIIT (85%-90% peak heart rate) with 3 minutes of active recovery in between bouts.[36] Most studies had patients perform HIIT three times per week for three to four months.[36] Based on seven systematic reviews, the patients in the HIIT groups had a statistically significant improvement in brachial artery flow–mediated dilation and a number of improvements in inflammation, insulin sensitivity, oxidative stress, and traditional cardiovascular risk factors when compared to the MICT groups.[36] Both HIIT and endurance training have been shown to result in improvements in VO2 max and other markers of fitness, but it appears that HIIT provides greater gains than endurance training.[37]

Research has yet to study the applicability of HIIT in populations prone to allergies or MCAD. However, one study evaluated six sessions of HIIT in an asthmatic population. They compared seven patients with asthma and seven healthy controls and found no adverse effects of HIIT; furthermore, a greater improvement in a number of measured factors including ventilation, carbon dioxide output, and time to exhaustion were noted in the group of patients who had asthma.[39]

Additional Considerations with Exercise

Histamine is the mast cell mediator most commonly studied with the human response to exercise. A 2017 study determined that histamine increases in skeletal muscle were due to both mast cell degranulation and *de novo* formulation of histamine, indicating that exercises produces an "anaphylactoid signal" that affects recovery and exercising muscle blood flow.[40] Post-exercise histamine appears to influence vasodilation of blood vessels, which has been associated with blood pressure drops and fainting or near-fainting in healthy subjects.[41]

While exercise may increase certain mast cell mediator levels, it appears that exercise-associated increases in histamine in tissues may play *less of a systemic role* than originally hypothesized. A 2017 review evaluated the mechanisms of histamine during exercise and concluded that histamine increases locally in muscle tissue, as opposed to systemically (in healthy subjects).[42] In addition, the physiological effects of histamine-related vasodilation may be most notable in the limb(s) that are being taxed; one study evaluated single-leg exercises and found that the post-exercise changes were localized to the exercising muscle groups and were not present in resting limbs.[43]

Histamine influences insulin sensitivity and glucose availability/utilization by skeletal muscle following exercise.[42] Histamine also appears to contribute to the pain and strength loss associated with Delayed Onset Muscle Soreness (DOMS).[42] However, a certain level of histamine during exercise facilitates important processes that affect everything from energy, endurance, and performance to post-exercise recovery.[42]

It's important to weigh the benefits of exercise in terms of long-term protective effects on physiological mechanisms, and not simply on an analysis of in-the-moment reactivity. While exercise is associated with short-term mast cell activation in some patients, there's also preliminary evidence in animal research that regular aerobic exercise may be a long-term protective factor for cardiac mast cell degranulation.[44]

Antihistamine Use and Exercise

Much of the research has focused on the use of antihistamines with exercise. In the post-exercise recovery window, systemic blockage of H1 and H2 receptors via medications may reduce skeletal muscle blood flow and glucose delivery, which could lead to glycogen depletion, increased potential for muscle tissue damage, and reduced exercise performance.[45] A 2017 review noted that blocking histamine receptors may reduce the body's ability to mediate inflammatory responses and the migration of immune system cells to damaged muscle tissue in post-exercise recovery.[42]

Despite potential tissue-level side effects of antihistamine use, these medications may attenuate the DOMS-type pain response and may assist in certain athletic scenarios. In one study, H1 and H2 receptor antagonists were associated with reduced pain scores 24 hours following intense downhill running exercise.[46] Animal studies support that antihistamines may have a more profound effect on longer endurance activities (greater than 2 hours).[42] The 2017 review noted that "blocking the action of histamine may be beneficial during longer-duration athletic performances (e.g., marathon), multi-event, or multi-day athletic events, when development of muscle soreness and the concurrent loss of muscle strength may otherwise impair athletic performance."[42]

Histamine has been shown to be responsible for drops in blood pressure up to 90 minutes post-exercise, and H1/H2 receptor antagonists (540 mg fexofenadine and 300 mg ranitidine) prevented the majority of these effects in both sedentary and endurance-trained subjects in a 2013 study.[47] Additional research compared head-up tilt test blood pressure readings in subjects with and without antihistamine (540 mg fexofenadine) use. The subjects were healthy participants who were prone to post-exercise syncope. Following moderate-intensity exercise in the heat, subjects who had premedication with antihistamines had no change in blood pressure, compared to drops in blood pressure observed in the control group.[48] The results of both studies[47,48] may have implications for patients with MCAS who experience potentially disabling fainting or near-fainting due to blood pressure drops from the vasodilatory effects of histamine following exercise.

In summary, while blood flow, muscle recovery, and energy factors may be generally negatively impacted by antihistamines, delayed-onset pain factors and excess hypotension following exercise may be improved with their use. *Anecdotally*, some patients find better results when timing their exercise within a certain window of taking their MCAS medications. None of the research evaluated the impacts of mast cells/their mediators and antihistamines for exercise *in the MCAD population*, so there are some obvious limitations to interpreting the available research as instructive for exercise management with these patients.

Breathing Exercises

Breathing exercises are important for patients with chronic illness and may be a useful routine adjunct for patients suffering with MCAS. Slow, deep breathing has been shown to increase parasympathetic nervous system function.[49] Breathing techniques, meditation, and relaxation exercises have been shown to reduce stress, negative emotions, and sympathetic dominance of the autonomic nervous system.[50] Regular practice of such techniques also appear to be effective in reducing symptom severity in patients suffering from Post-Traumatic Stress Disorder (PTSD).[51]

Most humans are shallow breathers, and it's important to periodically practice deeper breathing that stimulates the "rest and digest" functions of the autonomic nervous system and actively engages the lower muscles like the diaphragm instead of the "accessory muscles" of the neck and chest. Many physical therapists teach breathing exercises to patients who suffer from spine pain, rib issues, poor control of the muscles that control urination, chronic pain, anxiety, and many other conditions.

An example of a basic breathing exercise is "belly breathing" where inhalation occurs using the diaphragm muscle (belly bulges outward and lower ribs expand) for 3 seconds, the breath is held for 3 seconds, and then exhaled for 3 seconds. This type of breathing should be repeated for a few minutes. It's helpful to place one hand over the upper ribs/chest and one hand on the belly right below the ribcage to ensure that more of the motion is initiated from the abdomen (diaphragm) and not the neck/chest muscles. This exercise can easily be incorporated into the daily routine, for example, when starting the car, sitting at stoplights, during daily hygiene practices like flossing teeth or drying hair, or while lying face-up before bedtime.

Other types of exercises and treatments may assist in decreasing sympathetic nervous system tone. Home biofeedback monitors and apps that provide guided assistance with controlling heart rate and breathing may be of benefit. Gargling, gagging, and singing exercises may be prescribed to improve vagus nerve tone. Transcutaneous vagus nerve electrical stimulation is becoming increasingly popular. There are a number of additional web-based and book resources that provide tools for breathing and other exercises to enhance parasympathetic nervous system tone.

NEUROPSYCHOLOGICAL TREATMENT APPROACHES

Mental health resources are a huge priority for the patient newly diagnosed with a chronic condition. MCAS experts note that "Since both physical and psychological stress have long been known to activate MCs (mast cells), interventions aimed at stress reduction (e.g., psychotherapy) can be helpful."[26]

Clinically, it appears that some MCAS specialists encourage patients to address the psychological factors that can influence healing. Many people think of psychological trauma in the past as a potential trigger for the disease, but it can also work the other way around where patients with MCAS may experience trauma from emergency room visits or life-threatening allergic reactions associated with their disease after they've been diagnosed.

Establishing regular psychotherapy sessions is strongly encouraged for the newly diagnosed MCAS patient to assist in processing what one is going through, and therapy may also be a useful tool for long-term disease management. Letting go of past trauma and frustrations that inevitably surface with chronic, invisible illness can be empowering, and mental health specialists also offer great tools for stress reduction and trigger elimination. Don't let cost be a factor here—there are many nonprofits that provide counseling options and financial assistance.

In "Through the Shadowlands: A Science Writer's Odyssey into an Illness Science Doesn't Understand," Julie Rehmeyer described her experience with healing sessions that addressed past traumas that were theorized to be associated with sensitivities and allergens. Specifically, she worked with someone who believed that past trauma experienced in the presence of mold led to a mind-body association between mold and trauma.[52]

This is an interesting theory, especially in light of the patient with MCAS who may be reactive to dozens or even hundreds of triggers. Indeed, many patients with MCAS note that their baseline of symptoms worsened dramatically when they were re-exposed to a moldy environment later in life, and likewise many report a large relief of symptoms when moldy environments and belongings are eliminated. Mold is just one example, and perhaps the more prominent/devastating environmental triggers ought to be addressed with this approach on an individualized basis.

Some practitioners utilize a cognitive behavioral therapy approach that combines psychotherapy with nervous system stimulation. Other treatments can include physical contact with allergens in efforts to "rewire the brain." Dr. Tony Smith pioneered a technique called AllerTouch, which is an allergy desensitization program that involves manual stimulation of brain-related treatment points as an offending allergen is in contact with the body.[53] Dr. Smith later went on to create CranioBiotic Technique, which not only addresses allergies but also targets infections and chronic illnesses through brain stimulation and simultaneous stimulation of organ and infection points on the body.[53]

Similarly, Neuromodulation Technique (NT) is an approach that is sometimes used with patients who suffer from allergies, autoimmune conditions, bacterial and viral issues, gastrointestinal problems, and more.[54] Neuromodulation Technique combines autonomic nervous system muscle testing with corrective commands or statements, spinal or cranial nerve stimulation, and breathing techniques.[54]

Sound healing has been used since the times of ancient medicine and may also be of some benefit. In theory, certain sound frequencies are believed to help rewire the brain and connect the right and left hemispheres for healing of anxiety and depression that may stem from a history of trauma. The use of tuning forks, chanting, bowls, humming, and binaural beats are examples of techniques offered by practitioners for sound healing.

A number of additional neuropsychological treatments are available that may offer assistance with chronic disease. All patients are unique and respond differently to these types of approaches.

Regardless of what approach is taken, addressing psychological aspects of chronic disease should be at the top of the priority list for patients with MCAS. *In theory*, the combination of psychotherapy and other therapies that target autonomic nervous system regulation or allergen desensitization may offer an added benefit for patients who have both MCAS and POTS or other comorbidities, *though research has yet to address this area.*

STRATEGIES FOR EMOTIONAL HEALING

Mindset

When it comes to chronic illness, it's important to remember that "you can't ride a bike going backward" (author unknown). Too great of a focus on past wounds—on diagnoses and labels and symptom clusters, for example—can certainly be detrimental, but most patients are already so deeply embedded in the chronicity of their issues and their typically long-standing quest for answers (especially by the time they receive a diagnosis that best describes everything) that it seems impossible to *not* dwell on it.

That being said, progress is best facilitated when the patient is ready to let go of the past and move forward with a positive mindset for healing. Letting go of people who have wronged the patient in the past (including those in the medical system), releasing regrets pertaining to one's own actions, and ditching identities wrapped up in diagnostic labels are all key to getting back on that bicycle with forward momentum.

One helpful approach is to reframe the situation. Many websites depict mast cells in a negative manner in light of MCAS. Instead of thinking of the mast cell as an evil entity that is aggressively going into attack mode, it's important to have compassion and gratitude for its incredibly complex set of properties and functions. *MCAS reflects an intelligent immune system that is crying out for help, signaling an alarm system, and trying to get the body back to homeostasis.*

When mast cells flag the system to a buildup of underlying factors and toxicities that are detrimental to one's health, the patient can identify root issues and foster changes that, thanks to the sensitivity of the mast cell, should provide somewhat clear responses as to whether the change is effective over time.

Mast cells are like a home security system, but if the focus is solely on symptoms (or is too negatively embedded into the role of mast cells), the patient will likely remain stuck in a vicious cycle of surviving and reacting to crises (rather than thriving). Therefore, optimal management of MCAS goes far beyond medication management and far beyond the mast cell itself. Lifestyle changes needed to reduce inflammation/underlying root issues and promote healing should be continued for the long-term time frame; it's important that the patient is aware of this and is mentally prepared for the challenges and changes that are necessary to reap healing rewards.

There are a number of tools that can help keep a positive mindset while dealing with chronic illness. Journaling can be a powerful everyday resource, and it should be separate from a symptom log, which can be useful initially in identifying triggers but should not become all-consuming. Progress with MCAS often occurs in tiny steps, and journaling enables the patient to see the growth and the highs and lows over time in ways beyond a list of symptoms.

When practicing a mindset shift, it's important to have a dual mentality that involves aspects of both working hard and surrendering. Make sure that the focus of MCAS management is not on palliative care of putting Band-Aids on symptoms but, rather, on efforts for active rehabilitation of the root issues. On the same note, it's also helpful to acknowledge and accept the things out of one's control.

Practicing gratitude or finding ways to get involved in a community outside of the illness or to serve others in some way can be very helpful. "MCAS does not define me" is a phrase that can serve as a helpful reminder of the other aspects of life that are worth fighting for. And to take it a step further, the mindset that "this disease will open doors to new opportunities" can be even more powerful.

Dr. Sharon Meglathery offers some wonderful suggestions for patients suffering with chronic illness in her section of "The Driscoll Theory Newly Revised: The Cause of POTS in Ehlers-Danlos Syndrome and How to Reverse the Process."[55] She encourages patients to watch their thoughts and be aware of negative mindset patterns before they turn into a perseverated pattern.[55] "Practice watching your thoughts, without judgment. Study them like a

446

scientist."[55] The key, according to Meglathery, is becoming aware of emotions without becoming ruled by them.[55]

Meglathery recommends that patients utilize "state changing" techniques when they find themselves in a funk.[55] Music, creative projects, and visualization can help in moments where a negative mindset wants to take over.[55] She also recommends ground techniques, deep breathing and focusing on rational tasks as opposed to emotions for such scenarios.[55]

According to Meglathery, "Compassion for self is about making good self-care choices to nurture our sick bodies, while recognizing that it is now a reality that we rarely feel vigorous and a lot of the time, we feel terrible, despite good self-care. We need to make allowances for ourselves: allowing ourselves adequate rest, stress avoidance, asking for help when we need it. Just like it is a good idea not to judge our thoughts, emotions or other people to save energy, we should avoid judging ourselves."[55]

That balance is so important; it's essential to allow oneself the rest and self-care that is needed without being too hard on oneself. It's also important to remember that chronic disease does not equate to giving up on one's goals or passions, but it may mean rearranging one's life or time frame to make them possible. Meglathery says it best: "You can make good choices for yourself rooted in self-compassion and compassion for others. You can choose your battles and conserve your energy for the goals you can achieve."[55]

At the same time, painful decisions to change relationships or daily practices (or both) may be a necessary part of the process. In terms of cutting out aspects that may hinder healing, Meglathery writes that "...if the toxicity is clear, you must gather your spoons, cut your losses and sever your emotional ties. This goes for jobs, family members, healers and even foods."[55]

MCAS and other chronic diseases can be very hard on loved ones, who often feel helpless and can also grow frustrated with daily limitations, inconveniences, and stressors. Early on, family members may experience something called "research fatigue," which can also morph into sadness, grief, and "compassion fatigue." Solid communication is absolutely crucial in relationships between the patient with MCAS and loved ones. Mental health resources may also be important for family members and significant others.

Specific Exercises for Emotional Healing

Below are some tools that may assist the patient in emotional healing. Repression of emotions is discouraged as it may contribute to physical imbalances and stress, and it's important that the patient has some sort of outlets for the emotional struggles that, in some seasons, can occur on a daily basis.

These suggestions are experience-based and do not reflect professional medical advice; ultimately, patients with chronic illness ought to consider the utility of a mental health specialist.

1.   Self-Care Exercise

One of the important first steps in fostering healing is determining what adequate self-care looks like for the patient. The goal here is to very clearly write out what needs to happen on a daily basis for self-care, with the end goal of *thriving* (and not just surviving). The key to successful self-care is giving oneself permission to put oneself first. Not only is it possible to have good self-care as a parent or partner, but prioritizing self-care often carries over into better relationships with family and friends. When making the list, be specific about how much time would be ideal for each aspect and don't hold back from creating an ideal, perfect-scenario wish list.

Here's an example of a list of what a daily self-care list could look like:

- Adequate sleep (7-8 hours)
- Time to make juice every morning (10 mins.)
- Yoga class or time for walking or exercise (30-60 mins.)
- Daily sunshine, grounding, breathing exercises, and meditation (20 mins.)
- Quiet space to practice musical instrument (30 mins.)
- Food prep in the evening for the following day (30 mins.)
- Time for journaling, prayer, or reading before bed (15 mins.)

Some items may more realistically occur on a weekly or monthly basis, like:

- Epsom-salt baths
- Massage
- Time to chat with certain friends or family on the phone
- Acupuncture
- Coffee date with a friend
- Counseling session
- Getting outside for a hike
- Church group commitment

- Hobbies or passions: book club, photography, painting, etc.

For most people, on paper, the list may look unrealistic compared to the typical daily routine, particularly if caring for children, considering a demanding work or doctor visit schedule, or factoring in the levels of fatigue often experienced throughout the day. The next step is to determine which are the biggest "no-compromise" aspects and to make sure that these are consistently happening. (For example, most people rank sleep pretty high up there.)

Once the main priorities are identified and already in practice, the next step is to consider asking someone for help so that the other self-care components can be attained more easily. Working out a schedule so that a spouse or friend can share some cooking or childcare duties can free up time for exercise or meditation, for example, even if just a few times a week. Involving children in exercise routines or cooking may be another option for some people. Arranging for a babysitter once a week may free up time for meal prep, counseling, or a massage.

Working out some sort of bartering or exchange system may reduce financial stress. (For example, some parents have a rotating schedule where they watch the neighbors' kids for a few hours and the neighbors repeat the favor, freeing up time for both families.) Obviously, financial constraints and physical limitations can influence many of these decisions, but for some patients, adding in the cost of a babysitter or massage may provide long-term cost saving in terms of other health expenses. It's crucial to consider self-care an important *long-term investment*.

Lastly, take time to examine the current daily routine to see if there are certain activities that are overriding time for self-care. Perhaps that TV show can be watched while exercising or cooking, or perhaps 15 minutes of internet time can be replaced with journaling or meditation. Perhaps the phone call can occur while walking. Fast-paced Westernized cultures do not naturally offer a lot of down time, so self-care must be prioritized and facilitated as best as possible. Even five minutes per day is better than nothing!

With the realities of often-unpredictable flare-ups in symptoms, it's easy to get thrown off any sort of routine and to feel in constant survival mode. But the commitment to more regular time in the day that brings the nervous system into parasympathetic (rest and digest) dominance means it's less likely the patient will be stuck in a chronic cycle of stress and inflammation that negatively influences mast cells (and beyond). By clearly defining what optimal self-care looks like, the patient can identify a priority ranking of a) what needs to happen *no matter what* and b) what should be worked toward over time.

2. Boundary-Setting Exercise

Boundaries may need to be set in relationships in order to foster emotional healing. Boundaries serve as guidelines for what are reasonable ways for others to act and what are expected responses when the guidelines are not respected. Boundaries need to be communicated clearly; however, certain (physically or emotionally abusive) scenarios should *most certainly* be guided by the help of a professional.

Below are some important factors when evaluating whether boundaries need to be set or adjusted:

- What does the patient need for healing? What aspects of self-care and time constraints exist? What are things that need to be avoided? *Write out what is desired/required for healing.*

- What are the patient's core values, ethics, and morals? *Write out a list of the top five for each.* These should reflect what the patient feels is most true to them, not expectations placed on them by others.

- What barriers currently exist that may be untrue to the core values, ethics, and morals? *Write out areas where there is a conflict between theoretical values/ethics/morals and what is actually occurring.* Determine whether barriers are in place that prevent the patient from pursuing what is desired/required for healing.

- Once conflict areas have been determined, *create an action plan that has a solution for each area in terms of boundaries that can respect one's values/ethics/morals.*

- *Clearly and respectfully communicate the new boundaries with that person.* Make sure to include guidelines for what will happen if they are not willing to respect those needs and boundaries.

In some cases, patients may need to set up boundaries with themselves first. For example, Katie always experiences allergic reactions and flare-ups when she visits her brother's family for dinner because they forget about or are unwilling to accommodate her allergies and food sensitivities. Katie doesn't want to be a burden or to annoy them, so she prepares with extra mast cell medications and suffers through it. In this scenario, Katie needs to make changes within herself either 1) to better communicate her needs with her brother's family in terms of meals, or 2) to bring her own separate food for dinner. Often, more than one solution can be arranged, presuming it's communicated respectfully to everyone involved.

Another common example in the MCAS community is the scenario of patients who are odor- or chemical-sensitive. When family members or friends do not respect one's needs for a fragrance and perfume-free environment at planned events or get-togethers, boundaries need to be clearly communicated. For example, "I realize that it's easy to forget not to wear perfume or use certain products in the house when we spend time together. These types of triggers are really detrimental to my health and I must avoid them. I would really appreciate it if you could completely eliminate these triggers when we meet up or when I come over. If you're unable to do that, we will have to stop spending time together. This is not what I want, so hopefully we can work together to come up with a solution."

If boundaries are clearly and respectfully communicated and are still trampled all over, it may be an indicator of a toxic relationship that needs to be reassessed and potentially eliminated. Keep in mind that the way someone treats another person is *a reflection on them* and not on the person who is being mistreated. Chances are, that person will not change, but the patient may be able to change the way that they react to the situation and/or the way that they construct boundaries with that person.

3. Letter Exercise

It can be helpful to write out on paper the expression of emotions and frustrations with certain relationships, particularly if things that have happened in the past keep resurfacing with negative emotions. Writing a letter of exactly what could be said to that person can be very therapeutic, even if it's not sent to that person. Some patients find it helpful to do something symbolic to release the emotions (like burning the letter or visualizing releasing certain emotions in other ways).

2. Mindfulness Exercises

Certain strategies can help the patient to stay more present in the moment and avoid perseverating on negative emotions or experiences. When reactions, flares, or emotional stress are occurring, encourage experimentation with the following types of exercises (which, of course, should be preceded by appropriate care of physical symptoms):

- Find an object in the environment and mentally describe its appearance (color, texture, size, etc.) to help bring oneself back into the present moment.

- Write out frustrations in a journal or even as a note in the cell phone. Close the journal or consider deleting the note with a focus on release of frustrations and resetting oneself back in the present moment.

- Listen to short mindfulness meditation recordings or podcasts during the day.

- When frustrations arise, pause and take a series of deep belly breaths. On the inhale, think of characteristics that are desirable and life-giving (like peace, joy, love, healing) and envision those qualities increasing in the body. On the exhale, release the negative/frustrating emotions that are unhealthy in yourself or others (such as negativity, perfectionism, selfishness, ignorance, anger, etc.).

- Slow, rhythmic self-soothing tactics may help ease the system back into a parasympathetic state. Light movement of a hand over the arm or the slow repetitive making of a fist are some examples.

- Mantras can be useful inner self-talk methods to reduce negativity and stress and to change the mindset through repetitive brain retraining. They can be simple short phrases like "baby steps," "joy regardless of circumstances," "I am loved," or "cultivate calm." The easiest way to create personalized mantras is to make a list of thoughts that are "lies" repeated in one's head, such as "I will always feel terrible" and to then replace it with the opposite statement, like "this, too, shall pass." Every time the negative thought pops into the mind, it should be immediately replaced with its counterstatement. While it can seem daunting, over time this technique can truly make a difference on a healing mindset.

- A positivity board, gratitude wall or other artistic expressions with mantras or favorite quotations placed around the living space can serve as timely reminders for a mindset shift.

3. Outreach Exercise

This section is ordered last for a reason: *Self-care and achieving a stable baseline must be the initial priority*, even if it means de-committing to previously enjoyed activities or devoting less time to keeping up with friends. While life should be all about *who you are* and not *what you're doing*, there is certainly some therapeutic value to shifting one's perspective externally to the joy that comes from compassion toward others.

One of the most powerful ways to shift one's mindset away from a focus on one's situation is to actively engage in some sort of outreach to others. Some people find that regular volunteer work or community involvement can be great tools for this. However, many patients with MCAS may not find themselves physically able to make such commitments, especially early on in treatment. There are many other ways to reach out to others and to shift the focus externally, even if just for a few minutes at a time.

For this exercise, patients make a list of people and/or causes that are important to them. Determine what would be a realistic goal in terms of making efforts to reach out to another person or organization or to advocate for that particular cause. For example, "Every Sunday I will call one friend that I haven't spoken with in a long time" or "Every fall a local nonprofit puts on a 5K run. I will help them with marketing or logistics from home in the months prior to the event." Ultimately, this exercise should *not* add to the general stress level or feel like a burden but should serve as a source of joy and a sense of connectedness.

Joy vs. Happiness

In a culture that is fixated on the concept of happiness, it's easy to get derailed from mindsets that promote healing. But happiness is fleeting and circumstance-dependent. The pursuit of true, deep joy may be a better approach, particularly for patients with chronic illness. True joy ought to be cultivated in a manner that is *independent* of external factors and circumstances.

In "The Book of Joy: Lasting Happiness in a Changing World," Douglas Abrams described the interactions and dialogue between Archbishop Desmond Tutu and His Holiness the Dalai Lama, two men regarded as some of the world's wisest leaders.[56] The book is an excellent reference for perspectives on suffering and psychological healing.

True joy does not equate to less suffering but rather to a changed perspective on it.[56] According to Archbishop Tutu, "as we discover more joy, we can face suffering in a way that ennobles rather than embitters. We have hardship without becoming hard. We have heartbreak without becoming heartbroken."[56]

This is extremely difficult for the patient who is living moment to moment and with sometimes life-threatening symptoms, but it is possible. Even if daily (or monthly) social interactions are limited to emergency room or clinic staff, one can still strive to be the best version of oneself in difficult circumstances.

According to Abrams, in observation of the dialogue between His Holiness the Dalai Lama and Archbishop Tutu, "Suffering is inevitable, they said, but how we respond to that suffering is our choice. Not even oppression or occupation can take away this freedom to choose our response."[56] Abrams noted that the path to joy may lead right through suffering, and that the depth of suffering can contribute to the altitude of joy.[56]

Human interaction and connection form a foundation of joy, and that is what makes the isolation that can come along with MCAS so difficult. However, suffering can lead to increased compassion and connection with others in its own way. The reality is that many people are invisibly suffering and fighting their own battles, so the patient is never truly alone in this sentiment.

Not only is focusing on others helpful, but one's perspective on MCAS could be further changed by focusing on how to turn around and use the cards one's been dealt for something bigger. According to Archbishop Tutu, "The question is not, how do I escape? It is: How can I use this as something positive?"[56]

ADDITIONAL AT-HOME PRACTICES FOR HEALING
Meditation

It appears that as few as 5 minutes of meditation per day may improve stress levels.[57] Stress has been shown to activate heart mast cells, which can lead to cardiac events.[58] In theory, reduction of stress may reduce systemic levels of mast cell activation and prevent other health complications.

A 2014 meta-analysis of 47 studies determined that mindfulness meditation programs have moderate evidence of improvements in depression, pain, and anxiety.[59] Mindfulness training has been shown to be effective in patients with irritable bowel syndrome;[60] such progress with irritable bowel syndrome may be attributed to reduced stress levels, which decreases the likelihood of detrimental chronic inflammatory impacts on the gut barrier.[61]

There are a large number of great web-based and app-based programs that offer guided meditation programs of varying length and style. For gear junkies, EEG devices worn on the head (such as Muse) aim to provide feedback on what's going on in the brain, offering a novel approach to meditation.

Grounding

"Grounding" or "earthing" refers to direct physical contact through bare hands or feet with the earth's surface. Barefoot walking has been touted as a key to health for centuries. One theory for the beneficial impacts of this phenomenon has to do with the ground's electrically conductive free electrons that enter the human body through direct contact with the skin.

According to Oschman and colleagues, "Through this mechanism, every part of the body can equilibrate with the electrical potential of the earth, thereby stabilizing the electrical environment of all organs, tissues, cells and molecules, and providing a key ingredient needed for the operation of the immune system."[62]

This ties back to the studied effects of electromagnetic fields (EMFs) that were previously discussed. Direct earth contact has been suggested as a therapeutic antidote for people who are exposed to high levels of EMFs (such as following airplane travel or long periods of occupational exposure). Grounding may be a way for the body to recalibrate after exposure to the harmful effects of EMFs. Barefoot yoga on the earth's surface may be a way to enjoy the benefits of grounding and combine it with breathing techniques and exercise.

A 2015 publication connected increases in barefoot grounding with improvements in diabetes, osteoporosis, blood glucose regulation, sleep quality, pain, inflammation, cardiovascular function, aging, and cortisol levels.[62] In theory, daily grounding practices may be a beneficial consideration for healing in patients with MCAS who live in appropriate climates.

Binaural Beats

Binaural beats are a type of sound therapy that can be accessed using headphones and an internet connection. Two pitches of sounds are utilized that are different in each ear; these are close in pitch but are not quite identical. This fosters a brain-level interference that is akin to the brain waves that occur during certain states like meditation. Different frequencies are available that target different goals like relief of anxiety, reduction in depression, improved memory/concentration, or enhanced relaxation and sleeping.

Research has noted attention improvements in as little as three minutes of binaural beats exposure at certain frequencies, as well as reduced depression and improvements in heart rate variability and blood pressure in older adults who listened to 30 minutes of alpha binaural beats for five consecutive days.[63,64] The sounds have also been shown to significantly reduce preoperative dental anxiety.[65] It's plausible that regular use of binaural beats may assist patients with chronic illness, including patients who have MCAS.

Other Strategies to Restore Parasympathetic Nervous System Dominance

Eye Movement Desensitization and Reprocessing (EMDR) is a therapeutic technique used to alleviate the distress associated with traumatic injuries, and it may be beneficial for certain patients with MCAS.

Tension and Trauma Releasing Exercises (TRE) is a type of therapy that activates a natural shaking reflex that releases muscular trauma and subsequently calms the sympathetic nervous system of the impacts of repressed emotions and PTSD.

Treatments such as the Dynamic Neural Retraining System (DNRS) aim to rewire the limbic system to reduce the chronic stress response. Callahan Techniques thought field therapy (TFT) and the Emotional Freedom Technique (EFT) are examples of treatments that involve tapping. EFT focuses on acupressure meridians, and TFT focuses on sequential tapping as a code to balance the body's energy system.

Aromatherapy

Aromatherapy and the use of essential oils is gaining popularity and *may* be of assistance for some patients with MCAS, depending on odor reactivity. Special care should be taken in this area to procure products that are pure and not distilled with additives or exposed to pesticides or other chemicals. Each source ought to be considered carefully as oils can influence other medications and supplements.

SPIRITUALITY

Spirituality is a dimension of the human experience that looks different for each individual. For some, spirituality is accompanied by organized religion. For many, faith experiences know no physical boundaries.

Scientific research has attempted to uncover more information about spiritual healing—for example, the healing power of prayer.[66] While it's a difficult area to "research" and there are conflicting opinions on both ends of the spectrum, for many, spirituality cannot be adequately explained by science or quantified.

Forgiveness

Many public figures and speakers have described *unforgiveness* as a toxic poison that we drink in the hopes of hurting others. Often, the things that a person holds on to are most damaging to themselves. Regardless of one's religious perspective, many cultures and communities (and resources like Alcoholics Anonymous) incorporate forgiveness into the approach for physical and/or mental healing.

In order to foster deep emotional healing, forgiveness of self and others is a key foundation. Release of past hurts and wounds may have a benefit in assisting the body to release physical manifestations of toxins and disease. In some cases, a lifespan assessment of emotional baggage is followed by conversations with people who either 1) wronged the patient or 2) the patient wronged. This can be an especially powerful application of forgiveness. Some scenarios render a face-to-face conversation unsafe or impossible; journaling and prayer can also assist in this process. Exercises that involve the physical releasing of unforgiveness (such as letting balloons go or burying paper with words) offer another symbolic and unique way to express emotional release more literally.

Gratitude

Many patients with chronic illness find that daily gratitude practices assist in staying present in the moment and shifting the mindset to a more positive place. Some patients create a gratitude jar, while others may journal or formulate a form of prayer that expresses gratitude each day. Expressing gratitude for the supportive people in one's life can be especially important throughout all phases of healing.

Worship, Prayer, and Community

Worship in the form of music or organized gatherings, group and individual prayer, and community activities may be very beneficial for the patient suffering with chronic illness. In this digital age, there are many options for patients who are homebound. Podcasts, websites, books, and apps can help bring faith and spirituality resources into the home. Incorporating quiet time into one's daily routine for prayer and/or meditation can be challenging at first, but *anecdotally* many patients find that these practices serve as pillars for their individualized healing plan.

Spiritual Healers and Retreats

Some patients are open to visiting healers who may pray over them or include structured spiritual healing sessions. Holistic retreats that involve a period of isolation in nature or in other spiritual environments may provide resources for patients wanting to jumpstart the healing process with a more structured mind–body focus.

FINANCIAL AND ACCESSIBILITY CONSIDERATIONS

Some patients with MCAS are unable to work, while others may manage to maintain a regular job, a part-time job, or a work-from-home position, depending on the types of symptoms and the present "baseline" of stability.

Handicapped placards and accommodation cards may benefit this patient population, depending on the circumstances. Many patients with MCAS use support animals, particularly those who suffer from reactions that may cause intolerance to standing, loss of consciousness, anaphylaxis, or seizures.

In the United States, disability paperwork processes and decisions are difficult for this patient population, as the diagnosis is far from widely accepted and it can be difficult to "prove" a chronic debilitating (often invisible) illness such as MCAS, even though patients tend to be easily triggered by factors in the workplace that are outside of their control.

There are some *anecdotal* tips that can assist with applying for Social Security Disability Insurance (SSDI) and Supplemental Security Income (SSI). In answering questions in paperwork, adding written notes can help clarify details. For example, notes about the need for assistive devices (like a shower chair and handrail) or the need to rest for x amount of minutes after daily living tasks can accompany questions about personal hygiene abilities. The more a patient can paint a picture (instead of giving simple yes and no answers), the better someone will understand the reality of what ones' daily routine entails.

Patients with MCAS may want to include other comorbidities (as opposed to just MCAS alone) when applying for SSDI/SSI. Some doctors are unwilling to be involved with the paperwork or may have a personal bias against it. Others may be very helpful but should not be expected to remember all of one's medical details or to be aware of test results from other specialties. It may be helpful to draft up a sample document and a short, one-page summary of important (abnormal) tests, medical signs, and other findings that attest to abilities included on the Residual Functional Capacity Form. (Longer patient files like a huge binder of information can be overwhelming and may not be read in its entirety by doctors or individuals involved in the decision process.) Calling in advance to arrange a time to meet to focus on paperwork may facilitate a more thorough assessment with each doctor. An assortment of past and present medical specialists may assist in painting a picture of the chronicity and breadth of the disease.

Thorough documentation of symptoms, procedures, therapies, and hospital trips may also be useful. Photographic documentation may assist cases where patients experience physical symptoms during attacks. Some patients also recommend including information on published emergency room protocols and professional overviews of the disease to facilitate better understanding. The amount of paperwork can be overwhelming, and requests for additional time to meet deadlines may be arranged, if needed. Organizations such as the Job Accommodation Network for patients with disabilities may provide additional resources. There are also a number of informational websites and blogs that address questions about the process.

Certain nonprofit organizations may assist with medical visits and travel costs. Unfortunately, if the patient with suspected MCAS wants to see a well-known specialist, it typically entails out-of-state travel and out-of-pocket costs.

COMMUNITY-BASED RESOURCES

Online support (such as social media like Twitter or Facebook groups) can be a double-edged sword. There are many reliable pages and groups that offer accurate information, but one may also encounter fellow patients doling out inappropriate advice, venting negativity, or wrapping up their entire identity in the disease. It's helpful to connect with others who have the condition in order to feel better understood and less isolated, but it's unhealthy to revolve one's entire social world around it. A certain level of balance is warranted for all patients in this regard.

According to Meglathery, not everyone in social support is emotionally healthy.[55] It's possible to encounter angry, invalidated, aggressive, and narcissistic individuals in online support groups.[55] Meglathery offers the following advice: "Remember a saying we use in the mental health field, 'hurt people hurt people.' Remember that some of this online drama is unregulated misplaced aggression: don't let it invalidate you."[55]

In-person support groups are harder to find, though they do exist. Online support groups that occur via skype or other group-chatting platforms offer a nice alternative for many patients who are homebound or extra sensitive to new environments.

Some patients opt to write blogs, share their story with local media, organize walks and fundraisers, or get involved in other forms of advocacy and awareness. This can be another

459

useful tool for self-empowerment with MCAS. There are also periodic research studies and surveys that seek patients who have the diagnosis of MCAS, if one wishes to contribute in that manner.

Get connected to others for inspiration. There are many leaders in the MCAS community who have provided useful Facebook groups, blogs, and advocacy projects for certain topics. For example, Twilah Hiari is a patient who has created a fantastic blog resource that discusses the connection between autism spectrum disorders and MCAS.[67] Some patients openly share their journeys of troubleshooting through trials such as continual hospitalization or repeated anaphylaxis. Others have passed and have left a legacy, like Super T's Mast Cell Foundation, which honors Taylor Nearen's story and wishes for great unity, awareness, and resources for the MCAS community.[68] Healthy forms of inspiration are out there!

CHAPTER KEY POINTS

- The newly diagnosed patient can ease anxiety by preparing in advance for potential MCAS-related scenarios, such as how to handle emergency reactions and how to adapt to travel.

- Attention to mental health (facilitated with a professional) is a very important consideration for the patient newly diagnosed with MCAS, as well as for long-term chronic illness management.

- Widespread trigger elimination is an essential key to facilitate a stable baseline.

- Exercise is encouraged for patients with MCAS and should be part of a customized individual plan as determined by one's medical team.

- Attention to detoxification strategies, mitochondrial health, grounding and EMF-reduction, sleep hygiene, alternative therapies, healthy relationships, breathing exercises, mindset strategies, community resources, spirituality and prayer, and meditation techniques may be beneficial aspects of holistic management of MCAS.

- While the process can be lengthy and daunting, some patients with MCAS can qualify for disability, service animals, and handicapped-accessible accommodations as appropriate.

OVERALL CONCLUSIONS

Some say that living with a chronic debilitating illness rivals or even surpasses the weight of carrying the diagnosis of a serious acute medical condition. However, mainstream medical diagnoses tend to be acknowledged and socially accepted in our culture and often bring a flood of support and resources from both peers and organizations. Life with chronic (and often invisible) illness has a lot of similar challenges, but without a concrete remission status in sight and with a history that commonly reflects decades of disability and searching for answers. Patients with chronic conditions often lack the mental validation, support networks, employer understanding, or insurance coverage that the "mainstream" diagnoses are generally afforded.

The MCAS patient community is not universally supported by the system and must fight for many basic rights and overcome negative experiences where the system scoffs at symptoms or insinuates that the problem is mental. It's not an easy road to travel, and hopelessness and despair can be widespread. Socioeconomic stressors can weigh very heavily on patients living with MCAS. Many people with chronic illness lack ample support in their lives, and instead encounter great opposition and strife from loved ones and/or live in extreme isolation.

This reality has inspired me to take action for patient advocacy and support resources. Through the website "Mast Cells United" (www.mastcellsunited.com) I've attempted to provide useful MCAS-specific information for patients, families, and medical practitioners. The goal is to provide information about a holistic approach to wellness—a *united* effort, as opposed to efforts that villainize mast cells or focus on solely targeting mast cells without adequate attention to underlying root factors.

However, there are a number of helpful websites that already exist, so the bigger purpose of the site is to direct patients to helpful community-based resources. This dream includes a project to connect patients on a personal level with MCAS buddies in their geographical area as well as to create larger support groups in areas where other organizations lack a physical presence. I also hope to continue speaking and educating fellow physical therapists about MCAS, and am developing a novel model of care that I hope will reframe certain aspects of physical therapy clinical practice for the chronically ill patient.

As I've researched this book, I can't help but wonder whether MCAS is simply a label on top of a bunch of other labels. Inappropriate mast cell activation may explain labels like fibromyalgia and chronic fatigue, and could potentially contribute to the development/progression of many other diseases described in this book, but what is causing this surge in patients who are having increasing mast cell-associated problems? Is MCAS the next "thyroid disease"—a label for something that can be measured clinically, but sheds no

463

light onto *why* the system is out of whack in the first place? This book has revealed research that indicates a genetic component to MCAS, but it seems that many clinicians fail to address other aspects in the perfect storm of exposure to toxins, poor gut health, hidden viral and bacterial infections, inappropriate nervous system states, and so much more. For this reason, I believe that MCAS diagnosis should only serve as the *starting point* for a more detailed investigation into underlying factors.

Regardless of the etiology, mast cell activation syndrome is an inherently complex medical condition, but a holistic approach to diagnosis, treatment and prevention brings hope to this relatively newly coined patient population. A comprehensive medical team and an individualized approach are essential components of proper patient care. There is no one diet, medication or supplement that works wonders for all patients with MCAS. Instead of treating symptoms, an individualized root issue approach is paramount for healing.

> While living in Peru, my favorite local expression was:
> *"Poco a poco, se anda lejos." Little by little, one walks far.*

If we—as patient community and as a medical community—take it one step at a time, or maybe even three steps forward and two steps back, eventually, together, we will find a better place to improve the quality of life for patients with MCAS.

Hopefully this book has served as a useful starting resource for patients and medical practitioners alike. Despite full-time researching and writing for nearly two years, I feel like I've only gathered a small bit of information, truly the tip of the iceberg in this area. Over twenty studies were published on MCAS in 2018, [69-92] offering hope that the research will continue to investigate this condition more thoroughly. Hopefully the experts will fill in any gaps I missed along the way! I'm so grateful for the small but powerful groups of clinicians who are fighting tirelessly to move MCAS awareness, diagnosis and treatment options forward.

Whether a patient, a family member, a doctor, or a friend, never forget that patience and perseverance are the keys to success. The journey of MCAS diagnosis and treatment is truly an ultra-marathon distance, and…

> "The only failure is quitting. Everything else is just gathering information." [93]
>
> -Jen Sincero*

*From *You Are A Badass* ® by Jen Sincero, copyright ©2013. Reprinted by permission of Running Press, an imprint of Hachette Book Group, Inc.

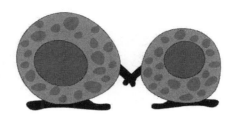

Please visit www.mastcellsunited.com for more MCAS resources:

PATIENT SUPPORT GROUPS

BUDDY PROGRAM

PATIENT SPOTLIGHT

ADVOCACY & AWARENESS OPPORTUNITIES

RECOMMENDED READING LIST

PODCAST SUGGESTIONS

BLOG ARTICLES

and much more!

Acknowledgments

Words won't ever suffice to adequately thank those who helped make this book happen. Jennifer Leopoldt Roop, my most patient editor, thank you so much for toiling away for months (nearly a year!) on end despite a lot on your plate (and amid sleep-deprived newborn life!). I learned so much from you! Special thanks also goes out to Ryan Biore, my fantastic cover art designer.

This process was significantly enhanced by the continual advice and mentoring of my bestselling author and dear friend, Ashley Mckee Leopoldt (pen name Ashley Mcleo). Ash, thank you so much for guiding me in the right direction! I'd also like to thank Elin Bandmann for proofreading sections of the book, providing valuable ideas, and agreeing to facetime at odd hours of the morning while on Australian time!

With deep gratitude, I'd like to give a shout out to the many experts who patiently answered my questions during interviews and follow-up communications, including:
Dr. Benoit Tano; Heidi Turner, MS, RDN; Dr. Jill Carnahan; Dr. Lawrence Afrin; Dr. Mariana Castells; Dr. Matthew Hamilton; and Dr. Sharon Meglathery.

I'd also like to thank additional individuals and organizations that granted me permission to share their perspectives, including:
Dr. Anthony Smith, Dr. Aviva Romm, Dr. Diana Driscoll, Dr. Gerhard Molderings, Dr. Gunnar Heuser, Dr. Joseph Pizzorno, Julie Rehmeyer, Lisa Klimas, Penguin Random House, Dr. Nichola McFadzean Ducharme, Rebecca Snow, Dr. Richard Horowitz, Dr. Ritchie Shoemaker, Saint Martin's Griffin Publishing, Sisters Media, Twilah Hiari, Warnick Publishing, and World Scientific Publishing Company.

A special thank you goes out to the medical professionals who gave me light and hope throughout the past five years of my patient journey, including Dr. Brown, Dr. Demain, Dr. Franco and the team at Sunridge Medical, Dr. Manning, Dr. Mclogan, Dr. Rose, and Dr. J. Smith. To Dr. Tony Smith and the team at Dynamic Health, my words are insufficient to express the depths of my gratitude for your expertise and generous care. Thank you for restoring my hope and sharing Craniobiotic Technique, an immensely valuable tool in patient care that has influenced me tremendously personally as well as in my career.

Finally, I must thank the family, friends and colleagues who supported me in this journey in so many different ways. Thank you to my parents Fred and Nancy, for supporting me during the writing of this book, sharing perspectives on the healing power of prayer, and for helping me to pursue more natural medical care options in Arizona—and with a roof over my head! I have no doubt that my story would have been very different had I not had those opportunities. To my sister, Britt, I am so grateful for you—thanks for lending a patient and compassionate listening ear when things got rough (and stayed rough for long periods of time). Sunnie and Larry, thank you for opening your home to me for so long, and for all of your generosity over the years. Uncle John, thank you for sending me so many interesting reads and resources! To my dear friend Jules, a wonderful partner in adventure, thank you for always being there, and for inspiring me to pursue more deeply rooted joy, gratitude, and presence in the moment throughout this journey. Nicole and Jan Deyong, thank you for supporting me in my housing situation while I was in transition. To my family at United Physical Therapy in Anchorage, thanks for your compassion and for helping me share information about MCAS with the community. And to the MCAS patient community, I am so grateful for your help and feedback in compiling this resource.

Lastly, to my love, Graham: Thank you for being you. Thank you for your unwavering support and positivity. Thank you for trying unconventional dietary changes with me, for moving several times (and states!) when the mold was too much for my system. Thank you for steering me clear of smokers on the street, for getting rid of personal belongings exposed to mold, for going above and beyond to remove triggers. Thank you for your calm acceptance when my symptoms derailed our plans. Thank you for bringing me tea, for listening without judgment, and being there with me through the lowest of lows. Thank you for believing in me and never doubting what I was experiencing. And thank you for your patience as I've toiled away on this book, taking up nights and weekends where we would otherwise be doing something together. My words certainly don't do justice to the immense gratitude I have for your sacrifices and selflessness, nor do they fully encompass the depths of love that I have for you. Maybe next time I'll write something *shorter* and more in your genre of choice! (But probably not, haha.)

With deep gratitude,

Amber

About the Author

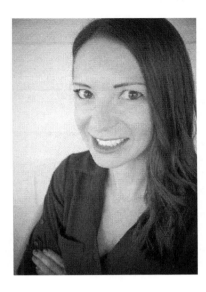

Amber Walker, PT, DPT, is a physical therapist graduate of Regis University. She began her career in northern Peru, where she worked with patients, conducted research and started a public health project for children with disabilities as a volunteer with Catholic Medical Mission Board. Upon returning to the U.S., she mainly focused her clinical practice on sports medicine and spine pain. Over the years, she gained valuable additional training in manual therapy, functional dry needling, and comprehensive strategies for the chronic pain and chronic fatigue patient populations.

Originally from Alaska, Amber thrives on being outdoors and is particularly drawn to mountain running and water sports. In the past she has held roles as a small business owner of a stand-up-paddling company, a swimming coach, a freelance photographer and writer, affiliate faculty of Regis DPT students in international immersion settings, and a leader in Christian groups and local community events.

Amber currently resides in Fort Collins, Colorado, where, as the owner of Origin Wellness (www.originwellnesscolorado.com), she encourages a "root issue" approach to patient care. Amber continues to advocate for the chronic illness population with speaking engagements and special projects via the MCAS resource website www.mastcellsunited.com.

Appendix 1: PROPOSED DIAGNOSTIC CRITERIA FOR MAST CELL ACTIVATION DISEASE

DIAGNOSTIC CRITERIA FOR SYSTEMIC MASTOCYTOSIS (SM)

The World Health Organization's Diagnostic Criteria for Systemic Mastocytosis (2016):

Major criterion:

- Multifocal, dense aggregates of mast cells (15 or more in aggregates) in sections of the bone marrow and/or other extracutaneous tissues, confirmed by tryptase immunohistochemistry or other special stains

Minor criteria:

- Atypical morphology or spindled appearance of at least 25% of the mast cells in the diagnostic biopsy or bone marrow aspirate smear

- Expression of CD2 and/or CD25 by mast cells in the marrow, blood, or extracutaneous organs

- *KIT* codon 816 mutation in the marrow, blood, or extracutaneous organs

- Persistent elevation of serum total tryptase >20 ng/ml

Diagnosis of SM made by either (1) the major criterion plus any one of the minor criteria or (2) any three minor criteria

From: Valent P, Akin C, Metcalfe DD. Mastocytosis: 2016 updated WHO classification and novel emerging treatment concepts. *Blood.* 2017;129:1420-1427. doi:10.1182/blood-2016-09-731893

DIAGNOSTIC CRITERIA FOR MAST CELL ACTIVATION SYNDROME (MCAS)

Note: The two published approaches for the diagnosis of MCAS are similar but slightly different. There is currently no universal standard for MCAS diagnosis.

Proposed MCAS Diagnostic Criteria by Valent et al. (2012), referred to as "Criteria X" in this book:

Major Criteria:

- Absence of any known disorder that can better account for symptoms

- Typical clinical symptoms (flushing, pruritus, urticaria, angioedema, nasal congestion, nasal pruritus, wheezing, throat swelling, headache, hypotension, diarrhea)

- Increase in serum total tryptase by at least 20% above baseline plus 2 ng/ml during or within 4 hours after a symptomatic period OR transient increase of another established mast cell mediator

- An objective response of clinical symptoms to anti-mediator drugs, such as histamine receptor blockers or 'mast cell targeting' agents, such as cromolyn*

All major criteria must be satisfied to meet diagnosis

*In regards to an objective response of symptoms to mast cell-targeting medications, the authors of this criteria agreed that H1/H2 blockers are most specific to mast cells and thus should be the medications of choice for fulfilling this criterion of MCAS. Other types of medications, such as leukotriene inhibitors and corticosteroids impact other cell types and would be less specific to rule in MCAS.

From: Valent P, Akin C, Arock M, et al. Definitions, criteria and global classification of mast cell disorders with special reference to mast cell activation syndromes: A consensus proposal. *Int Arch Allergy Immunol.* 2012;157(3):215-225. doi:10.1159/000328760

Proposed MCAS Diagnostic Criteria by Molderings et al., referred to as "Criteria Y" in this book – developed in 2011, modified in 2014, updated version published in 2016:

Major Criterion:

1. Unique constellation of clinical complaints as a result of a pathologically increased mast cell activity (mast cell mediator release syndrome)

Minor Criteria:

1. Multifocal or disseminated dense infiltrates of mast cells in bone marrow biopsies and/or in sections of other extracutaneous organ(s) (e.g., gastrointestinal tract biopsies; CD117-, tryptase- and CD25-stained)

2. Mast cells in bone marrow or other extracutaneous organ(s) show an abnormal morphology (>25%) in bone marrow smears or in histologies (minor criterion 1 for SM)

3. Mast cells in bone marrow express CD2 and/or CD25 (minor criterion 2 for SM)

4. Detection of genetic changes in mast cells from blood, bone marrow, or extracutaneous organs for which an impact on the state of activity of affected mast cells in terms of an increased activity has been proven

5. Evidence of a pathologically increased release of mast cell mediators by determination of the content of tryptase in blood, N-methylhistamine in urine, heparin in blood, chromogranin A in blood, or other mast cell-specific mediators (e.g., eicosanoids including prostaglandin PGD2, its metabolite 11-β-PGF2α, or leukotriene E4)

6. Symptomatic response to inhibitors of mast cell activation or mast cell mediator production or action (e.g., histamine H1 and/or H2 receptor antagonists, cromolyn)

Diagnosis of MCAS made by either (1) the major criterion plus any one of the minor criteria or (2) any three minor criteria

From: Molderings GJ, Haenisch B, Brettner S, et al. Pharmacological treatment options for mast cell activation disease. *Naunyn Schmiedebergs Arch Pharmacol.* 2016;389(7):671-694. doi:10.1007/s00210-016-1247-1

Appendix 2: CLINICAL RESOURCES

Clinical Decision-Making Algorithm Resources for Clinicians

- Afrin L, Molderings GJ. A concise, practical guide to diagnostic assessment for mast cell activation disease. *World J Hematol.* 2014;3(1):1-7. doi:10.5315
  - Link to full text: https://www.wjgnet.com/2218-6204/full/v3/i1/1.htm
- Picard M, Giavina-Bianchi P, Mezzano V, Castells M. Expanding Spectrum of Mast Cell Activation Disorders: Monoclonal and Idiopathic Mast Cell Activation Syndromes. *Clin Ther.* 2013;35(5):548-562. doi:10.1016/J.CLINTHERA.2013.04.001
  - Link to full text: http://www.clinicaltherapeutics.com/article/S0149-2918(13)00171-9/fulltext
  - see Table IV in article for stepwise prophylactic medication recommendations
- Molderings GJ, Brettner S, Homann J, Afrin LB. Mast cell activation disease: A concise practical guide for diagnostic workup and therapeutic options. *J Hematol Oncol.* 2011;4:10. doi:10.1186/1756-8722-4-10
  - Link to full text: https://www.ncbi.nlm.nih.gov/pmc/articles/PMC3069946/

Questionnaire for Clinician Use

- Mast Cell Mediator Release Syndrome Questionnaire
  - Original source:
    Alfter K, von Kügelgen I, Haenisch B, et al. New aspects of liver abnormalities as part of the systemic mast cell activation syndrome. *Liver Int.* 2009;29(2):181-186. doi:10.1111/j.1478-3231.2008.01839.x
  - Link to article: https://europepmc.org/abstract/med/18662284
- Link to access questionnaire:
  - ***Instead of clicking on the link below, for most browsers it works best to enter a Google search of "University of Bonn AND Mast Cell Mediator Release Syndrome Questionnaire." From the Google search page, you can then download the word document directly.
  - https://www.humangenetics.unibonn.de/de/forschung/forschungsprojekte/mastzellerkrankungen/validatedquestionnaire

Pharmacological Treatment Guidelines

- Molderings GJ, Haenisch B, Brettner S, et al. Pharmacological treatment options for mast cell activation disease. *Naunyn Schmiedebergs Arch Pharmacol*. 2016;389(7):671-694. doi:10.1007/s00210-016-1247-1
  - Link to full text: https://link.springer.com/article/10.1007/s00210-016-1247-1

- Wirz S, Molderings GJ. A practical guide for treatment of pain in patients with systemic mast cell activation disease. *Pain Physician*. 2017;20:E849-E861.
  - Link to full text: http://www.mastcelldisease.com/wp-content/uploads/2018/01/201720E849-E861.pdf

Emergency Tools

- Anaphylaxis Emergency Action Plan – customizable version provided by the American Academy of Allergy Asthma & Immunology
  - http://www.aaaai.org/Aaaai/media/MediaLibrary/PDF%20Documents/Libraries/Anaphylaxis-Emergency-Action-Plan.pdf

- The Mastocytosis Society Emergency Room Protocol
  - https://tmsforacure.org/anaphylaxis/ → click on "emergency room guide" on right hand side

Other Clinical Resources

- Ehlers-Danlos Society: Hypermobile EDS Diagnostic Criteria
  - https://www.ehlers-danlos.com/heds-diagnostic-checklist/

- Mold Illness: Dr. Shoemaker's Surviving Mold Diagnostic Lab Information
  - http://www.survivingmold.com/diagnosis/lab-orders

BIBLIOGRAPHY

References Chapter 1: My MCAS Story

1. Paz Soldan CO, Vargas Vásquez F, Gonzalez Varas A, et al. Intestinal parasitism in Peruvian children and molecular characterization of Cryptosporidium species. *Parasitol Res.* 2006;98(6):576-581. doi:10.1007/s00436-005-0114-7

2. Afrin LB. *Never Bet Against Occam: Mast Cell Activation Disease and the Modern Epidemics of Chronic Illness and Medical Complexity.* Bethesda, Maryland: Sisters Media; 2016.

3. Zanichelli A, Magerl M, Longhurst H, Fabien V, Maurer M. Hereditary angioedema with C1 inhibitor deficiency: delay in diagnosis in Europe. *Allergy, Asthma Clin Immunol.* 2013;9(1):29. doi:10.1186/1710-1492-9-29

4. Stevens C, Biedenkapp JC, Mensah R, Chyung YH, Adelman B. Hereditary Angioedema Is Associated with Neuropathic Pain, Systemic Lupus Erythematosis and Systemic Mastocytosis in an Analysis of a Health Analytics Claims Database. *J Allergy Clin Immunol.* 2016;137(2):AB75. doi:10.1016/j.jaci.2015.12.255

5. United States Hereditary Angioedema Association. https://www.haea.org. Accessed February 23, 2018.

6. Bork K, Meng G, Staubach P, Hardt J. Hereditary Angioedema: New Findings Concerning Symptoms, Affected Organs, and Course. *Am J Med.* 2006;119(3):267-274. doi:10.1016/J.AMJMED.2005.09.064

7. Mark 5:24-34. *The Bible, NIV Version.* https://www.biblegateway.com/passage/?search=Mark+5. Accessed March 3, 2018.

References Chapter 2: The Mast Cell

1. Walker ME, Hatfield JK, Brown MA. New insights into the role of mast cells in autoimmunity: Evidence for a common mechanism of action? *Biochim Biophys Acta - Mol Basis Dis.* 2012;1822(1):57-65. doi:10.1016/j.bbadis.2011.02.009

2. Kraneveld AD, Sagar S, Garssen J, Folkerts G. The two faces of mast cells in food allergy and allergic asthma: The possible concept of Yin Yang. *Biochim Biophys Acta - Mol Basis Dis.* 2012;1822(1):93-99. doi:10.1016/j.bbadis.2011.06.013

3. Ryan JJ, Morales JK, Falanga YT, Fernando JFA, Macey MR. Mast Cell Regulation of the Immune Response. *World Allergy Organ J.* 2009;2(10):224-232. doi:10.1097/WOX.0b013e3181c2a95e

4. St. John AL, Abraham SN. Innate Immunity and Its Regulation by Mast Cells. *J Immunol.* 2013;190:4458–4463. doi:10.4049/jimmunol.1203420

5. Mecheri S. Contribution of allergic inflammatory response to the pathogenesis of malaria disease. *Biochim Biophys Acta - Mol Basis Dis.* 2012;1822(1):49-56. doi:10.1016/j.bbadis.2011.02.005

6. Marshall JS, King C a, McCurdy JD. Mast cell cytokine and chemokine responses to bacterial and viral infection. *Curr Pharm Des.* 2003;9(1):11-24. doi:10.2174/1381612033392413

7. Theoharides TC, Valent P, Akin C. Mast Cells, Mastocytosis, and Related Disorders. Ingelfinger JR, ed. *N Engl J Med.* 2015;373(2):163-172. doi:10.1056/NEJMra1409760

8. Ribatti D. The development of human mast cells. An historical reappraisal. *Exp Cell Res.* 2016;342(2):210-215. doi:10.1016/j.yexcr.2016.03.013

9. Theoharides TC. Neuroendocrinology of mast cells: Challenges and controversies. *Exp Dermatol.* 2017;26(9):751-9. doi:10.1111/exd.13288

10. Żelechowska P, Agier J, Kozłowska E, Brzezińska-Błaszczyk E. Mast cells participate in chronic low-grade inflammation within adipose tissue. *Obes Rev.* 2018;19(5):686-97. doi:10.1111/obr.12670

11. Soderberg M. The Mast Cell Activation Syndrome: A Mini Review. *MOJ Immunol.* 2015;2(1). doi:10.15406/moji.2015.02.00032

12. Stone KD, Prussin C, Metcalfe DD. IgE, mast cells, basophils, and eosinophils. *J Allergy Clin Immunol.* 2010;111(2 Suppl):S486–94. doi:10.1016/j.jaci.2009.11.017

13. Theoharides TC, Bielory L. Mast cells and mast cell mediators as targets of dietary supplements. In: *Annals of Allergy, Asthma and Immunology.* 2004;93:S24. doi:10.1016/S1081-1206(10)61484-6

14. Polyzoidis S, Koletsa T, Panagiotidou S, Ashkan K, Theoharides TC. Mast cells in meningiomas and brain inflammation. *J Neuroinflammation.* 2015;12(1):170. doi:10.1186/s12974-015-0388-3

15. Theoharides TC, Kalogeromitros D. The critical role of mast cells in allergy and inflammation. *Ann N Y Acad Sci.* 2006;1088(1):78-99. doi:10.1196/annals.1366.025

16. Nautiyal KM, Ribeiro AC, Pfaff DW, Silver R. Brain mast cells link the immune system to anxiety-like behavior. *Proceedings of the National Academy of Sciences.* 2008;105(46):18053-18057.

17. Dunn AJ. Cytokine Activation of the HPA Axis. *Ann N Y Acad Sci.* 2000;917(1):608-617. doi:10.1111/j.1749-6632.2000.tb05426.x

18. Conti B, Tabarean I, Andrei C, Bartfai T, Dorris HL. Cytokines and fever. *Front Biosci.* 2004;9:1433-1449.

19. Krueger JM, Obál F, Fang J, Kubota T, Taishi P. The Role of Cytokines in Physiological Sleep Regulation. *Ann N Y Acad Sci.* 2006;933(1):211-221. doi:10.1111/j.1749-6632.2001.tb05826.x

20. Sigal LH. Basic science for the clinician 53: Mast cells. *J Clin Rheumatol.* 2011;17(7):395-400. doi:10.1097/RHU.0b013e31823150b5

21. Seneviratne SL, Maitland A, Afrin L. Mast cell disorders in Ehlers–Danlos syndrome. *Am J Med Genet Part C Semin Med Genet.* 2017;175(1):226-236. doi:10.1002/ajmg.c.31555

22. Galli SJ, Borregaard N, Wynn TA. Phenotypic and functional plasticity of cells of innate immunity: macrophages, mast cells and neutrophils. *Nat Immunol.* 2011;12(11):1035. doi:10.1038/ni.2109

23. Okayama Y, Benyon RC, Rees PH, Lowman MA, Hillier K, Church MK. Inhibition profiles of sodium cromoglycate and nedocromil sodium on mediator release from mast cells of human skin, lung, tonsil, adenoid and intestine. *Clin Exp Allergy.* 1992;22(3):401-409. doi:10.1111/j.1365-2222.1992.tb03102.x

24. Theoharides TC, Cochrane DE. Critical role of mast cells in inflammatory diseases and the effect of acute stress. *J Neuroimmunol.* 2004;146(1-2):1-12. doi:S0165572803004636 [pii]

25. Theoharides TC, Alysandratos KD, Angelidou A, et al. Mast cells and inflammation. *Biochim Biophys Acta - Mol Basis Dis.* 2012;1822:21-33. doi:10.1016/j.bbadis.2010.12.014

26. Marshall JS. Mast-cell responses to pathogens. *Nat Rev Immunol.* 2004;4(10):787. doi:10.1038/nri1460

27. Ratner V. Mast cell activation syndrome. *Transl Androl Urol.* 2015;4(5):587-588. doi:10.3978/j.issn.2223-4683.2015.09.03

28. Valent P, Akin C, Arock M, et al. Definitions, criteria and global classification of mast cell disorders with special reference to mast cell activation syndromes: A consensus proposal. *Int Arch Allergy Immunol.* 2012;157(3):215-225. doi:10.1159/000328760

29. Parsons ME, Ganellin CR. Histamine and its receptors. *Br J Pharmacol.* 2006;147(S1):S127-35. doi:10.1038/sj.bjp.0706440

30. Reese I, Ballmer-Weber B, Beyer K, et al. German guideline for the management of adverse reactions to ingested histamine. *Allergo J Int.* 2017;26(2):72-79. doi:10.1007/s40629-017-0011-5

31. Goldschmidt RC, Hough LB, Glick SD. Rat Brain Mast Cells: Contribution to Brain Histamine Levels. *J Neurochem.* 1985;44(6):1943-1947. doi:10.1111/j.1471-4159.1985.tb07191.x

32. Wirz S, Molderings GJ. A practical guide for treatment of pain in patients with systemic mast cell activation disease. *Pain Physician.* 2017;20:E849-E861.

33. Maintz L, Novak N. Histamine and histamine intolerance. *Am J Clin Nutr.* 2007;85(5):1185-1196. doi:10.1093/ajcn/85.5.1185

34. Wöhrl S, Hemmer W, Focke M, Rappersberger K, Jarisch R. Histamine intolerance-like symptoms in healthy volunteers after oral provocation with liquid histamine. *Allergy asthma Proc.* 25(5):305-311. http://www.ncbi.nlm.nih.gov/pubmed/15603203. Accessed September 17, 2018.

35. Jarisch R. Histamine Intolerance in Women. In: *Histamine Intolerance.* Berlin, Heidelberg: Springer Berlin Heidelberg; 2015:109-115. doi:10.1007/978-3-642-55447-6_6

36. He S, Gaça MD, Walls a F. A role for tryptase in the activation of human mast cells: modulation of histamine release by tryptase and inhibitors of tryptase. *J Pharmacol Exp Ther.* 1998;286(1):289-297.

37. Schwartz, B. L. Tryptase from human mast cells : biochemistry, biology and clinical utility. *Monogr Allergy.* 1990;27:90-113. https://ci.nii.ac.jp/naid/10029051057/. Accessed July 18, 2018.

38. Austen KF, Akin C. Clonal and non-clonal mast cell activation disorders. Clinical Pain Advisor: Oncology Section. 2016. http://www.clinicalpainadvisor.com/oncology/clonal-and-non-clonal-mast-cell-activation-disorders/article/619291/?utm_source=TrendMD&DCMP=OTC-CPA_trendmd&dl=0. Accessed June 23, 2017.

39. Blair RJ, Meng H, Marchese MJ, et al. Human mast cells stimulate vascular tube formation. Tryptase is a novel, potent angiogenic factor. *J Clin Invest.* 1997;99(11):2691. doi:10.1172/JCI119458

40. Krueger JM, Obál FJ, Fang J, Kubota T, Taishi P. The role of cytokines in physiological sleep regulation. *Ann N Y Acad Sci.* 2001;933:211-221. http://www.ncbi.nlm.nih.gov/pubmed/12000022. Accessed July 18, 2018.

41. Ueno R, Honda K, Inoué S, Hayaishi O. Prostaglandin D2, a cerebral sleep-inducing substance in rats. *Proc Natl Acad Sci U S A.* 1983;80(6):1735-1737. doi:10.1073/PNAS.80.6.1735

42. Ueno R, Narumiya S, Ogorochi T, Nakayama T, Ishikawa Y, Hayaishi O. Role of prostaglandin D2 in the hypothermia of rats caused by bacterial lipopolysaccharide. *Proc Natl Acad Sci.* 1982;79(19):6093-6097. doi:10.1073/pnas.79.19.6093

478

43. Mong J a, Devidze N, Frail DE, et al. Estradiol differentially regulates lipocalin-type prostaglandin D synthase transcript levels in the rodent brain: Evidence from high-density oligonucleotide arrays and in situ hybridization. *Proc Natl Acad Sci U S A*. 2003;100:318-323. doi:10.1073/pnas.262663799

44. Sivridis E, Giatromanolaki A, Agnantis N, Anastasiadis P. Mast cell distribution and density in the normal uterus - Metachromatic staining using lectins. *Eur J Obstet Gynecol Reprod Biol*. 2001;98(1):109-113. doi:10.1016/S0301-2115(00)00564-9

45. Koullapis EN, Collins WP. The concentration of 13,14-dihydro-15-oxo-prostaglandin F2 alpha in peripheral venous plasma throughout the normal ovarian and menstrual cycle. *Acta Endocrinol (Copenh)*. 1980;93(1):123-128.

46. Ricciotti E, FitzGerald GA. Prostaglandins and inflammation. *Arterioscler Thromb Vasc Biol*. 2011;31(5):986-1000. doi:10.1161/ATVBAHA.110.207449

47. Dharmananda S. Reducing Inflammation with Diet and Supplements: The Story of Eicosanoid Inhibition. Institute for Traditional Medicine. http://www.itmonline.org/arts/lox.htm. Accessed July 18, 2018.

48. Klimas L. Mast cell mediators: Prostaglandin D2 (PGD2). Mast Attack. http://www.mastattack.org/2015/04/mast-cell-mediators-prostaglandin-d2-pgd2/. Accessed July 18, 2018.

49. Funk CD. Prostaglandins and leukotrienes: Advances in eicosanoid biology. *Science*. 2001;294:1871-1875. doi:10.1126/science.294.5548.1871

50. Berger A. What are leukotrienes and how do they work in asthma? *BMJ*. 1999;319(7):7202. doi:10.1136/bmj.319.7202.90

51. Miligkos M, Bannuru RR, Alkofide H, Kher SR, Schmid CH, Balk EM. Leukotriene receptor antagonists versus placebo in the treatment of asthma in adults and adolescents: a systematic review and meta-analysis. *Ann Intern Med*. 2015;163(10):756-767. doi:10.1161/CIRCRESAHA.116.303790.The

52. Klimas L. The MastAttack 107: The Layperson's Guide to Understanding Mast Cell Diseases, Part 76. Mast Attack. http://www.mastattack.org/2017/11/mastattack-107-laypersons-guide-understanding-mast-cell-diseases-part-76/. Accessed July 18, 2018.

53. Kim T, Tao-Cheng J-H, Eiden LE, Loh YP. Chromogranin A, an "On/Off" Switch Controlling Dense-Core Secretory Granule Biogenesis. *Cell*. 2001;106(4):499-509. doi:10.1016/S0092-8674(01)00459-7

54. Patcharatrakul T, El-Salhy M, Hatlebakk JG, Hausken T, Gilja OH, Gonlachanvit S. Difference of Chromogranin a Cell Density in the Large Intestine Between Asian and European Patients with Irritable Bowel Syndrome (IBS). *Gastroenterology*. 2017;152(5):S728. doi:10.1016/S0016-5085(17)32532-5

55. Hanjra P, Lee C-CR, Maric I, et al. Chromogranin A is not a biomarker of mastocytosis. *J allergy Clin Immunol Pract*. 2018;6(2):687-689.e4. doi:10.1016/j.jaip.2017.08.022

56. Afrin L, Molderings GJ. A concise, practical guide to diagnostic assessment for mast cell activation disease. *World J Hematol*. 2014;3(1):1-7. doi:10.5315

57. Lucki I. The spectrum of behaviors influenced by serotonin. *Biol Psychiatry*. 1998;44:151–162. doi:10.1016/S0006-3223(98)00139-5

58. Gould E. Serotonin and hippocampal neurogenesis. *Neuropsychopharmacology*. 1999;21:46S–51S. doi:10.1016/S0893-133X(99)00045-7

59. Gaspar P, Cases O, Maroteaux L. The developmental role of serotonin: news from mouse molecular genetics. *Nat Rev Neurosci*. 2003;4(12):1002-1012. doi:10.1038/nrn1256

60. Kushnir-Sukhov NM, Brown JM, Wu Y, Kirshenbaum A, Metcalfe DD. Human mast cells are capable of serotonin synthesis and release. *J Allergy Clin Immunol*. 2007;119, no. 2(2):498-499. doi:10.1016/j.jaci.2006.09.003

61. Kritas SK, Saggini A, Cerulli G, et al. Relationship between serotonin and mast cells: Inhibitory effect of anti-serotonin. *J Biol Regul Homeost Agents*. 2014;28:377-380.

62. Young SN, Leyton M. The role of serotonin in human mood and social interaction: Insight from altered tryptophan levels. *Pharmacol Biochem Behav*. 2002;71(4):857-865. doi:10.1016/S0091-3057(01)00670-0

63. Markus CR, Olivier B, Panhuysen GEM, et al. The bovine protein α-lactalbumin increases the plasma ratio of tryptophan to the other large neutral amino acids, and in vulnerable subjects raises brain serotonin activity, reduces cortisol concentration, and improves mood under stress. *Am J Clin Nutr*. 2000;71(6):1536-1544. doi:10.1093/ajcn/71.6.1536

64. Porter RJ, Gallagher P, Watson S, Young AH. Corticosteroid-serotonin interactions in depression: A review of the human evidence. *Psychopharmacology (Berl)*. 2004;173(1-2):1-17. doi:10.1007/s00213-004-1774-1

65. Zhang X, Beaulieu JM, Sotnikova TD, Gainetdinov RR, Caron MG. Tryptophan hydroxylase-2 controls brain serotonin synthesis. *Science*. 2004;5681:217. doi:10.1126/science.1097540

66. Liu Y, Ho RC-M, Mak A. Interleukin (IL)-6, tumour necrosis factor alpha (TNF-α) and soluble interleukin-2 receptors (sIL-2R) are elevated in patients with major depressive disorder: A meta-analysis and meta-regression. *J Affect Disord*. 2012;139(3):230-239. doi:10.1016/j.jad.2011.08.003

67. Feldman JM. Urinary serotonin in the diagnosis of carcinoid tumors. *Clin Chem*. 1986;32(5):840-844.

68. Spiller R. Recent advances in understanding the role of serotonin in gastrointestinal motility in functional bowel disorders: Alterations in 5-HT signalling and metabolism in human disease. *Neurogastroenterol Motil*. 2007;19(S2):25-31. doi:10.1111/j.1365-2982.2007.00965.x

69. Klimas L. Mood disorders and inflammation: High cortisol and low serotonin (Part 2 of 4). Mast Attack. http://www.mastattack.org/2016/05/mood-disorders-and-inflammation-high-cortisol-and-low-serotonin-part-2-of-4/. Accessed July 18, 2018.

70. Buhner S, Schemann M. Mast cell-nerve axis with a focus on the human gut. *Biochim Biophys Acta - Mol Basis Dis*. 2012;1822(1):85-92. doi:10.1016/j.bbadis.2011.06.004

71. Kushnir-Sukhov NM, Brittain E, Scott L, Metcalfe DD. Clinical correlates of blood serotonin levels in patients with mastocytosis. *Eur J Clin Invest*. 2008;38:953-958. doi:10.1111/j.1365-2362.2008.02047.x

72. Butterfield J, Weiler C. Whole bood serotonin levels in cutaneous mastocytosis, systemic mastocytosis and mast cell activation syndrome. *J Allergy Clin Immunol*. 2011;127:AB132. doi:10.1016/j.jaci.2010.12.528

73. da Silva EZM, Jamur MC, Oliver C. Mast Cell Function: A New Vision of an Old Cell. *J Histochem Cytochem*. 2014;62(10):698–738. doi:10.1369/0022155414545334

74. Polyzoidis S, Koletsa T, Panagiotidou S, Ashkan K, Theoharides TC. Mast cells in meningiomas and brain inflammation. *J Neuroinflammation*. 2015;12(1):170. doi:10.1186/s12974-015-0388-3

75. Piliponsky AM, Romani L. The contribution of mast cells to bacterial and fungal infection immunity. *Immunol Rev*. 2018;282(1):188-197. doi:10.1111/imr.12623

76. Molderings GJ. The genetic basis of mast cell activation disease - looking through a glass darkly. *Crit Rev Oncol Hematol*. 2015;93(2):75-89. doi:10.1016/j.critrevonc.2014.09.001

77. Li X, Ehrlich H. *Traditional Chinese Medicine, Western Science, and the Fight Against Allergic Disease*. World Scientific Publishing Co.; 2016.

78. Lee J, Veatch SL, Baird B, Holowka D. Molecular mechanisms of spontaneous and directed mast cell motility. *J Leukoc Biol*. 2012;92(5):1029-1041. doi:10.1189/jlb.0212091

79. Kambayashi T, Allenspach EJ, Chang JT, et al. Inducible MHC class II expression by mast cells supports effector and regulatory T cell activation. *J Immunol*. 2009;182(8):4686-4695. doi:10.4049/jimmunol.0803180

80. Horowitz R. *How Can I Get Better? An Action Plan for Treating Resistant Lyme and Chronic Disease*. New York, NY: St. Martin's Griffin; 2017.

81. Malbec O, Daëron M. The mast cell IgG receptors and their roles in tissue inflammation. *Immunol Rev*. 2007;217(1):206-221. doi:10.1111/j.1600-065X.2007.00510.x

82. Jennings S V., Slee VM, Zack RM, et al. Patient Perceptions in Mast Cell Disorders. *Immunol Allergy Clin North Am*. 2018;38(3):505-525. doi:10.1016/j.iac.2018.04.006

83. González-de-Olano D, Domínguez-Ortega J, Sánchez-García S. Mast Cell Activation Syndromes and Environmental Exposures. *Curr Treat Options Allergy*. 2018;5(1):41-51. doi:10.1007/s40521-018-0151-y

84. Coop CA, Schapira RS, Freeman TM. Are ACE Inhibitors and Beta-blockers Dangerous in Patients at Risk for Anaphylaxis? *J Allergy Clin Immunol Pract*. 2017;5(5):1207-1211. doi:10.1016/j.jaip.2017.04.033

85. Tsai YT, Zhou J, Weng H, Tang EN, Baker DW, Tang L. Optical imaging of fibrin deposition to elucidate participation of mast cells in foreign body responses. *Biomaterials*. 2014;35(7):2089-2096. doi:10.1016/j.biomaterials.2013.11.040

86. Jennings S, Russell N, Jennings B, et al. The Mastocytosis Society Survey on Mast Cell Disorders: Patient Experiences and Perceptions. *J Allergy Clin Immunol Pract*. 2014;2(1):70-76. doi:10.1016/j.jaip.2013.09.004

References Chapter 3: Mast Cell Activation Disease

1. Molderings GJ, Brettner S, Homann J, Afrin LB. Mast cell activation disease: A concise practical guide for diagnostic workup and therapeutic options. *J Hematol Oncol*. 2011;4:10. doi:10.1186/1756-8722-4-10

2. Afrin L. Episode 10 - Understanding Mast Cell Activation Disorder with Dr. Afrin. In: Unbound Healing Podcast by Anne Marie Garland and Michelle Hoover on Apple Podcasts. Aired on 8/31/17. https://itunes.apple.com/us/podcast/unbound-healing-podcast/id1253479733?mt=2.

3. Soderberg M. The Mast Cell Activation Syndrome: A Mini Review. *MOJ Immunol*. 2015;2(1). doi:10.15406/moji.2015.02.00032

4. Theoharides TC, Valent P, Akin C. Mast Cells, Mastocytosis, and Related Disorders. Ingelfinger JR, ed. *N Engl J Med*. 2015;373(2):163-172. doi:10.1056/NEJMra1409760

5. Afrin LB. *Never Bet Against Occam: Mast Cell Activation Disease and the Modern Epidemics of Chronic Illness and Medical Complexity*. Bethesda, Maryland: Sisters Media; 2016.

6. Shan L, Publication O, Dauvilliers Y, Siegel JM. Interactions of the histamine and hypocretin systems in CNS disorders. *Nat Rev Neurol*. 2015. doi:10.1038/nrneurol.2015.99

7. Olsson A, Kayhan G, Lagercrantz H, Herlenius E. IL-1β Depresses Respiration and Anoxic Survival via a Prostaglandin-Dependent Pathway in Neonatal Rats. *Pediatr Res*. 2003;54(3):326-331. doi:10.1203/01.PDR.0000076665.62641.A2

8. Valent P, Akin C, Arock M, et al. Definitions, criteria and global classification of mast cell disorders with special reference to mast cell activation syndromes: A consensus proposal. *Int Arch Allergy Immunol*. 2012;157(3):215-225. doi:10.1159/000328760

9. Valent P, Akin C, Metcalfe DD. Mastocytosis: 2016 updated WHO classification and novel emerging treatment concepts. *Blood*. 2017;129:1420-1427. doi:10.1182/blood-2016-09-731893

10. Yung A. Mastocytosis. DermNet New Zealand. https://www.dermnetnz.org/topics/mastocytosis/. Accessed September 20, 2018.

11. Castells MC, Akin C. Mastocytosis (cutaneous and systemic): Epidemiology, pathogenesis, and clinical manifestations. Up to Date. https://www.uptodate.com/contents/mastocytosis-cutaneous-and-systemic-epidemiology-pathogenesis-and-clinical-manifestations. Published 2015. Accessed July 17, 2018.

12. Seneviratne SL, Maitland A, Afrin L. Mast cell disorders in Ehlers–Danlos syndrome. *Am J Med Genet Part C Semin Med Genet*. 2017;175(1):226-236. doi:10.1002/ajmg.c.31555

13. Koyamangalat K. Systemic Mastocytosis. Medscape. http://emedicine.medscape.com/article/203948-workup#showall. Published 2016.

14. Garcia-Montero AC, Jara-Acevedo M, Teodosio C, et al. KIT mutation in mast cells and other bone marrow hematopoietic cell lineages in systemic mast cell disorders: A prospective study of the Spanish Network on Mastocytosis (REMA) in a series of 113 patients. *Blood*. 2006;108:2366–2372. doi:10.1182/blood-2006-04-015545

15. Arber DA, Orazi A, Hasserjian R, et al. The 2016 revision to the World Health Organization classification of myeloid neoplasms and acute leukemia. *Blood*. 2016;127(20):2391-2405. doi:10.1182/blood-2016-03-643544

16. Horny H, Akin C, Arber D, Al E. Mastocytosis. In: Swerdlow S, Campo E, Harris N, Al E, eds. *World Health Organization (WHO) Classification of Tumours. Pathology & Genetics. Tumours of Haematopoietic and Lymphoid Tissues*. Lyon, France: IARC Press; 2016.

17. Austen KF, Akin C. Clonal and non-clonal mast cell activation disorders. Clinical Pain Advisor: Oncology Section. 2016. http://www.clinicalpainadvisor.com/oncology/clonal-and-non-clonal-mast-cell-activation-disorders/article/619291/?utm_source=TrendMD&DCMP=OTC-CPA_trendmd&dl=0. Accessed June 23, 2017.

18. Valent P, Sperr WR, Samorapoompichit P, et al. Myelomastocytic overlap syndromes: biology, criteria, and relationship to mastocytosis. *Leuk Res*. 2001;25(7):595-602. doi:10.1016/S0145-2126(01)00040-6

19. Lichtman MA, Segel GB. Uncommon phenotypes of acute myelogenous leukemia: Basophilic, mast cell, eosinophilic, and myeloid dendritic cell subtypes: A review. *Blood Cells, Mol Dis*. 2005;35(3):370-383. doi:10.1016/J.BCMD.2005.08.006

20. Sperr WR, Jordan J-H, Fiegl M, et al. Serum tryptase levels in patients with mastocytosis: correlation with mast cell burden and implication for defining the category of disease. *Int Arch Allergy Immunol*. 2002;128(2):136-141. doi:10.1159/000059404

21. Monnier J, Georgin-Lavialle S, Canioni D, et al. Mast cell sarcoma: new cases and literature review. *Oncotarget*. 2016;40:662-699. doi:10.18632/oncotarget.11812

22. Álvarez-Twose I, González de Olano D, Sánchez-Muñoz L, et al. Clinical, biological, and molecular characteristics of clonal mast cell disorders presenting with systemic mast cell activation symptoms. *J Allergy Clin Immunol*. 2010;125:1269-1278. doi:10.1016/j.jaci.2010.02.019

23. Afrin L, Molderings GJ. A concise, practical guide to diagnostic assessment for mast cell activation disease. *World J Hematol*. 2014;3(1):1-7. doi:10.5315

24. Picard M, Giavina-Bianchi P, Mezzano V, Castells M. Expanding Spectrum of Mast Cell Activation Disorders: Monoclonal and Idiopathic Mast Cell Activation Syndromes. *Clin Ther*. 2013;35(5):548-562. doi:10.1016/J.CLINTHERA.2013.04.001

25. Hamilton MJ, Hornick JL, Akin C, Castells MC, Greenberger NJ. Mast cell activation syndrome: A newly recognized disorder with systemic clinical manifestations. *J Allergy Clin Immunol*. 2011;128(1)(1):147-152. doi:10.1016/j.jaci.2011.04.037

26. Haenisch B, Nöthen MM, Molderings, Gerhard J. Systemic mast cell activation disease: The role of molecular genetic alterations in pathogenesis, heritability and diagnostics. *Immunology*. 2012;137:197–205. doi:10.1111/j.1365-2567.2012.03627.x

27. Molderings GJ, Haenisch B, Bogdanow M, Fimmers R, Nöthen MM. Familial Occurrence of Systemic Mast Cell Activation Disease. *PLoS One*. 2013;8(9):e76241. doi:10.1371/journal.pone.0076241

28. Afrin L, Self S, Menk J, Lazarchick J. Characterization of mast cell activation syndrome. *Am J Med Sci*. 2017;353(3):207-215.

29. Arndt KK, Viswanathan RK, Mathur SK. Clinical Characteristics of Patients in Allergy Clinic with Presumed Diagnosis of Mast Cell Activation Syndrome (MCAS). *J Allergy Clin Immunol*. 2018;141(2):AB50. doi:10.1016/J.JACI.2017.12.162

30. Mackey E, Ayyadurai S, Pohl CS, D'Costa S, Li Y, Moeser AJ. Sexual dimorphism in the mast cell transcriptome and the pathophysiological responses to immunological and psychological stress. *Biol Sex Differ*. 2016;7(1):60. doi:10.1186/s13293-016-0113-7

31. Li X, Ehrlich H. *Traditional Chinese Medicine, Western Science, and the Fight Against Allergic Disease*. World Scientific Publishing Co.; 2016.

32. Zblewski D, Abdelrahman RA, Chen D, Butterfield JH, Tefferi A, Pardanani A. Patient Reported Symptoms and Tryptase Levels in WHO-Defined Systemic Mastocytosis (SM) Versus Mast Cell Activation Syndrome (MCAS) Versus Neither. *Blood*. 2014;124(21). http://www.bloodjournal.org/content/124/21/3204?sso-checked=true. Accessed July 17, 2018.

33. Roberts LJ, Oates JA. Biochemical Diagnosis of Systemic Mast Cell Disorders. *J Invest Dermatol*. 1991;96(3):S19-S25. doi:10.1111/1523-1747.ep12468945

34. Sonneck K, Florian S, Müllauer L, et al. Diagnostic and Subdiagnostic Accumulation of Mast Cells in the Bone Marrow of Patients with Anaphylaxis: Monoclonal Mast Cell Activation Syndrome. *Int Arch Allergy Immunol*. 2007;142(2):158-164. doi:10.1159/000096442

35. Akin C, Valent P, Metcalfe DD, et al. Mast cell activation syndrome: Proposed diagnostic criteria. *J Allergy Clin Immunol*. 2010;126(6):1099-1104. doi:10.1016/j.jaci.2010.08.035

36. Molderings GJ, Haenisch B, Brettner S, et al. Pharmacological treatment options for mast cell activation disease. *Naunyn Schmiedebergs Arch Pharmacol*. 2016;389(7):671-694. doi:10.1007/s00210-016-1247-1

37. Talkington J, Nickell SP. Borrelia burgdorferi spirochetes induce mast cell activation and cytokine release. *Infect Immun*. 1999;67:1107-1115.

38. Quintás-Cardama A, Sever M, Cortes J, Kantarjian H, Verstovsek S. Bone marrow mast cell burden and serum tryptase level as markers of response in patients with systemic mastocytosis. *Leuk Lymphoma*. 2013;54(9):1959-1964. doi:10.3109/10428194.2012.763121

39. Butterfield JH, Li CY. Bone Marrow Biopsies for the Diagnosis of Systemic Mastocytosis: Is One Biopsy Sufficient? *Am J Clin Pathol*. 2004;121:264–267. doi:10.1309/2EWQKN00PG02JKY0

40. Molderings GJ. The genetic basis of mast cell activation disease - looking through a glass darkly. *Crit Rev Oncol Hematol*. 2015;93(2):75-89. doi:10.1016/j.critrevonc.2014.09.001

41. Afrin LB, Khoruts A. Mast Cell Activation Disease and Microbiotic Interactions. *Clin Ther*. 2015;37(5):941-953. doi:10.1016/j.clinthera.2015.02.008

42. Valent P. Mast cell activation syndromes: definition and classification. *Allergy*. 2013;68(4):417-424. doi:10.1111/all.12126

43. Petra AI, Panagiotidou S, Stewart JM, Conti P, Theoharides TC. Spectrum of mast cell activation disorders. *Expert Rev Clin Immunol*. 2014;10(6):729-739. doi:10.1586/1744666X.2014.906302

44. Sotlar K, Horny HP, Simonitsch I, et al. CD25 indicates the neoplastic phenotype of mast cells: A novel immunohistochemical marker for the diagnosis of systemic mastocytosis (SM) in routinely processed bone marrow biopsy specimens. *Am J Surg Pathol*. 2004;10:1319-1325. doi:10.1097/01.pas.0000138181.89743.7b

45. Reichard KK, Chen D, Pardanani A, et al. Morphologically occult systemic mastocytosis in bone marrow: Clinicopathologic features and an algorithmic approach to diagnosis. *Am J Clin Pathol*. 2015;144(3):493-502. doi:10.1309/AJCPSGQ71GJQQACL

46. Van den Poel B, Kochuyt A-M, Del Biondo E, et al. Highly sensitive assays are mandatory for the differential diagnosis of patients presenting with symptoms of mast cell activation: diagnostic work-up of 38 patients. *Acta Clin Belg*. 2017;72(2):123-129. doi:10.1080/17843286.2017.1293312

47. Hahn HP, Hornick JL. Immunoreactivity for CD25 in gastrointestinal mucosal mast cells is specific for systemic mastocytosis. *Am J Surg Pathol*. 2007;31(11):1669-1676. doi:10.1097/PAS.0b013e318078ce7a

48. Morgado JMT, Sánchez-Muñoz L, Teodósio CG, et al. Immunophenotyping in systemic mastocytosis diagnosis: 'CD25 positive' alone is more informative than the 'CD25 and/or CD2' WHO criterion. *Mod Pathol*. 2012;25(4):516-521. doi:10.1038/modpathol.2011.192

49. van Daele PL, Beukenkamp BS, Geertsma-Kleinekoort WM, et al. Immunophenotyping of mast cells: a sensitive and specific diagnostic tool for systemic mastocytosis. *Neth J Med*. 2009;67:142-146.

50. Pozdnyakova O, Kondtratiev S, Li B, Charest K, Dorfman DM. High-sensitivity flow cytometric analysis for the evaluation of systemic mastocytosis including the identification of a new flow cytometric criterion for bone marrow involvement. *Am J Clin Pathol*. 2012;138:416-424. doi:10.1309/AJCP5PJWK4QFHWHM

51. Del Biondo E, Bouckx N. Critically Appraised Topic: Diagnosis of Systemic Mastocytosis. *Lab Geneeskd*. 2013:1-15. http://www.uzleuven.be/sites/default/files/Laboratoriumgeneeskunde/CAT_140320_mastocytose.pdf.

52. Hamilton M. Phone interview conducted on 6-22-18.

53. Klimas L. The MastAttack 107: The Layperson's Guide to Understanding Mast Cell Diseases, Part 14. Mast Attack. http://www.mastattack.org/2017/04/mastattack-107-laypersons-guide-understanding-mast-cell-diseases-part-14/. Accessed July 18, 2018.

54. Cohen SS, Skovbo S, Vestergaard H, et al. Epidemiology of systemic mastocytosis in Denmark. *Br J Haematol*. 2014;166:5218. doi:10.1111/bjh.12916

55. Theoharides TC, Kalogeromitros D. The critical role of mast cells in allergy and inflammation. *Ann N Y Acad Sci*. 2006;1088(1):78-99. doi:10.1196/

56. Barbara G, Stanghellini V, de giorgio R, Corinaldesi R. Functional gastrointestinal disorders and mast cells: implications for therapy. *Neurogastroenterol Motil*. 2006;18(1):6-17. doi:10.1111/j.1365-2982.2005.00685.x

57. Ratner V. Mast cell activation syndrome. *Transl Androl Urol.* 2015;4(5):587-588. doi:10.3978/j.issn.2223-4683.2015.09.03
58. Enestrom S, Bengtsson A, Frodin T. Dermal IgG deposits and increase of mast cells in patients with fibromyalgia--relevant findings or epiphenomena? *Scand J Rheumatol.* 1997;26:308-313.

References Chapter 4: Special Topics in MCAD

1. Voehringer D. Protective and pathological roles of mast cells and basophils. *Nat Rev Immunol.* 2013;13(5):362. doi:10.1038/nri3427
2. Akin C, Valent P, Metcalfe DD, et al. Mast cell activation syndrome: Proposed diagnostic criteria. *J Allergy Clin Immunol.* 2010;126(6):1099-1104. doi:10.1016/j.jaci.2010.08.035
3. Afrin LB. Episode 10 - Understanding Mast Cell Activation Disorder with Dr. Afrin. In: Unbound Healing Podcast by Anne Marie Garland and Michelle Hoover on Apple Podcasts. Aired on 8/31/17. https://itunes.apple.com/us/podcast/unbound-healing-podcast/id1253479733?mt=2.
4. Afrin LB. Personal email correspondence on October 3rd, 2018.
5. Polyzoidis S, Koletsa T, Panagiotidou S, Ashkan K, Theoharides TC. Mast cells in meningiomas and brain inflammation. *J Neuroinflammation.* 2015;12(1):170. doi:10.1186/s12974-015-0388-3
6. Benoist C, Mathis D. Mast cells in autoimmune disease. *Nature.* 2002;420(6917):875-878. doi:10.1038/nature01324
7. Johansson O. Disturbance of the immune system by electromagnetic fields—A potentially underlying cause for cellular damage and tissue repair reduction which could lead to disease and impairment. *Pathophysiology.* 2009;16(2-3):157-177. doi:10.1016/J.PATHOPHYS.2009.03.004
8. Theoharides TC, Kalogeromitros D. The critical role of mast cells in allergy and inflammation. *Ann N Y Acad Sci.* 2006;1088(1):78-99. doi:10.1196/annals.1366.025
9. Gregory GD, Bickford A, Robbie-Ryan M, Tanzola M, Brown MA. MASTering the immune response: mast cells in autoimmunity. *Novartis Found Symp.* 2005;271:215-225. doi:10.1002/9780470033449.ch18
10. Walker ME, Hatfield JK, Brown MA. New insights into the role of mast cells in autoimmunity: Evidence for a common mechanism of action? *Biochim Biophys Acta - Mol Basis Dis.* 2012;1822(1):57-65. doi:10.1016/j.bbadis.2011.02.009
11. Kim DY, Jeoung D, Ro JY. Signaling Pathways in the Activation of Mast Cells Cocultured with Astrocytes and Colocalization of Both Cells in Experimental Allergic Encephalomyelitis. *J Immunol.* 2010;185:273–283. doi:10.4049/jimmunol.1000991
12. Sayed BA, Christy A, Quirion MR, Brown MA. The Master Switch: The Role of Mast Cells in Autoimmunity and Tolerance. *Annu Rev Immunol.* 2008;26:705–739. doi:10.1146/annurev.immunol.26.021607.090320
13. Pilartz M, Jess T, Indefrei D, Schröder JM. Adoptive transfer-experimental allergic neuritis in newborn Lewis rats results in inflammatory infiltrates, mast cell activation, and increased Ia expression with only minor nerve fiber degeneration. *Acta Neuropathol.* 2002;104:513–524. doi:10.1007/s00401-002-0586-9
14. Ryan JJ, Morales JK, Falanga YT, Fernando JFA, Macey MR. Mast Cell Regulation of the Immune Response. *World Allergy Organ J.* 2009;2(10):224-232. doi:10.1097/WOX.0b013e3181c2a95e
15. St. John AL, Abraham SN. Innate Immunity and Its Regulation by Mast Cells. *J Immunol.* 2013;190:4458–4463. doi:10.4049/jimmunol.1203420
16. Kinet J-P. The essential role of mast cells in orchestrating inflammation. *Immunol Rev.* 2007;217(1):5-7. doi:10.1111/j.1600-065X.2007.00528.x
17. Proal AD, Marshall TG. Re-framing the theory of autoimmunity in the era of the microbiome: persistent pathogens, autoantibodies, and molecular mimicry. *Discov Med.* 2018;26(144).
18. Afrin LB. Presentation, diagnosis, and management of mast cell activation syndrome. In: *Mast Cells: Phenotypic Features, Biological Functions and Role in Immunity.* Nova Science Publishers, Inc.; 2013:155-232.
19. Afrin LB, Khoruts A. Mast Cell Activation Disease and Microbiotic Interactions. *Clin Ther.* 2015;37(5):941-953. doi:10.1016/j.clinthera.2015.02.008
20. Molderings GJ, Brettner S, Homann J, Afrin LB. Mast cell activation disease: A concise practical guide for diagnostic workup and therapeutic options. *J Hematol Oncol.* 2011;4:10. doi:10.1186/1756-8722-4-10
21. Valent P, Akin C, Arock M, et al. Definitions, criteria and global classification of mast cell disorders with special reference to mast cell activation syndromes: A consensus proposal. *Int Arch Allergy Immunol.* 2012;157(3):215-225. doi:10.1159/000328760
22. Broesby-Olsen S, Kristensen T, Vestergaard H, Brixen K, Møller MB, Bindslev-Jensen C. KIT D816V mutation burden does not correlate to clinical manifestations of indolent systemic mastocytosis. *J Allergy Clin Immunol.* 2013;132(3):723-728. doi:10.1016/j.jaci.2013.02.019
23. Molderings GJ. The genetic basis of mast cell activation disease - looking through a glass darkly. *Crit Rev Oncol Hematol.* 2015;93(2):75-89. doi:10.1016/j.critrevonc.2014.09.001

24. Theoharides TC, Valent P, Akin C. Mast Cells, Mastocytosis, and Related Disorders. Ingelfinger JR, ed. *N Engl J Med*. 2015;373(2):163-172. doi:10.1056/NEJMra1409760

25. Afrin L. Not All Mast Cell Disease is Systemic Mastocytosis: Mast Cell Activation Disorder. Welapalooza Presentation 4-30-17. 2017. http://mastcellresearch.com/wp-content/uploads/2017/06/MCAD-Overview-2017-Wellapalooza-General.pptx.

26. Gotlib J, Berubé C, Growney JD, et al. Activity of the tyrosine kinase inhibitor PKC412 in a patient with mast cell leukemia with the D816V KIT mutation. *Blood*. 2005;106(8):2865-2870. doi:10.1182/blood-2005-04-1568

27. Molderings GJ, Kolck UW, Scheurlen C, Brüss M, Homann J, Von Kügelgen I. Multiple novel alterations in Kit tyrosine kinase in patients with gastrointestinally pronounced systemic mast cell activation disorder. *Scand J Gastroenterol*. 2007;42(8):1045-1053. doi:10.1080/00365520701245744

28. Molderings GJ, Meis K, Kolck UW, Homann J, Frieling T. Comparative analysis of mutation of tyrosine kinase kit in mast cells from patients with systemic mast cell activation syndrome and healthy subjects. *Immunogenetics*. 2010;62:721-727. doi:10.1007/s00251-010-0474-8

29. Hermine O, Lortholary O, Leventhal PS, et al. Case-Control Cohort Study of Patients' Perceptions of Disability in Mastocytosis. Soyer HP, ed. *PLoS One*. 2008;3(5):e2266. doi:10.1371/journal.pone.0002266

30. Milner J. Research update: POTS, EDS, MCAS Genetics. In: Dysautonomia International Conference & CME, Washington DC; 2015. https://vimeo.com/142039306.

31. Afrin L. Ask the Expert: Mast Cell Activation Syndrome. https://www.drtaniadempsey.com/single-post/Ask-The-Expert-Mast-Cell-Activation-Syndrome. Accessed July 20, 2018.

32. Molderings GJ, Haenisch B, Bogdanow M, Fimmers R, Nöthen MM. Familial Occurrence of Systemic Mast Cell Activation Disease. *PLoS One*. 2013;8(9):e76241. doi:10.1371/journal.pone.0076241

33. Chen G-L, Xu Z-H, Wang W, et al. Analysis of the C314T and A595G mutations in histamine N-methyltransferase gene in a Chinese population. *Clin Chim Acta*. 2002;326(1-2):163-167. doi:10.1016/S0009-8981(02)00299-1

34. Yang X, Liu C, Zhang J, et al. Association of Histamine N-Methyltransferase Thr105Ile Polymorphism with Parkinson's Disease and Schizophrenia in Han Chinese: A Case-Control Study. Wu Z-Y, ed. *PLoS One*. 2015;10(3):e0119692. doi:10.1371/journal.pone.0119692

35. Lyons JJ, Yu X, Hughes JD, et al. Elevated basal serum tryptase identifies a multisystem disorder associated with increased TPSAB1 copy number. *Nat Genet*. 2016;48(12):1564-1569. doi:10.1038/ng.3696

36. Vitte J. Human mast cell tryptase in biology and medicine. *Mol Immunol*. 2014;63(1):18-24. doi:10.1016/j.molimm.2014.04.001

37. Altmüller J, Haenisch B, Kawalia A, et al. Mutational profiling in the peripheral blood leukocytes of patients with systemic mast cell activation syndrome using next-generation sequencing. *Immunogenetics*. 2017;69(6):359-369. doi:10.1007/s00251-017-0981-y

38. Epigenetics: Fundamentals, History, and Examples | What is Epigenetics? https://www.whatisepigenetics.com/fundamentals/. Accessed July 20, 2018.

39. Kresser C. RHR: Methylation 101. https://chriskresser.com/methylation-101/. Published 2015. Accessed July 20, 2018.

40. Haenisch B, Frohlich H, Herms S, Molderings GJ. Evidence for contribution of epigenetic mechanisms in the pathogenesis of systemic mast cell activation disease. *Immunogenetics*. 2014;66(5):287-297. doi:10.1007/s00251-014-0768-3

41. Meglathery S. RCCX and Illness. https://www.rccxandillness.com/. Accessed September 27, 2017.

42. Meglathery S. In-person interview conducted in Tucson, Arizona on 7-25-18.

43. Driscoll D, De A, Doherty C, Ferreira JP, Meglathery S, Pazun J. *The Driscoll Theory Newly Revised: The Cause of POTS in Ehlers-Danlos Syndrome and How to Reverse the Process*. Warnick Publishing; 2015.

44. Naviaux RK. Metabolic features and regulation of the healing cycle—A new model for chronic disease pathogenesis and treatment. *Mitochondrion*. August 2018. doi:10.1016/J.MITO.2018.08.001

45. Afrin L, Self S, Menk J, Lazarchick J. Characterization of mast cell activation syndrome. *Am J Med Sci*. 2017;353(3):207-215.

46. Zenker N, Afrin L. Utilities of various mast cell mediators in diagnosing mast cell activation syndrome. *Blood*. 2015;126:51-74.

47. Zblewski D, Abdelrahman RA, Chen D, Butterfield JH, Tefferi A, Pardanani A. Patient Reported Symptoms and Tryptase Levels in WHO-Defined Systemic Mastocytosis (SM) Versus Mast Cell Activation Syndrome (MCAS) Versus Neither. *Blood*. 2014;124(21).

48. Gonzalez-Quintela A, Vizcaino L, Gude F, et al. Factors influencing serum total tryptase concentrations in a general adult population. *Clin Chem Lab Med*. 2010;48:701-706. doi:10.1515/CCLM.2010.124

49. Fellinger C, Hemmer W, Wohrl S, Sesztak-Greinecker G, Jarisch R, Wantke F. Clinical characteristics and risk profile of patients with elevated baseline serum tryptase. *Allergol Immunopathol (Madr)*. 2014;42:544–552. doi:10.1016/j.aller.2014.05.002

50. Lyons JJ, Sun G, Stone KD, et al. Mendelian inheritance of elevated serum tryptase associated with atopy and connective tissue abnormalities. *J Allergy Clin Immunol*. 2014;133(5):1471-1474. doi:10.1016/j.jaci.2013.11.039

51. Lyons JJ, Yu X, Hughes JD, et al. Elevated basal serum tryptase identifies a multisystem disorder associated with increased TPSAB1 copy number. *Nature genetics*. 2016;48(12):1564.

52. Sabato V, Van De Vijver E, Hagendorens M, et al. Familial hypertryptasemia with associated mast cell activation syndrome. *J Allergy Clin Immunol*. 2014;134(6):1448-1450.e3. doi:10.1016/j.jaci.2014.06.007

53. Sabato V, Chovanec J, Faber M, et al. First identification of an inherited TPSAB1 quintuplication in patient with clonal mast cell disease. *J Clin Immunol*. 2018;1-3.

54. Austen KF, Akin C. Clonal and non-clonal mast cell activation disorders. Clinical Pain Advisor: Oncology Section. 2016. http://www.clinicalpainadvisor.com/oncology/clonal-and-non-clonal-mast-cell-activation-disorders/article/619291/?utm_source=TrendMD&DCMP=OTC-CPA_trendmd&dl=0. Accessed June 23, 2017.

55. Myers A. Everything You Need To Know About Histamine Intolerance - mindbodygreen. Mind Body Green Health. https://www.mindbodygreen.com/0-11175/everything-you-need-to-know-about-histamine-intolerance.html. Accessed July 20, 2018.

56. Lynch B. Histamine Intolerance, MTHFR and Methylation. MTHFR.net. http://mthfr.net/histamine-intolerance-mthfr-and-methylation/2015/06/11/. Published 2015. Accessed July 20, 2018.

57. Pinzer TC, Tietz E, Waldmann E, Schink M, Neurath MF, Zopf Y. Circadian profiling reveals higher histamine plasma levels and lower diamine oxidase serum activities in 24% of patients with suspected histamine intolerance compared to food allergy and controls. *Allergy*. 2018;73(4):949-957. doi:10.1111/all.13361

58. Brockow K, Jofer C, Behrendt H, Ring J. Anaphylaxis in patients with mastocytosis: a study on history, clinical features and risk factors in 120 patients. *Allergy*. 2008;63:226-232. doi:10.1111/j.1398-9995.2007.01569.x

59. Van Anrooij B, Van Der Veer E, De Monchy JGR, et al. Higher mast cell load decreases the risk of Hymenoptera venom-induced anaphylaxis in patients with mastocytosis. *J Allergy Clin Immunol*. 2013;132(1):125-130. doi:10.1016/j.jaci.2012.12.1578

60. Akin C, Scott LM, Kocabas CN, et al. Demonstration of an aberrant mast-cell population with clonal markers in a subset of patients with "idiopathic" anaphylaxis. *Blood*. 2007;110:2331-2333. doi:10.1182/blood-2006-06-028100

61. Bonadonna P, Perbellini O, Passalacqua G, et al. Clonal mast cell disorders in patients with systemic reactions to Hymenoptera stings and increased serum tryptase levels. *J Allergy Clin Immunol*. 2009;123(3):680-686. doi:10.1016/J.JACI.2008.11.018

62. Zanotti R, Lombardo C, Passalacqua G, et al. Clonal mast cell disorders in patients with severe Hymenoptera venom allergy and normal serum tryptase levels. *J Allergy Clin Immunol*. 2015;136(1):135-139. doi:10.1016/j.jaci.2014.11.035

63. Álvarez-Twose I, González de Olano D, Sánchez-Muñoz L, et al. Clinical, biological, and molecular characteristics of clonal mast cell disorders presenting with systemic mast cell activation symptoms. *J Allergy Clin Immunol*. 2010;125:1269-1278. doi:10.1016/j.jaci.2010.02.019

64. Li X, Ehrlich H. *Traditional Chinese Medicine, Western Science, and the Fight Against Allergic Disease*. World Scientific Publishing Co.; 2016.

65. Hamilton MJ, Hornick JL, Akin C, Castells MC, Greenberger NJ. Mast cell activation syndrome: A newly recognized disorder with systemic clinical manifestations. *J Allergy Clin Immunol*. 2011;128(1)(1):147-152. doi:10.1016/j.jaci.2011.04.037

66. Afrin L. Conference round table discussion as part of "Often Seen, Rarely Recognized" continuing education event on 9-16-17. CentraCare Health Plaza. St. Cloud, Minnesota. 2017.

67. Arndt KK, Viswanathan RK, Mathur SK. Clinical Characteristics of Patients in Allergy Clinic with Presumed Diagnosis of Mast Cell Activation Syndrome (MCAS). *J Allergy Clin Immunol*. 2018;141(2):AB50. doi:10.1016/J.JACI.2017.12.162

68. Weiler CR, Alhurani RE, Butterfield JH, Divekar R. Systemic Mastocytosis (SM) and Mast Cell Activation Syndrome (MCAS); How Do They Differ? *J Allergy Clin Immunol*. 2018;141(2):AB275. doi:10.1016/j.jaci.2017.12.875

69. Russell N, Jennings S, Jennings B, et al. The Mastocytosis Society Survey on Mast Cell Disorders: Part 2- Patient Clinical Experiences and Beyond. *J allergy Clin Immunol Pract*. 2018. doi:10.1016/j.jaip.2018.07.032

70. Hamilton M. Phone interview conducted on 6-22-18.

71. Lee D, Mueller E. Mast Cell Activation Features in Ehlers-Danlos/Joint Hypermobility Patients: A Retrospective Analysis in Light of an Emerging Disease Cluster [abstract]. *Arthritis Rheumatol*. 2017;69(suppl 10). https://acrabstracts.org/abstract/mast-cell-activation-features-in-ehlers-danlosjoint-hypermobility-patients-a-retrospective-analysis-in-light-of-an-emerging-disease-cluster/. Accessed September 19, 2018.

72. Afrin L. In-person interview conducted in St. Cloud, Minnesota on 9-16-17.

References Chapter 5: Many Systems, One Diagnosis

1. Bot I, Shi G-P, Kovanen PT. Mast cells as effectors in atherosclerosis. Arterioscler Thromb Vasc Biol. 2015 February ; 35(2): 265–271. doi:10.1161/ATVBAHA.114.303570

2. Alfter K, von Kügelgen I, Haenisch B, et al. New aspects of liver abnormalities as part of the systemic mast cell activation syndrome. *Liver Int.* 2009;29(2):181-186. doi:10.1111/j.1478-3231.2008.01839.x

3. Arac A, Grimbaldeston MA, Nepomuceno ARB, et al. Evidence that meningeal mast cells can worsen stroke pathology in mice. *Am J Pathol.* 2014;184(9):2493-2504. doi:10.1016/j.ajpath.2014.06.003

4. Solmazgul E, Kutlu A, Dogru S, et al. Anaphylactic reactions presenting with hypertension. *Springerplus.* 2016;5:12-23. doi:10.1186/s40064-016-2913-y

5. Shibao C, Arzubiaga C, Roberts ILJ, et al. Hyperadrenergic postural tachycardia syndrome in mast cell activation disorders. *Hypertension.* 2005;45(3):385-390. doi:http://dx.doi.org/10.1161/01.HYP.0000158259.68614.40

6. Raj SR. The Postural Tachycardia Syndrome (POTS): pathophysiology, diagnosis & management. *Indian Pacing Electrophysiol J.* 2006;6(2):84-99. http://www.ncbi.nlm.nih.gov/pubmed/16943900. Accessed July 20, 2018.

7. Afrin LB. *Never Bet Against Occam: Mast Cell Activation Disease and the Modern Epidemics of Chronic Illness and Medical Complexity.* Bethesda, Maryland: Sisters Media; 2016.

8. Steinsvoll S, Helgeland K, Schenck K. Mast cells--a role in periodontal diseases? *J Clin Periodontol.* 2004;31(6):413-419. doi:10.1111/j.1600-051X.2004.00516.x

9. Batista AC, Rodini CO, Lara VS. Quantification of mast cells in different stages of human periodontal disease. *Oral Dis.* 2005. doi:10.1111/j.1601-0825.2005.01113.x

10. Divoux A, Moutel S, Poitou C, et al. Mast cells in human adipose tissue: link with morbid obesity, inflammatory status, and diabetes. *J Clin Endocrinol Metab.* 2012;97(9):E1677–E1685. doi:10.1210/jc.2012-1532

11. Zhang J, Shi G-P. Mast cells and metabolic syndrome. *Biochim Biophys Acta.* 2012;1822:14-20. doi:10.1016/j.bbadis.2010.12.012

12. Donath MY, Shoelson SE. Type 2 diabetes as an inflammatory disease. *Nat Rev Immunol.* 2011;11(2). doi:10.1038/nri2925

13. Tellechea A, Leal EC, Kafanas A, et al. Mast cells regulate wound healing in diabetes. *Diabetes.* 2016;65(7):2006-2019. doi:10.2337/db15-0340

14. Geoffrey R, Jia S, Kwitek AE, et al. Evidence of a functional role for mast cells in the development of type 1 diabetes mellitus in the BioBreeding rat. *J Immunol.* 2006;177:7275-7286. doi:10.4049/jimmunol.177.10.7275

15. Bottini N, Fontana L. Asthma and diabetes. *Lancet.* 1999;354:515–516.

16. Cavalher-Machado SC, de Lima WT, Damazo a S, et al. Down-regulation of mast cell activation and airway reactivity in diabetic rats: role of insulin. *Eur Respir J.* 2004;24(4):552-558. doi:10.1183/09031936.04.00130803

17. Carvalho VF, Barreto EO, Diaz BL, et al. Systemic anaphylaxis is prevented in alloxan-diabetic rats by a mechanism dependent on glucocorticoids. *Eur J Pharmacol.* 2003;472(3):221-227. doi:10.1016/S0014-2999(03)01934-4

18. Siebenhaar F, Kühn W, Zuberbier T, Maurer M. Successful treatment of cutaneous mastocytosis and Ménière disease with anti-IgE therapy. *J Allergy Clin Immunol.* 2007;120(1):213-215. doi:10.1016/j.jaci.2007.05.011

19. Afrin LB. Personal email correspondence on October 3rd, 2018.

20. Elieh Ali Komi D, Rambasek T, Bielory L. Clinical implications of mast cell involvement in allergic conjunctivitis. *Allergy.* 2018;73(3):528-539. doi:10.1111/all.13334

21. Chang L, Wong T, Ohbayashi M, et al. Increased mast cell numbers in the conjunctiva of glaucoma patients: a possible indicator of preoperative glaucoma surgery inflammation. *Eye.* 2009;23(9):1859-1865. doi:10.1038/eye.2008.330

22. Lee CH, Lang LS, Orr EL. Changes in ocular mast cell numbers and histamine distribution during experimental autoimmune uveitis. *Reg Immunol.* 1993;5(2):106-113. http://www.ncbi.nlm.nih.gov/pubmed/8217552. Accessed July 20, 2018.

23. Bianco AC, Nunes MT, Douglas CR. Influence of mast cells on thyroid function. *Endocrinol Exp.* 1983;17(2):99-106. http://www.ncbi.nlm.nih.gov/pubmed/6411454. Accessed July 20, 2018.

24. Baccari GC, Monteforte R, Pinelli C, Santillo A, Polese G, Rastogi RK. Thyroid Status Can Influence Brain Mast Cell Population. *Ann N Y Acad Sci.* 2009;1163(1):369-371. doi:10.1111/j.1749-6632.2008.03656.x

25. Rojas J, José Calvo Delgado M, Chávez C, et al. *Mast Cell Activation Disease Associated with Autoimmune Thyroid Disease: Case Report and Review of Literature Abstract.* https://search.proquest.com/openview/80710b354d4241277a0af33246106b24/1?pq-origsite=gscholar&cbl=1216408. Accessed September 21, 2018.

26. Benucci M, Bettazzi C, Bracci S, et al. Systemic mastocytosis with skeletal involvement: a case report and review of the literature. *Clin Cases Miner Bone Metab.* 2009;6(1):66-70. http://www.ncbi.nlm.nih.gov/pubmed/22461100. Accessed September 21, 2018.

27. Guo N, Baglole CJ, O'Loughlin CW, Feldon SE, Phipps RP. Mast Cell-derived Prostaglandin D$_2$ Controls Hyaluronan Synthesis in Human Orbital Fibroblasts via DP1 Activation. *J Biol Chem*. 2010;285(21):15794-15804. doi:10.1074/jbc.M109.074534

28. Khong JJ, McNab AA, Ebeling PR, Craig JE, Selva D. Pathogenesis of thyroid eye disease: review and update on molecular mechanisms. *Br J Ophthalmol*. 2016;100(1):142-150. doi:10.1136/bjophthalmol-2015-307399

29. Rumbyrt JS, Schocket AL. Chronic urticaria and thyroid disease. *Immunol Allergy Clin North Am*. 2004;24(2):215-223. doi:10.1016/j.iac.2004.01.009

30. Leznoff A, Sussman GL. Syndrome of idiopathic chronic urticaria and angioedema with thyroid autoimmunity: a study of 90 patients. *J Allergy Clin Immunol*. 1989;84(1):66-71. http://www.ncbi.nlm.nih.gov/pubmed/2754146. Accessed September 21, 2018.

31. Rottem M. Chronic urticaria and autoimmune thyroid disease: is there a link? *Autoimmun Rev*. 2003;2(2):69-72. http://www.ncbi.nlm.nih.gov/pubmed/12848961. Accessed September 21, 2018.

32. Musilli C, De Siena G, Manni ME, et al. Histamine mediates behavioural and metabolic effects of 3-iodothyroacetic acid, an endogenous end product of thyroid hormone metabolism. *Br J Pharmacol*. 2014;171(14):3476-3484. doi:10.1111/bph.12697

33. Edwards O, Yakish ED, Wang L-M, Wu Q, Hoffman JM, Morton KA. Histamine Receptor 1 and 2 Antagonists Alter Biodistribution of Radioiodine. *J Nucl Med Technol*. 2015;43(3):214-219. doi:10.2967/jnmt.115.160697

34. Melillo RM, Guarino V, Avilla E, et al. Mast cells have a protumorigenic role in human thyroid cancer. *Oncogene*. 2010;29(47):6203-6215. doi:10.1038/onc.2010.348

35. Theoharides TC. Neuroendocrinology of mast cells: Challenges and controversies. *Exp Dermatol*. 2017;26(9):751-9. doi:10.1111/exd.13288

36. Bugajski AJ, Chłap Z, Gadek-Michalska, Bugajski J. Effect of isolation stress on brain mast cells and brain histamine levels in rats. *Agents Actions*. 1994;41:C75-6. http://www.ncbi.nlm.nih.gov/pubmed/7526664. Accessed July 20, 2018.

37. Cirulli F, Pistillo L, de Acetis L, Alleva E, Aloe L. Increased Number of Mast Cells in the Central Nervous System of Adult Male Mice Following Chronic Subordination Stress. *Brain Behav Immun*. 1998;12(2):123-133. doi:10.1006/brbi.1998.0505

38. Nautiyal KM, Ribeiro AC, Pfaff DW, Silver R. Brain mast cells link the immune system to anxiety-like behavior. *Proceedings of the National Academy of Sciences*. 2008;105(46):18053-18057.

39. Theoharides TC, Alysandratos KD, Angelidou A, et al. Mast cells and inflammation. *Biochim Biophys Acta - Mol Basis Dis*. 2012;1822:21-33. doi:10.1016/j.bbadis.2010.12.014

40. Hamilton MJ, Hornick JL, Akin C, Castells MC, Greenberger NJ. Mast cell activation syndrome: A newly recognized disorder with systemic clinical manifestations. *J Allergy Clin Immunol*. 2011;128(1)(1):147-152. doi:10.1016/j.jaci.2011.04.037

41. Barbara G, Stanghellini V, de giorgio R, Corinaldesi R. Functional gastrointestinal disorders and mast cells: implications for therapy. *Neurogastroenterol Motil*. 2006;18(1):6-17. doi:10.1111/j.1365-2982.2005.00685.x

42. Barbara G, De Giorgio R, Stanghellini V, Cremon C, Corinaldesi R. A role for inflammation in irritable bowel syndrome? *Gut*. 2002;51(Suppl 1):i41-4. doi:10.1136/GUT.51.SUPPL_1.I41

43. Weinstock LB, Klutke CG, Lin HC. Small Intestinal Bacterial Overgrowth in Patients with Interstitial Cystitis and Gastrointestinal Symptoms. *Dig Dis Sci*. 2008;53(5):1246-1251. doi:10.1007/s10620-007-0022-z

44. McCarthy DO, Daun JM. The role of prostaglandins in interleukin-1 induced gastroparesis. *Physiol Behav*. 1992;52(2):351-353. http://www.ncbi.nlm.nih.gov/pubmed/1523264. Accessed July 20, 2018.

45. Hasler WL, Soudah HC, Dulai G, Owyang C. Mediation of hyperglycemia-evoked gastric slow-wave dysrhythmias by endogenous prostaglandins. *Gastroenterology*. 1995;108(3):727-736. http://www.ncbi.nlm.nih.gov/pubmed/7875475. Accessed July 20, 2018.

46. Doi H, Sakakibara R, Sato M, et al. Nizatidine ameliorates gastroparesis in Parkinson's disease: a pilot study. *Mov Disord*. 2014;29(4):562-566. doi:10.1002/mds.25777

47. Jakate S, Demeo M, John R, Tobin M, Keshavarzian A. Mastocytic enterocolitis: increased mucosal mast cells in chronic intractable diarrhea. Arch Pathol Lab Med. 2006;130:362–367. doi: 10.1043/1543-2165(2006)130[362:MEIMMC]2.0.CO;2.

48. Farhadi A, Fields J-Z, Keshavarzian A. Mucosal mast cells are pivotal elements in inflammatory bowel disease that connect the dots: stress, intestinal hyperpermeability and inflammation. *World J Gastroenterol*. 2007;13(22):3027-3030. doi:10.3748/WJG.V13.I22.3027

49. Cianferoni A, Spergel J. Eosinophilic Esophagitis: A Comprehensive Review. *Clin Rev Allergy Immunol*. 2016;50(2):159-174. doi:10.1007/s12016-015-8501-z

50. Arias Á, Lucendo AJ, Martínez-Fernández P, et al. Dietary treatment modulates mast cell phenotype, density, and activity in adult eosinophilic oesophagitis. *Clin Exp Allergy*. 2016;46(1):78-91. doi:10.1111/cea.12504

51. Kirchhoff D, Kaulfuss S, Fuhrmann U, Maurer M, Zollner TM. Mast cells in endometriosis: guilty or innocent bystanders? *Expert Opin Ther Targets*. 2012;16(3):237-241. doi:10.1517/14728222.2012.661415

52. Hart DA. Curbing Inflammation in Multiple Sclerosis and Endometriosis: Should Mast Cells Be Targeted? *Int J Inflam*. 2015:1-10. doi:10.1155/2015/452095

53. Anaf V, Chapron C, Elnakadi I, Demoor V, Simonart T, Noel J. Pain, mast cells, and nerves in peritoneal, ovarian, and deep infiltrating endometriosis. *Fertil Steril*. 2006;86(5):1336-1343. doi:10.1016/j.fertnstert.2006.03.057

54. Kempuraj D, Papadopoulou N, Stanford EJ, et al. Increased Numbers of Activated Mast Cells in Endometriosis Lesions Positive for Corticotropin-Releasing Hormone and Urocortin. *Am J Reprod Immunol*. 2004;52(4):267-275. doi:10.1111/j.1600-0897.2004.00224.x

55. Fujiwara H, Konno R, Netsu S, et al. Localization of Mast Cells in Endometrial Cysts. *Am J Reprod Immunol*. 2004;51(5):341-344. doi:10.1111/j.1600-0897.2004.00166.x

56. Zhu T-H, Ding S-J, Li T-T, Zhu L-B, Huang X-F, Zhang X-M. Estrogen is an important mediator of mast cell activation in ovarian endometriomas. *Reproduction*. 2018;155(1):73-83. doi:10.1530/REP-17-0457

57. French LM, Bhambore N. Interstitial cystitis/painful bladder syndrome. *Am Fam Physician*. 2011;83(10):1175-1181. http://www.ncbi.nlm.nih.gov/pubmed/21568251. Accessed July 20, 2018.

58. Ratner V. Mast cell activation syndrome. *Transl Androl Urol*. 2015;4(5):587-588. doi:10.3978/j.issn.2223-4683.2015.09.03

59. Wilhelm M, King B, Silverman A-J, Silver R. Gonadal Steroids Regulate the Number and Activational State of Mast Cells in the Medial Habenula [1]. *Endocrinology*. 2000;141(3):1178-1186. doi:10.1210/endo.141.3.7352

60. Yang M, Chien C, Lu K. Morphological, immunohistochemical and quantitative studies of murine brain mast cells after mating. *Brain Res*. 1999;846(1):30-39. http://www.ncbi.nlm.nih.gov/pubmed/10536211. Accessed July 20, 2018.

61. Asarian L, Yousefzadeh E, Silverman A-J, Silver R. Stimuli from conspecifics influence brain mast cell population in male rats. *Horm Behav*. 2002;42(1):1-12. http://www.ncbi.nlm.nih.gov/pubmed/12191642. Accessed July 20, 2018.

62. Donoso AO, Broitman ST. Effects of a histamine synthesis inhibitor and antihistamines on the sexual behavior of female rats. *Psychopharmacology (Berl)*. 1979;66(3):251-255. http://www.ncbi.nlm.nih.gov/pubmed/43551. Accessed July 20, 2018.

63. Ikarashi Y, Yuzurihara M. Experimental anxiety induced by histaminergics in mast cell-deficient and congenitally normal mice. *Pharmacol Biochem Behav*. 2002;72(1-2):437-441. http://www.ncbi.nlm.nih.gov/pubmed/11900817. Accessed August 9, 2018.

64. Devidze N, Lee AW, Zhou J, Pfaff DW. CNS arousal mechanisms bearing on sex and other biologically regulated behaviors. *Physiol Behav*. 2006;88(3):283-293. doi:10.1016/j.physbeh.2006.05.030

65. Meston CM, Frohlich PF. The neurobiology of sexual function. *Arch Gen Psychiatry*. 2000;57(11):1012-1030. http://www.ncbi.nlm.nih.gov/pubmed/11074867. Accessed August 9, 2018.

66. Rudolph MI, Oviedo C, Vega E, et al. Oxytocin inhibits the uptake of serotonin into uterine mast cells. *J Pharmacol Exp Ther*. 1998;287(1):389-394. http://www.ncbi.nlm.nih.gov/pubmed/9765360. Accessed August 9, 2018.

67. Theoharides TC, Stewart JM. Genitourinary mast cells and survival. *Transl Androl Urol*. 2015;4(5):579-586. doi:10.3978/j.issn.2223-4683.2015.10.04

68. Done JD, Rudick CN, Quick ML, Schaeffer AJ, Thumbikat P. Role of mast cells in male chronic pelvic pain. *J Urol*. 2012;187(4):1473-1482. doi:10.1016/j.juro.2011.11.116

69. Dickerson LM, Mazyck PJ, Hunter MH. Premenstrual syndrome. *Am Fam Physician*. 2003;67(8):1743-1752. http://www.ncbi.nlm.nih.gov/pubmed/12725453. Accessed August 9, 2018.

70. Menzies FM, Shepherd MC, Nibbs RJ, Nelson SM. The role of mast cells and their mediators in reproduction, pregnancy and labour. *Hum Reprod Update*. 2011;17(3):383-396. doi:10.1093/humupd/dmq053

71. Jin X, Zhao W, Kirabo A, et al. Elevated Levels of Mast Cells Are Involved in Pruritus Associated with Polycythemia Vera in JAK2V617F Transgenic Mice. *J Immunol*. 2014;193(2):477-484. doi:10.4049/jimmunol.1301946

72. Vincent L, Vang D, Nguyen J, et al. Mast cell activation contributes to sickle cell pathobiology and pain in mice. *Blood*. 2013;122(11):1853-1862. doi:10.1182/blood-2013-04-498105

73. Afrin LB. Mast cell activation syndrome as a significant comorbidity in sickle cell disease. *Am J Med Sci*. 2014;348(6):460-464. doi:10.1097/MAJ.0000000000000325

74. Cara DC, Ebbert KVJ, McCafferty D-M. Mast cell-independent mechanisms of immediate hypersensitivity: a role for platelets. *J Immunol*. 2004;172(8):4964-4971. http://www.ncbi.nlm.nih.gov/pubmed/15067077. Accessed August 9, 2018.

75. Kasperska-Zając A, Rogala B. Platelet function in anaphylaxis. *J Investig Allergol Clin Immunol*. 2006;16(1):1-4. http://www.ncbi.nlm.nih.gov/pubmed/16599241. Accessed August 9, 2018.

76. Roizen G, Peruffo C, Maitland AL. Mast Cell Activation Disorders In The Setting Of Idiopathic CD4 Lymphopenia. *J Allergy Clin Immunol*. 2018;141(2):AB23. doi:10.1016/J.JACI.2017.12.072

77. Pappa CA, Tsirakis G, Stavroulaki E, et al. Mast Cells Influence the Proliferation Rate of Myeloma Plasma Cells. *Cancer Invest*. 2015;33(4):137-141. doi:10.3109/07357907.2015.1008639

78. Vyzoukaki R, Tsirakis G, Pappa CA, Devetzoglou M, Tzardi M, Alexandrakis MG. The Impact of Mast Cell Density on the Progression of Bone Disease in Multiple Myeloma Patients. *Int Arch Allergy Immunol*. 2015;168(4):263-268. doi:10.1159/000443275

79. Filanovsky K, Lev S, Haran M, et al. Systemic mastocytosis associated with smoldering multiple myeloma: an unexpected diagnosis in a patient with a rash. *Leuk Lymphoma*. 2010;51(6):1152-1154. doi:10.3109/10428191003743452

80. Devetzoglou M, Vyzoukaki R, Kokonozaki M, et al. High density of tryptase-positive mast cells in patients with multiple myeloma: correlation with parameters of disease activity. *Tumor Biol*. 2015;36(11):8491-8497. doi:10.1007/s13277-015-3586-9

81. Douaiher J, Succar J, Lancerotto L, et al. Development of mast cells and importance of their tryptase and chymase serine proteases in inflammation and wound healing. *Adv Immunol*. 2014;122:211-252. doi:10.1016/B978-0-12-800267-4.00006-7

82. Navi D, Saegusa J, Liu F-T. Mast cells and immunological skin diseases. *Clin Rev Allergy Immunol*. 2007;33(1-2):144-155. doi:10.1007/s12016-007-0029-4

83. Mashiko S, Bouguermouh S, Rubio M, Baba N, Bissonnette R, Sarfati M. Human mast cells are major IL-22 producers in patients with psoriasis and atopic dermatitis. *J Allergy Clin Immunol*. 2015;136(2):351-359.e1. doi:10.1016/j.jaci.2015.01.033

84. Muto Y, Wang Z, Vanderberghe M, Two A, Gallo RL, Di Nardo A. Mast cells are key mediators of cathelicidin-initiated skin inflammation in rosacea. *J Invest Dermatol*. 2014;134(11):2728-2736. doi:10.1038/jid.2014.222

85. Lin AM, Rubin CJ, Khandpur R, et al. Mast cells and neutrophils release IL-17 through extracellular trap formation in psoriasis. *J Immunol*. 2011;187(1):490-500. doi:10.4049/jimmunol.1100123

86. Toruniowa B, Jabłońska S. Mast cells in the initial stages of psoriasis. *Arch Dermatol Res*. 1988;280(4):189-193. http://www.ncbi.nlm.nih.gov/pubmed/3233011. Accessed August 9, 2018.

87. Afrin L. Mast Cell Activation Disease: Basic Concepts. In: Discussion in PowerPoint Presentation in "Often Seen, Rarely Recognized" Conference on 9-16-17 in St. Cloud, Minnesota.

88. Schor J. The Multifaceted Role of Mast Cells in Cancer. *Nat Med J*. 2011;3(2). https://www.naturalmedicinejournal.com/journal/2011-02/multifaceted-role-mast-cells-cancer. Accessed August 9, 2018.

89. Skwarczynski M, Tóth I. *Micro- and Nanotechnology in Vaccine Development*. Elsevier. 2017. Page 92.

90. Theoharides TC, Asadi S, Patel AB. Focal brain inflammation and autism. *J Neuroinflammation*. 2013;10(1):815. doi:10.1186/1742-2094-10-46

91. Theoharides TC. Autism Spectrum Disorders and Mastocytosis. *Int J Immunopathol Pharmacol*. 2009;22(4):859-865. doi:10.1177/039463200902200401

92. Hendriksen E, van Bergeijk D, Oosting RS, Redegeld FA. Mast cells in neuroinflammation and brain disorders. *Neurosci Biobehav Rev*. 2017;79:119-133. doi:10.1016/j.neubiorev.2017.05.001

93. Butterfield J, Weiler C. Whole bood serotonin levels in cutaneous mastocytosis, systemic mastocytosis and mast cell activation syndrome. *J Allergy Clin Immunol*. 2011;127:AB132. doi:10.1016/j.jaci.2010.12.528

94. Ito C. The role of brain histamine in acute and chronic stresses. *Biomed Pharmacother*. 2000;54(5):263-267. doi:10.1016/S0753-3322(00)80069-4

95. Llorca P-M, Spadone C, Sol O, et al. Efficacy and safety of hydroxyzine in the treatment of generalized anxiety disorder: a 3-month double-blind study. *J Clin Psychiatry*. 2002;63(11):1020-1027. http://www.ncbi.nlm.nih.gov/pubmed/12444816. Accessed August 9, 2018.

96. Metabolic Syndrome. National Heart, Lung, and Blood Institute (NHLBI). https://www.nhlbi.nih.gov/health-topics/metabolic-syndrome. Accessed August 9, 2018.

97. Chiappetta N, Gruber B. The Role of Mast Cells in Osteoporosis. *Semin Arthritis Rheum*. 2006;36(1):32-36. doi:10.1016/j.semarthrit.2006.03.004

98. Johansson C, Roupe G, Lindstedt G, Mellström D. Bone density, bone markers and bone radiological features in mastocytosis. *Age Ageing*. 1996;25(1):1-7. http://www.ncbi.nlm.nih.gov/pubmed/8670521. Accessed August 9, 2018.

99. Rossini M, Zanotti R, Viapiana O, et al. Bone Involvement and Osteoporosis in Mastocytosis. *Immunol Allergy Clin North Am*. 2014;34(2):383-396. doi:10.1016/j.iac.2014.01.011

100. Lee JHP, Sharma N, Young S, et al. Aberrant mast cell activation promotes chronic recurrent multifocal osteomyelitis. *bioRxiv*. February 2018:259275. doi:10.1101/259275

101. de Lange-Brokaar BJE, Ioan-Facsinay A, Yusuf E, et al. Association of Pain in Knee Osteoarthritis With Distinct Patterns of Synovitis. *Arthritis Rheumatol*. 2015;67(3):733-740. doi:10.1002/art.38965

102. Elias-Jones CJ, Farrow L, Reilly JH, et al. Inflammation and Neovascularization in Hip Impingement. *Am J Sports Med*. 2015;43(8):1875-1881. doi:10.1177/0363546515588176

103. Tüfek A, Kaya S, Tokgöz O, et al. The protective effect of dexmedetomidine on bupivacaine-induced sciatic nerve inflammation is mediated by mast cells. *Clin Invest Med*. 2013;36(2):E95-102. http://www.ncbi.nlm.nih.gov/pubmed/23544611. Accessed August 9, 2018.

104. Brisby H, Olmarker K, Larsson K, Nutu M, Rydevik B. Proinflammatory cytokines in cerebrospinal fluid and serum in patients with disc herniation and sciatica. *Eur Spine J*. 2002;11(1):62-66. doi:10.1007/S005860100306

489

105. Ma W, Eisenach JC. Four PGE2 EP receptors are up-regulated in injured nerve following partial sciatic nerve ligation. *Exp Neurol*. 2003;183(2):581-592. http://www.ncbi.nlm.nih.gov/pubmed/14552899. Accessed August 9, 2018.

106. Freemont AJ, Jeziorska M, Hoyland JA, Rooney P, Kumar S. Mast cells in the pathogenesis of chronic back pain: a hypothesis. *J Pathol*. 2002;197(3):281-285. doi:10.1002/path.1107

107. Lindenlaub T, Sommer C. Partial sciatic nerve transection as a model of neuropathic pain: a qualitative and quantitative neuropathological study. *Pain*. 2000;89(1):97-106. http://www.ncbi.nlm.nih.gov/pubmed/11113298. Accessed August 9, 2018.

108. Scholz J, Woolf CJ. The neuropathic pain triad: neurons, immune cells and glia. *Nat Neurosci*. 2007;10(11):1361-1368. doi:10.1038/nn1992

109. Monk KR, Wu J, Williams JP, et al. Mast cells can contribute to axon-glial dissociation and fibrosis in peripheral nerve. *Neuron Glia Biol*. 2007;3(3):233-244. doi:10.1017/S1740925X08000021

110. Li X, Ehrlich H. *Traditional Chinese Medicine, Western Science, and the Fight Against Allergic Disease*. World Scientific Publishing Co.; 2015.

111. Luzgina NG, Potapova O V, Shkurupiy VA. Structural and functional peculiarities of mast cells in undifferentiated connective tissue dysplasia. *Bull Exp Biol Med*. 2011;150(6):676-678. http://www.ncbi.nlm.nih.gov/pubmed/22235414. Accessed August 9, 2018.

112. Behzad H, Sharma A, Mousavizadeh R, Lu A, Scott A. Mast cells exert pro-inflammatory effects of relevance to the pathophyisology of tendinopathy. *Arthritis Res Ther*. 2013;15(6):R184. doi:10.1186/ar4374

113. Millar NL, Hueber AJ, Reilly JH, et al. Inflammation is Present in Early Human Tendinopathy. *Am J Sports Med*. 2010;38(10):2085-2091. doi:10.1177/0363546510372613

114. Pingel J, Wienecke J, Kongsgaard M, et al. Increased mast cell numbers in a calcaneal tendon overuse model. *Scand J Med Sci Sports*. 2013;23(6):e353-60. doi:10.1111/sms.12089

115. Neeck G. Pathogenic mechanisms of fibromyalgia. *Ageing Res Rev*. 2002;1(2):243-255. http://www.ncbi.nlm.nih.gov/pubmed/12039441. Accessed August 9, 2018.

116. Lucas HJ, Brauch CM, Settas L, Theoharides TC. Fibromyalgia--new concepts of pathogenesis and treatment. *Int J Immunopathol Pharmacol*. 19(1):5-10. http://www.ncbi.nlm.nih.gov/pubmed/16569342. Accessed August 9, 2018.

117. Eneström S, Bengtsson A, Frödin T. Dermal IgG deposits and increase of mast cells in patients with fibromyalgia--relevant findings or epiphenomena? *Scand J Rheumatol*. 1997;26(4):308-313. http://www.ncbi.nlm.nih.gov/pubmed/9310112. Accessed August 9, 2018.

118. Ang DC, Hilligoss J, Stump T. Mast Cell Stabilizer (Ketotifen) in Fibromyalgia: Phase 1 Randomized Controlled Clinical Trial. *Clin J Pain*. 2015;31(9):836-842. doi:10.1097/AJP.0000000000000169

119. Theoharides TC, Bielory L. Mast cells and mast cell mediators as targets of dietary supplements. *Ann Allergy Asthma Immunol*. 2004;93(2 Suppl 1):S24-34. http://www.ncbi.nlm.nih.gov/pubmed/15330009. Accessed August 9, 2018.

120. Lin JT, Lachmann E, Nagler W. Low back pain and myalgias in acute and relapsed mast cell leukemia: a case report. *Arch Phys Med Rehabil*. 2002;83(6):860-863. http://www.ncbi.nlm.nih.gov/pubmed/12048668. Accessed August 9, 2018.

121. Theoharides TC. Mast cells: the immune gate to the brain. *Life Sci*. 1990;46(9):607-617. http://www.ncbi.nlm.nih.gov/pubmed/2407920. Accessed August 9, 2018.

122. Adams S, Dorris S. Urticaria Pigmentosa and Epilepsy... Or is it something more? *of Aller Asthm Immunol*. 2017;119(5):S85.

123. Pehlivanidis C, Fotoulaki M, Boucher W, et al. Acute stress-induced seizures and loss of consciousness in a ten-year-old boy with cutaneous mastocytosis. *J Clin Psychopharmacol*. 2002;22(2):221-224. http://www.ncbi.nlm.nih.gov/pubmed/11910271. Accessed August 9, 2018.

124. Boncoraglio GB, Brucato A, Carriero MR, et al. Systemic mastocytosis: A potential neurologic emergency. *Neurology*. 2005;65(2):332-333. doi:10.1212/01.wnl.0000168897.35545.61

125. Akin C, Scott LM, Metcalfe DD. Slowly progressive systemic mastocytosis with high mast-cell burden and no evidence of a non-mast-cell hematologic disorder: an example of a smoldering case? *Leuk Res*. 2001;25(7):635-638. http://www.ncbi.nlm.nih.gov/pubmed/11377688. Accessed August 9, 2018.

126. Sarrot-Reynauld F, Massot C, Amblard P, et al. Systemic mastocytosis: incidence and risks of vasomotor seizures. *La Rev Med interne*. 1993;14(10):1034. http://www.ncbi.nlm.nih.gov/pubmed/7516568. Accessed August 9, 2018.

127. Krowchuk DP, Williford PM, Jorizzo JL, Kandt RS. Solitary Mastocytoma Producing Symptoms Mimicking Those of a Seizure Disorder. *J Child Neurol*. 1994;9(4):451-453. doi:10.1177/088307389400900428

128. Theoharides TC, Zhang B. Neuro-inflammation, blood-brain barrier, seizures and autism. *J Neuroinflammation*. 2011;8:168. doi:10.1186/1742-2094-8-168

129. Rehni AK, Singh TG, Singh N, Arora S. Tramadol-induced seizurogenic effect: a possible role of opioid-dependent histamine (H1) receptor activation-linked mechanism. *Naunyn Schmiedebergs Arch Pharmacol*. 2010;381(1):11-19. doi:10.1007/s00210-009-0476-y

490

130. Valle-Dorado MG, Santana-Gómez CE, Orozco-Suárez SA, Rocha L. The mast cell stabilizer sodium cromoglycate reduces histamine release and status epilepticus-induced neuronal damage in the rat hippocampus. *Neuropharmacology*. 2015;92:49-55. doi:10.1016/j.neuropharm.2014.12.032

131. Truong DD, Sandroni P, van den Noort S, Matsumoto RR. Diphenhydramine is effective in the treatment of idiopathic dystonia. *Arch Neurol*. 1995;52(4):405-407. http://www.ncbi.nlm.nih.gov/pubmed/7710376. Accessed August 9, 2018.

132. van't Groenewout JL, Stone MR, Vo VN, Truong DD, Matsumoto RR. Evidence for the Involvement of Histamine in the Antidystonic Effects of Diphenhydramine. *Exp Neurol*. 1995;134(2):253-260. doi:10.1006/exnr.1995.1055

133. Phillips A, Hoyte FCL, Leung DYM. Dystonia as an unusual presentation of systemic mastocytosis: Possible link between histamine release and movement disorders. *J Allergy Clin Immunol Pract*. 2018;6(1):269-271.e1. doi:10.1016/j.jaip.2017.06.005

134. Brown RE, Stevens DR, Haas HL. The physiology of brain histamine. *Prog Neurobiol*. 2001;63(6):637-672. http://www.ncbi.nlm.nih.gov/pubmed/11164999. Accessed August 9, 2018.

135. Valko PO, Gavrilov Y V., Yamamoto M, et al. Increase of histaminergic tuberomammillary neurons in narcolepsy. *Ann Neurol*. 2013;74(6):794-804. doi:10.1002/ana.24019

136. Hayaishi O. Molecular mechanisms of sleep-wake regulation: roles of prostaglandins D2 and E2. *FASEB J*. 1991;5(11):2575-2581. http://www.ncbi.nlm.nih.gov/pubmed/1907936. Accessed August 9, 2018.

137. Hayaishi O. Prostaglandins and sleep. *Nihon Rinsho*. 1998;56(2):285-289. http://www.ncbi.nlm.nih.gov/pubmed/9503823. Accessed August 9, 2018.

138. Theoharides TC, Cochrane DE. Critical role of mast cells in inflammatory diseases and the effect of acute stress. *J Neuroimmunol*. 2004;146(1-2):1-12. doi:S0165572803004636 [pii]

139. Haenisch B, Molderings G. White matter abnormalities are also repeatedly present in patients with systemic mast cell activation syndrome. *Transl Psychiatry*. 2018;8(1):95. doi:10.1038/s41398-018-0143-5

140. Afrin LB. Burning mouth syndrome and mast cell activation disorder. *Oral Surgery, Oral Med Oral Pathol Oral Radiol Endodontology*. 2011;111(4):465-472. doi:10.1016/j.tripleo.2010.11.030

141. Afrin L. Mast Cell Activation Disease: Current Concepts. PowerPoint Presentation as Part of Wellapalooza Conference on 4-30-17.

142. Afrin LB. Presentation, diagnosis, and management of mast cell activation syndrome. In: *Mast Cells: Phenotypic Features, Biological Functions and Role in Immunity*. Nova Science Publishers, Inc.; 2013:155-232.

143. Diez-Arias JA, Aller MA, Palma MD, et al. Increased Duodenal Mucosa Infiltration by Mast Cells in Rats with Portal Hypertension. *Dig Surg*. 2001;18(1):34-40. doi:10.1159/000050094

144. Aller M-A, Arias J-L, Arias J. The mast cell integrates the splanchnic and systemic inflammatory response in portal hypertension. *J Transl Med*. 2007;5:44. doi:10.1186/1479-5876-5-44

145. Capron JP, Lebrec D, Degott C, Chivrac D, Coevoet B, Delobel J. Portal hypertension in systemic mastocytosis. *Gastroenterology*. 1978;74(3):595-597. http://www.ncbi.nlm.nih.gov/pubmed/631492. Accessed August 9, 2018.

146. Grundfest S, Cooperman AM, Ferguson R, Benjamin S. Portal hypertension associated with systemic mastocytosis and splenomegaly. *Gastroenterology*. 1980;78(2):370-373. http://www.ncbi.nlm.nih.gov/pubmed/6965282. Accessed August 9, 2018.

147. Esposito I, Friess H, Kappeler A, et al. Mast cell distribution and activation in chronic pancreatitis. *Hum Pathol*. 2001;32(11):1174-1183. http://www.ncbi.nlm.nih.gov/pubmed/11727255. Accessed August 9, 2018.

148. Francis T, Graf A, Hodges K, et al. Histamine regulation of pancreatitis and pancreatic cancer: a review of recent findings. *Hepatobiliary Surg Nutr*. 2013;2(4):216-226. doi:10.3978/j.issn.2304-3881.2013.08.06

149. Lopez-Font I, Gea-Sorlí S, de-Madaria E, Gutiérrez LM, Pérez-Mateo M, Closa D. Pancreatic and pulmonary mast cells activation during experimental acute pancreatitis. *World J Gastroenterol*. 2010;16(27):3411-3417. doi:10.3748/WJG.V16.I27.3411

150. Theoharides TC. Mast Cells and Pancreatic Cancer. *N Engl J Med*. 2008;358(17):1860-1861. doi:10.1056/NEJMcibr0801519

151. Holdsworth SR, Summers SA. Role of Mast Cells in Progressive Renal Diseases. *J Am Soc Nephrol*. 2008;19(12):2254-2261. doi:10.1681/ASN.2008010015

152. Blank U, Essig M, Scandiuzzi L, Benhamou M, Kanamaru Y. Mast cells and inflammatory kidney disease. *Immunol Rev*. 2007;217(1):79-95. doi:10.1111/j.1600-065X.2007.00503.x

153. Abdel-Hafez M, Shimada M, Lee PY, Johnson RJ, Garin EH. Idiopathic nephrotic syndrome and atopy: is there a common link? *Am J Kidney Dis*. 2009;54(5):945-953. doi:10.1053/j.ajkd.2009.03.019

154. Rau B, Friesen CA, Daniel JF, et al. Gallbladder wall inflammatory cells in pediatric patients with biliary dyskinesia and cholelithiasis: a pilot study. *J Pediatr Surg*. 2006;41(9):1545-1548. doi:10.1016/j.jpedsurg.2006.05.015

155. Jennings LJ, Salido GM, Pozo MJ, et al. The source and action of histamine in the isolated guinea-pig gallbladder. *Inflamm Res*. 1995;44(10):447-453. http://www.ncbi.nlm.nih.gov/pubmed/8564521. Accessed August 9, 2018.

156. Freedman SM, Wallace JL, Shaffer EA. Characterization of leukotriene-induced contraction of the guinea-pig gallbladder in vitro. *Can J Physiol Pharmacol*. 1993;71(2):145-150. http://www.ncbi.nlm.nih.gov/pubmed/8391373. Accessed August 9, 2018.

157. Friesen CA, Neilan N, Daniel JF, et al. Mast cell activation and clinical outcome in pediatric cholelithiasis and biliary dyskinesia. *BMC Res Notes*. 2011;4(1):322. doi:10.1186/1756-0500-4-322

158. Theoharides TC, Kalogeromitros D. The critical role of mast cells in allergy and inflammation. *Ann N Y Acad Sci*. 2006;1088(1):78-99. doi:10.1196/annals.1366.025

159. Matsunaga K, Yanagisawa S, Ichikawa T, et al. Airway cytokine expression measured by means of protein array in exhaled breath condensate: Correlation with physiologic properties in asthmatic patients. *J Allergy Clin Immunol*. 2006;118(1):84-90. doi:10.1016/J.JACI.2006.04.020

160. Chipps BE, Lanier B, Milgrom H, et al. Omalizumab in children with uncontrolled allergic asthma: Review of clinical trial and real-world experience. *J Allergy Clin Immunol*. 2017;139(5):1431-1444. doi:10.1016/j.jaci.2017.03.002

161. Abraham I, Alhossan A, Lee CS, Kutbi H, MacDonald K. 'Real-life' effectiveness studies of omalizumab in adult patients with severe allergic asthma: systematic review. *Allergy*. 2016;71(5):593-610. doi:10.1111/all.12815

162. Lai T, Wang S, Xu Z, et al. Long-term efficacy and safety of omalizumab in patients with persistent uncontrolled allergic asthma: a systematic review and meta-analysis. *Sci Rep*. 2015;5(1):8191. doi:10.1038/srep08191

163. Xu X, Zhang D, Lyubynska N, et al. Mast Cells Protect Mice from Mycoplasma Pneumonia. *Am J Respir Crit Care Med*. 2006;173(2):219-225. doi:10.1164/rccm.200507-1034OC

164. Medina JL, Brooks EG, Chaparro A, Dube PH. Mycoplasma pneumoniae CARDS toxin elicits a functional IgE response in Balb/c mice. Balish MF, ed. *PLoS One*. 2017;12(2):e0172447. doi:10.1371/journal.pone.0172447

165. COPD - Symptoms and causes - Mayo Clinic. https://www.mayoclinic.org/diseases-conditions/copd/symptoms-causes/syc-20353679. Accessed August 9, 2018.

166. Wygrecka M, Dahal BK, Kosanovic D, et al. Mast Cells and Fibroblasts Work in Concert to Aggravate Pulmonary Fibrosis: role of transmembrane SCF and the PAR-2/PKC-alpha/Raf-1/p44/42 signaling pathway. *Am J Pathol*. 2013;182(6):2094-2108. doi:10.1016/j.ajpath.2013.02.013

167. Overed-Sayer C, Rapley L, Mustelin T, Clarke DL. Are mast cells instrumental for fibrotic diseases? *Front Pharmacol*. 2013;4:174. doi:10.3389/fphar.2013.00174

168. Molderings GJ, Zienkiewicz T, Homann J, Menzen M, Afrin LB. Risk of solid cancer in patients with mast cell activation syndrome: Results from Germany and USA. *F1000Research*. 2017;6:1889. doi:10.12688/f1000research.12730.1

169. Slipicevic A, Herlyn M. KIT in melanoma: many shades of gray. *J Invest Dermatol*. 2015;135(2):337-338. doi:10.1038/jid.2014.417

170. Phung B, Kazi JU, Lundby A, et al. KITD816V Induces SRC-Mediated Tyrosine Phosphorylation of MITF and Altered Transcription Program in Melanoma. *Mol Cancer Res*. 2017;15(9):1265-1274. doi:10.1158/1541-7786.MCR-17-0149

171. Hägglund H, Sander B, Gülen T, Lindelöf B, Nilsson G. Increased Risk of Malignant Melanoma in Patients with Systemic Mastocytosis? *Acta Derm Venereol*. 2014;94(5):583-584. doi:10.2340/00015555-1788

172. Tóth-Jakatics R, Jimi S, Takebayashi S, Kawamoto N. Cutaneous malignant melanoma: correlation between neovascularization and peritumor accumulation of mast cells overexpressing vascular endothelial growth factor. *Hum Pathol*. 2000;31(8):955-960. http://www.ncbi.nlm.nih.gov/pubmed/10987256. Accessed August 9, 2018.

173. Broesby-Olsen S, Farkas DK, Vestergaard H, et al. Risk of solid cancer, cardiovascular disease, anaphylaxis, osteoporosis and fractures in patients with systemic mastocytosis: A nationwide population-based study. *Am J Hematol*. 2016;91(11):1069-1075. doi:10.1002/ajh.24490

174. Afrin L, Self S, Menk J, Lazarchick J. Characterization of mast cell activation syndrome. *Am J Med Sci*. 2017;353(3):207-215.

175. Molderings GJ, Knüchel-Clarke R, Hertfelder H-J, Kuhl C. Mast Cell Activation Syndrome Mimicking Breast Cancer: Case Report With Pathophysiologic Considerations. *Clin Breast Cancer*. 2018;18(3):e271-e276. doi:10.1016/j.clbc.2017.12.004

176. Ryan JJ, Morales JK, Falanga YT, Fernando JFA, Macey MR. Mast cell regulation of the immune response. *World Allergy Organ J*. 2009;2(10):224-232. doi:10.1097/WOX.0b013e3181c2a95e

177. Galdiero MR, Varricchi G, Seaf M, Marone G, Levi-Schaffer F, Marone G. Bidirectional Mast Cell–Eosinophil Interactions in Inflammatory Disorders and Cancer. *Front Med*. 2017;4:103. doi:10.3389/FMED.2017.00103

178. Heijmans J, Büller NV, Muncan V, van den Brink GR. Role of mast cells in colorectal cancer development, the jury is still out. *Biochim Biophys Acta - Mol Basis Dis*. 2012;1822(1):9-13. doi:10.1016/j.bbadis.2010.12.001

179. Ribatti D, Crivellato E. Mast cells, angiogenesis, and tumour growth. *Biochim Biophys Acta - Mol Basis Dis*. 2012;1822(1):2-8. doi:10.1016/j.bbadis.2010.11.010

180. Menzies FM, Shepherd MC, Nibbs RJ, Nelson SM. The role of mast cells and their mediators in reproduction, pregnancy and labour. *Hum Reprod Update*. 2011;17(3):383-396. doi:10.1093/humupd/dmq053

181. Weinstock LB, Walters AS, Paueksakon P. Restless legs syndrome – Theoretical roles of inflammatory and immune mechanisms. *Sleep Med Rev.* 2012;16(4):341-354. doi:10.1016/j.smrv.2011.09.003

182. The MCS illness makes women allergic to the modern world | Daily Mail Online. http://www.dailymail.co.uk/health/article-5014369/The-illness-makes-women-allergic-modern-world.html#ixzz4weWXRZl5. Accessed August 9, 2018.

183. Multiple Chemical Sensitivity – what is multiple chemical sensitivity. https://www.multiplechemicalsensitivity.org/. Accessed August 9, 2018.

184. The Role of the Brain and Mast Cells in MCS. http://www.tldp.com/issue/210/roleoftheb.htm. Accessed August 9, 2018.

References Chapter 6: Clinical Considerations for Diagnosis

1. Driscoll D, De A, Doherty C, Ferreira JP, Meglathery S, Pazun J. *The Driscoll Theory Newly Revised: The Cause of POTS in Ehlers-Danlos Syndrome and How to Reverse the Process.* Warnick Publishing; 2015.

2. Molderings GJ, Brettner S, Homann J, Afrin LB. Mast cell activation disease: A concise practical guide for diagnostic workup and therapeutic options. *J Hematol Oncol.* 2011;4:10. doi:10.1186/1756-8722-4-10

3. Picard M, Giavina-Bianchi P, Mezzano V, Castells M. Expanding Spectrum of Mast Cell Activation Disorders: Monoclonal and Idiopathic Mast Cell Activation Syndromes. *Clin Ther.* 2013;35(5):548-562. doi:10.1016/J.CLINTHERA.2013.04.001

4. Izikson L, English JC, Zirwas MJ. The flushing patient: Differential diagnosis, workup, and treatment. *J Am Acad Dermatol.* 2006;55(2):193-208. doi:10.1016/J.JAAD.2005.07.057

5. Valent P, Akin C, Arock M, et al. Definitions, criteria and global classification of mast cell disorders with special reference to mast cell activation syndromes: A consensus proposal. *Int Arch Allergy Immunol.* 2012;157(3):215-225. doi:10.1159/000328760

6. Afrin L, Molderings GJ. A concise, practical guide to diagnostic assessment for mast cell activation disease. *World J Hematol.* 2014;3(1):1-7. doi:10.5315

7. Molderings GJ, Haenisch B, Bogdanow M, Fimmers R, Nöthen MM. Familial Occurrence of Systemic Mast Cell Activation Disease. *PLoS One.* 2013;8(9):e76241. doi:10.1371/journal.pone.0076241

8. Molderings GJ. Personal Email Correspondence on October 7th, 2018.

9. Alfter K, von Kügelgen I, Haenisch B, et al. New aspects of liver abnormalities as part of the systemic mast cell activation syndrome. *Liver Int.* 2009;29(2):181-186. doi:10.1111/j.1478-3231.2008.01839.x

10. van Anrooij B, Kluin-Nelemans JC, Safy M, Flokstra-de Blok BMJ, Oude Elberink JNG. Patient-reported disease-specific quality-of-life and symptom severity in systemic mastocytosis. *Allergy.* 2016;71(11):1585-1593. doi:10.1111/all.12920

11. Mazar, Evans E, Taylor F, et al. Development and Content Validity of the Advanced Systemic Mastocytosis Symptom Assessment Form (ADVSM-SAF). *Value Heal.* 2016;19(7):A386. doi:10.1016/j.jval.2016.09.224

12. The Mastocytosis Society. ICD-10-CM Codes for Mast Cell Activation Syndrome and Mastocytosis. https://tmsforacure.org/icd-10-cm/. Published 2017. Accessed September 20, 2018.

13. Theoharides TC, Valent P, Akin C. Mast Cells, Mastocytosis, and Related Disorders. Ingelfinger JR, ed. *N Engl J Med.* 2015;373(2):163-172. doi:10.1056/NEJMra1409760

14. Afrin L. Mast Cell Activation Disease: Basic Concepts. In: Discussion in PowerPoint Presentation in "Often Seen, Rarely Recognized" Conference on 9-16-17 in St. Cloud, Minnesota.

15. Austen KF, Akin C. Clonal and non-clonal mast cell activation disorders. *Clin Pain Advis Oncol Sect.* 2016. http://www.clinicalpainadvisor.com/oncology/clonal-and-non-clonal-mast-cell-activation-disorders/article/619291/?utm_source=TrendMD&DCMP=OTC-CPA_trendmd&dl=0. Accessed June 23, 2017.

16. Butterfield JH, Li CY. Bone Marrow Biopsies for the Diagnosis of Systemic Mastocytosis: Is One Biopsy Sufficient? *Am J Clin Pathol.* 2004;121:264–267. doi:10.1309/2EWQKN00PG02JKY0

17. Quintás-Cardama A, Sever M, Cortes J, Kantarjian H, Verstovsek S. Bone marrow mast cell burden and serum tryptase level as markers of response in patients with systemic mastocytosis. *Leuk Lymphoma.* 2013;54(9):1959-1964. doi:10.3109/10428194.2012.763121

18. Seneviratne SL, Maitland A, Afrin L. Mast cell disorders in Ehlers–Danlos syndrome. *Am J Med Genet Part C Semin Med Genet.* 2017;175(1):226-236. doi:10.1002/ajmg.c.31555

19. Afrin L. In-person interview conducted in St. Cloud, Minnesota on 9-16-17.

20. Soderberg M. The Mast Cell Activation Syndrome: A Mini Review. *MOJ Immunol.* 2015;2(1). doi:10.15406/moji.2015.02.00032

21. Álvarez-Twose I, González de Olano D, Sánchez-Muñoz L, et al. Clinical, biological, and molecular characteristics of clonal mast cell disorders presenting with systemic mast cell activation symptoms. *J Allergy Clin Immunol.* 2010;125:1269-1278. doi:10.1016/j.jaci.2010.02.019

22. Kristensen T, Vestergaard H, Møller MB. Improved detection of the KIT D816V mutation in patients with systemic mastocytosis using a quantitative and highly sensitive real-time qPCR assay. *J Mol Diagnostics*. 2011. doi:10.1016/j.jmoldx.2010.10.004

23. Ratner V. Mast cell activation syndrome. *Transl Androl Urol*. 2015;4(5):587-588. doi:10.3978/j.issn.2223-4683.2015.09.03

24. Afrin L. Mast Cell Activation Syndrome & Autoimmunity: Episode 133 of CoreBrain Journal Podcast with Dr. Charles Parker. https://www.corebrainjournal.com/2017/07/133-mast-cell-activation-syndrome.

25. Afrin LB. Mast cell activation syndrome as a significant comorbidity in sickle cell disease. *Am J Med Sci*. 2014;348(6):460-464. doi:10.1097/MAJ.0000000000000325

26. Vysniauskaite M, Hertfelder HJ, Oldenburg J, et al. Determination of plasma heparin level improves identification of systemic mast cell activation disease. *PLoS One*. 2015. doi:10.1371/journal.pone.0124912

27. Afrin L, Self S, Menk J, Lazarchick J. Characterization of mast cell activation syndrome. *Am J Med Sci*. 2017;353(3):207-215.

28. Afrin L. *Collection of 24-Hour Urine Sample for Mast Cell Mediator Testing*. http://mastcellresearch.com/wp-content/uploads/2016/05/Afrin-Instructions-for-24hr-urine-collection-for-mast-cell-mediator-testing.pdf. Accessed September 22, 2018.

29. Afrin L. Personal email correspondence on October 3rd, 2018.

30. Koyamangalath K. Systemic Mastocytosis. Medscape. http://emedicine.medscape.com/article/203948-workup#showall. Published 2016.

31. Lin RY, Schwartz LB, Curry A, et al. Histamine and tryptase levels in patients with acute allergic reactions: An emergency department–based study. *J Allergy Clin Immunol*. 2000;106(1):65-71. doi:10.1067/mai.2000.107600

32. Ohtsuka T, Matsumaru S, Uchida K, et al. Time course of plasma histamine and tryptase following food challenges in children with suspected food allergy. *Ann Allergy*. 1993;71(2):139-146. http://www.ncbi.nlm.nih.gov/pubmed/8346867. Accessed August 10, 2018.

33. Dua S, Dowey J, Foley L, et al. Diagnostic Value of Tryptase in Food Allergic Reactions: A Prospective Study of 160 Adult Peanut Challenges. *J Allergy Clin Immunol Pract*. 2018;6(5):1692-1698.e1. doi:10.1016/j.jaip.2018.01.006

34. Afrin L. Episode 10 - Understanding Mast Cell Activation Disorder with Dr. Afrin. In: Unbound Healing Podcast by Anne Marie Garland and Michelle Hoover on Apple Podcasts. Aired 8/31/17. https://itunes.apple.com/us/podcast/unbound-healing-podcast/id1253479733?mt=2.

35. Afrin L. Emergency Information - Mast Cell Research. http://mastcellresearch.com/emergency-information/. Accessed August 10, 2018.

36. Bonadonna P, Lombardo C, Zanotti R. Mastocytosis and allergic diseases. *J Investig Allergol Clin Immunol*. 2014;24(5):288-97; quiz 3 p preceding 297.

37. Gülen T, Hägglund H, Dahlén B, Nilsson G. High prevalence of anaphylaxis in patients with systemic mastocytosis - a single-centre experience. *Clin Exp Allergy*. 2014;44(1):121-129. doi:10.1111/cea.12225

38. Sampson HA, Muñoz-Furlong A, Campbell RL, et al. Second Symposium on the Definition and Management of Anaphylaxis: Summary Report—Second National Institute of Allergy and Infectious Disease/Food Allergy and Anaphylaxis Network Symposium. *Ann Emerg Med*. 2006;47(4):373-380. doi:10.1016/j.annemergmed.2006.01.018

39. Campbell RL, Hagan JB, Manivannan V, et al. Evaluation of National Institute of Allergy and Infectious Diseases/Food Allergy and Anaphylaxis Network criteria for the diagnosis of anaphylaxis in emergency department patients. *J Allergy Clin Immunol*. 2012;129(3):748-752. doi:10.1016/j.jaci.2011.09.030

40. Campbell RL, Li JTC, Nicklas RA, Sadosty AT, Members of the Joint Task Force, Practice Parameter Workgroup. Emergency department diagnosis and treatment of anaphylaxis: a practice parameter. *Ann Allergy, Asthma Immunol*. 2014;113(6):599-608. doi:10.1016/j.anai.2014.10.007

41. American College of Asthma A and I. Experts agree: Even if severe allergic reaction is in doubt, epinephrine should be used | Experts agree it's best to use epinephrine in all emergency situations. | ACAAI Public Website. https://acaai.org/news/experts-agree-even-if-severe-allergic-reaction-doubt-epinephrine-should-be-used. Published 2015. Accessed August 10, 2018.

42. Memon S, Chhabra L, Masrur S, Parker MW. Allergic acute coronary syndrome (Kounis syndrome). *Proc (Bayl Univ Med Cent)*. 2015;28(3):358-362. http://www.ncbi.nlm.nih.gov/pubmed/26130889. Accessed August 10, 2018.

43. Coop CA, Schapira RS, Freeman TM. Are ACE Inhibitors and Beta-blockers Dangerous in Patients at Risk for Anaphylaxis? *J Allergy Clin Immunol Pract*. 2017;5(5):1207-1211. doi:10.1016/j.jaip.2017.04.033

44. Stoevesandt J, Hain J, Kerstan A, Trautmann A. Over- and underestimated parameters in severe Hymenoptera venom–induced anaphylaxis: Cardiovascular medication and absence of urticaria/angioedema. *J Allergy Clin Immunol*. 2012;130(3):698-704.e1. doi:10.1016/J.JACI.2012.03.024

45. Lieberman P. Biphasic anaphylactic reactions. *Ann Allergy, Asthma Immunol*. 2005;95(3):217-226. doi:10.1016/S1081-1206(10)61217-3

494

46. Kemp SF, Lockey RF, Simons FER, World Allergy Organization ad hoc Committee on Epinephrine in Anaphylaxis. Epinephrine: the drug of choice for anaphylaxis-a statement of the world allergy organization. *World Allergy Organ J.* 2008;1(7 Suppl):S18-26. doi:10.1097/WOX.0b013e31817c9338

47. Heilborn H, Hjemdahl P, Daleskog M, Adamsson U. Comparison of subcutaneous injection and high-dose inhalation of epinephrine--implications for self-treatment to prevent anaphylaxis. *J Allergy Clin Immunol.* 1986;78(6):1174-1179. http://www.ncbi.nlm.nih.gov/pubmed/3782679. Accessed August 10, 2018.

48. Simons FE, Gu X, Johnston LM, Simons KJ. Can epinephrine inhalations be substituted for epinephrine injection in children at risk for systemic anaphylaxis? *Pediatrics.* 2000;106(5):1040-1044. http://www.ncbi.nlm.nih.gov/pubmed/11061773. Accessed August 10, 2018.

49. Robinson M, Greenhawt M, Stukus DR. Factors associated with epinephrine administration for anaphylaxis in children before arrival to the emergency department. *Ann Allergy, Asthma Immunol.* 2017;119(2):164-169. doi:10.1016/j.anai.2017.06.001

50. Romm A. Overcoming Survival Overdrive Syndrome with Dr. Aviva Romm. In: The Good Life Project Podcast with Jonathan Fields on Apple Podcasts. Aired on 2/5/17. http://www.goodlifeproject.com/podcast/dr-aviva-romm/.

51. Romm A. *The Adrenal Thyroid Revolution: A Proven 4-Week Program to Rescue Your Metabolism, Hormones, Mind & Mood.* Harper Collins; 2017.

52. Horowitz R. *How Can I Get Better: An Action Plan for Treating Resistant Lyme & Chronic Disease.* New York: St. Martin's Griffin; 2017.

53. Forsgren S, Klinghardt D. Kryptopyrroluria (aka Hemopyrrollactamuria): A Major Piece of the Puzzle in Overcoming Chronic Lyme Disease. *Townsend Lett.* 2017:29-37. http://www.townsendletter.com/July2017/krypto0717.html. Accessed August 10, 2018.

54. Klinghardt D. Biotoxins: Supporting removal via intrinsic pathways. In: Ingrid Kohlstadt, ed. *Advancing Medicine with Food and Nutrients.* 2nd edition. Boca Raton, FL: CRC Press; 2012. http://klinghardtinstitute.com/wp-content/uploads/2015/06/1.-Biotoxin-chapter.pdf. Accessed August 10, 2018.

55. Hoffmann K. Cryptopyrroluria–The most common form of porphyria: A typical example of a mitochondrial dysfunction. 1-9. Accessed 3-19-18. http://www.omundernaehrung.com/media/documents/en/Hoffmann_Kyra_Cryptopyrroluria_The_most_common_form_of_porphyria_A_typical_example_of_a_mitochondrial_dysfunction.pdf.

56. Pizzorno J. *The Toxin Solution: How Hidden Poisons in the Air, Water, Food and Products We Use Are Destroying Our Health.* Harper Collins; 2017.

57. Arbuckle J. Severe allergic rhinitis, perennial sinusitis and antihistamine dependence resolved with naturopathic treatment: A case study and short literature review. *Aust J Herb Med.* 2017;29(4):142. www.mediherb.com.au. Accessed August 10, 2018.

58. Hodson Wendy, Hampilos K. Mast Cell Activation Syndrome. Naturopathic Doctor News and Review. April 11, 2016. Accessed March 1, 2018. http://ndnr.com/autoimmuneallergy-medicine/mast-cell-activation-syndrome/.

59. Richmond Natural Medicine. Functional Medicine and Naturopathic Medicine: What's the difference? http://richmondnaturalmed.com/functional-medicine-naturopathic-medicine/. Accessed August 10, 2018.

60. Ducharme N. Functional Medicine Testing - Top 5 General Blood Tests. RestorMedicine. https://restormedicine.com/functional-medicine-testing/. Accessed August 10, 2018.

61. Afrin LB, Khoruts A. Mast Cell Activation Disease and Microbiotic Interactions. *Clin Ther.* 2015;37(5):941-953. doi:10.1016/j.clinthera.2015.02.008

62. Carnahan, J. In-person interview conduction on 1-3-18 in Louisville, Colorado.

63. Snow R. "Mast Cell Activation Syndrome: ID, Explanation and Treatment" presented at the 27th Annual American Herbalists Guild Symposium, September 29 – October 2, 2016, Seven Springs, PA. Accessed February 19, 2018.

64. Bahri R, Custovic A, Korosec P, et al. Mast cell activation test in the diagnosis of allergic disease and anaphylaxis. *J Allergy Clin Immunol.* 2018;142(2):485-496.e16. doi:10.1016/J.JACI.2018.01.043

References Chapter 7: Coexisting Conditions

1. Beighton P, De Paepe A, Steinmann B, Tsipouras P, Wenstrup RJ. Ehlers-Danlos syndromes: revised nosology, Villefranche, 1997. Ehlers-Danlos National Foundation (USA) and Ehlers-Danlos Support Group (UK). *Am J Med Genet.* 1998;77(1):31-37. http://www.ncbi.nlm.nih.gov/pubmed/9557891. Accessed August 31, 2018.

2. Malfait F, Francomano C, Byers P, et al. The 2017 international classification of the Ehlers-Danlos syndromes. *Am J Med Genet C Semin Med Genet.* 2017;175(1):8-26. doi:10.1002/ajmg.c.31552

3. Tilstra D. Ehlers-Danlos Syndrome Hypermobility Type (hEDS). PowerPoint Presentation in "Often Seen, Rarely Recognized" Conference on 9-16-17 in St. Cloud, Minnesota.

4. Lee D, Mueller E. Mast Cell Activation Features in Ehlers-Danlos/Joint Hypermobility Patients: A Retrospective Analysis in Light of an Emerging Disease Cluster [abstract]. *Arthritis Rheumatol.* 2017;69(suppl 10). https://acrabstracts.org/abstract/mast-cell-activation-features-in-ehlers-danlosjoint-hypermobility-patients-a-retrospective-analysis-in-light-of-an-emerging-disease-cluster/. Accessed September 19, 2018.

5. Chopra P. Complex Regional Pain Syndrome (CRPS) Diagnosis and Management. PowerPoint Presentation in "Often Seen, Rarely Recognized" Conference on 9-16-17 in St. Cloud, Minnesota.

6. Henderson FC, Austin C, Benzel E, et al. Neurological and spinal manifestations of the Ehlers-Danlos syndromes. *Am J Med Genet Part C Semin Med Genet.* 2017;175(1):195-211. doi:10.1002/ajmg.c.31549

7. Milhorat TH, Bolognese PA, Nishikawa M, McDonnell NB, Francomano CA. Syndrome of occipitoatlantoaxial hypermobility, cranial settling, and Chiari malformation Type I in patients with hereditary disorders of connective tissue. *J Neurosurg Spine.* 2007;7(6):601-609. doi:10.3171/SPI-07/12/601

8. Mathias CJ, Low DA, Iodice V, Owens AP, Kirbis M, Grahame R. Postural tachycardia syndrome—current experience and concepts. *Nat Rev Neurol.* 2012;8(1):22-34. doi:10.1038/nrneurol.2011.187

9. Raj SR. The Postural Tachycardia Syndrome (POTS): pathophysiology, diagnosis & management. *Indian Pacing Electrophysiol J.* 2006;6(2):84-99. http://www.ncbi.nlm.nih.gov/pubmed/16943900. Accessed July 20, 2018.

10. Klimas L. The MastAttack 107: The Layperson's Guide to Understanding Mast Cell Diseases, Part 31 - Mast Attack. https://www.mastattack.org/2017/06/mastattack-107-laypersons-guide-understanding-mast-cell-diseases-part-31/. Accessed September 22, 2018.

11. Conner R, Sheikh M, Grubb B. Postural Orthostatic Tachycardia Syndrome (POTS): evaluation and management. *Br J Med Pract.* 2012;5(4):12-18. http://go.galegroup.com/ps/anonymous?id=GALE%7CA321462577&sid=googleScholar&v=2.1&it=r&linkaccess=abs&issn=17578515&p=AONE&sw=w. Accessed August 31, 2018.

12. Raj V, Haman KL, Raj SR, et al. Psychiatric profile and attention deficits in postural tachycardia syndrome. *J Neurol Neurosurg Psychiatry.* 2009;80(3):339-344. doi:10.1136/jnnp.2008.144360

13. Raj SR, Garland EM, Biaggioni I, Black BK, Robertson D. Morning heart rate surge in postural tachycardia syndrome. *Circulation.* 2005;112:U810.

14. Raj SR, Biaggioni I, Yamhure PC, et al. Renin-Aldosterone Paradox and Perturbed Blood Volume Regulation Underlying Postural Tachycardia Syndrome. *Circulation.* 2005;111(13):1574-1582. doi:10.1161/01.CIR.0000160356.97313.5D

15. Shibao C, Arzubiaga C, Roberts ILJ, et al. Hyperadrenergic postural tachycardia syndrome in mast cell activation disorders. *Hypertension.* 2005;45(3):385-390. doi:http://dx.doi.org/10.1161/01.HYP.0000158259.68614.40

16. Jacob G, Costa F, Shannon JR, et al. The Neuropathic Postural Tachycardia Syndrome. *N Engl J Med.* 2000;343(14):1008-1014. doi:10.1056/NEJM200010053431404

17. Strasheim C. Chapter One: Wayne Anderson, ND. In: *New Paradigms in Lyme Disease Treatment: 10 Top Doctors Reveal Healing Strategies That Work.* BioMed Publishing Group; 2016:40.

18. Wikipedia. Median Arcuate Ligament Syndrome. https://en.wikipedia.org/wiki/Median_arcuate_ligament_syndrome. Accessed September 22, 2018.

19. Brinth LS, Pors K, Theibel AC, Mehlsen J. Orthostatic intolerance and postural tachycardia syndrome as suspected adverse effects of vaccination against human papilloma virus. *Vaccine.* 2015;33(22):2602-2605. doi:10.1016/j.vaccine.2015.03.098

20. Ykelenstam Y. Dr. Diana Driscoll interview: vagus nerve and POTS/mast cell activation. Healing Histamine. https://healinghistamine.com/dr-diana-driscoll-interview-vagus-nerve-and-potsmast-cell-activation/. Accessed September 22, 2018.

21. Theoharides TC, Kalogeromitros D. The critical role of mast cells in allergy and inflammation. *Ann N Y Acad Sci.* 2006;1088(1):78-99. doi:10.1196/annals.1366.025

22. Theoharides TC, Valent P, Akin C. Mast Cells, Mastocytosis, and Related Disorders. Ingelfinger JR, ed. *N Engl J Med.* 2015;373(2):163-172. doi:10.1056/NEJMra1409760

23. Zadourian A, Doherty TA, Swiatkiewicz I, Taub PR. Postural Orthostatic Tachycardia Syndrome: Prevalence, Pathophysiology, and Management. *Drugs.* 2018;78(10):983-994. doi:10.1007/s40265-018-0931-5

24. Brooks JK, Francis LAP. Postural orthostatic tachycardia syndrome: Dental treatment considerations. *J Am Dent Assoc.* 2006;137(4):488-493. http://www.ncbi.nlm.nih.gov/pubmed/16637478. Accessed August 31, 2018.

25. Kanjwal K, Saeed B, Karabin B, Kanjwal Y, Grubb BP. Comparative clinical profile of postural orthostatic tachycardia patients with and without joint hypermobility syndrome. *Indian Pacing Electrophysiol J.* 2010;10(4):173-178. http://www.ncbi.nlm.nih.gov/pubmed/20376184. Accessed August 31, 2018.

26. Cheung I, Vadas P. A New Disease Cluster: Mast Cell Activation Syndrome, Postural Orthostatic Tachycardia Syndrome, and Ehlers-Danlos Syndrome. *J Allergy Clin Immunol.* 2015;135(2):AB65. doi:10.1016/j.jaci.2014.12.1146

27. Hoffman-Snyder C, Lewis J, Harris L, Dhawan P GB. Evidence of Mast Cell Activation Disorder in Postural Tachycardia Syndrome. *Neurology*. 2015;84(14 Supplement):P1.277. http://n.neurology.org/content/84/14_Supplement/P1.277.short. Accessed August 31, 2018.

28. Goodman B, Hoffman-Snyder C, Dhawan P. Joint Hypermobility Syndrome in a Postural Orthostatic Tachycardia Syndrome (POTS) Cohort. *Neurology*. 2016;86(16 Supplement):P5.116. http://n.neurology.org/content/86/16_Supplement/P5.116.short. Accessed August 31, 2018.

29. Klimas L. The MastAttack 107: The Layperson's Guide to Understanding Mast Cell Diseases, Part 32 - Mast Attack. https://www.mastattack.org/2017/06/mastattack-107-laypersons-guide-understanding-mast-cell-diseases-part-32/. Accessed September 22, 2018.

30. Driscoll D, De A, Doherty C, Ferreira JP, Meglathery S, Pazun J. *The Driscoll Theory Newly Revised: The Cause of POTS in Ehlers-Danlos Syndrome and How to Reverse the Process*. Warnick Publishing; 2015.

31. Borovikova L V., Ivanova S, Zhang M, et al. Vagus nerve stimulation attenuates the systemic inflammatory response to endotoxin. *Nature*. 2000;405(6785):458-462. doi:10.1038/35013070

32. Ben-Menachem E, Mañon-Espaillat R, Ristanovic R, et al. Vagus nerve stimulation for treatment of partial seizures: 1. A controlled study of effect on seizures. First International Vagus Nerve Stimulation Study Group. *Epilepsia*. 35(3):616-626. http://www.ncbi.nlm.nih.gov/pubmed/8026408. Accessed August 31, 2018.

33. George R, Sonnen A, Upton A, et al. A randomized controlled trial of chronic vagus nerve stimulation for treatment of medically intractable seizures. The Vagus Nerve Stimulation Study Group. *Neurology*. 1995;45(2):224-230. http://www.ncbi.nlm.nih.gov/pubmed/7854516. Accessed August 31, 2018.

34. DeGiorgio CM, Schachter SC, Handforth A, et al. Prospective long-term study of vagus nerve stimulation for the treatment of refractory seizures. *Epilepsia*. 2000;41(9):1195-1200. http://www.ncbi.nlm.nih.gov/pubmed/10999559. Accessed August 31, 2018.

35. Armstrong S, Look J, Christie L, Allen R. *Sound Ideas: Lymphedema Therapy for the Treatment of Complex Regional Pain Syndrome*; Vol 23.; 2016. http://soundideas.pugetsound.edu/ptsymposium/23. Accessed August 31, 2018.

36. Chang C, McDonnell P, Gershwin ME. Complex regional pain syndrome – False hopes and miscommunications. *Autoimmun Rev*. January 2019. doi:10.1016/J.AUTREV.2018.10.003

37. Huygen FJPM, Ramdhani N, van Toorenenbergen A, Klein J, Zijlstra FJ. Mast cells are involved in inflammatory reactions during Complex Regional Pain Syndrome type 1. *Immunol Lett*. 2004;91(2-3):147-154. doi:10.1016/j.imlet.2003.11.013

38. Chatterjea D, Martinov T. Mast cells: versatile gatekeepers of pain. *Mol Immunol*. 2015;63(1):38-44. doi:10.1016/j.molimm.2014.03.001

39. Aich A, Afrin LB, Gupta K. Mast Cell-Mediated Mechanisms of Nociception. *Int J Mol Sci*. 2015;16(12):29069-29092. doi:10.3390/ijms161226151

40. Theoharides TC, Alysandratos KD, Angelidou A, et al. Mast cells and inflammation. *Biochim Biophys Acta - Mol Basis Dis*. 2012;1822:21-33. doi:10.1016/j.bbadis.2010.12.014

41. Wirz S, Molderings GJ. A practical guide for treatment of pain in patients with systemic mast cell activation disease. *Pain Physician*. 2017;20:E849-E861.

42. Hamilton M. Phone interview conducted on 6-22-18.

43. Weinstock LB, Brook JB, Myers TL, Goodman B. Successful treatment of postural orthostatic tachycardia and mast cell activation syndromes using naltrexone, immunoglobulin and antibiotic treatment. *BMJ Case Rep*. 2018. doi:10.1136/bcr-2017-221405

44. Turner H. Episode 6: SIBO and Mast Cell Activation Syndrome with Heidi Turner. In: The SIBO Doctor Podcast with Dr. Nirala Jacobi on Apple Podcasts. Aired on 2/22/17. https://www.thesibodoctor.com/the-sibo-doctor-podcast-heidi-turner/.

45. Park JH, Rhee P-L, Kim HS, et al. Mucosal mast cell counts correlate with visceral hypersensitivity in patients with diarrhea predominant irritable bowel syndrome. *J Gastroenterol Hepatol*. 2006;21(1):71-78. doi:10.1111/j.1440-1746.2005.04143.x

46. Goral V, Kucukoner M, Buyukbayram H. Mast cells count and serum cytokine levels in patients with irritable bowel syndrome. *Hepatogastroenterology*. 2010;57(101):751-754. http://www.ncbi.nlm.nih.gov/pubmed/21033222. Accessed August 31, 2018.

47. O'Sullivan M, Clayton N, Breslin NP, et al. Increased mast cells in the irritable bowel syndrome. *Neurogastroenterol Motil*. 2000;12(5):449-457. http://www.ncbi.nlm.nih.gov/pubmed/11012945. Accessed August 31, 2018.

48. Guilarte M, Santos J, de Torres I, et al. Diarrhoea-predominant IBS patients show mast cell activation and hyperplasia in the jejunum. *Gut*. 2007;56(2):203-209. doi:10.1136/gut.2006.100594

49. Frieling T, Meis K, Kolck U, et al. Evidence for Mast Cell Activation in Patients with Therapy-Resistant Irritable Bowel Syndrome. *Z Gastroenterol*. 2011;49(02):191-194. doi:10.1055/s-0029-1245707

50. Ramsay DB, Stephen S, Borum M, Voltaggio L, Doman DB. Mast cells in gastrointestinal disease. *Gastroenterol Hepatol (N Y)*. 2010;6(12):772-777. http://www.ncbi.nlm.nih.gov/pubmed/21301631. Accessed August 31, 2018.

51. Cremon C, Carini G, Wang B, et al. Intestinal Serotonin Release, Sensory Neuron Activation and Abdominal Pain in Irritable Bowel Syndrome. *Am J Gastroenterol*. 2011;106(7):1290-1298. doi:10.1038/ajg.2011.86

52. Kushnir-Sukhov NM, Brittain E, Scott L, Metcalfe DD. Clinical correlates of blood serotonin levels in patients with mastocytosis. *Eur J Clin Invest.* 2008;38:953-958. doi:10.1111/j.1365-2362.2008.02047.x

53. Klooker TK, Braak B, Koopman KE, et al. The mast cell stabiliser ketotifen decreases visceral hypersensitivity and improves intestinal symptoms in patients with irritable bowel syndrome. *Gut.* 2010;59(9):1213-1221. doi:10.1136/gut.2010.213108

54. Behdad A, Owens SR. Systemic Mastocytosis Involving the Gastrointestinal Tract: Case Report and Review. *Arch Pathol Lab Med.* 2013;137(9):1220-1223. doi:10.5858/arpa.2013-0271-CR

55. Buhner S, Schemann M. Mast cell-nerve axis with a focus on the human gut. *Biochim Biophys Acta - Mol Basis Dis.* 2012;1822(1):85-92. doi:10.1016/j.bbadis.2011.06.004

56. Weston AP, Biddle WL, Bhatia PS, Miner PB. Terminal ileal mucosal mast cells in irritable bowel syndrome. *Dig Dis Sci.* 1993;38(9):1590-1595. http://www.ncbi.nlm.nih.gov/pubmed/8359068. Accessed August 31, 2018.

57. De Winter BY, van den Wijngaard RM, de Jonge WJ. Intestinal mast cells in gut inflammation and motility disturbances. *Biochim Biophys Acta - Mol Basis Dis.* 2012;1822(1):66-73. doi:10.1016/j.bbadis.2011.03.016

58. Wood JD. Enteric neuroimmunophysiology and pathophysiology. *Gastroenterology.* 2004;127(2):635-657. http://www.ncbi.nlm.nih.gov/pubmed/15300595. Accessed August 31, 2018.

59. Coelho AM, Fioramonti J, Bueno L. Mast cell degranulation induces delayed rectal allodynia in rats: role of histamine and 5-HT. *Dig Dis Sci.* 1998;43(4):727-737. http://www.ncbi.nlm.nih.gov/pubmed/9558027. Accessed August 31, 2018.

60. Bonaz B, Sinniger V, Pellissier S. Vagus nerve stimulation: a new promising therapeutic tool in inflammatory bowel disease. *J Intern Med.* 2017;282(1):46-63. doi:10.1111/joim.12611

61. Schoenen J, Romain N, D'Ostilio K, Sava S, Magis D. Non-Invasive Vagus Nerve Stimulation with the gammaCore in Healthy Subjects: Is There Electrophysiological Evidence for Activation of Vagal Afferents? (P2. 202). *Neurology.* 2016;86(16 Supplement):P2.202. http://n.neurology.org/content/86/16_Supplement/P2.202.short. Accessed August 31, 2018.

62. Mattarelli P, Brandi G, Calabrese C, et al. Occurrence of Bifidobacteriaceae in human hypochlorhydria stomach. *Microb Ecol Heal Dis.* 2014;25(0). doi:10.3402/mehd.v25.21379

63. Nosál R. Histamine release from isolated rat mast cells due to glycoprotein from Candida albicans in vitro. *J Hyg Epidemiol Microbiol Immunol.* 1974;18(3):377-378. http://www.ncbi.nlm.nih.gov/pubmed/4138120. Accessed August 31, 2018.

64. Yamaguchi N, Sugita R, Miki A, et al. Gastrointestinal Candida colonisation promotes sensitisation against food antigens by affecting the mucosal barrier in mice. *Gut.* 2006;55(7):954-960. doi:10.1136/gut.2005.084954

65. Bennet SMP, Ohman L, Simren M. Gut microbiota as potential orchestrators of irritable bowel syndrome. *Gut Liver.* 2015;9(3):318-331. doi:10.5009/gnl14344

66. Noverr MC, Noggle RM, Toews GB, Huffnagle GB. Role of antibiotics and fungal microbiota in driving pulmonary allergic responses. *Altern Med Rev.* 2005;10(1):68-69. http://go.galegroup.com/ps/anonymous?id=GALE%7CA131086158&sid=googleScholar&v=2.1&it=r&link access=abs&issn=10895159&p=AONE&sw=w. Accessed August 31, 2018.

67. Afrin LB, Khoruts A. Mast Cell Activation Disease and Microbiotic Interactions. *Clin Ther.* 2015;37(5):941-953. doi:10.1016/j.clinthera.2015.02.008

68. Oksaharju A, Kooistra T, Kleemann R, et al. Effects of probiotic Lactobacillus rhamnosus GG and Propionibacterium freudenreichii ssp. shermanii JS supplementation on intestinal and systemic markers of inflammation in ApoE*3Leiden mice consuming a high-fat diet. *Br J Nutr.* 2013;110(01):77-85. doi:10.1017/S0007114512004801

69. Luyer MD, Greve JWM, Hadfoune M, Jacobs JA, Dejong CH, Buurman WA. Nutritional stimulation of cholecystokinin receptors inhibits inflammation via the vagus nerve. *J Exp Med.* 2005;202(8):1023-1029. doi:10.1084/jem.20042397

70. Lubbers T, de Haan JJ, Luyer MDP, et al. Cholecystokinin/Cholecystokinin-1 receptor-mediated peripheral activation of the afferent vagus by enteral nutrients attenuates inflammation in rats. *Ann Surg.* 2010;252(2):376-382. doi:10.1097/SLA.0b013e3181dae411

71. de Haan JJ, Thuijls G, Lubbers T, et al. Protection against early intestinal compromise by lipid-rich enteral nutrition through cholecystokinin receptors. *Crit Care Med.* 2010;38(7):1592-1597. doi:10.1097/CCM.0b013e3181e2cd4d

72. Luyer MDP, Buurman WA, Hadfoune M, et al. Pretreatment with High-Fat Enteral Nutrition Reduces Endotoxin and Tumor Necrosis Factor-?? and Preserves Gut Barrier Function Early After Hemorrhagic Shock. *Shock.* 2004;21(1):65-71. doi:10.1097/01.shk.0000101671.49265.cf

73. Vadlamudi RS, Chi DS, Krishnaswamy G. Intestinal strongyloidiasis and hyperinfection syndrome. *Clin Mol Allergy.* 2006;4:8. doi:10.1186/1476-7961-4-8

74. Askenase PW. Immunopathology of parasitic diseases: Involvement of basophils and mast cells. *Springer Semin Immunopathol.* 1980;2(4):417-442. doi:10.1007/BF01857177

75. McDermott JR, Bartram RE, Knight PA, Miller HRP, Garrod DR, Grencis RK. Mast cells disrupt epithelial barrier function during enteric nematode infection. *Proc Natl Acad Sci U S A*. 2003;100(13):7761-7766. doi:10.1073/pnas.1231488100

76. Crowle PK, Reed ND. Rejection of the intestinal parasite Nippostrongylus brasiliensis by mast cell-deficient W/Wv anemic mice. *Infect Immun*. 1981;33(1):54-58. http://www.ncbi.nlm.nih.gov/pubmed/7263072. Accessed August 31, 2018.

77. Mukai K, Karasuyama H, Kabashima K, Kubo M, Galli SJ. Differences in the Importance of Mast Cells, Basophils, IgE, and IgG versus That of CD4+ T Cells and ILC2 Cells in Primary and Secondary Immunity to Strongyloides venezuelensis. *Infect Immun*. 2017;85(5). doi:10.1128/IAI.00053-17

78. Galli SJ, Maurer M, Lantz CS. Mast cells as sentinels of innate immunity. *Curr Opin Immunol*. 1999;11(1):53-59. http://www.ncbi.nlm.nih.gov/pubmed/10047539. Accessed August 31, 2018.

79. Abraham SN, Malaviya R. Mast cells in infection and immunity. 1997;65(9):3501.

80. Galli SJ, Kalesnikoff J, Grimbaldeston MA, Piliponsky AM, Williams CMM, Tsai M. Mast Cells as "Tunable" Effector and Immunoregulatory Cells: Recent Advances. *Annu Rev Immunol*. 2005;23(1):749-786. doi:10.1146/annurev.immunol.21.120601.141025

81. Abraham SN, St John AL. Mast cell-orchestrated immunity to pathogens. *Nat Rev Immunol*. 2010;10(6):440-452. doi:10.1038/nri2782

82. Potts RA, Tiffany CM, Pakpour N, et al. Mast cells and histamine alter intestinal permeability during malaria parasite infection. *Immunobiology*. 2016;221(3):468-474. doi:10.1016/j.imbio.2015.11.003

83. Chau JY, Tiffany CM, Nimishakavi S, et al. Malaria-associated L-arginine deficiency induces mast cell-associated disruption to intestinal barrier defenses against nontyphoidal Salmonella bacteremia. *Infect Immun*. 2013;81(10):3515-3526. doi:10.1128/IAI.00380-13

84. Jakate S, Demeo M, John R, Tobin M, Keshavarzian A. Mastocytic enterocolitis: increased mucosal mast cells in chronic intractable diarrhea. *Arch Pathol Lab Med*. 2006;130(3):362-367. doi:10.1043/1543-2165(2006)130[362:MEIMMC]2.0.CO;2

85. Kurashima Y, Amiya T, Nochi T, et al. Extracellular ATP mediates mast cell-dependent intestinal inflammation through P2X7 purinoceptors. *Nat Commun*. 2012;3:1034. doi:10.1038/ncomms2023

86. Andoh A, Deguchi Y, Inatomi O, et al. Immunohistochemical study of chymase-positive mast cells in inflammatory bowel disease. *Oncol Rep*. 2006;16(1):103-107. http://www.ncbi.nlm.nih.gov/pubmed/16786130. Accessed August 31, 2018.

87. Vivinus-Nébot M, Frin-Mathy G, Bzioueche H, et al. Functional bowel symptoms in quiescent inflammatory bowel diseases: role of epithelial barrier disruption and low-grade inflammation. *Gut*. 2014;63(5):744-752. doi:10.1136/gutjnl-2012-304066

88. Raithel M, Schneider HT, Hahn EG. Effect of substance P on histamine secretion from gut mucosa in inflammatory bowel disease. *Scand J Gastroenterol*. 1999;34(5):496-503. http://www.ncbi.nlm.nih.gov/pubmed/10423066. Accessed August 31, 2018.

89. Raithel M, Winterkamp S, Pacurar A, Ulrich P, Hochberger J, Hahn EG. Release of mast cell tryptase from human colorectal mucosa in inflammatory bowel disease. *Scand J Gastroenterol*. 2001;36(2):174-179. http://www.ncbi.nlm.nih.gov/pubmed/11252410. Accessed August 31, 2018.

90. Winterkamp S, Weidenhiller M, Otte P, et al. Urinary excretion of N-methylhistamine as a marker of disease activity in inflammatory bowel disease. *Am J Gastroenterol*. 2002;97(12):3071-3077. doi:10.1111/j.1572-0241.2002.07028.x

91. Baratelli F, Le M, Gershman GB, French SW. Do mast cells play a pathogenetic role in neurofibromatosis type 1 and ulcerative colitis? *Exp Mol Pathol*. 2014;96(2):230-234. doi:10.1016/j.yexmp.2014.02.006

92. Adams W, Mitchell L, Candelaria-Santiago R, Hefner J, Gramling J. Concurrent Ulcerative Colitis and Neurofibromatosis Type 1: The Question of a Common Pathway. *Pediatrics*. 2016;137(2):e20150973-e20150973. doi:10.1542/peds.2015-0973

93. Mannan R, Syed AA, Shen B, et al. Systemic Mastocytosis Mimicking Pouchitis in a Patient With Ulcerative Colitis. *Am J Clin Pathol*. 2015;144:325. https://search.proquest.com/openview/d3fecfeedbd7dd35b4b2090808bd33e4/1?pq-origsite=gscholar&cbl=586299. Accessed August 31, 2018.

94. Shih AR, Deshpande V, Ferry JA, Zukerberg L. Clinicopathological characteristics of systemic mastocytosis in the intestine. *Histopathology*. 2016;69(6):1021-1027. doi:10.1111/his.13033

95. Bedeir A, Jukic DM, Wang L, Mullady DK, Regueiro M, Krasinskas AM. Systemic Mastocytosis Mimicking Inflammatory Bowel Disease: A Case Report and Discussion of Gastrointestinal Pathology in Systemic Mastocytosis. *Am J Surg Pathol*. 2006;30(11):1478-1482. doi:10.1097/01.pas.0000213310.51553.d7

96. Söderholm JD, Perdue MH. II. Stress and intestinal barrier function. *Am J Physiol Liver Physiol*. 2001;280(1):G7-G13. doi:10.1152/ajpgi.2001.280.1.G7

97. Bernstein CN, Singh S, Graff LA, Walker JR, Miller N, Cheang M. A Prospective Population-Based Study of Triggers of Symptomatic Flares in IBD. *Am J Gastroenterol*. 2010;105(9):1994-2002. doi:10.1038/ajg.2010.140

98. Brzozowski B, Mazur-Bialy A, Pajdo R, et al. Mechanisms by which Stress Affects the Experimental and Clinical Inflammatory Bowel Disease (IBD): Role of Brain-Gut Axis. *Curr Neuropharmacol.* 2016;14(8):892-900. doi:10.2174/1570159X14666160404124127

99. Vivinus-Nébot M, Frin-Mathy G, Bzioueche H, et al. Functional bowel symptoms in quiescent inflammatory bowel diseases: role of epithelial barrier disruption and low-grade inflammation. *Gut.* 2014;63(5):744-752. doi:10.1136/gutjnl-2012-304066

100. Roblin X, Rinaudo M, Del Tedesco E, et al. Development of an Algorithm Incorporating Pharmacokinetics of Adalimumab in Inflammatory Bowel Diseases. *Am J Gastroenterol.* 2014;109(8):1250-1256. doi:10.1038/ajg.2014.146

101. Sanders KM, Koh SD, Ward SM. Interstitial cells of cajal as pacemakers in the gastrointestinal tract. *Annu Rev Physiol.* 2006;68(1):307-343. doi:10.1146/annurev.physiol.68.040504.094718

102. Beckett EAH, Sanders KM, Ward SM. Inhibitory responses mediated by vagal nerve stimulation are diminished in stomachs of mice with reduced intramuscular interstitial cells of Cajal. *Sci Rep.* 2017;7:44759. doi:10.1038/srep44759

103. Wouters MM, Vicario M, Santos J. The role of mast cells in functional GI disorders. *Gut.* 2016;65(1):155-168. doi:10.1136/gutjnl-2015-309151

104. Bischoff SC. Role of mast cells in allergic and non-allergic immune responses: comparison of human and murine data. *Nat Rev Immunol.* 2007;7(2):93-104. doi:10.1038/nri2018

105. Klimas L. Third spacing - Mast Attack. https://www.mastattack.org/2014/07/third-spacing/. Accessed September 23, 2018.

106. Mutnuri S, Khan A, Variyam EP. Visceral angioedema: an under-recognized complication of angiotensin-converting enzyme inhibitors. *Postgrad Med.* 2015;127(2):215-217. doi:10.1080/00325481.2015.1001305

107. Afrin L. In-person interview conducted in St. Cloud, Minnesota on 9-16-17.

108. Molderings GJ, Brettner S, Homann J, Afrin LB. Mast cell activation disease: A concise practical guide for diagnostic workup and therapeutic options. *J Hematol Oncol.* 2011;4:10. doi:10.1186/1756-8722-4-10

109. United States Hereditary Angioedema Association. https://www.haea.org. Accessed February 23, 2018.

110. Bork K, Staubach P, Eckardt AJ, Hardt J. Symptoms, Course, and Complications of Abdominal Attacks in Hereditary Angioedema Due to C1 Inhibitor Deficiency. *Am J Gastroenterol.* 2006;101(3):619-627. doi:10.1111/j.1572-0241.2006.00492.x

111. Cicardi M, Aberer W, Banerji A, et al. Classification, diagnosis, and approach to treatment for angioedema: consensus report from the Hereditary Angioedema International Working Group. *Allergy.* 2014;69(5):602-616. doi:10.1111/all.12380

112. Banerji A. Hereditary angioedema: Classification, pathogenesis, and diagnosis. *Allergy Asthma Proc.* 2011;32(6):403-407. doi:10.2500/aap.2011.32.3492

113. Stevens C, Biedenkapp JC, Mensah R, Chyung YH, Adelman B. Hereditary Angioedema Is Associated with Neuropathic Pain, Systemic Lupus Erythematosis and Systemic Mastocytosis in an Analysis of a Health Analytics Claims Database. *J Allergy Clin Immunol.* 2016;137(2):AB75. doi:10.1016/j.jaci.2015.12.255

114. Oschatz C, Maas C, Lecher B, et al. Mast Cells Increase Vascular Permeability by Heparin-Initiated Bradykinin Formation In Vivo. *Immunity.* 2011;34(2):258-268. doi:10.1016/j.immuni.2011.02.008

115. Humphries DE, Wong GW, Friend DS, et al. Heparin is essential for the storage of specific granule proteases in mast cells. *Nature.* 1999;400(6746):769-772. doi:10.1038/23481

116. Dai H, Korthuis RJ. Mast Cell Proteases and Inflammation. *Drug Discov Today Dis Models.* 2011;8(1):47-55. doi:10.1016/j.ddmod.2011.06.004

117. Tsilioni I, Russell IJ, Stewart JM, Gleason RM, Theoharides TC. Neuropeptides CRH, SP, HK-1, and Inflammatory Cytokines IL-6 and TNF Are Increased in Serum of Patients with Fibromyalgia Syndrome, Implicating Mast Cells. *J Pharmacol Exp Ther.* 2016;356(3):664-672. doi:10.1124/jpet.115.230060

118. Mandel D, Askari AD, Malemud CJ, Kaso A. Joint Hypermobility Syndrome and Postural Orthostatic Tachycardia Syndrome (HyPOTS). *Res Artic Biomed Res Clin Pract Biomed Res Clin Pr.* 2017;2(1):1-4. doi:10.15761/BRCP.1000132

119. Erdogan KH, Sas S, Acer E, Bulur I, Altunay IK, Erdem HR. Cutaneous findings in fibromyalgia syndrome and their effect on quality of life. *Dermatologica Sin.* 2016;34(3):131-134. doi:10.1016/J.DSI.2016.01.006

120. Eneström S, Bengtsson A, Frödin T. Dermal IgG deposits and increase of mast cells in patients with fibromyalgia--relevant findings or epiphenomena? *Scand J Rheumatol.* 1997;26(4):308-313. http://www.ncbi.nlm.nih.gov/pubmed/9310112. Accessed August 31, 2018.

121. Blanco I, Béritze N, Argüelles M, et al. Abnormal overexpression of mastocytes in skin biopsies of fibromyalgia patients. *Clin Rheumatol.* 2010;29(12):1403-1412. doi:10.1007/s10067-010-1474-7

122. Afrin LB, Butterfield JH, Raithel M, Molderings GJ. Often seen, rarely recognized: mast cell activation disease – a guide to diagnosis and therapeutic options. *Ann Med.* 2016;48(3):190-201. doi:10.3109/07853890.2016.1161231

123. Jones KD, Gelbart T, Whisenant TC, et al. Genome-wide expression profiling in the peripheral blood of patients with fibromyalgia. *Clin Exp Rheumatol.* 2016;34(2 Suppl 96):S89-98. http://www.ncbi.nlm.nih.gov/pubmed/27157394. Accessed August 31, 2018.

124. Ang DC, Hilligoss J, Stump T. Mast Cell Stabilizer (Ketotifen) in Fibromyalgia: Phase 1 Randomized Controlled Clinical Trial. *Clin J Pain*. 2015;31(9):836-842. doi:10.1097/AJP.0000000000000169

125. Lakhan SE, Kirchgessner A. Gut inflammation in chronic fatigue syndrome. *Nutr Metab (Lond)*. 2010;7:79. doi:10.1186/1743-7075-7-79

126. Theoharides TC, Papaliodis D, Tagen M, Konstantinidou A, Kempuraj D, Clemons A. Chronic fatigue syndrome, mast cells, and tricyclic antidepressants. *J Clin Psychopharmacol*. 2005;25(6):515-520. http://www.ncbi.nlm.nih.gov/pubmed/16282830. Accessed September 22, 2018.

127. Theoharides TC, Asadi S, Weng Z, Zhang B. Serotonin-Selective Reuptake Inhibitors and Nonsteroidal Anti-Inflammatory Drugs-Important Considerations of Adverse Interactions Especially for the Treatment of Myalgic Encephalomyelitis/Chronic Fatigue Syndrome. *J Clin Psychopharmacol*. 2011;31(4):403-405. doi:10.1097/JCP.0b013e318225848c

128. Kuo Y-H, Tsai W-J, Loke S-H, Wu T-S, Chiou W-F. Astragalus membranaceus flavonoids (AMF) ameliorate chronic fatigue syndrome induced by food intake restriction plus forced swimming. *J Ethnopharmacol*. 2009;122(1):28-34. doi:10.1016/j.jep.2008.11.025

129. Singh A, Naidu PS, Gupta S, Kulkarni SK. Effect of Natural and Synthetic Antioxidants in a Mouse Model of Chronic Fatigue Syndrome. *J Med Food*. 2002;5(4):211-220. doi:10.1089/109662002763003366

130. Afrin LB, Pöhlau D, Raithel M, et al. Mast cell activation disease: An underappreciated cause of neurologic and psychiatric symptoms and diseases. *Brain Behav Immun*. 2015;50:314-321. doi:10.1016/j.bbi.2015.07.002

131. Kõlves K, Barker E, De Leo D. Allergies and suicidal behaviors: A systematic literature review. *Allergy Asthma Proc*. 2015;36(6):433-438. doi:10.2500/aap.2015.36.3887

132. O'Donovan A, Epel E, Lin J, et al. Childhood Trauma Associated with Short Leukocyte Telomere Length in Posttraumatic Stress Disorder. *Biol Psychiatry*. 2011;70(5):465-471. doi:10.1016/J.BIOPSYCH.2011.01.035

133. Kempuraj D, Selvakumar GP, Thangavel R, et al. Mast Cell Activation in Brain Injury, Stress, and Post-traumatic Stress Disorder and Alzheimer's Disease Pathogenesis. *Front Neurosci*. 2017;11:703. doi:10.3389/fnins.2017.00703

134. Holman DM, Ports KA, Buchanan ND, et al. The Association Between Adverse Childhood Experiences and Risk of Cancer in Adulthood: A Systematic Review of the Literature. *Pediatrics*. 2016;138(Suppl 1):S81-S91. doi:10.1542/peds.2015-4268L

135. Lindqvist D, Janelidze S, Hagell P, et al. Interleukin-6 Is Elevated in the Cerebrospinal Fluid of Suicide Attempters and Related to Symptom Severity. *Biol Psychiatry*. 2009;66(3):287-292. doi:10.1016/J.BIOPSYCH.2009.01.030

136. Pandey GN, Rizavi HS, Ren X, et al. Proinflammatory cytokines in the prefrontal cortex of teenage suicide victims. *J Psychiatr Res*. 2012;46(1):57-63. doi:10.1016/j.jpsychires.2011.08.006

137. Serafini G, Pompili M, Elena Seretti M, et al. The role of inflammatory cytokines in suicidal behavior: A systematic review. *Eur Neuropsychopharmacol*. 2013;23(12):1672-1686. doi:10.1016/j.euroneuro.2013.06.002

138. Piche T, Saint-Paul MC, Dainese R, et al. Mast cells and cellularity of the colonic mucosa correlated with fatigue and depression in irritable bowel syndrome. *Gut*. 2008;57(4):468-473. doi:10.1136/gut.2007.127068

139. Addolorato G, Marsigli L, Capristo E, Caputo F, Dall'Aglio C, Baudanza P. Anxiety and depression: a common feature of health care seeking patients with irritable bowel syndrome and food allergy. *Hepatogastroenterology*. 45(23):1559-1564. http://www.ncbi.nlm.nih.gov/pubmed/9840105. Accessed August 31, 2018.

140. Graziottin A, Skaper SD, Fusco M. Mast cells in chronic inflammation, pelvic pain and depression in women. *Gynecol Endocrinol*. 2014;30(7):472-477. doi:10.3109/09513590.2014.911280

141. Theoharides TC, Cochrane DE. Critical role of mast cells in inflammatory diseases and the effect of acute stress. *J Neuroimmunol*. 2004;146(1-2):1-12. doi:S0165572803004636 [pii]

142. Esposito P, Chandler N, Kandere K, et al. Corticotropin-Releasing Hormone and Brain Mast Cells Regulate Blood-Brain-Barrier Permeability Induced by Acute Stress. *J Pharmacol Exp Ther*. 2002;303(3):1061-1066. doi:10.1124/jpet.102.038497

143. Roberts F, Calcutt CR. Histamine and the hypothalamus. *Neuroscience*. 1983;9(4):721-739. http://www.ncbi.nlm.nih.gov/pubmed/6312374. Accessed August 31, 2018.

144. Kjaer A, Larsen PJ, Knigge U, Jørgensen H, Warberg J. Neuronal histamine and expression of corticotropin-releasing hormone, vasopressin and oxytocin in the hypothalamus: relative importance of H1 and H2 receptors. *Eur J Endocrinol*. 1998;139(2):238-243. http://www.ncbi.nlm.nih.gov/pubmed/9724083. Accessed August 31, 2018.

145. Kempuraj D, Papadopoulou N, Stanford EJ, et al. Increased Numbers of Activated Mast Cells in Endometriosis Lesions Positive for Corticotropin-Releasing Hormone and Urocortin. *Am J Reprod Immunol*. 2004;52(4):267-275. doi:10.1111/j.1600-0897.2004.00224.x

146. Sun Y, Hunt S, Sah P. Norepinephrine and Corticotropin-Releasing Hormone: Partners in the Neural Circuits that Underpin Stress and Anxiety. *Neuron*. 2015;87(3):468-470. doi:10.1016/J.NEURON.2015.07.022

147. Costa-Pinto FA, Basso AS, Russo M. Role of mast cell degranulation in the neural correlates of the immediate allergic reaction in a murine model of asthma. *Brain Behav Immun*. 2007;21(6):783-790. doi:10.1016/j.bbi.2007.01.002

148. Costa-Pinto FA, Basso AS, De Sa-Rocha LC, Britto LRG, Russo M, Palermo-Neto J. Neural Correlates of IgE-Mediated Allergy. *Ann N Y Acad Sci*. 2006;1088(1):116-131. doi:10.1196/annals.1366.028

149. Bealer SL. Histamine releases norepinephrine in the paraventricular nucleus/anterior hypothalamus of the conscious rat. *J Pharmacol Exp Ther*. 1993;264(2):734-738. http://www.ncbi.nlm.nih.gov/pubmed/8437121. Accessed August 31, 2018.

150. Imamura M, Poli E, Omoniyi AT, Levi R. Unmasking of activated histamine H3-receptors in myocardial ischemia: their role as regulators of exocytotic norepinephrine release. *J Pharmacol Exp Ther*. 1994;271(3):1259-1266. http://www.ncbi.nlm.nih.gov/pubmed/7527852. Accessed August 31, 2018.

151. Nautiyal KM, Ribeiro AC, Pfaff DW, Silver R. Brain mast cells link the immune system to anxiety-like behavior. *Proc Natl Acad Sci*. 2008;105(46):18053-18057. https://pdfs.semanticscholar.org/aeff/46af642e59961b8557e7ff444acf6cd6b73c.pdf. Accessed July 17, 2018.

152. Theoharides TC. Autism Spectrum Disorders and Mastocytosis. *Int J Immunopathol Pharmacol*. 2009;22(4):859-865. doi:10.1177/039463200902200401

153. Tsilioni I, Dodman N, Petra AI, et al. Elevated serum neurotensin and CRH levels in children with autistic spectrum disorders and tail-chasing Bull Terriers with a phenotype similar to autism. *Transl Psychiatry*. 2014;4(10):e466-e466. doi:10.1038/tp.2014.106

154. Gamakaranage C. Heavy Metals and Autism. *J Heavy Met Toxic Dis*. 2016;01(03). doi:10.21767/2473-6457.100012

155. Ornoy A, Weinstein-Fudim L, Ergaz Z. Prenatal factors associated with autism spectrum disorder (ASD). *Reprod Toxicol*. 2015;56:155-169. doi:10.1016/j.reprotox.2015.05.007

156. Nuttall JR. The plausibility of maternal toxicant exposure and nutritional status as contributing factors to the risk of autism spectrum disorders. *Nutr Neurosci*. 2017;20(4):209-218. doi:10.1080/1028415X.2015.1103437

157. Tabatadze T, Zhorzholiani L, Kherkheulidze M, Kandelaki E, Ivanashvili T. Hair Heavy Metal and Essential Trace Element Concentration with Autism Spectrum Disorder. *Georgian Med News*. 2015;(248):77-82. http://www.ncbi.nlm.nih.gov/pubmed/26656556. Accessed August 31, 2018.

158. Vela G, Stark P, Socha M, Sauer AK, Hagmeyer S, Grabrucker AM. Zinc in gut-brain interaction in autism and neurological disorders. *Neural Plast*. 2015;2015:972791. doi:10.1155/2015/972791

159. Mohamed FEB, Zaky EA, El-Sayed AB, et al. Assessment of Hair Aluminum, Lead, and Mercury in a Sample of Autistic Egyptian Children: Environmental Risk Factors of Heavy Metals in Autism. *Behav Neurol*. 2015;2015:545674. doi:10.1155/2015/545674

160. Theoharides TC, Angelidou A, Alysandratos K-D, et al. Mast cell activation and autism. *Biochim Biophys Acta - Mol Basis Dis*. 2012;1822(1):34-41. doi:10.1016/j.bbadis.2010.12.017

161. Dickerson AS, Rahbar MH, Han I, et al. Autism spectrum disorder prevalence and proximity to industrial facilities releasing arsenic, lead or mercury. *Sci Total Environ*. 2015;536:245-251. doi:10.1016/j.scitotenv.2015.07.024

162. Koyuncu OO, Hogue IB, Enquist LW. Virus infections in the nervous system. *Cell Host Microbe*. 2013;13(4):379-393. doi:10.1016/j.chom.2013.03.010

163. Matsushima K, Matsubayashi J, Toichi M, et al. Unusual sensory features are related to resting-state cardiac vagus nerve activity in autism spectrum disorders. *Res Autism Spectr Disord*. 2016;25(25):37-46. doi:10.1016/j.rasd.2015.12.006

164. Filcikova D, Mravec B. Alterations in autonomic nervous system in autism spectrum disorders: Means of detection and intervention. *Act Nerv Super Rediviva*. 2016;58(4):115-117. https://pdfs.semanticscholar.org/184f/98f0a972e08354276b5e128872d7d043361d.pdf. Accessed August 31, 2018.

165. Colzato LS, Sellaro R, Beste C. Darwin revisited: The vagus nerve is a causal element in controlling recognition of other's emotions. *Cortex*. 2017;92:95-102. doi:10.1016/j.cortex.2017.03.017

166. Magalhães ES, Pinto-Mariz F, Bastos-Pinto S, Pontes AT, Prado EA, deAzevedo LC. Immune allergic response in Asperger syndrome. *J Neuroimmunol*. 2009;216(1-2):108-112. doi:10.1016/j.jneuroim.2009.09.015

167. Sacco R, Curatolo P, Manzi B, et al. Principal pathogenetic components and biological endophenotypes in autism spectrum disorders. *Autism Res*. 2010;3(5):237-252. doi:10.1002/aur.151

168. Gurney JG, McPheeters ML, Davis MM. Parental Report of Health Conditions and Health Care Use Among Children With and Without Autism. *Arch Pediatr Adolesc Med*. 2006;160(8):825. doi:10.1001/archpedi.160.8.825

169. Croen LA, Grether JK, Yoshida CK, Odouli R, Van de Water J. Maternal Autoimmune Diseases, Asthma and Allergies, and Childhood Autism Spectrum Disorders. *Arch Pediatr Adolesc Med*. 2005;159(2):151-157. doi:10.1001/archpedi.159.2.151

170. Angelidou A, Francis K, Vasiadi M, et al. Neurotensin is increased in serum of young children with autistic disorder. *J Neuroinflammation*. 2010;7:48. doi:10.1186/1742-2094-7-48

171. Zhang B, Angelidou A, Alysandratos K-D, et al. Mitochondrial DNA and anti-mitochondrial antibodies in serum of autistic children. *J Neuroinflammation*. 2010;7:80. doi:10.1186/1742-2094-7-80

172. Kempuraj D, Asadi S, Zhang B, et al. Mercury induces inflammatory mediator release from human mast cells. *J Neuroinflammation*. 2010;7:20. doi:10.1186/1742-2094-7-20

173. Akhondzadeh S, Erfani S, Mohammadi MR, et al. Cyproheptadine in the treatment of autistic disorder: a double-blind placebo-controlled trial. *J Clin Pharm Ther*. 2004;29(2):145-150. doi:10.1111/j.1365-2710.2004.00546.x

174. Theoharides TC, Kempuraj D, Redwood L. Autism: an emerging 'neuroimmune disorder' in search of therapy. *Expert Opin Pharmacother*. 2009;10(13):2127-2143. doi:10.1517/14656560903107789

175. Theoharides TC, Asadi S, Panagiotidou S. A Case Series of a Luteolin Formulation (Neuroprotek®) in Children with Autism Spectrum Disorders. *Int J Immunopathol Pharmacol*. 2012;25(2):317-323. doi:10.1177/039463201202500201

176. Vieira dos Santos R, Magerl M, Martus P, et al. Topical sodium cromoglicate relieves allergen- and histamine-induced dermal pruritus. *Br J Dermatol*. 2010;162(3):674-676. doi:10.1111/j.1365-2133.2009.09516.x

177. Asadi S, Zhang B, Weng Z, et al. Luteolin and Thiosalicylate Inhibit HGCL $_2$ and Thimerosal-Induced VEGF Release from Human Mast Cells. *Int J Immunopathol Pharmacol*. 2010;23(4):1015-1020. doi:10.1177/039463201002300406

178. Kempuraj D, Castellani ML, Petrarca C, et al. Inhibitory effect of quercetin on tryptase and interleukin-6 release, and histidine decarboxylase mRNA transcription by human mast cell-1 cell line. *Clin Exp Med*. 2006;6(4):150-156. doi:10.1007/s10238-006-0114-7

179. Kempuraj D, Madhappan B, Christodoulou S, et al. Flavonols inhibit proinflammatory mediator release, intracellular calcium ion levels and protein kinase C theta phosphorylation in human mast cells. *Br J Pharmacol*. 2005;145(7):934-944. doi:10.1038/sj.bjp.0706246

180. Weng Z, Zhang B, Asadi S, et al. Quercetin Is More Effective than Cromolyn in Blocking Human Mast Cell Cytokine Release and Inhibits Contact Dermatitis and Photosensitivity in Humans. Taube C, ed. *PLoS One*. 2012;7(3):e33805. doi:10.1371/journal.pone.0033805

References Chapter 8: Common Root Issues

1. Hoffman TILT Program. What is TILT? https://tiltresearch.org/about-tilt/. Accessed September 3, 2018.

2. Pizzorno J. *The Toxin Solution: How Hidden Poisons in the Air, Water, Food and Products We Use Are Destroying Our Health*. Harper Collins; 2017.

3. Environmental Working Group. *A Benchmark Investigation of Industrial Chemicals, Pollutants and Pesticides in Umbilical Cord Blood. Body Burden: The Pollution in Newborns.*; 2005. http://www.ewg.org/research/body-burden-pollution-newborns.

4. Lang CJ. The use of neuroimaging techniques for clinical detection of neurotoxicity: a review. *Neurotoxicology*. 2000;21(5):847-855. http://www.ncbi.nlm.nih.gov/pubmed/11130290. Accessed September 3, 2018.

5. Swedenborg E, Rüegg J, Mäkelä S, Pongratz I. Endocrine disruptive chemicals: mechanisms of action and involvement in metabolic disorders. *J Mol Endocrinol*. 2009;43(1):1-10. doi:10.1677/JME-08-0132

6. Corsini E, Sokooti M, Galli CL, Moretto A, Colosio C. Pesticide induced immunotoxicity in humans: A comprehensive review of the existing evidence. *Toxicology*. 2013;307:123-135. doi:10.1016/j.tox.2012.10.009

7. Schon EA, DiMauro S, Hirano M. Human mitochondrial DNA: roles of inherited and somatic mutations. *Nat Rev Genet*. 2012;13(12):878-890. doi:10.1038/nrg3275

8. Diaz-Sanchez D, Penichet-Garcia M, Saxon A. Diesel exhaust particles directly induce activated mast cells to degranulate and increase histamine levels and symptom severity. *J Allergy Clin Immunol*. 2000;106(6):1140-1146. doi:10.1067/mai.2000.111144

9. Kempuraj D, Asadi S, Zhang B, et al. Mercury induces inflammatory mediator release from human mast cells. *J Neuroinflammation*. 2010;7:20. doi:10.1186/1742-2094-7-20

10. Natural Resources Defense Council. NRDC Web Page. https://www.nrdc.org/. Accessed September 3, 2018.

11. Agency for Toxic Substances and Disease Registry. Set It Up Safe: A Planning Tool | Safe Places for Child Care | ATSDR. https://www.atsdr.cdc.gov/safeplacesforECE/set_it_up_safe.html. Accessed October 1, 2018.

12. Centers for Disease Control. Agency for Toxic Substances and Disease Registry. https://www.atsdr.cdc.gov/. Accessed October 1, 2018.

13. Chan K. Some aspects of toxic contaminants in herbal medicines. *Chemosphere*. 2003;52(9):1361-1371. doi:10.1016/S0045-6535(03)00471-5

14. Agency for Toxic Substances and Disease Registry. Per- and Polyfluoroalkyl Substances (PFAS) and Your Health. https://www.atsdr.cdc.gov/pfas/index.html. Accessed October 1, 2018.

15. Agency for Toxic Substances and Disease Registry. Substance Priority List | ATSDR. https://www.atsdr.cdc.gov/spl/. Accessed September 30, 2018.

16. Ly T, Lee S. If you think you can safely ink, beware of the masking effects of tattoos. *Hong Kong J Dermatol Venereol*. 2012;20:106-110. http://medcomhk.com/hkdvb/pdf/2012v20n106-110.pdf. Accessed September 3, 2018.

17. Sweeney SM. Tattoos: a review of tattoo practices and potential treatment options for removal. *Curr Opin Pediatr.* 2006;18(4):391-395. doi:10.1097/01.mop.0000236388.64333.cd

18. Watson R. Tattooists use pigments designed as car paint. *BMJ.* 2003;327(7408):182. doi:10.1136/bmj.327.7408.182-b

19. Juhas E, English JC. Tattoo-Associated Complications. *J Pediatr Adolesc Gynecol.* 2013;26(2):125-129. doi:10.1016/J.JPAG.2012.08.005

20. Goldenberg A, Jacob SE. Paraphenylenediamine in black henna temporary tattoos: 12-year Food and Drug Administration data on incidence, symptoms, and outcomes. *J Am Acad Dermatol.* 2015;72(4):724-726. doi:10.1016/j.jaad.2014.11.031

21. Li Z, Zhang H, Li S-H, Byard RW. Fatal Phenol Toxicity Following Attempted Tattoo Removal. *J Forensic Sci.* 2016;61(4):1143-1145. doi:10.1111/1556-4029.13106

22. Jaishankar M, Tseten T, Anbalagan N, Mathew BB, Beeregowda KN. Toxicity, mechanism and health effects of some heavy metals. *Interdiscip Toxicol.* 2014;7(2):60-72. doi:10.2478/intox-2014-0009

23. Sterritt RM, Lester JN. Interactions of heavy metals with bacteria. *Sci Total Environ.* 1980;14(1):5-17. http://www.ncbi.nlm.nih.gov/pubmed/6988964. Accessed September 3, 2018.

24. Natural Resources Defense Council. Electromagnetic Fields Fact Sheet. https://www.cancer.gov/about-cancer/causes-prevention/risk/radiation/electromagnetic-fields-fact-sheet. Accessed September 3, 2018.

25. Lindén V, Rolfsen S. Video computer terminals and occupational dermatitis. *Scand J Work Environ Health.* 1981;7(1):62-64. http://www.ncbi.nlm.nih.gov/pubmed/6458886. Accessed September 3, 2018.

26. Nilsen A. Facial rash in visual display unit operators. *Contact Dermatitis.* 1982;8(1):25-28. http://www.ncbi.nlm.nih.gov/pubmed/6461488. Accessed September 3, 2018.

27. Cox R. *Electromagnetic hypersensitivity – human studies in the UK. Proceedings from the International Workshop in EMF Hypersensitivity in Prague on October 24-25, 2004.* Published in 2006 by the World Health Organization. http://www.who.int/peh-emf/publications/reports/EHS_Proceedings_June2006.pdf.

28. Mueller C, Schierz C. *Project NEMESIS: Double Blind Study on Effects of 50 Hz EMF on Sleep Quality, Physiological Parameters and Field Perception in People Suffering from Electrical Hypersensitivity. Proceedings of International Workshop on EMF Hypersensitivity in Prague on October 24-25, 2004.* http://www.who.int/peh-emf/publications/reports/EHS_Proceedings_June2006.pdf#page=121. Accessed September 3, 2018.

29. Vecchio F, Babiloni C, Ferreri F, et al. Mobile phone emission modulates interhemispheric functional coupling of EEG alpha rhythms. *Eur J Neurosci.* 2007;25(6):1908-1913. doi:10.1111/j.1460-9568.2007.05405.x

30. Belyaev IY, Markovà E, Hillert L, Malmgren LOG, Persson BRR. Microwaves from UMTS/GSM mobile phones induce long-lasting inhibition of 53BP1/γ-H2AX DNA repair foci in human lymphocytes. *Bioelectromagnetics.* 2009;30(2):129-141. doi:10.1002/bem.20445

31. Khurana VG, Teo C, Kundi M, Hardell L, Carlberg M. Cell phones and brain tumors: a review including the long-term epidemiologic data. *Surg Neurol.* 2009;72(3):205-214. doi:10.1016/j.surneu.2009.01.019

32. Kesari KK, Siddiqui MH, Meena R, Verma HN, Kumar S. Cell phone radiation exposure on brain and associated biological systems. *Indian J Exp Biol.* 2013;51(3):187-200. http://www.ncbi.nlm.nih.gov/pubmed/23678539. Accessed September 3, 2018.

33. Lamech F. Self-reporting of symptom development from exposure to radiofrequency fields of wireless smart meters in Victoria, Australia: a case series. *Altern Ther Health Med.* 20(6):28-39. http://www.ncbi.nlm.nih.gov/pubmed/25478801. Accessed September 3, 2018.

34. Carpenter DO. Excessive exposure to radiofrequency electromagnetic fields may cause the development of electrohypersensitivity. *Altern Ther Health Med.* 20(6):40-42. http://www.ncbi.nlm.nih.gov/pubmed/25478802. Accessed September 3, 2018.

35. Carpenter DO. Human disease resulting from exposure to electromagnetic fields1). *Rev Environ Health.* 2013;28(4):159-172. doi:10.1515/reveh-2013-0016

36. Milham S, Morgan LL. A new electromagnetic exposure metric: High frequency voltage transients associated with increased cancer incidence in teachers in a california school. *Am J Ind Med.* 2008;51(8):579-586. doi:10.1002/ajim.20598

37. Johansson O. Disturbance of the immune system by electromagnetic fields—A potentially underlying cause for cellular damage and tissue repair reduction which could lead to disease and impairment. *Pathophysiology.* 2009;16(2-3):157-177. doi:10.1016/j.pathophys.2009.03.004

38. Sandström M, Lyskov E, Berglund A, Medvedev S, Mild KH. Neurophysiological effects of flickering light in patients with perceived electrical hypersensitivity. *J Occup Environ Med.* 1997;39(1):15-22. http://www.ncbi.nlm.nih.gov/pubmed/9029427. Accessed September 3, 2018.

39. Johansson O, Gangi S, Liang Y, Yoshimura K, Jing C, Liu P-Y. Cutaneous mast cells are altered in normal healthy volunteers sitting in front of ordinary TVs/PCs - results from open-field provocation experiments. *J Cutan Pathol.* 2001;28(10):513-519. doi:10.1034/j.1600-0560.2001.281004.x

40. Johansson O, Hilliges M, Han SW. A screening of skin changes, with special emphasis on neurochemical marker antibody evaluation, in patients claiming to suffer from "screen dermatitis" as compared to normal healthy controls. *Exp Dermatol.* 1996;5(5):279-285. http://www.ncbi.nlm.nih.gov/pubmed/8981027. Accessed September 3, 2018.

41. Johannson O, Liu P. "Electrohypersensitivity," "electrosupersensitivity" and "screen dermatitis": preliminary observations from on-going studies in the human skin. Proceedings of the COST 244: Biomedical Effects of Electromagnetic Fields Workshop Works. In: Simunic D, editor.; 1995:52-57.

42. Vorhees D, Zielinski S, Ottoson C, Bourgeios N. Commonwealth of Massachusetts. Special Legislative Committee on Indoor Air Pollution: Indoor Air Pollution in Massachusetts. 1989.

43. Hope J. A review of the mechanism of injury and treatment approaches for illness resulting from exposure to water-damaged buildings, mold, and mycotoxins. *ScientificWorldJournal*. 2013;2013:767482. doi:10.1155/2013/767482

44. Theoharides T. Better Health Guy Blogcast with Scott Forsgren. Interview for episode 58: Mast Cell Master with Dr. T.C. Theoharides, PhD, MD. Aired January 30, 2018.

45. Curtis L, Lieberman A, Stark M, Rea W, Vetter M. Adverse Health Effects of Indoor Molds. *J Nutr Environ Med*. 2004;14(3):261-274. doi:10.1080/13590840400010318

46. Rea WJ, Didriksen N, Simon TR, Pan Y, Fenyves EJ, Griffiths B. Effects of toxic exposure to molds and mycotoxins in building-related illnesses. *Arch Environ Health*. 2003;58(7):399-405. http://www.ncbi.nlm.nih.gov/pubmed/15143852. Accessed September 3, 2018.

47. Forsgren S, Nathan N, Anderson W. Mold and Mycotoxins: Often Overlooked Factors in Chronic Lyme Disease. *Townsend Lett*. 2014:62-73.

48. Shoemaker R. Mold Illness: Surviving Mold Website. https://www.survivingmold.com/. Accessed September 3, 2018.

49. Agag BI. *Mycotoxins in Foods and Feeds 1-Aflatoxins*. Vol 7.; 2004. https://pdfs.semanticscholar.org/1823/f0c7c5fe283999c0c24a452febd88f557e73.pdf. Accessed September 3, 2018.

50. Rehmeyer J. *Through the Shadowlands: A Science Writer's Odyssey into an Illness Science Doesn't Understand*. Rodale; 2017.

51. Wang X, Lien K-W, Ling M-P. Probabilistic health risk assessment for dietary exposure to aflatoxin in peanut and peanut products in Taiwan. *Food Control*. 2018;91:372-380. doi:10.1016/J.FOODCONT.2018.04.021

52. Schwartzbord J, Brown D. Aflatoxin contamination in Haitian peanut products and maize and the safety of oil processed from contaminated peanuts. *Food Control*. 2015;56:114-118. https://www.cabdirect.org/cabdirect/abstract/20153232082. Accessed September 3, 2018.

53. Martins LM, Sant'Ana AS, Iamanaka BT, Berto MI, Pitt JI, Taniwaki MH. Kinetics of aflatoxin degradation during peanut roasting. *Food Res Int*. 2017;97:178-183. doi:10.1016/J.FOODRES.2017.03.052

54. Nehad EA, Farag MM, Kawther MS, Abdel-Samed AKM, Naguib K. Stability of ochratoxin A (OTA) during processing and decaffeination in commercial roasted coffee beans. *Food Addit Contam*. 2005;22(8):761-767. doi:10.1080/02652030500136852

55. Vieira T, Cunha S, Casal S. Mycotoxins in Coffee. *Coffee Heal Dis Prev*. January 2015:225-233. doi:10.1016/B978-0-12-409517-5.00025-5

56. Paterson RRM, Lima N, Taniwaki MH. Coffee, mycotoxins and climate change. *Food Res Int*. 2014;61:1-15. doi:10.1016/J.FOODRES.2014.03.037

57. García-Moraleja A, Font G, Mañes J, Ferrer E. Simultaneous determination of mycotoxin in commercial coffee. *Food Control*. 2015;57:282-292. doi:10.1016/J.FOODCONT.2015.04.031

58. Jeszka-Skowron M, Zgoła-Grześkowiak A, Waśkiewicz A, Stępień Ł, Stanisz E. Positive and negative aspects of green coffee consumption - antioxidant activity versus mycotoxins. *J Sci Food Agric*. 2017;97(12):4022-4028. doi:10.1002/jsfa.8269

59. Martins ML, Martins HM, Gimeno A. Incidence of microflora and of ochratoxin A in green coffee beans (*Coffea arabica*). *Food Addit Contam*. 2003;20(12):1127-1131. doi:10.1080/02652030310001620405

60. Micco C, Grossi M, Miraglia M, Brera C. A study of the contamination by ochratoxin A of green and roasted coffee beans. *Food Addit Contam*. 1989;6(3):333-339. doi:10.1080/02652038909373788

61. Studer-Rohr I, Dietrich DR, Schlatter J, Schlatter C. The occurrence of ochratoxin A in coffee. *Food Chem Toxicol*. 1995;33(5):341-355. http://www.ncbi.nlm.nih.gov/pubmed/7759018. Accessed September 17, 2018.

62. Vaclavik L, Vaclavikova M, Begley TH, Krynitsky AJ, Rader JI. Determination of Multiple Mycotoxins in Dietary Supplements Containing Green Coffee Bean Extracts Using Ultrahigh-Performance Liquid Chromatography–Tandem Mass Spectrometry (UHPLC-MS/MS). *J Agric Food Chem*. 2013;61(20):4822-4830. doi:10.1021/jf401139u

63. Brewer JH, Thrasher JD, Straus DC, Madison RA, Hooper D. Detection of mycotoxins in patients with chronic fatigue syndrome. *Toxins (Basel)*. 2013;5(4):605-617. doi:10.3390/toxins5040605

64. Underhill RA. Myalgic encephalomyelitis, chronic fatigue syndrome: An infectious disease. *Med Hypotheses*. 2015;85(6):765-773. doi:10.1016/J.MEHY.2015.10.011

65. Osterman JW. Comment on Detection of Mycotoxins in Patients with Chronic Fatigue Syndrome: Toxins 2013, 5, 605–617. *Toxins (Basel)*. 2016;8(11):322. doi:10.3390/toxins8110322

66. Brewer J, Thrasher JD, Hooper D. Reply to Comment on Detection of Mycotoxins in Patients with Chronic Fatigue Syndrome Toxins 2013, 5, 605-617 by John W. Osterman, M.D. *Toxins (Basel)*. 2016;8(11). doi:10.3390/toxins8110323

67. Gray MR, Thrasher JD, Hooper D, Crago R. A Case of Reye's-Like Syndrome in a 68-Day Old Infant: Water Damaged Home, Mold, Bacteria and Aflatoxins. *Int J Clin Toxicol.* 2014;2:42-54. https://pdfs.semanticscholar.org/50b1/8ae921d988b7f3bb92642bb744ad49838058.pdf. Accessed September 3, 2018.

68. Berndtson K, Mcmahon S, Ackerley M, Rapaport S, Gupta S, Shoemaker RC. *CONSENSUS STATEMENT Part I: Medically Sound Investigation and Remediation of Water-Damaged Buildings in Cases of CIRS-WDB.*; 2016. https://www.survivingmold.com/MEDICAL_CONSENSUS_STATEMENT_10_30_15.PDF. Accessed September 3, 2018.

69. Thrasher JD, Prokop C, Roberts C, Hooper D. A Family with ME/CFS Following Exposure to Molds, Mycotoxins and Bacteria in a Water-Damaged Home: A Case Report. *Int J Clin Toxicol.* 2016;4. https://www.researchgate.net/publication/297920408. Accessed September 3, 2018.

70. Valtonen V. Clinical Diagnosis of the Dampness and Mold Hypersensitivity Syndrome: Review of the Literature and Suggested Diagnostic Criteria. 2017;8:951. doi:10.3389/fimmu.2017.00951

71. Gunn SR, Gunn GG, Mueller FW. Reversal of Refractory Ulcerative Colitis and Severe Chronic Fatigue Syndrome Symptoms Arising from Immune Disturbance in an HLA-DR/DQ Genetically Susceptible Individual with Multiple Biotoxin Exposures. *Am J Case Rep.* 2016;17:320-325. doi:10.12659/AJCR.896949

72. Morris G, Berk M, Walder K, Maes M. The Putative Role of Viruses, Bacteria, and Chronic Fungal Biotoxin Exposure in the Genesis of Intractable Fatigue Accompanied by Cognitive and Physical Disability. *Mol Neurobiol.* 2016;53(4):2550-2571. doi:10.1007/s12035-015-9262-7

73. Deville L. Lyme and Mold: they go together. In: Christian Natural Health Podcast on Apple Podcasts. Aired on 1/13/17. https://itunes.apple.com/us/podcast/christian-natural-health/id1087096284?mt=2.

74. Shoemaker R. Personal Email Correspondence on 11-28-18.

75. Centers for Disease Control and Prevention. Lyme Disease | CDC. https://www.cdc.gov/lyme/index.html. Accessed September 3, 2018.

76. Schlesinger PA, Duray PH, Burke BA, Steere AC, Stillman MT. Maternal-fetal transmission of the Lyme disease spirochete, Borrelia burgdorferi. *Ann Intern Med.* 1985;103(1):67-68. http://www.ncbi.nlm.nih.gov/pubmed/4003991. Accessed September 3, 2018.

77. Cook MJ, Puri BK. Commercial test kits for detection of Lyme borreliosis: a meta-analysis of test accuracy. *Int J Gen Med.* 2016;9:427-440. doi:10.2147/IJGM.S122313

78. Steere AC, Dhar A, Hernandez J, et al. Systemic symptoms without erythema migrans as the presenting picture of early Lyme disease. *Am J Med.* 2003;114(1):58-62. http://www.ncbi.nlm.nih.gov/pubmed/12543291. Accessed September 3, 2018.

79. Seltzer EG, Gerber MA, Cartter ML, Freudigman K, Shapiro ED. Long-term outcomes of persons with Lyme disease. *JAMA.* 2000;283(5):609-616. http://www.ncbi.nlm.nih.gov/pubmed/10665700. Accessed September 3, 2018.

80. Ingels D. Episode 43: Overcoming Lyme with Dr. Darin Ingels, ND. In: Better Health Guy Blogcasts with Scott Forsgren on Apple Podcasts. Aired on 9/11/17. http://www.betterhealthguy.com/episode43.

81. Goossens HA, Nohlmans MK, van den Bogaard AE. Epstein-Barr virus and cytomegalovirus infections cause false-positive results in IgM two-test protocol for early Lyme borreliosis. *Infection.* 27(3):231. http://www.ncbi.nlm.nih.gov/pubmed/10378140. Accessed September 3, 2018.

82. Wilson A. *Film — Under Our Skin.* Open Eye Pictures. http://underourskin.com/uos1/#film. Accessed September 3, 2017.

83. Hinckley AF, Connally NP, Meek JI, et al. Lyme Disease Testing by Large Commercial Laboratories in the United States. *Clin Infect Dis.* 2014;59(5):676-681. doi:10.1093/cid/ciu397

84. Branda JA, Strle K, Nigrovic LE, et al. Evaluation of Modified 2-Tiered Serodiagnostic Testing Algorithms for Early Lyme Disease. *Clin Infect Dis.* 2017;64(8):1074-1080. doi:10.1093/cid/cix043

85. Leeflang MMG, Ang CW, Berkhout J, et al. The diagnostic accuracy of serological tests for Lyme borreliosis in Europe: a systematic review and meta-analysis. *BMC Infect Dis.* 2016;16(1):140. doi:10.1186/s12879-016-1468-4

86. Commins SP, Platts-Mills TAE. Delayed anaphylaxis to red meat in patients with IgE specific for galactose alpha-1,3-galactose (alpha-gal). *Curr Allergy Asthma Rep.* 2013;13(1):72-77. doi:10.1007/s11882-012-0315-y

87. Talkington J, Nickell SP. Borrelia burgdorferi spirochetes induce mast cell activation and cytokine release. *Infect Immun.* 1999;67(3):1107-1115. http://www.ncbi.nlm.nih.gov/pubmed/10024550. Accessed September 3, 2018.

88. Afrin L. In-person interview conducted in St. Cloud, Minnesota on 9-16-17.

89. Dai J, Narasimhan S, Zhang L, Liu L, Wang P, Fikrig E. Tick histamine release factor is critical for Ixodes scapularis engorgement and transmission of the lyme disease agent. *PLoS Pathog.* 2010;6(11):e1001205. doi:10.1371/journal.ppat.1001205

90. Bowman AS, Dillwith JW, Sauer JR. Tick salivary prostaglandins: Presence, origin and significance. *Parasitol Today.* 1996;12(10):388-396. http://www.ncbi.nlm.nih.gov/pubmed/15275289. Accessed September 3, 2018.

91. Steere AC, Brinckerhoff CE, Miller DJ, Drinker H, Harris ED, Malawista SE. Elevated levels of collagenase and prostaglandin E2 from synovium associated with erosion of cartilage and bone in a patient with chronic Lyme arthritis. *Arthritis Rheum.* 1980;23(5):591-599. http://www.ncbi.nlm.nih.gov/pubmed/6246904. Accessed September 3, 2018.

92. Urioste S, Hall LR, Telford SR, Titus RG. Saliva of the Lyme disease vector, Ixodes dammini, blocks cell activation by a nonprostaglandin E2-dependent mechanism. *J Exp Med*. 1994;180(3):1077-1085. http://www.ncbi.nlm.nih.gov/pubmed/8064226. Accessed September 3, 2018.

93. Rahbar F. Episode 8: SIBO and Lyme Disease. In: The SIBO Doctor Podcast with Dr. Nirala Jacobi on Apple Podcasts. Aired on 4/2/17. https://itunes.apple.com/us/podcast/the-sibo-doctor-podcast/id1199274329?mt=2.

94. Hutt-Fletcher L. Epstein–Barr Virus. In: *Cancers in People with HIV and AIDS*. New York, NY: Springer New York; 2014:75-85. doi:10.1007/978-1-4939-0859-2_6

95. Pembrey L, Waiblinger D, Griffiths P, Patel M, Azad R, Wright J. Cytomegalovirus, Epstein-Barr virus and varicella zoster virus infection in the first two years of life: a cohort study in Bradford, UK. *BMC Infect Dis*. 2017;17(1):220. doi:10.1186/s12879-017-2319-7

96. Cohen JI. Epstein–Barr Virus Infection. *N Engl J Med*. 2000;343(7):481-492. doi:10.1056/NEJM200008173430707

97. Sarwari NM, Khoury JD, Hernandez CMR. Chronic Epstein Barr virus infection leading to classical Hodgkin lymphoma. *BMC Hematol 2016 161*. 2016;16(1):19. doi:10.1186/s12878-016-0059-3

98. Cohen JI. Optimal treatment for chronic active Epstein-Barr virus disease. *Pediatr Transplant*. 2009;13(4):393-396. doi:10.1111/j.1399-3046.2008.01095.x

99. Taylor GS, Long HM, Brooks JM, Rickinson AB, Hislop AD. The Immunology of Epstein-Barr Virus–Induced Disease. *http://dx.doi.org/101146/annurev-immunol-032414-112326*. April 2015. doi:10.1146/ANNUREV-IMMUNOL-032414-112326

100. Kimura H, Hoshino Y, Kanegane H, et al. Clinical and virologic characteristics of chronic active Epstein-Barr virus infection. *Blood*. 2001;98(2):280-286. http://www.ncbi.nlm.nih.gov/pubmed/11435294. Accessed September 28, 2018.

101. Vockerodt M, Yap L-F, Shannon-Lowe C, et al. The Epstein-Barr virus and the pathogenesis of lymphoma. *J Pathol*. 2015;235(2):312-322. doi:10.1002/path.4459

102. Shen Z-J, Hu J, Kashi VP, et al. Epstein-Barr Virus–induced Gene 2 Mediates Allergen-induced Leukocyte Migration into Airways. *Am J Respir Crit Care Med*. 2017;195(12):1576-1585. doi:10.1164/rccm.201608-1580OC

103. Gil A, Mishra R, Song I, Aslan N, Luzuriaga K, Selin LK. Influenza A virus (IAV) infection in humans leads to expansion of highly diverse CD8 T cell repertoires cross-reactive with Epstein Barr virus (EBV). *J Immunol*. 1950;198(1 Supplement):203.11-203.11. http://www.jimmunol.org/content/198/1_Supplement/203.11. Accessed September 3, 2018.

104. Janegova A, Janega P, Rychly B, Kuracinova K, Babal P. The role of Epstein-Barr virus infection in the development of thyroid diseases. *Endokrynol Pol*. 2015;66(2):132-136. doi:10.5603/EP.2015.0020

105. Englund A, Molin D, Enblad G, et al. The role of tumour-infiltrating eosinophils, mast cells and macrophages in Classical and Nodular Lymphocyte Predominant Hodgkin Lymphoma in children. *Eur J Haematol*. 2016;97(5):430-438. doi:10.1111/ejh.12747

References Chapter 9: Conventional Treatment Approaches

1. Afrin L. In-person interview conducted in St. Cloud, Minnesota on 9-16-17.

2. Austen KF, Akin C. Clonal and non-clonal mast cell activation disorders. *Clin Pain Advis Oncol Sect*. 2016. http://www.clinicalpainadvisor.com/oncology/clonal-and-non-clonal-mast-cell-activation-disorders/article/619291/?utm_source=TrendMD&DCMP=OTC-CPA_trendmd&dl=0. Accessed June 23, 2017.

3. Afrin L. Mast Cell Activation Disease: Current Concepts. Powerpoint Presentation as Part of Wellapalooza Conference on 4-30-17.

4. Molderings GJ, Haenisch B, Brettner S, et al. Pharmacological treatment options for mast cell activation disease. *Naunyn Schmiedebergs Arch Pharmacol*. 2016;389(7):671-694. doi:10.1007/s00210-016-1247-1

5. Afrin L. Personal email correspondence on October 3rd, 2018.

6. Malik F, Ali N, Jafri SIM, et al. Continuous diphenhydramine infusion and imatinib for KIT-D816V-negative mast cell activation syndrome: a case report. *J Med Case Rep*. 2017;11(1):119. doi:10.1186/s13256-017-1278-3

7. da Silva EN, Randall KL. Omalizumab mitigates anaphylaxis during ultrarush honey bee venom immunotherapy in monoclonal mast cell activation syndrome. *J Allergy Clin Immunol Pract*. 2013;1(6):687-688. doi:10.1016/j.jaip.2013.07.004

8. Bell MC, Jackson DJ. Prevention of anaphylaxis related to mast cell activation syndrome with omalizumab. *Ann Allergy Asthma Immunol*. 2012;108(5):383-384. doi:10.1016/j.anai.2012.02.021

9. Wirz S, Molderings GJ. A practical guide for treatment of pain in patients with systemic mast cell activation disease. *Pain Physician*. 2017;20:E849-E861.

10. Molderings GJ, Brettner S, Homann J, Afrin LB. Mast cell activation disease: A concise practical guide for diagnostic workup and therapeutic options. *J Hematol Oncol*. 2011;4:10. doi:10.1186/1756-8722-4-10

11. Afrin L. Ask The NY MCAS Expert: Mast Cell Activation Syndrome Questions Answered. Posted on October 16, 2017. https://www.drtaniadempsey.com/single-post/Ask-The-NY-MCAS-Expert-Mast-Cell-Activation-Syndrome-Questions-Answered. Accessed September 22, 2018.

12. Seneviratne SL, Maitland A, Afrin L. Mast cell disorders in Ehlers–Danlos syndrome. *Am J Med Genet Part C Semin Med Genet.* 2017;175(1):226-236. doi:10.1002/ajmg.c.31555

13. Theoharides T. Better Health Guy Blogcast with Scott Forsgren. Interview for episode 58: Mast Cell Master with Dr. T.C. Theoharides, PhD, MD. Aired on 1-30-18. http://www.betterhealthguy.com/episode58.

14. Afrin L. Conference round table discussion as part of "Often Seen, Rarely Recognized" continuing education event on 9-16-17. CentraCare Health Plaza. St. Cloud, Minnesota.

15. Afrin LB, Khoruts A. Mast Cell Activation Disease and Microbiotic Interactions. *Clin Ther.* 2015;37(5):941-953. doi:10.1016/j.clinthera.2015.02.008

16. Soderberg M. The Mast Cell Activation Syndrome: A Mini Review. *MOJ Immunol.* 2015;2(1). doi:10.15406/moji.2015.02.00032

17. Kemp SF, Lockey RF, Simons FER, World Allergy Organization ad hoc Committee on Epinephrine in Anaphylaxis. Epinephrine: the drug of choice for anaphylaxis-a statement of the world allergy organization. *World Allergy Organ J.* 2008;1(7 Suppl):S18-26. doi:10.1097/WOX.0b013e31817c9338

18. Afrin LB. Utility of Continuous Diphenhydramine Infusion in Severe Mast Cell Activation Syndrome. *Blood.* 2015;126(23). http://www.bloodjournal.org/content/126/23/5194?sso-checked=true. Accessed September 4, 2018.

19. Yanai K, Yoshikawa T, Yanai A, et al. The clinical pharmacology of non-sedating antihistamines. *Pharmacol Ther.* 2017;178:148-156. doi:10.1016/j.pharmthera.2017.04.004

20. The Mastocytosis Society. Medications to Treat Mast Cell Disorders - TMS. https://tmsforacure.org/treatments-2/medications-treat-mast-cell-disorders/. Accessed September 4, 2018.

21. Handley DA, Magnetti A, Higgins AJ. Therapeutic advantages of third generation antihistamines. *Expert Opin Investig Drugs.* 1998;7(7):1045-1054. doi:10.1517/13543784.7.7.1045

22. Carson S, Lee N, Thakurta S. *Drug Class Review: Newer Antihistamines: Final Report Update 2.* Oregon Health & Science University, Portland (OR); 2010. http://www.ncbi.nlm.nih.gov/pubmed/21348045. Accessed September 4, 2018.

23. Campbell N, Boustani M, Limbil T, et al. The cognitive impact of anticholinergics: a clinical review. *Clin Interv Aging.* 2009;4:225-233. http://www.ncbi.nlm.nih.gov/pubmed/19554093. Accessed September 4, 2018.

24. Monthly Prescribing Reference. Medications with Significant Anticholinergic Properties. https://www.empr.com/clinical-charts/medications-with-significant-anticholinergic-properties/article/123667/. Accessed September 4, 2018.

25. Zuberbier T, Bindslev-Jensen C, Canonica W, et al. EAACI/GA2LEN/EDF guideline: definition, classification and diagnosis of urticaria. *Allergy.* 2006;61(3):316-320. doi:10.1111/j.1398-9995.2005.00964.x

26. Gray SL, Anderson ML, Dublin S, et al. Cumulative use of strong anticholinergics and incident dementia: a prospective cohort study. *JAMA Intern Med.* 2015;175(3):401-407. doi:10.1001/jamainternmed.2014.7663

27. Risacher SL, McDonald BC, Tallman EF, et al. Association Between Anticholinergic Medication Use and Cognition, Brain Metabolism, and Brain Atrophy in Cognitively Normal Older Adults. *JAMA Neurol.* 2016;73(6):721. doi:10.1001/jamaneurol.2016.0580

28. Green AJ, Gelfand JM, Cree BA, et al. Clemastine fumarate as a remyelinating therapy for multiple sclerosis (ReBUILD): a randomised, controlled, double-blind, crossover trial. *Lancet.* 2017;390(10111):2481-2489. doi:10.1016/S0140-6736(17)32346-2

29. Phanuphak P, Schocket A, Kohler PF. Treatment of chronic idiopathic urticaria with combined H1 and H2 blockers. *Clin Allergy.* 1978;8(5):429-433. http://www.ncbi.nlm.nih.gov/pubmed/30546. Accessed September 5, 2018.

30. Harvey RP, Schocket AL. The effect of H1 and H2 blockade on cutaneous histamine response in man. *J Allergy Clin Immunol.* 1980;65(2):136-139. http://www.ncbi.nlm.nih.gov/pubmed/6101337. Accessed September 5, 2018.

31. Lippert U, Möller A, Welker P, Artuc M, Henz BM. Inhibition of cytokine secretion from human leukemic mast cells and basophils by H1- and H2-receptor antagonists. *Exp Dermatol.* 2000;9(2):118-124. http://www.ncbi.nlm.nih.gov/pubmed/10772385. Accessed September 5, 2018.

32. Lin RY, Curry A, Pesola GR, et al. Improved outcomes in patients with acute allergic syndromes who are treated with combined H1 and H2 antagonists. *Ann Emerg Med.* 2000;36(5):462-468. doi:10.1067/mem.2000.109445

33. Sanada S, Tanaka T, Kameyoshi Y, Hide M. The effectiveness of montelukast for the treatment of anti-histamine-resistant chronic urticaria. *Arch Dermatol Res.* 2005;297(3):134-138. doi:10.1007/s00403-005-0586-4

34. Fedorowicz Z, van Zuuren EJ, Hu N. Histamine H2-receptor antagonists for urticaria. *Cochrane Database Syst Rev.* 2012;(3):CD008596. doi:10.1002/14651858.CD008596.pub2

35. Nurmatov UB, Rhatigan E, Simons FER, Sheikh A. H2-antihistamines for the treatment of anaphylaxis with and without shock: a systematic review. *Ann Allergy, Asthma Immunol.* 2014;112(2):126-131. doi:10.1016/j.anai.2013.11.010

36. Lam JR, Schneider JL, Zhao W, Corley DA. Proton Pump Inhibitor and Histamine 2 Receptor Antagonist Use and Vitamin B$_{12}$ Deficiency. *JAMA*. 2013;310(22):2435. doi:10.1001/jama.2013.280490

37. Valuck RJ, Ruscin JM. A case-control study on adverse effects: H2 blocker or proton pump inhibitor use and risk of vitamin B12 deficiency in older adults. *J Clin Epidemiol*. 2004;57(4):422-428. doi:10.1016/j.jclinepi.2003.08.015

38. Ruscin JM, Lee Page R, Valuck RJ. Vitamin B$_{12}$ Deficiency Associated with Histamine$_2$-Receptor Antagonists and a Proton-Pump Inhibitor. *Ann Pharmacother*. 2002;36(5):812-816. doi:10.1345/aph.10325

39. Jung SB, Nagaraja V, Kapur A, Eslick GD. Association between vitamin B12 deficiency and long-term use of acid-lowering agents: a systematic review and meta-analysis. *Intern Med J*. 2015;45(4):409-416. doi:10.1111/imj.12697

40. Force RW, Nahata MC. Effect of Histamine H$_2$-Receptor Antagonists on Vitamin B$_{12}$ Absorption. Hartshorn EA, ed. *Ann Pharmacother*. 1992;26(10):1283-1286. doi:10.1177/106002809202601018

41. Varughese GI, Scarpello JHB. Metformin and vitamin B12 deficiency: the role of H2 receptor antagonists and proton pump inhibitors. *Age Ageing*. 2007;36(1):110-111. doi:10.1093/ageing/afl139

42. Ting RZ-W, Szeto CC, Chan MH-M, Ma KK, Chow KM. Risk Factors of Vitamin B12 Deficiency in Patients Receiving Metformin. *Arch Intern Med*. 2006;166(18):1975. doi:10.1001/archinte.166.18.1975

43. Zandi PP, Anthony JC, Hayden KM, et al. Reduced incidence of AD with NSAID but not H2 receptor antagonists: the Cache County Study. *Neurology*. 2002;59(6):880-886. http://www.ncbi.nlm.nih.gov/pubmed/12297571. Accessed September 5, 2018.

44. Boustani M, Hall KS, Lane KA, et al. The association between cognition and histamine-2 receptor antagonists in African Americans. *J Am Geriatr Soc*. 2007;55(8):1248-1253. doi:10.1111/j.1532-5415.2007.01270.x

45. Weller CL, Collington SJ, Brown JK, et al. Leukotriene B4, an activation product of mast cells, is a chemoattractant for their progenitors. *J Exp Med*. 2005;201(12):1961-1971. doi:10.1084/jem.20042407

46. Tintinger GR, Feldman C, Theron AJ, Anderson R. Montelukast: More than a Cysteinyl Leukotriene Receptor Antagonist? *Sci World J*. 2010;10:2403-2413. doi:10.1100/tsw.2010.229

47. Shiota N, Shimoura K, Okunishi H. Pathophysiological role of mast cells in collagen-induced arthritis: Study with a cysteinyl leukotriene receptor antagonist, montelukast. *Eur J Pharmacol*. 2006;548(1-3):158-166. doi:10.1016/j.ejphar.2006.07.046

48. Riccioni G, Di Ilio C, Conti P, Theoharides TC, D'Orazio N. Advances in therapy with antileukotriene drugs. *Ann Clin Lab Sci*. 2004;34(4):379-387. http://www.ncbi.nlm.nih.gov/pubmed/15648777. Accessed September 5, 2018.

49. Tolar J, Tope WD, Neglia JP. Leukotriene-Receptor Inhibition for the Treatment of Systemic Mastocytosis. *N Engl J Med*. 2004;350(7):735-736. doi:10.1056/NEJM200402123500723

50. Turner PJ, Kemp AS, Rogers M, Mehr S. Refractory Symptoms Successfully Treated with Leukotriene Inhibition in a Child with Systemic Mastocytosis. *Pediatr Dermatol*. 2012;29(2):222-223. doi:10.1111/j.1525-1470.2011.01576.x

51. Di Lernia V, Ricci C, Lallas A, Ficarelli E. Clinical predictors of non-response to any tumor necrosis factor (TNF) blockers: a retrospective study. *J Dermatolog Treat*. 2014;25(1):73-74. doi:10.3109/09546634.2013.800184

52. Diak P, Siegel J, La Grenade L, Choi L, Lemery S, McMahon A. Tumor necrosis factor α blockers and malignancy in children: Forty-eight cases reported to the food and drug administration. *Arthritis Rheum*. 2010;62(8):2517-2524. doi:10.1002/art.27511

53. Askling J, Fahrbach K, Nordstrom B, Ross S, Schmid CH, Symmons D. Cancer risk with tumor necrosis factor alpha (TNF) inhibitors: meta-analysis of randomized controlled trials of adalimumab, etanercept, and infliximab using patient level data. *Pharmacoepidemiol Drug Saf*. 2011;20(2):119-130. doi:10.1002/pds.2046

54. Jacobsson LTH, Turesson C, Gülfe A, et al. Treatment with tumor necrosis factor blockers is associated with a lower incidence of first cardiovascular events in patients with rheumatoid arthritis. *J Rheumatol*. 2005;32(7):1213-1218. http://www.ncbi.nlm.nih.gov/pubmed/15996054. Accessed September 5, 2018.

55. Dinarello CA, Simon A, van der Meer JWM. Treating inflammation by blocking interleukin-1 in a broad spectrum of diseases. *Nat Rev Drug Discov*. 2012;11(8):633-652. doi:10.1038/nrd3800

56. Steinke JW, Borish L. Th2 cytokines and asthma. Interleukin-4: its role in the pathogenesis of asthma, and targeting it for asthma treatment with interleukin-4 receptor antagonists. *Respir Res*. 2001;2(2):66-70. doi:10.1186/RR40

57. Thurmond RL, Venable J, Savall B, et al. Clinical Development of Histamine H4 Receptor Antagonists. In: *Handbook of Experimental Pharmacology*. Vol 241. ; 2017:301-320. doi:10.1007/164_2016_130

58. Theoharides TC, Sieghart W, Greengard P, Douglas WW. Antiallergic drug cromolyn may inhibit histamine secretion by regulating phosphorylation of a mast cell protein. *Science*. 1980;207(4426):80-82. http://www.ncbi.nlm.nih.gov/pubmed/6153130. Accessed September 5, 2018.

59. Barrett KE, Metcalfe DD. The histologic and functional characterization of enzymatically dispersed intestinal mast cells of nonhuman primates: effects of secretagogues and anti-allergic drugs on histamine secretion. *J Immunol*. 1985;135(3):2020-2026. http://www.ncbi.nlm.nih.gov/pubmed/2410511. Accessed September 5, 2018.

60. Pearce FL, Befus AD, Gauldie J, Bienenstock J. Mucosal mast cells. II. Effects of anti-allergic compounds on histamine secretion by isolated intestinal mast cells. *J Immunol.* 1982;128(6):2481-2486. http://www.ncbi.nlm.nih.gov/pubmed/6176639. Accessed September 5, 2018.

61. Okayama Y, Benyon RC, Rees PH, Lowman MA, Hillier K, Church MK. Inhibition profiles of sodium cromoglycate and nedocromil sodium on mediator release from mast cells of human skin, lung, tonsil, adenoid and intestine. *Clin Exp Allergy.* 1992;22(3):401-409. http://www.ncbi.nlm.nih.gov/pubmed/1375128. Accessed September 5, 2018.

62. Edwards AM, Stevens MT, Church MK. The effects of topical sodium cromoglicate on itch and flare in human skin induced by intradermal histamine: a randomised double-blind vehicle controlled intra-subject design trial. *BMC Res Notes.* 2011;4:47. doi:10.1186/1756-0500-4-47

63. Camarasa JG, Serra-Baldrich E, Monreal P, Soller J. Contact dermatitis from sodium-cromoglycate-containing eyedrops. *Contact Dermatitis.* 1997;36(3):160-161. http://www.ncbi.nlm.nih.gov/pubmed/9145269. Accessed September 5, 2018.

64. Kudo H, Tanaka T, Miyachi Y, Imamura S. Contact dermatitis from sodium cromoglycate eyedrops. *Contact Dermatitis.* 1988;19(4):312. http://www.ncbi.nlm.nih.gov/pubmed/3146462. Accessed September 5, 2018.

65. Davydov L. Omalizumab (Xolair) for treatment of asthma. *Am Fam Physician.* 2005;71(2):341-342. http://www.ncbi.nlm.nih.gov/pubmed/15686303. Accessed September 5, 2018.

66. Fanta CH. Asthma. *N Engl J Med.* 2009;360(10):1002-1014. doi:10.1056/NEJMra0804579

67. Molderings GJ, Raithel M, Kratz F, et al. Omalizumab Treatment of Systemic Mast Cell Activation Disease: Experiences from Four Cases. *Intern Med.* 2011;50(6):611-615. doi:10.2169/internalmedicine.50.4640

68. Kibsgaard L, Skjold T, Deleuran M, Vestergaard C. Omalizumab Induced Remission of Idiopathic Anaphylaxis in a Patient Suffering from Indolent Systemic Mastocytosis. *Acta Derm Venereol.* 2014;94(3):363-364. doi:10.2340/00015555-1687

69. Douglass JA, Carroll K, Voskamp A, Bourke P, Wei A, O'Hehir RE. Omalizumab is effective in treating systemic mastocytosis in a nonatopic patient. *Allergy.* 2009;65(7):926-927. doi:10.1111/j.1398-9995.2009.02259.x

70. Carter MC, Robyn JA, Bressler PB, Walker JC, Shapiro GG, Metcalfe DD. Omalizumab for the treatment of unprovoked anaphylaxis in patients with systemic mastocytosis. *J Allergy Clin Immunol.* 2007;119(6):1550-1551. doi:10.1016/j.jaci.2007.03.032

71. Broesby-Olsen S, Vestergaard H, Mortz CG, et al. Omalizumab prevents anaphylaxis and improves symptoms in systemic mastocytosis: Efficacy and safety observations. *Allergy.* 2018;73(1):230-238. doi:10.1111/all.13237

72. Sokol KC, Ghazi A, Kelly BC, Grant JA. Omalizumab as a Desensitizing Agent and Treatment in Mastocytosis: A Review of the Literature and Case Report. *J Allergy Clin Immunol Pract.* 2014;2(3):266-270. doi:10.1016/j.jaip.2014.03.009

73. Lieberoth S, Thomsen SF. Cutaneous and gastrointestinal symptoms in two patients with systemic mastocytosis successfully treated with omalizumab. *Case Rep Med.* 2015;2015:903541. doi:10.1155/2015/903541

74. Bidri M, Royer B, Averlant G, Bismuth G, Guillosson JJ, Arock M. Inhibition of mouse mast cell proliferation and proinflammatory mediator release by benzodiazepines. *Immunopharmacology.* 1999;43(1):75-86. http://www.ncbi.nlm.nih.gov/pubmed/10437659. Accessed September 6, 2018.

75. Suzuki-Nishimura T, Sano T, Uchida MK. Effects of benzodiazepines on serotonin release from rat mast cells. *Eur J Pharmacol.* 1989;167(1):75-85. http://www.ncbi.nlm.nih.gov/pubmed/2550260. Accessed September 6, 2018.

76. Ramirez K, Niraula A, Sheridan JF. GABAergic modulation with classical benzodiazepines prevent stress-induced neuro-immune dysregulation and behavioral alterations. *Brain Behav Immun.* 2016;51:154-168. doi:10.1016/j.bbi.2015.08.011

77. van der Weide HY, van Westerloo DJ, van den Bergh WM. Critical care management of systemic mastocytosis: when every wasp is a killer bee. *Crit Care.* 2015;19(1):238. doi:10.1186/s13054-015-0956-z

78. Zermati Y, De Sepulveda P, Féger F, et al. Effect of tyrosine kinase inhibitor STI571 on the kinase activity of wild-type and various mutated c-kit receptors found in mast cell neoplasms. *Oncogene.* 2003;22(5):660-664. doi:10.1038/sj.onc.1206120

79. Pardanani A, Tefferi A. Systemic mastocytosis in adults: a review on prognosis and treatment based on 342 Mayo Clinic patients and current literature. *Curr Opin Hematol.* 2010;17(2):125-132. doi:10.1097/MOH.0b013e3283366c59

80. Akin C, Brockow K, D'Ambrosio C, et al. Effects of tyrosine kinase inhibitor STI571 on human mast cells bearing wild-type or mutated c-kit. *Exp Hematol.* 2003;31(8):686-692. http://www.ncbi.nlm.nih.gov/pubmed/12901973. Accessed September 6, 2018.

81. Gotlib J, Berubé C, Growney JD, et al. Activity of the tyrosine kinase inhibitor PKC412 in a patient with mast cell leukemia with the D816V KIT mutation. *Blood.* 2005;106(8):2865-2870. doi:10.1182/blood-2005-04-1568

82. Valent P, Akin C, Hartmann K, et al. Midostaurin: a magic bullet that blocks mast cell expansion and activation. *Ann Oncol.* 2017;28(10):2367-2376. doi:10.1093/annonc/mdx290

83. Dispenza MC, Regan JA, Bochner BS. Potential applications of Bruton's tyrosine kinase inhibitors for the prevention of allergic reactions. *Expert Rev Clin Immunol*. 2017;13(10):921-923. doi:10.1080/1744666X.2017.1370374

84. Latar I, Koufany M, Hablot J, et al. Association between rheumatoid arthritis and systemic mastocytosis: a case report and literature review. *Clin Rheumatol*. 2016;35(10):2619-2623. doi:10.1007/s10067-016-3368-9

85. Nwaru BI, Dhami S, Sheikh A. Idiopathic Anaphylaxis. *Curr Treat options allergy*. 2017;4(3):312-319. doi:10.1007/s40521-017-0136-2

86. Ustun C, Reiter A, Scott BL, et al. Hematopoietic Stem-Cell Transplantation for Advanced Systemic Mastocytosis. *J Clin Oncol*. 2014;32(29):3264-3274. doi:10.1200/JCO.2014.55.2018

87. Valent P, Akin C, Metcalfe DD. Mastocytosis: 2016 updated WHO classification and novel emerging treatment concepts. *Blood*. 2017;129:1420-1427. doi:10.1182/blood-2016-09-731893

88. Hurd YL, Yoon M, Manini AF, et al. Early Phase in the Development of Cannabidiol as a Treatment for Addiction: Opioid Relapse Takes Initial Center Stage. *Neurotherapeutics*. 2015;12(4):807-815. doi:10.1007/s13311-015-0373-7

89. Devinsky O, Cilio MR, Cross H, et al. Cannabidiol: pharmacology and potential therapeutic role in epilepsy and other neuropsychiatric disorders. *Epilepsia*. 2014;55(6):791-802. doi:10.1111/epi.12631

90. De Filippis D, D'Amico A, Iuvone T. Cannabinomimetic Control of Mast Cell Mediator Release: New Perspective in Chronic Inflammation. *J Neuroendocrinol*. 2008;20(s1):20-25. doi:10.1111/j.1365-2826.2008.01674.x

91. Pini A, Mannaioni G, Pellegrini-Giampietro D, et al. The role of cannabinoids in inflammatory modulation of allergic respiratory disorders, inflammatory pain and ischemic stroke. *Curr Drug Targets*. 2012;13(7):984-993. http://www.ncbi.nlm.nih.gov/pubmed/22420307. Accessed September 6, 2018.

92. Ständer S, Schmelz M, Metze D, Luger T, Rukwied R. Distribution of cannabinoid receptor 1 (CB1) and 2 (CB2) on sensory nerve fibers and adnexal structures in human skin. *J Dermatol Sci*. 2005;38(3):177-188. doi:10.1016/j.jdermsci.2005.01.007

93. Srivastava MD, Srivastava BI, Brouhard B. Delta9 tetrahydrocannabinol and cannabidiol alter cytokine production by human immune cells. *Immunopharmacology*. 1998;40(3):179-185. http://www.ncbi.nlm.nih.gov/pubmed/9858061. Accessed September 6, 2018.

94. Badiner A. High on Health: CBD in the Food Supply - Reality Sandwich. http://realitysandwich.com/171680/high_health_cbd_food_supply/. Accessed September 6, 2018.

95. Afrin LB. Utility of hydroxyurea in mast cell activation syndrome. *Exp Hematol Oncol*. 2013;2(1):28. doi:10.1186/2162-3619-2-28

96. Lim K-H, Pardanani AD, Butterfield JH, Li CY, Tefferi A. Cytoreductive Therapy in Systemic Mastocytosis: Outcome Analysis and Response Prediction in 134 Consecutive Patients. *Blood*. 2008;112(11). http://www.bloodjournal.org/content/112/11/1759?sso-checked=true. Accessed September 6, 2018.

97. Sheikh J, Drews RE, Nunez R, et al. Management of Type II Systemic Mastocytosis (SM-AHNMD) with Hydroxyurea. *J Allergy Clin Immunol*. 2006;117(2):S70. doi:10.1016/j.jaci.2005.12.282

98. Shaik-Dasthagirisaheb YB, Varvara G, Murmura G, et al. Role of vitamins D, E and C in immunity and inflammation. *J Biol Regul Homeost Agents*. 27(2):291-295. http://www.ncbi.nlm.nih.gov/pubmed/23830380. Accessed September 6, 2018.

99. Meister A. Glutathione-ascorbic acid antioxidant system in animals. *J Biol Chem*. 1994;269(13):9397-9400. http://www.ncbi.nlm.nih.gov/pubmed/8144521. Accessed September 6, 2018.

100. Johnston CS, Meyer CG, Srilakshmi JC. Vitamin C elevates red blood cell glutathione in healthy adults. *Am J Clin Nutr*. 1993;58(1):103-105. doi:10.1093/ajcn/58.1.103

101. Tecklenburg SL, Mickleborough TD, Fly AD, Bai Y, Stager JM. Ascorbic acid supplementation attenuates exercise-induced bronchoconstriction in patients with asthma. *Respir Med*. 2007;101(8):1770-1778. doi:10.1016/j.rmed.2007.02.014

102. Jarisch R, Weyer D, Ehlert E, et al. Impact of oral vitamin C on histamine levels and seasickness. *J Vestib Res*. 2014;24(4):281-288. doi:10.3233/VES-140509

103. Hickey S, Roberts HJ, Miller NJ. Pharmacokinetics of oral vitamin C. *J Nutr Environ Med*. 2008;17(3):169-177. doi:10.1080/13590840802305423

104. Hagel AF, Layritz CM, Hagel WH, et al. Intravenous infusion of ascorbic acid decreases serum histamine concentrations in patients with allergic and non-allergic diseases. *Naunyn Schmiedebergs Arch Pharmacol*. 2013;386(9):789-793. doi:10.1007/s00210-013-0880-1

105. Carr A, Maggini S. Vitamin C and Immune Function. *Nutrients*. 2017;9(11):1211. doi:10.3390/nu9111211

106. Klooker TK, Braak B, Koopman KE, et al. The mast cell stabiliser ketotifen decreases visceral hypersensitivity and improves intestinal symptoms in patients with irritable bowel syndrome. *Gut*. 2010;59(9):1213-1221. doi:10.1136/gut.2010.213108

107. Cap JP, Schwanitz HJ, Czarnetzki BM. Effect of ketotifen in urticaria factitia and urticaria cholinergica in a crossover double-blind trial. *Hautarzt*. 1985;36(9):509-511. http://www.ncbi.nlm.nih.gov/pubmed/3905713. Accessed September 6, 2018.

108. St-Pierre JP, Kobric M, Rackham A. Effect of ketotifen treatment on cold-induced urticaria. *Ann Allergy.* 1985;55(6):840-843. http://www.ncbi.nlm.nih.gov/pubmed/3907425. Accessed September 6, 2018.

109. Kamide R, Niimura M, Ueda H, et al. Clinical evaluation of ketotifen for chronic urticaria: multicenter double-blind comparative study with clemastine. *Ann Allergy.* 1989;62(4):322-325. http://www.ncbi.nlm.nih.gov/pubmed/2650586. Accessed September 6, 2018.

110. McClean SP, Arreaza EE, Lett-Brown MA, Grant JA. Refractory cholinergic urticaria successfully treated with ketotifen. *J Allergy Clin Immunol.* 1989;83(4):738-741. http://www.ncbi.nlm.nih.gov/pubmed/2651507. Accessed September 6, 2018.

111. Czarnetzki BM. A double-blind cross-over study of the effect of ketotifen in urticaria pigmentosa. *Dermatologica.* 1983;166(1):44-47. http://www.ncbi.nlm.nih.gov/pubmed/6341102. Accessed September 6, 2018.

112. Nurmatov UB, Rhatigan E, Simons FER, Sheikh A. H$_1$-antihistamines for primary mast cell activation syndromes: a systematic review. *Allergy.* 2015;70(9):1052-1061. doi:10.1111/all.12672

113. González-de-Olano D, Matito A, Orfao A, Escribano L. Advances in the understanding and clinical management of mastocytosis and clonal mast cell activation syndromes. *F1000Research.* 2016;5:2666. doi:10.12688/f1000research.9565.1

114. Ting S. Ketotifen and systemic mastocytosis. *J Allergy Clin Immunol.* 1990;85(4):818. http://www.ncbi.nlm.nih.gov/pubmed/2324420. Accessed September 6, 2018.

115. Póvoa P, Ducla-Soares J, Fernandes A, Palma-Carlos AG. A case of systemic mastocytosis; therapeutic efficacy of ketotifen. *J Intern Med.* 1991;229(5):475-477. http://www.ncbi.nlm.nih.gov/pubmed/2040876. Accessed September 6, 2018.

116. Graves L, Stechschulte DJ, Morris DC, Lukert BP. Inhibition of mediator release in systemic mastocytosis is associated with reversal of bone changes. *J Bone Miner Res.* 2009;5(11):1113-1119. doi:10.1002/jbmr.5650051104

117. Theoharides TC. Mast Cell Master. http://www.mastcellmaster.com/research.php. Accessed September 6, 2018.

118. Degboé Y, Eischen M, Nigon D, et al. Prevalence and risk factors for fragility fracture in systemic mastocytosis. *Bone.* 2017;105:219-225. doi:10.1016/j.bone.2017.09.005

119. Broesby-Olsen S, Farkas DK, Vestergaard H, et al. Risk of solid cancer, cardiovascular disease, anaphylaxis, osteoporosis and fractures in patients with systemic mastocytosis: A nationwide population-based study. *Am J Hematol.* 2016;91(11):1069-1075. doi:10.1002/ajh.24490

120. Chiappetta N, Gruber B. The Role of Mast Cells in Osteoporosis. *Semin Arthritis Rheum.* 2006;36(1):32-36. doi:10.1016/j.semarthrit.2006.03.004

121. Seitz S, Barvencik F, Koehne T, et al. Increased osteoblast and osteoclast indices in individuals with systemic mastocytosis. *Osteoporos Int.* 2013;24(8):2325-2334. doi:10.1007/s00198-013-2305-x

122. Veer E, Goot W, Monchy JGR, Kluin-Nelemans HC, Doormaal JJ. High prevalence of fractures and osteoporosis in patients with indolent systemic mastocytosis. *Allergy.* 2012;67(3):431-438. doi:10.1111/j.1398-9995.2011.02780.x

123. Lim C, Leondar J, Abbara A, Forbes P, Cox J, Comninos A. Systemic Mastocytosis: A Rare but Important Cause of Osteoporosis. *Endocr Abstr.* 2017;50(EP032). doi:10.1530/endoabs.50.EP032

124. Wirz S, Hertfelder H-J, Seidel H, Homann J, Molderings G. Lower prevalence of vitamin D insufficiency in German patients with systemic mast cell activation syndrome compared with the general population. *Z Gastroenterol.* 2017;55(12):1297-1306. doi:10.1055/s-0043-121346

125. Aich A, Afrin LB, Gupta K. Mast Cell-Mediated Mechanisms of Nociception. *Int J Mol Sci.* 2015;16(12):29069-29092. doi:10.3390/ijms161226151

126. Uygun DS, Ye Z, Zecharia AY, et al. Bottom-Up versus Top-Down Induction of Sleep by Zolpidem Acting on Histaminergic and Neocortex Neurons. *J Neurosci.* 2016;36(44):11171-11184. doi:10.1523/JNEUROSCI.3714-15.2016

References Chapter 10: Natural Treatment Options

1. Galloway T, Handy R. Immunotoxicity of organophosphorous pesticides. *Ecotoxicology.* 12(1-4):345-363. http://www.ncbi.nlm.nih.gov/pubmed/12739880. Accessed September 10, 2018.

2. Rohr U, König W, Selenka F. Effect of pesticides on the release of histamine, chemotactic factors and leukotrienes from rat mast cells and human basophils. *Zentralbl Bakteriol Mikrobiol Hyg B.* 1985;181(6):469-486. http://www.ncbi.nlm.nih.gov/pubmed/2420099. Accessed September 10, 2018.

3. Teshima R, Nakamura R, Nakajima O, Hachisuka A, Sawada J-I. Effect of two nitrogenous diphenyl ether pesticides on mast cell activation. *Toxicol Lett.* 2004;150(3):277-283. doi:10.1016/j.toxlet.2004.02.001

4. Park KR, Monsky WL, Lee CG, et al. Mast Cells Contribute to Radiation-Induced Vascular Hyperpermeability. *Radiat Res.* 2016;185(2):182-189. doi:10.1667/RR14190.1

5. Tsunoda M, Sharma RP. Modulation of tumor necrosis factor alpha expression in mouse brain after exposure to aluminum in drinking water. *Arch Toxicol.* 1999;73(8-9):419-426. http://www.ncbi.nlm.nih.gov/pubmed/10650912. Accessed September 10, 2018.

6. Schedle A, Samorapoompichit P, Füreder W, et al. Metal ion-induced toxic histamine release from human basophils and mast cells. *J Biomed Mater Res.* 1998;39(4):560-567. http://www.ncbi.nlm.nih.gov/pubmed/9492216. Accessed September 10, 2018.

7. Anogeianaki A, Castellani ML, Tripodi D, et al. Vitamins and Mast Cells. *Int J Immunopathol Pharmacol.* 2010;23(4):991-996. doi:10.1177/039463201002300403

8. Weng Z, Zhang B, Asadi S, et al. Quercetin Is More Effective than Cromolyn in Blocking Human Mast Cell Cytokine Release and Inhibits Contact Dermatitis and Photosensitivity in Humans. Taube C, ed. *PLoS One.* 2012;7(3):e33805. doi:10.1371/journal.pone.0033805

9. Basu A, Sarkar A, Basak P. Nutraceuticals for Human Health and Hypersensitivity Reaction. In: Verma, Amit Srivastava K, Singh S, Singh H, eds. *Nutraceuticals and Innovative Food Products for Healthy Living and Preventive Care.* 2018. doi:10.4018/978-1-5225-2970-5.ch015

10. Theoharides T. Better Health Guy Blogcast with Scott Forsgren. Interview for episode 58: Mast Cell Master with Dr. T.C. Theoharides, PhD, MD. Aired January 30, 2018.

11. Theoharides TC, Asadi S, Panagiotidou S. A Case Series of a Luteolin Formulation (Neuroprotek®) in Children with Autism Spectrum Disorders. *Int J Immunopathol Pharmacol.* 2012;25(2):317-323. doi:10.1177/039463201202500201

12. Theoharides TC, Angelidou A, Alysandratos K-D, et al. Mast cell activation and autism. *Biochim Biophys Acta - Mol Basis Dis.* 2012;1822(1):34-41. doi:10.1016/j.bbadis.2010.12.017

13. Theoharides TC, Kempuraj D, Redwood L. Autism: an emerging 'neuroimmune disorder' in search of therapy. *Expert Opin Pharmacother.* 2009;10(13):2127-2143. doi:10.1517/14656560903107789

14. Theoharides TC, Asadi S, Patel AB. Focal brain inflammation and autism. *J Neuroinflammation.* 2013;10(1):815. doi:10.1186/1742-2094-10-46

15. Theoharides TC, Asadi S, Panagiotidou S, Weng Z. The "missing link" in autoimmunity and autism: Extracellular mitochondrial components secreted from activated live mast cells. *Autoimmun Rev.* 2013;12(12):1136-1142. doi:10.1016/J.AUTREV.2013.06.018

16. Kanazawa LKS, Vecchia DD, Wendler EM, et al. Quercetin reduces manic-like behavior and brain oxidative stress induced by paradoxical sleep deprivation in mice. *Free Radic Biol Med.* 2016;99:79-86. doi:10.1016/j.freeradbiomed.2016.07.027

17. Kumar A, Goyal R. Quercetin Protects Against Acute Immobilization Stress-Induced Behaviors and Biochemical Alterations in Mice. *J Med Food.* 2008;11(3):469-473. doi:10.1089/jmf.2006.0207

18. Foreman JC. Mast cells and the actions of flavonoids. *J Allergy Clin Immunol.* 1984;73(6):769-774. http://www.ncbi.nlm.nih.gov/pubmed/6202730. Accessed September 10, 2018.

19. Middleton E. Effect of plant flavonoids on immune and inflammatory cell function. *Adv Exp Med Biol.* 1998;439:175-182. http://www.ncbi.nlm.nih.gov/pubmed/9781303. Accessed September 10, 2018.

20. Kimata M, Shichijo M, Miura T, Serizawa I, Inagaki N, Nagai H. Effects of luteolin, quercetin and baicalein on immunoglobulin E-mediated mediator release from human cultured mast cells. *Clin Exp Allergy.* 2000;30(4):501-508. http://www.ncbi.nlm.nih.gov/pubmed/10718847. Accessed September 10, 2018.

21. Pearce FL, Befus AD, Bienenstock J. Mucosal mast cells. III. Effect of quercetin and other flavonoids on antigen-induced histamine secretion from rat intestinal mast cells. *J Allergy Clin Immunol.* 1984;73(6):819-823. http://www.ncbi.nlm.nih.gov/pubmed/6202731. Accessed September 10, 2018.

22. Beretz A, Cazenave JP, Anton R. Inhibition of aggregation and secretion of human platelets by quercetin and other flavonoids: structure-activity relationships. *Agents Actions.* 1982;12(3):382-387. http://www.ncbi.nlm.nih.gov/pubmed/6182778. Accessed September 10, 2018.

23. Kempuraj D, Madhappan B, Christodoulou S, et al. Flavonols inhibit proinflammatory mediator release, intracellular calcium ion levels and protein kinase C theta phosphorylation in human mast cells. *Br J Pharmacol.* 2005;145(7):934-944. doi:10.1038/sj.bjp.0706246

24. Park H-H, Lee S, Son H-Y, et al. Flavonoids inhibit histamine release and expression of proinflammatory cytokines in mast cells. *Arch Pharm Res.* 2008;31(10):1303-1311. doi:10.1007/s12272-001-2110-5

25. Fox CC, Wolf EJ, Kagey-Sobotka A, Lichtenstein LM. Comparison of human lung and intestinal mast cells. *J Allergy Clin Immunol.* 1988;81(1):89-94. http://www.ncbi.nlm.nih.gov/pubmed/2448357. Accesse

26. Theoharides TC. Mast Cell Master: Research. http://www.mastcellmaster.com/research.php.d September 10, 2018.

27. Ennis M, Truneh A, White JR, Pearce FL. Inhibition of histamine secretion from mast cells. *Nature.* 1981;289(5794):186-187. http://www.ncbi.nlm.nih.gov/pubmed/6161310. Accessed September 10, 2018.

28. Formica J V, Regelson W. Review of the biology of Quercetin and related bioflavonoids. *Food Chem Toxicol.* 1995;33(12):1061-1080. http://www.ncbi.nlm.nih.gov/pubmed/8847003. Accessed September 10, 2018.

29. Katsarou A, Davoy E, Xenos K, Armenaka M, Theoharides TC. Effect of an antioxidant (quercetin) on sodium-lauryl-sulfate-induced skin irritation. *Contact Dermatitis.* 2000;42(2):85-89. http://www.ncbi.nlm.nih.gov/pubmed/10703630. Accessed September 10, 2018.

30. Theoharides TC, Patra P, Boucher W, et al. Chondroitin sulphate inhibits connective tissue mast cells. *Br J Pharmacol.* 2000;131(6):1039-1049. doi:10.1038/sj.bjp.0703672

31. Weinstock LB, Brook JB, Myers TL, Goodman B. Successful treatment of postural orthostatic tachycardia and mast cell activation syndromes using naltrexone, immunoglobulin and antibiotic treatment. *BMJ Case Rep.* 2018;2018. doi:10.1136/bcr-2017-221405

32. Seneviratne SL, Maitland A, Afrin L. Mast cell disorders in Ehlers–Danlos syndrome. *Am J Med Genet Part C Semin Med Genet.* 2017;175(1):226-236. doi:10.1002/ajmg.c.31555

33. Holick MF. Vitamin D Deficiency. *N Engl J Med.* 2007;357(3):266-281. doi:10.1056/NEJMra070553

34. Wang T-T, Tavera-Mendoza LE, Laperriere D, et al. Large-Scale *in Silico* and Microarray-Based Identification of Direct 1,25-Dihydroxyvitamin D 3 Target Genes. *Mol Endocrinol.* 2005;19(11):2685-2695. doi:10.1210/me.2005-0106

35. Kamen DL, Tangpricha V. Vitamin D and molecular actions on the immune system: modulation of innate and autoimmunity. *J Mol Med.* 2010;88(5):441-450. doi:10.1007/s00109-010-0590-9

36. Chinellato I, Piazza M, Sandri M, et al. Serum vitamin D levels and exercise-induced bronchoconstriction in children with asthma. *Eur Respir J.* 2011;37(6):1366-1370. doi:10.1183/09031936.00044710

37. Gupta A, Sjoukes A, Richards D, et al. Relationship between Serum Vitamin D, Disease Severity, and Airway Remodeling in Children with Asthma. *Am J Respir Crit Care Med.* 2011;184(12):1342-1349. doi:10.1164/rccm.201107-1239OC

38. Barete S, Assous N, de Gennes C, et al. Systemic mastocytosis and bone involvement in a cohort of 75 patients. *Ann Rheum Dis.* 2010;69(10):1838-1841. doi:10.1136/ard.2009.124511

39. Johansson C, Roupe G, Lindstedt G, Mellström D. Bone density, bone markers and bone radiological features in mastocytosis. *Age Ageing.* 1996;25(1):1-7. http://www.ncbi.nlm.nih.gov/pubmed/8670521. Accessed September 10, 2018.

40. Guillaume N, Desoutter J, Chandesris O, et al. Bone Complications of Mastocytosis: A Link between Clinical and Biological Characteristics. *Am J Med.* 2013;126(1):75.e1-75.e7. doi:10.1016/j.amjmed.2012.07.018

41. Wirz S, Hertfelder H-J, Seidel H, Homann J, Molderings G. Lower prevalence of vitamin D insufficiency in German patients with systemic mast cell activation syndrome compared with the general population. *Z Gastroenterol.* 2017;55(12):1297-1306. doi:10.1055/s-0043-121346

42. Conti P, Kempuraj D. Impact of Vitamin D on Mast Cell Activity, Immunity and Inflammation. *J Food Nutr Res.* 2016;4(1):33-39. doi:10.12691/jfnr-4-1-6

43. Biggs L, Yu C, Fedoric B, Lopez AF, Galli SJ, Grimbaldeston MA. Evidence that vitamin D(3) promotes mast cell-dependent reduction of chronic UVB-induced skin pathology in mice. *J Exp Med.* 2010;207(3):455-463. doi:10.1084/jem.20091725

44. Yip K-H, Kolesnikoff N, Yu C, et al. Mechanisms of vitamin D3 metabolite repression of IgE-dependent mast cell activation. *J Allergy Clin Immunol.* 2014;133(5):1356-1364.e14. doi:10.1016/J.JACI.2013.11.030

45. Takemoto S, Yamamoto A, Tomonaga S, Funaba M, Matsui T. Magnesium deficiency induces the emergence of mast cells in the liver of rats. *J Nutr Sci Vitaminol (Tokyo).* 2013;59(6):560-563. http://www.ncbi.nlm.nih.gov/pubmed/24477254. Accessed September 10, 2018.

46. Nishio A, Ishiguro S, Miyao N. Specific change of histamine metabolism in acute magnesium-deficient young rats. *Drug Nutr Interact.* 1987;5(2):89-96. http://www.ncbi.nlm.nih.gov/pubmed/3111814. Accessed September 10, 2018.

47. Mazur A, Maier JAM, Rock E, Gueux E, Nowacki W, Rayssiguier Y. Magnesium and the inflammatory response: Potential physiopathological implications. *Arch Biochem Biophys.* 2007;458(1):48-56. doi:10.1016/j.abb.2006.03.031

48. Broitman SA, McCray RS, May JC, et al. Mastocytosis and intestinal malabsorption. *Am J Med.* 1970;48(3):382-389. http://www.ncbi.nlm.nih.gov/pubmed/5435650. Accessed September 10, 2018.

49. Horan RF, Austen KF. Systemic mastocytosis: retrospective review of a decade's clinical experience at the Brigham and Women's Hospital. *J Invest Dermatol.* 1991;96(3):5S-13S; discussion 13S-14S. http://www.ncbi.nlm.nih.gov/pubmed/2002264. Accessed September 10, 2018.

50. Martner-Hewes PM, Hunt IF, Murphy NJ, Swendseid ME, Settlage RH. Vitamin B-6 nutriture and plasma diamine oxidase activity in pregnant Hispanic teenagers. *Am J Clin Nutr.* 1986;44(6):907-913. doi:10.1093/ajcn/44.6.907

51. Molderings GJ, Haenisch B, Brettner S, et al. Pharmacological treatment options for mast cell activation disease. *Naunyn Schmiedebergs Arch Pharmacol.* 2016;389(7):671-694. doi:10.1007/s00210-016-1247-1

52. Monastra G, De Grazia S, Cilaker Micili S, Goker A, Unfer V. Immunomodulatory activities of alpha lipoic acid with a special focus on its efficacy in preventing miscarriage. *Expert Opin Drug Deliv.* 2016;13(12):1695-1708. doi:10.1080/17425247.2016.1200556

53. Kucukgoncu S, Zhou E, Lucas KB, Tek C. Alpha-lipoic acid (ALA) as a supplementation for weight loss: results from a meta-analysis of randomized controlled trials. *Obes Rev.* 2017;18(5):594-601. doi:10.1111/obr.12528

54. Diken Allahverdi T, Allahverdi E, Yayla S, et al. Effects of alpha lipoic acid on intra-abdominal adhesion: an experimental study in a rat model. *Ulus Travma Acil Cerrahi Derg*. 2015;21(1):9-14. http://www.ncbi.nlm.nih.gov/pubmed/25779706. Accessed September 10, 2018.

55. Sztanek F, Seres I, Lorincz H, Molnar A, Paragh G. Effect of alpha-lipoic acid supplementation on oxidative stress markers and antioxidative defense in patients with diabetic neuropathy. *Atherosclerosis*. 2017;263:e263. doi:10.1016/J.ATHEROSCLEROSIS.2017.06.852

56. Shinto L, Quinn J, Montine T, et al. A Randomized Placebo-Controlled Pilot Trial of Omega-3 Fatty Acids and Alpha Lipoic Acid in Alzheimer's Disease. *J Alzheimers Dis*. 2014;38(1):111-120. doi:10.3233/JAD-130722

57. Mahboob A, Farhat SM, Iqbal G, et al. Alpha-lipoic acid-mediated activation of muscarinic receptors improves hippocampus- and amygdala-dependent memory. *Brain Res Bull*. 2016;122:19-28. doi:10.1016/j.brainresbull.2016.02.014

58. Ekiz A, Özdemir-Kumral ZN, Erşahin M, et al. Functional and structural changes of the urinary bladder following spinal cord injury; treatment with alpha lipoic acid. *Neurourol Urodyn*. 2017;36(4):1061-1068. doi:10.1002/nau.23083

59. Murina F, Graziottin A, Felice R, Gambini D. Alpha Lipoic Acid Plus Omega-3 Fatty Acids for Vestibulodynia Associated With Painful Bladder Syndrome. *J Obstet Gynaecol Canada*. 2017;39(3):131-137. doi:10.1016/j.jogc.2016.12.035

60. Palacios-Sánchez B, Moreno-López L-A, Cerero-Lapiedra R, Llamas-Martínez S, Esparza-Gómez G. Alpha lipoic acid efficacy in burning mouth syndrome. A controlled clinical trial. *Med Oral Patol Oral Cir Bucal*. 2015;20(4):e435-40. doi:10.4317/MEDORAL.20410

61. Femiano F, Gombos F, Buscuilano M, Scully C, De Luca P. Burning mouth syndrome (BMS):controlled open trial of the efficacy of alpha-lipoic acid on symptomatology. *Oral Dis*. 2000;6(5):274-277. https://iris.unicampania.it/handle/11591/212151#.W5lYEOhKjIU. Accessed September 12, 2018.

62. Femiano F, Scully C. Burning mouth syndrome (BMS): double blind controlled study of alpha-lipoic acid (thioctic acid) therapy. *J Oral Pathol Med*. 2002;31(5):267-269. http://www.ncbi.nlm.nih.gov/pubmed/12110042. Accessed September 12, 2018.

63. López-D'alessandro E, Escovich L. Combination of alpha lipoic acid and gabapentin, its efficacy in the treatment of Burning Mouth Syndrome: a randomized, double-blind, placebo controlled trial. *Med Oral Patol Oral Cir Bucal*. 2011;16(5):e635-40. http://www.ncbi.nlm.nih.gov/pubmed/20711135. Accessed September 12, 2018.

64. Carbone M, Pentenero M, Carrozzo M, Ippolito A, Gandolfo S. Lack of efficacy of alpha-lipoic acid in burning mouth syndrome: A double-blind, randomized, placebo-controlled study. *Eur J Pain*. 2009;13(5):492-496. doi:10.1016/j.ejpain.2008.06.004

65. Lopez-Jornet P, Camacho-Alonso F, Leon-Espinosa S. Efficacy of alpha lipoic acid in burning mouth syndrome: a randomized, placebo-treatment study. *J Oral Rehabil*. 2009;36(1):52-57. doi:10.1111/j.1365-2842.2008.01914.x

66. Cavalcanti DR, Da Silveira FRX. Alpha lipoic acid in burning mouth syndrome - a randomized double-blind placebo-controlled trial. *J Oral Pathol Med*. 2009;38(3):254-261. doi:10.1111/j.1600-0714.2008.00735.x

67. Miziara I, Chagury A, Vargas C, Freitas L, Mahmoud A. Therapeutic options in idiopathic burning mouth syndrome: literature review. *Int Arch Otorhinolaryngol*. 2015;19(1):86-89. doi:10.1055/s-0034-1378138

68. Bradley P. *Bromelain Containing Enzyme-Rutosid Combination Therapy Is as Effective as Nonsteroidal Antiinflammatory Agents for Treatment of Osteoarthritis*.; 2014. http://commons.pacificu.edu/pa/475. Accessed September 12, 2018.

69. Horowitz R. *How Can I Get Better? An Action Plan for Treating Resistant Lyme and Chronic Disease*. New York, NY: St. Martin's Griffin; 2017.

70. van Zanten ARH, Dhaliwal R, Garrel D, Heyland DK. Enteral glutamine supplementation in critically ill patients: a systematic review and meta-analysis. *Crit Care*. 2015;19(1):294. doi:10.1186/s13054-015-1002-x

71. Mokhtari V, Afsharian P, Shahhoseini M, Kalantar SM, Moini A. A Review on Various Uses of N-Acetyl Cysteine. *Cell J*. 19(1):11-17. http://www.ncbi.nlm.nih.gov/pubmed/28367412. Accessed September 12, 2018.

72. Gao X, Lampraki E-M, Al-Khalidi S, Qureshi MA, Desai R, Wilson JB. N-acetylcysteine (NAC) ameliorates Epstein-Barr virus latent membrane protein 1 induced chronic inflammation. *PLoS One*. 2017;12(12):e0189167. doi:10.1371/journal.pone.0189167

73. Sekhar R V, Patel SG, Guthikonda AP, et al. Deficient synthesis of glutathione underlies oxidative stress in aging and can be corrected by dietary cysteine and glycine supplementation. *Am J Clin Nutr*. 2011;94(3):847-853. doi:10.3945/ajcn.110.003483

74. Mirzaei H, Shakeri A, Rashidi B, Jalili A, Banikazemi Z, Sahebkar A. Phytosomal curcumin: A review of pharmacokinetic, experimental and clinical studies. *Biomed Pharmacother*. 2017;85:102-112. doi:10.1016/j.biopha.2016.11.098

75. Lee JH, Kim JW, Ko NY, et al. Curcumin, a constituent of curry, suppresses IgE-mediated allergic response and mast cell activation at the level of Syk. *J Allergy Clin Immunol*. 2008;121(5):1225-1231. doi:10.1016/J.JACI.2007.12.1160

76. Li X, Lu Y, Jin Y, Son J-K, Lee SH, Chang HW. Curcumin inhibits the activation of immunoglobulin e-mediated mast cells and passive systemic anaphylaxis in mice by reducing serum eicosanoid and histamine levels. *Biomol Ther (Seoul)*. 2014;22(1):27-34. doi:10.4062/biomolther.2013.092

77. Sharma RA, McLelland HR, Hill KA, et al. Pharmacodynamic and pharmacokinetic study of oral Curcuma extract in patients with colorectal cancer. *Clin Cancer Res*. 2001;7(7):1894-1900. doi:10.1158/1078-0432.ccr-04-0744

78. Koeberle A, Northoff H, Werz O. Curcumin blocks prostaglandin E2 biosynthesis through direct inhibition of the microsomal prostaglandin E2 synthase-1. *Mol Cancer Ther*. 2009;8(8):2348-2355. doi:10.1158/1535-7163.MCT-09-0290

79. Choi Y-H, Yan G-H, Chai OH, Song CH. Inhibitory effects of curcumin on passive cutaneous anaphylactoid response and compound 48/80-induced mast cell activation. *Anat Cell Biol*. 2010;43(1):36-43. doi:10.5115/acb.2010.43.1.36

80. Basu A, Sarkar A, Basak P. Nutraceuticals for Human Health and Hypersensitivity Reaction. In: Verma, Amit Srivastava K, Singh S, Singh H, eds. *Nutraceuticals and Innovative Food Products for Healthy Living and Preventive Care*.; 2018. doi:10.4018/978-1-5225-2970-5.ch015

81. Chae H-S, Oh S-R, Lee H-K, Joo SH, Chin Y-W. Mangosteen xanthones, α-and γ-mangostins, inhibit allergic mediators in bone marrow-derived mast cell. *Food Chem*. 2012;134(1):397-400. doi:10.1016/J.FOODCHEM.2012.02.075

82. Nakatani K, Atsumi M, Arakawa T, et al. Inhibitions of histamine release and prostaglandin E2 synthesis by mangosteen, a Thai medicinal plant. *Biol Pharm Bull*. 2002;25(9):1137-1141. http://www.ncbi.nlm.nih.gov/pubmed/12230104. Accessed September 12, 2018.

83. Wang M-H, Zhang K-J, Gu Q-L, Bi X-L, Wang J-X. Pharmacology of mangostins and their derivatives: A comprehensive review. *Chin J Nat Med*. 2017;15(2):81-93. doi:10.1016/S1875-5364(17)30024-9

84. Higuchi H, Tanaka A, Nishikawa S, et al. Suppressive effect of mangosteen rind extract on the spontaneous development of atopic dermatitis in NC/Tnd mice. *J Dermatol*. 2013;40(10):n/a-n/a. doi:10.1111/1346-8138.12250

85. Jang H-Y, Kwon O-K, Oh S-R, Lee H-K, Ahn K-S, Chin Y-W. Mangosteen xanthones mitigate ovalbumin-induced airway inflammation in a mouse model of asthma. *Food Chem Toxicol*. 2012;50(11):4042-4050. doi:10.1016/j.fct.2012.08.037

86. Finn DF, Walsh JJ. Twenty-first century mast cell stabilizers. *Br J Pharmacol*. 2013;170(1):23-37. doi:10.1111/bph.12138

87. Al-Snafi AE. Chemical constituents and pharmacological activities of Ammi majus and Ammi visnaga. A review. *Int J Pharm Ind Res*. 2013;3(3):257-265. www.ijpir.com. Accessed September 12, 2018.

88. Yang T, Wang L, Zhu M, Zhang L, Yan L. Properties and molecular mechanisms of resveratrol: a review. *Pharmazie*. 2015;70(8):501-506. http://www.ncbi.nlm.nih.gov/pubmed/26380517. Accessed September 12, 2018.

89. Cottart C-H, Nivet-Antoine V, Beaudeux J-L. Review of recent data on the metabolism, biological effects, and toxicity of resveratrol in humans. *Mol Nutr Food Res*. 2014;58(1):7-21. doi:10.1002/mnfr.201200589

90. Kang O-H, Jang H-J, Chae H-S, et al. Anti-inflammatory mechanisms of resveratrol in activated HMC-1 cells: Pivotal roles of NF-κB and MAPK. *Pharmacol Res*. 2009;59(5):330-337. doi:10.1016/J.PHRS.2009.01.009

91. Shirley D, McHale C, Gomez G. Resveratrol preferentially inhibits IgE-dependent PGD2 biosynthesis but enhances TNF production from human skin mast cells. *Biochim Biophys Acta - Gen Subj*. 2016;1860(4):678-685. doi:10.1016/j.bbagen.2016.01.006

92. Huang X, Zhao W, Hu D, et al. Resveratrol efficiently improves pulmonary function via stabilizing mast cells in a rat intestinal injury model. *Life Sci*. 2017;185:30-37. doi:10.1016/j.lfs.2017.07.018

93. Zeng H, He Y, Yu Y, et al. Resveratrol improves prostate fibrosis during progression of urinary dysfunction in chronic prostatitis by mast cell suppression. *Mol Med Rep*. 2018;17(1):918-924. doi:10.3892/mmr.2017.7960

94. Raina K, Kumar S, Dhar D, Agarwal R. Silibinin and colorectal cancer chemoprevention: a comprehensive review on mechanisms and efficacy. *J Biomed Res*. 2016;30(6):452-465. doi:10.7555/JBR.30.20150111

95. Polachi N, Bai G, Li T, et al. Modulatory effects of silibinin in various cell signaling pathways against liver disorders and cancer – A comprehensive review. *Eur J Med Chem*. 2016;123:577-595. doi:10.1016/j.ejmech.2016.07.070

96. Alfonso-Moreno V, López-Serrano A, Moreno-Osset E. Chemoprevention of polyp recurrence with curcumin followed by silibinin in a case of multiple colorectal adenomas. *Rev Española Enfermedades Dig*. 2017;109(12):875. doi:10.17235/reed.2017.5178/2017

97. Bosch-Barrera J, Menendez JA. Silibinin and STAT3: A natural way of targeting transcription factors for cancer therapy. *Cancer Treat Rev*. 2015;41(6):540-546. doi:10.1016/J.CTRV.2015.04.008

98. Zheng W, Feng Z, Lou Y, et al. Silibinin protects against osteoarthritis through inhibiting the inflammatory response and cartilage matrix degradation in vitro and in vivo. *Oncotarget*. 2017;8(59):99649-99665. doi:10.18632/oncotarget.20587

99. Thakur P, Hem Raj V, Sharma R. A review on pharmacological aspects of milk thistle. *World J Pharm Pharm Sci*. 2016;6(1):247-263.

516

100. Posadzki PP, Bajpai R, Kyaw BM, et al. Melatonin and health: an umbrella review of health outcomes and biological mechanisms of action. *BMC Med.* 2018;16(1):18. doi:10.1186/s12916-017-1000-8

101. Theoharides TC. Neuroendocrinology of mast cells: Challenges and controversies. *Exp Dermatol.* 2017;26(9):751-759. doi:10.1111/exd.13288

102. Rossi SP, Windschuettl S, Matzkin ME, et al. Melatonin in testes of infertile men: evidence for anti-proliferative and anti-oxidant effects on local macrophage and mast cell populations. *Andrology.* 2014;2(3):436-449. doi:10.1111/j.2047-2927.2014.00207.x

103. Izzo G, d'Istria M, Serino I, Minucci S. Inhibition of the increased 17beta-estradiol-induced mast cell number by melatonin in the testis of the frog Rana esculenta, in vivo and in vitro. *J Exp Biol.* 2004;207(Pt 3):437-441. http://www.ncbi.nlm.nih.gov/pubmed/14691091. Accessed September 13, 2018.

104. Catini C, Legnaioli M. Role of mast cells in health: daily rhythmic variations in their number, exocytotic activity, histamine and serotonin content in the rat thyroid gland. *Eur J Histochem.* 1992;36(4):501-516. http://www.ncbi.nlm.nih.gov/pubmed/1283837. Accessed September 13, 2018.

105. Nakao A, Nakamura Y, Shibata S. The circadian clock functions as a potent regulator of allergic reaction. *Allergy.* 2015;70(5):467-473. doi:10.1111/all.12596

106. Gao Y, Hou R, Fei Q, et al. The Three-Herb Formula Shuang-Huang-Lian stabilizes mast cells through activation of mitochondrial calcium uniporter. *Sci Rep.* 2017;7:38736. doi:10.1038/srep38736

107. Toi M, Bando H, Ramachandran C, et al. Preliminary studies on the anti-angiogenic potential of pomegranate fractions in vitro and in vivo. *Angiogenesis.* 2003;6(2):121-128. doi:10.1023/B:AGEN.0000011802.81320.e4

108. Dharmananda S. Reducing Inflammation with Diet and Supplements: The Story of Eicosanoid Inhibition. Institution for Traditional Medicine. http://www.itmonline.org/arts/lox.htm. Accessed September 13, 2018.

109. Gerges Geagea A, Rizzo M, Eid A, et al. Tea catechins induce crosstalk between signaling pathways and stabilize mast cells in ulcerative colitis. *J Biol Regul Homeost Agents.* 31(4):865-877. http://www.ncbi.nlm.nih.gov/pubmed/29254289. Accessed September 13, 2018.

110. Nguyet TMN, Lomunova M, Le BV, et al. The mast cell stabilizing activity of Chaga mushroom critical for its therapeutic effect on food allergy is derived from inotodiol. *Int Immunopharmacol.* 2018;54:286-295. doi:10.1016/j.intimp.2017.11.025

111. Hawrelak J. Episode 24 - Microbiota and SIBO with Dr. Jason Hawrelak. In: The Healthy Gut Podcast by Rebecca Coomes on Apple Podcasts. Aired on 3/27/17. https://itunes.apple.com/us/podcast/the-healthy-gut/id1170766921?mt=2.

112. Afrin LB, Khoruts A. Mast Cell Activation Disease and Microbiotic Interactions. *Clin Ther.* 2015;37(5):941-953. doi:10.1016/j.clinthera.2015.02.008

113. Gao C, Major A, Rendon D, et al. Histamine H2 Receptor-Mediated Suppression of Intestinal Inflammation by Probiotic Lactobacillus reuteri. *MBio.* 2015;6(6):e01358-15. doi:10.1128/mBio.01358-15

114. Oksaharju A, Kooistra T, Kleemann R, et al. Effects of probiotic Lactobacillus rhamnosus GG and Propionibacterium freudenreichii ssp. shermanii JS supplementation on intestinal and systemic markers of inflammation in ApoE*3Leiden mice consuming a high-fat diet. *Br J Nutr.* 2013;110(01):77-85. doi:10.1017/S0007114512004801

115. Hamilton M. Phone interview conducted on 6-22-18.

116. Snow R. "Mast Cell Activation Syndrome: ID, Explanation and Treatment" presented at the 27th Annual American Herbalists Guild Symposium, September 29 – October 2, 2016, Seven Springs, PA. Accessed February 19, 2018.

117. Carnahan J. Mold is a Major Trigger of Mast Activation Cell Syndrome - Jill Carnahan, MD. https://www.jillcarnahan.com/2018/03/12/mold-is-a-major-trigger-of-mast-activation-cell-syndrome/. Accessed September 13, 2018.

118. Turner H. Phone interview conducted on 7-13-18.

119. Guéniche A, Bastien P, Ovigne JM, et al. Bifidobacterium longum lysate, a new ingredient for reactive skin. *Exp Dermatol.* 2009;19(8):e1-e8. doi:10.1111/j.1600-0625.2009.00932.x

120. Klimas L. The use of intravenous fluids for management of mast cell disease - Mast Attack. https://www.mastattack.org/2017/10/use-intravenous-fluids-management-mast-cell-disease/. Accessed September 13, 2018.

121. Pang X, Cotreau-Bibbo MM, Sant GR, Theoharides TC. Bladder mast cell expression of high affinity oestrogen receptors in patients with interstitial cystitis. *Br J Urol.* 1995;75(2):154-161. http://www.ncbi.nlm.nih.gov/pubmed/7850318. Accessed September 13, 2018.

122. Menzies FM, Shepherd MC, Nibbs RJ, Nelson SM. The role of mast cells and their mediators in reproduction, pregnancy and labour. *Hum Reprod Update.* 2011;17(3):383-396. doi:10.1093/humupd/dmq053

123. Tano B. In-person interview conducted in St. Cloud, Minnesota on 9-16-17.

124. Zhang D, Ding G, Shen X, et al. Role of Mast Cells in Acupuncture Effect: A Pilot Study. *Explor J Sci Heal.* 2008;4(3):170-177. doi:10.1016/j.explore.2008.02.002

125. Centers for Disease Control and Prevention. Thimerosal in Vaccines Thimerosal | Concerns | Vaccine Safety | CDC. https://www.cdc.gov/vaccinesafety/concerns/thimerosal/index.html. Accessed September 13, 2018.

126. Kempuraj D, Asadi S, Zhang B, et al. Mercury induces inflammatory mediator release from human mast cells. *J Neuroinflammation*. 2010;7(1):20. doi:10.1186/1742-2094-7-20

127. Huszti Z, Balogh I. Effects of lead and mercury on histamine uptake by glial and endothelial cells. *Pharmacol Toxicol*. 1995;76(6):339-342.

128. Fujimaki H, Kawagoe A, Bissonnette E, Befus D. Mast cell response to formaldehyde. 1. Modulation of mediator release. *Int Arch Allergy Immunol*. 1992;98(4):324-331. doi:10.1159/000236206http://www.ncbi.nlm.nih.gov/pubmed/7479572. Accessed September 13, 2018.

129. Tomljenovic L, Shaw CA. Aluminum vaccine adjuvants: are they safe? *Curr Med Chem*. 2011;18(17):2630-2637. http://www.ncbi.nlm.nih.gov/pubmed/21568886. Accessed September 13, 2018.

130. Lai Y-L, Lin T-Y. Mast cells in citric acid-induced cough of guinea pigs. *Toxicol Appl Pharmacol*. 2005;202(1):18-24. doi:10.1016/j.taap.2004.05.012

131. Knott L. Mastocytosis and Mast Cell Disorders. Patient: Health Information You Can Trust. https://patient.info/doctor/mastocytosis-and-mast-cell-disorders#ref-10. Published 2015.

132. Canadian Mastocytosis Society. Symptom Management & Triggers. https://www.mastocytosis.ca/en/treatment/symptom-management-triggers. Accessed September 13, 2018.

133. Klimas L. Immunity, vaccination and disease transmission - Mast Attack. https://www.mastattack.org/2014/12/immunity-vaccination-disease-transmission/. Accessed September 13, 2018.

134. Wirz S, Molderings GJ. A practical guide for treatment of pain in patients with systemic mast cell activation disease. *Pain Physician*. 2017;20:E849-E861.

135. Bonadonna P, Passalacqua G, Reccardini F, et al. Severe Anaphylactic Reactions after Stopping Hymenoptera Venom Immunotherapy. a Clonal Mast Cell Disorder Should be Suspected. *J Allergy Clin Immunol*. 2017;139(2):AB229. doi:10.1016/j.jaci.2016.12.738

136. Álvarez-Twose I, González de Olano D, Sánchez-Muñoz L, et al. Clinical, biological, and molecular characteristics of clonal mast cell disorders presenting with systemic mast cell activation symptoms. *J Allergy Clin Immunol*. 2010;125:1269-1278. doi:10.1016/j.jaci.2010.02.019

137. Bonadonna P, Zanotti R, Pagani M, et al. Anaphylactic Reactions After Discontinuation of Hymenoptera Venom Immunotherapy: A Clonal Mast Cell Disorder Should Be Suspected. *J Allergy Clin Immunol Pract*. 2018;6(4):1368-1372. doi:10.1016/J.JAIP.2017.11.025

138. Afrin L. In-person interview conducted in St. Cloud, Minnesota on 9-16-17.

139. Oliva A, Multigner L. Ketotifen improves sperm motility and sperm morphology in male patients with leukocytospermia and unexplained infertility. *Fertil Steril*. 2006;85(1):240-243. doi:10.1016/j.fertnstert.2005.06.047

140. Weidinger S, Mayerhofer A, Frungieri MB, Meineke V, Ring J, Kohn FM. Mast cell-sperm interaction: evidence for tryptase and proteinase-activated receptors in the regulation of sperm motility. *Hum Reprod*. 2003;18(12):2519-2524. http://www.ncbi.nlm.nih.gov/pubmed/14645166. Accessed September 12, 2018.

141. Cincik M, Sezen SC. The mast cells in semen: their effects on sperm motility. *Arch Androl*. 49(4):307-311. http://www.ncbi.nlm.nih.gov/pubmed/12851033. Accessed September 12, 2018.

142. Maseki Y, Miyake K, Mitsuya H, Kitamura H, Yamada K. Mastocytosis occurring in the testes from patients with idiopathic male infertility. *Fertil Steril*. 1981;36(6):814-817. http://www.ncbi.nlm.nih.gov/pubmed/7308527. Accessed September 12, 2018.

143. Nagai T, Takaba H, Miyake K, Hirabayashi Y, Yamada K. Testicular mast cell heterogeneity in idiopathic male infertility. *Fertil Steril*. 1992;57(6):1331-1336. http://www.ncbi.nlm.nih.gov/pubmed/1376286. Accessed September 12, 2018.

144. Yamanaka K, Fujisawa M, Tanaka H, Okada H, Arakawa S, Kamidono S. Significance of human testicular mast cells and their subtypes in male infertility. *Hum Reprod*. 2000;15(7):1543-1547. http://www.ncbi.nlm.nih.gov/pubmed/10875863. Accessed September 12, 2018.

145. Bytautiene E, Vedernikov YP, Saade GR, Romero R, Garfield RE. Degranulation of uterine mast cell modifies contractility of isolated myometrium from pregnant women. *Am J Obstet Gynecol*. 2004;191(5):1705-1710. doi:10.1016/j.ajog.2004.04.008

146. Woidacki K, Zenclussen AC, Siebenhaar F. Mast cell-mediated and associated disorders in pregnancy: a risky game with an uncertain outcome? *Front Immunol*. 2014;5:231. doi:10.3389/fimmu.2014.00231

147. Maintz L, Schwarzer V, Bieber T, van der Ven K, Novak N. Effects of histamine and diamine oxidase activities on pregnancy: a critical review. *Hum Reprod Update*. 2008;14(5):485-495. doi:10.1093/humupd/dmn014

148. McLaren J, Taylor DJ, Bell SC. Prostaglandin E(2)-dependent production of latent matrix metalloproteinase-9 in cultures of human fetal membranes. *Mol Hum Reprod*. 2000;6(11):1033-1040. http://www.ncbi.nlm.nih.gov/pubmed/11044467. Accessed September 12, 2018.

149. Keirse MJ. Prostaglandins in preinduction cervical ripening. Meta-analysis of worldwide clinical experience. *J Reprod Med*. 1993;38(1 Suppl):89-100. http://www.ncbi.nlm.nih.gov/pubmed/8429533. Accessed September 12, 2018.

150. Mitani R, Maeda K, Fukui R, et al. Production of human mast cell chymase in human myometrium and placenta in cases of normal pregnancy and preeclampsia. *Eur J Obstet Gynecol Reprod Biol.* 2002;101(2):155-160. http://www.ncbi.nlm.nih.gov/pubmed/11858891. Accessed September 12, 2018.

151. Madhappan B, Kempuraj D, Christodoulou S, et al. High Levels of Intrauterine Corticotropin-Releasing Hormone, Urocortin, Tryptase, and Interleukin-8 in Spontaneous Abortions. *Endocrinology.* 2003;144(6):2285-2290. doi:10.1210/en.2003-0063

152. Cruz MA, Gonzalez C, Acevedo CG, Sepulveda WH, Rudolph MI. Effects of Histamine and Serotonin on the Contractility of Isolated Pregnant and Nonpregnant Human Myometrium. *Gynecol Obstet Invest.* 1989;28(1):1-4. doi:10.1159/000293482

153. Rudolph MI, Oviedo C, Vega E, et al. Oxytocin inhibits the uptake of serotonin into uterine mast cells. *J Pharmacol Exp Ther.* 1998;287(1):389-394. http://www.ncbi.nlm.nih.gov/pubmed/9765360. Accessed August 9, 2018.

154. Saito H. Role of Mast Cell Proteases in Tissue Remodeling. In: *Mast Cells in Allergic Diseases.* Vol 87. Basel: KARGER; 2005:80-84. doi:10.1159/000087572

155. Caughey GH. Mast cell tryptases and chymases in inflammation and host defense. *Immunol Rev.* 2007;217:141-154. doi:10.1111/j.1600-065X.2007.00509.x

156. Schwartz LB, Bradford TR, Littman BH, Wintroub BU. The fibrinogenolytic activity of purified tryptase from human lung mast cells. *J Immunol.* 1985;135(4):2762-2767. http://www.ncbi.nlm.nih.gov/pubmed/3161948. Accessed September 12, 2018.

157. Bytautiene E, Vedernikov YP, Saade GR, Romero R, Garfield RE. Degranulation of uterine mast cell modifies contractility of isolated myometrium from pregnant women. *Am J Obstet Gynecol.* 2004;191(5):1705-1710. doi:10.1016/j.ajog.2004.04.008

158. Bytautiene E, Romero R, Vedernikov YP, El-Zeky F, Saade GR, Garfield RE. Induction of premature labor and delivery by allergic reaction and prevention by histamine H1 receptor antagonist. *Am J Obstet Gynecol.* 2004;191(4):1356-1361. doi:10.1016/j.ajog.2004.06.092

159. Romero R, Kusanovic JP, Muñoz H, Gomez R, Lamont RF, Yeo L. Allergy-induced preterm labor after the ingestion of shellfish. *J Matern Fetal Neonatal Med.* 2010;23(4):351-359. doi:10.3109/14767050903177193

160. Tsuzuki Y, Narita M, Nawa M, Nakagawa U, Wakai T. Management of maternal anaphylaxis in pregnancy: a case report. *Acute Med Surg.* 2017;4(2):202-204. doi:10.1002/ams2.238

161. Soh JY, Chiang WC, Huang CH, et al. An unusual cause of food-induced anaphylaxis in mothers. *World Allergy Organ J.* 2017;10(1):3. doi:10.1186/s40413-016-0136-x

162. Kibriya SZ, Fatima N, Rakhshan S, Rokadia S. Ant Bite: A Rare Cause of Anaphylaxis in Pregnancy. *J Evol Med Dent Sci.* 2015;4(01):123-126. doi:10.14260/jemds/2015/19

163. Mccall S, Bunch K, Brocklehurst P, et al. The incidence and outcomes of anaphylaxis in pregnancy: a UK population-based descriptive study. *Bjog An Int J Obstet Gynaecol.* 2016;123:49-60. http://oaawebcast.info/assets/20-may-1215-knight.pdf. Accessed September 12, 2018.

164. Truong HT, Browning RM. Anaphylaxis-induced hyperfibrinolysis in pregnancy. *Int J Obstet Anesth.* 2015;24(2):180-184. doi:10.1016/j.ijoa.2014.12.009

165. Oykhman P, Kim HL, Ellis AK. Allergen immunotherapy in pregnancy. *Allergy Asthma Clin Immunol.* 2015;11:31. doi:10.1186/s13223-015-0096-7

166. Pali-Schöll I, Namazy J, Jensen-Jarolim E. Allergic diseases and asthma in pregnancy, a secondary publication. *World Allergy Organ J.* 2017;10(1):10. doi:10.1186/s40413-017-0141-8

167. Purcell WM, Hanahoe TH. A novel source of mast cells: the human placenta. *Agents Actions.* 1991;33(1-2):8-12. http://www.ncbi.nlm.nih.gov/pubmed/1716842. Accessed September 12, 2018.

168. Szewczyk G, Pyzlak M, Smiertka W, Klimkiewicz J, Szukiewicz D. Does histamine influence differentiation of trophoblast in preeclampsia? *Inflamm Res.* 2008;57(S1):71-72. doi:10.1007/s00011-007-0635-x

169. Dey SK. Role of histamine in implantation: inhibition of histidine decarboxylase induces delayed implantation in the rabbit. *Biol Reprod.* 1981;24(4):867-869. http://www.ncbi.nlm.nih.gov/pubmed/7248415. Accessed September 12, 2018.

170. Vasiadi M, Kempuraj D, Boucher W, Kalogeromitros D, Theoharides TC. Progesterone Inhibits Mast Cell Secretion. *Int J Immunopathol Pharmacol.* 2006;19(4):787-794. doi:10.1177/039463200601900408

171. Roby KF, Hunt JS. Myometrial tumor necrosis factor alpha: cellular localization and regulation by estradiol and progesterone in the mouse. *Biol Reprod.* 1995;52(3):509-515. http://www.ncbi.nlm.nih.gov/pubmed/7756446. Accessed September 12, 2018.

172. Abrahams VM, Kim YM, Straszewski SL, Romero R, Mor G. Macrophages and Apoptotic Cell Clearance During Pregnancy. *Am J Reprod Immunol.* 2004;51(4):275-282. doi:10.1111/j.1600-0897.2004.00156.x

173. Koga K, Mor G. Toll-like receptors at the maternal-fetal interface in normal pregnancy and pregnancy disorders. *Am J Reprod Immunol.* 2010;63(6):587-600. doi:10.1111/j.1600-0897.2010.00848.x

174. Mor G, Cardenas I, Abrahams V, Guller S. Inflammation and pregnancy: the role of the immune system at the implantation site. *Ann N Y Acad Sci.* 2011;1221(1):80-87. doi:10.1111/j.1749-6632.2010.05938.x

175. Piccinni MP, Scaletti C, Maggi E, Romagnani S. Role of hormone-controlled Th1- and Th2-type cytokines in successful pregnancy. *J Neuroimmunol.* 2000;109(1):30-33. http://www.ncbi.nlm.nih.gov/pubmed/10969178. Accessed September 12, 2018.

176. Schatz M, Harden K, Forsythe A, et al. The course of asthma during pregnancy, post partum, and with successive pregnancies: a prospective analysis. *J Allergy Clin Immunol.* 1988;81(3):509-517. http://www.ncbi.nlm.nih.gov/pubmed/3346481. Accessed September 12, 2018.

177. Matito A, Álvarez-Twose I, Morgado JM, Sánchez-Muñoz L, Orfao A, Escribano L. Clinical Impact of Pregnancy in Mastocytosis: A Study of the Spanish Network on Mastocytosis (REMA) in 45 Cases. *Int Arch Allergy Immunol.* 2011;156(1):104-111. doi:10.1159/000321954

178. Worobec AS, Akin C, Scott LM, Metcalfe DD. Mastocytosis complicating pregnancy. *Obstet Gynecol.* 2000;95(3):391-395. http://www.ncbi.nlm.nih.gov/pubmed/10711550. Accessed September 12, 2018.

179. Ciach K, Niedoszytko M, Abacjew-Chmylko A, et al. Pregnancy and Delivery in Patients with Mastocytosis Treated at the Polish Center of the European Competence Network on Mastocytosis (ECNM). Ribatti D, ed. *PLoS One.* 2016;11(1):e0146924. doi:10.1371/journal.pone.0146924

180. Watson KD, Arendt KW, Watson WJ, Volcheck GW. Systemic Mastocytosis Complicating Pregnancy. *Obstet Gynecol.* 2012;119(Part 2):486-489. doi:10.1097/AOG.0b013e318242d3c5

181. Yitshak-Sade M, Gorodischer R, Aviram M, Novack L. Prenatal exposure to H$_2$ blockers and to proton pump inhibitors and asthma development in offspring. *J Clin Pharmacol.* 2016;56(1):116-123. doi:10.1002/jcph.574

182. Devine RE, McCleary N, Sheikh A, Nwaru BI. Acid-suppressive medications during pregnancy and risk of asthma and allergy in children: A systematic review and meta-analysis. *J Allergy Clin Immunol.* 2017;139(6):1985-1988.e12. doi:10.1016/j.jaci.2016.09.046

183. Perlow JH, Montgomery D, Morgan MA, Towers C V, Porto M. Severity of asthma and perinatal outcome. *Am J Obstet Gynecol.* 1992;167(4 Pt 1):963-967. http://www.ncbi.nlm.nih.gov/pubmed/1415433. Accessed September 12, 2018.

184. Ulbrich F, Engelstädter H, Wittau N, Steinmann D. Anaesthetic management of emergency caesarean section in a parturient with systemic mastocytosis. *Int J Obstet Anesth.* 2013;22(3):243-246. doi:10.1016/j.ijoa.2013.03.011

185. Castells MC. Phone interview conducted on 7-20-18.

186. Afrin L. Personal email correspondence on October 3rd, 2018.

187. Broesby-Olsen S, Carter M, Kjaer HF, et al. Pediatric Expression of Mast Cell Activation Disorders. *Immunol Allergy Clin North Am.* 2018;38(3):365-377. doi:10.1016/J.IAC.2018.04.009

188. Ravi A, Meeusen J, Divekar R, Donato L, Hartz MF, Butterfield JH. Pediatric Mast Cell Activation Syndrome. *J Allergy Clin Immunol.* 2018;141(2):AB275. doi:10.1016/j.jaci.2017.12.876

References Chapter 11: Dietary Considerations for MCAS

1. Laher AE, Moolla M, McDonald M. Successful desensitisation of non-immune type symptoms secondary to salicylate hypersensitivity/intolerance. *Curr Allergy Clin Immunol.* 2017;30(4):284-286. http://www.webmd.com/allergies/salicylate-allergy. Accessed September 17, 2018.

2. Bolweg M. *The Three-Week Salicylate Exclusion Diet.* University of Otago, Dunedin, New Zealand.; 2010.

3. Gunsalus KTW, Tornberg-Belanger SN, Matthan NR, Lichtenstein AH, Kumamoto CA. Manipulation of Host Diet To Reduce Gastrointestinal Colonization by the Opportunistic Pathogen Candida albicans. *mSphere.* 2016;1(1). doi:10.1128/mSphere.00020-15

4. Teodoro GR, Ellepola K, Seneviratne CJ, Koga-Ito CY. Potential Use of Phenolic Acids as Anti-Candida Agents: A Review. *Front Microbiol.* 2015;6:1420. doi:10.3389/fmicb.2015.01420

5. Steinke JW, Platts-Mills TAE, Commins SP. The alpha-gal story: lessons learned from connecting the dots. *J Allergy Clin Immunol.* 2015;135(3):589-96; quiz 597. doi:10.1016/j.jaci.2014.12.1947

6. Afrin LB, Khoruts A. Mast Cell Activation Disease and Microbiotic Interactions. *Clin Ther.* 2015;37(5):941-953. doi:10.1016/j.clinthera.2015.02.008

7. Halmos EP, Power VA, Shepherd SJ, Gibson PR, Muir JG. A Diet Low in FODMAPs Reduces Symptoms of Irritable Bowel Syndrome. *Gastroenterology.* 2014;146(1):67-75.e5. doi:10.1053/j.gastro.2013.09.046

8. Lomer MCE. Review article: the aetiology, diagnosis, mechanisms and clinical evidence for food intolerance. *Aliment Pharmacol Ther.* 2015;41(3):262-275. doi:10.1111/apt.13041

9. Vieira T, Cunha S, Casal S. Mycotoxins in Coffee. *Coffee Heal Dis Prev.* January 2015:225-233. doi:10.1016/B978-0-12-409517-5.00025-5

10. Micco C, Grossi M, Miraglia M, Brera C. A study of the contamination by ochratoxin A of green and roasted coffee beans. *Food Addit Contam.* 1989;6(3):333-339. doi:10.1080/02652038909373788

11. Tsubouchi H, Yamamoto K, Hisada K, Sakabe Y, Udagawa S. Effect of roasting on ochratoxin A level in green coffee beans inoculated with Aspergillus ochraceus. *Mycopathologia.* 1987;97(2):111-115. http://www.ncbi.nlm.nih.gov/pubmed/3574430. Accessed September 17, 2018.

12. Horowitz R. *How Can I Get Better? An Action Plan for Treating Resistant Lyme and Chronic Disease*. New York, NY: St. Martin's Griffin; 2017.

13. U.S. Food & Drug Administration. Food Additives and Ingredients - Overview of Food Ingredients, Additives and Colors. 2010. https://www.fda.gov/Food/IngredientsPackagingLabeling/FoodAdditivesIngredients/ucm094211.htm. Accessed September 17, 2018.

14. Hamilton M. Phone interview conducted on 6-22-18.

15. Seneviratne SL, Maitland A, Afrin L. Mast cell disorders in Ehlers–Danlos syndrome. *Am J Med Genet Part C Semin Med Genet*. 2017;175(1):226-236. doi:10.1002/ajmg.c.31555

16. Maintz L, Novak N. Histamine and histamine intolerance. *Am J Clin Nutr*. 2007;85(5):1185-1196. doi:10.1093/ajcn/85.5.1185

17. San Mauro Martin I, Brachero S, Garicano Vilar E. Histamine intolerance and dietary management: A complete review. *Allergol Immunopathol (Madr)*. 2016;44(5):475-483. doi:10.1016/j.aller.2016.04.015

18. Reese I, Ballmer-Weber B, Beyer K, et al. German guideline for the management of adverse reactions to ingested histamine. *Allergo J Int*. 2017;26(2):72-79. doi:10.1007/s40629-017-0011-5

19. Ede G. Histamine Intolerance: Why Freshness Matters. *J Evol Heal*. 2016;2(1):11. doi:10.15310/2334-3591.1054

20. Duelo A. Dietistas nutricionistas especialistas en Déficit DAO - AD Dietistas. http://www.adrianaduelo.com/. Accessed September 17, 2018.

21. Ykelenstam Y. Histamine in Foods (list) | Healing Histamine. https://healinghistamine.com/histamine-in-foods-list/. Accessed September 17, 2018.

22. de Wild-Scholten M. *Understanding Histamine Intolerance & Mast Cell Activation: 3rd Edition*. Create Space; 2015.

23. Paramasivam, Sadayan, Balachandar, Balakrishnan Arulkumar A. Change in Histamine Levels and Microbial Load in the Eviscerated and Uneviscerated Indian Mackerel Fish (Rastrelliger kanagurta) at Different Storage Temperatures. *Am J Adv Food Sci Technol*. 2015;3(2):94-106.

24. Auerswald L, Morren C, Lopata AL. Histamine levels in seventeen species of fresh and processed South African seafood. *Food Chem*. 2006;98(2):231-239. doi:10.1016/J.FOODCHEM.2005.05.071

25. Cilliers JD, Van Wyk CJ. Histamine and Tyramine Content of South African Wine. *South African J Enol Vitic*. 2017;6(2):35-40. doi:10.21548/6-2-2349

26. Swiss Interest Group Histamine Intolerance (SIGHI). HIT and Introduction. https://www.histaminintoleranz.ch/en/introduction.html. Accessed September 17, 2018.

27. Ykelenstam Y. Healing Histamine | Histamine Intolerance Research and Recipes. https://healinghistamine.com/. Accessed September 17, 2018.

28. Komericki P, Klein G, Reider N, et al. Histamine intolerance: lack of reproducibility of single symptoms by oral provocation with histamine: A randomised, double-blind, placebo-controlled cross-over study. *Wien Klin Wochenschr*. 2011;123(1-2):15-20. doi:10.1007/s00508-010-1506-y

29. Ykelenstam Y. *The Anti-Cookbook, 4th Edition*. LHC Productions; 2013.

30. Wöhrl S, Hemmer W, Focke M, Rappersberger K, Jarisch R. Histamine intolerance-like symptoms in healthy volunteers after oral provocation with liquid histamine. *Allergy asthma Proc*. 25(5):305-311. http://www.ncbi.nlm.nih.gov/pubmed/15603203. Accessed September 17, 2018.

31. Schwelberger HG. Histamine intolerance: a metabolic disease? *Inflamm Res*. 2010;59(S2):219-221. doi:10.1007/s00011-009-0134-3

32. Hoffmann KM, Gruber E, Deutschmann A, Jahnel J, Hauer AC. Histamine intolerance in children with chronic abdominal pain. *Arch Dis Child*. 2013;98(10):832-833. doi:10.1136/archdischild-2013-305024

33. Afrin L. In-person interview conducted in St. Cloud, Minnesota on 9-16-17.

34. Castells MC. Phone interview conducted on 7-20-18.

35. Simopoulos AP. The importance of the ratio of omega-6/omega-3 essential fatty acids. *Biomed Pharmacother*. 2002;56(8):365-379. http://www.ncbi.nlm.nih.gov/pubmed/12442909. Accessed September 17, 2018.

36. Hibi M, Hachimura S, Hashizume S, Obata T, Kaminogawa S. Amaranth Grain Inhibits Antigen-Specific IgE Production Through Augmentation of the IFN-gamma Response in vivo and in vitro. *Cytotechnology*. 2003;43(1-3):33-40. doi:10.1023/B: CYTO.0000039908.34387.d3

37. Patil SD, Patel MR, Patel SR, Surana SJ. *Amaranthus spinosus* Linn. inhibits mast cell-mediated anaphylactic reactions. *J Immunotoxicol*. 2012;9(1):77-84. doi:10.3109/1547691X.2011.631609

38. Shealy N. *Illustrated Encyclopedia of Healing Rememedies*. Harper Collins; 2018.

39. Tokura T, Nakano N, Ito T, et al. Inhibitory effect of polyphenol-enriched apple extracts on mast cell degranulation in vitro targeting the binding between IgE and FcepsilonRI. *Biosci Biotechnol Biochem*. 2005;69(10):1974-1977. doi:10.1271/bbb.69.1974

40. Kanda T, Akiyama H, Yanagida A, et al. Inhibitory Effects of Apple Polyphenol on Induced Histamine Release from RBL-2H3 Cells and Rat Mast Cells. *Biosci Biotechnol Biochem*. 1998;62(7):1284-1289. doi:10.1271/bbb.62.1284

41. Fratianni F, Pepe R, Nazzaro F. Polyphenol Composition, Antioxidant, Antimicrobial and Quorum Quenching Activity of the "Carciofo di Montoro" (Cynara cardunculus var. scolymus) Global Artichoke of the Campania Region, Southern Italy. *Food Nutr Sci*. 2014;5:2053-2062. doi:10.4236/fns.2014.521217

42. Jain S, Garg VK, Sharma PK. Anti-inflammatory activity of aqueous extract of Beta vulgaris L. *J basic Clin Pharm*. 2011;2(2):83-86. http://www.ncbi.nlm.nih.gov/pubmed/24826006. Accessed September 17, 2018.

43. Nagase H, Hojima Y, Moriwaki C, Moriya H. Anti-bradykinin activity found in beet (Beta vulgaris L. var rapa Dumort. f. rubra DC.). *Chem Pharm Bull (Tokyo)*. 1975;23(5):971-979. doi:10.1248/CPB.23.971

44. Martinez RM, Longhi-Balbinot DT, Zarpelon AC, et al. Anti-inflammatory activity of betalain-rich dye of Beta vulgaris: effect on edema, leukocyte recruitment, superoxide anion and cytokine production. *Arch Pharm Res*. 2015;38(4):494-504. doi:10.1007/s12272-014-0473-7

45. Choi SP, Kim SP, Kang MY, Nam SH, Friedman M. Protective effects of black rice bran against chemically-induced inflammation of mouse skin. *J Agric Food Chem*. 2010;58(18):10007-10015. doi:10.1021/jf102224b

46. Kim CD, Lee W-K, No K-O, et al. Anti-allergic action of buckwheat (Fagopyrum esculentum Moench) grain extract. *Int Immunopharmacol*. 2003;3(1):129-136. http://www.ncbi.nlm.nih.gov/pubmed/12538043. Accessed September 17, 2018.

47. Imaoka K, Ushijima H, Inouye S, Takahashi T, Kojima Y. Effects of Celosia argentea and Cucurbita moschata extracts on anti-DNP IgE antibody production in mice. *Arerugi*. 1994;43(5):652-659. http://www.ncbi.nlm.nih.gov/pubmed/8031259. Accessed September 17, 2018.

48. Trombetta D, Occhiuto F, Perri D, et al. Antiallergic and antihistaminic effect of two extracts of Capparis spinosa L. flowering buds. *Phyther Res*. 2005;19(1):29-33. doi:10.1002/ptr.1591

49. Das S, Vasudeva N, Sharma S. Cichorium intybu : A concise report on its ethnomedicinal, botanical, and phytopharmacological aspects. *Drug Dev Ther*. 2016;7(1):1. doi:10.4103/2394-6555.180157

50. Verma C. Applications and Utilization of Coriander-A. *Int J Res Eng Appl Sci*. 2014;4(3):85-94. http://www.euroasiapub.orghttp//www.euroasiapub.org86. Accessed September 17, 2018.

51. Kumar D, Kumar S, Singh J, et al. Free Radical Scavenging and Analgesic Activities of Cucumis sativus L. Fruit Extract. *J Young Pharm*. 2010;2(4):365-368. doi:10.4103/0975-1483.71627

52. Agatemor UM-M, Okwesili FCN, Anosike CA. Anti-inflammatory Activity of Cucumis sativus L. *Br J Pharm Res*. 2015;8(2):1-8. doi:10.9734/BJPR/2015/19700

53. Kyo E, Uda N, Kasuga S, Itakura Y. Immunomodulatory Effects of Aged Garlic Extract. *J Nutr*. 2001;131(3):1075S-1079S. doi:10.1093/jn/131.3.1075S

54. Kim JH, Nam SH, Rico CW, Kang MY. A comparative study on the antioxidative and anti-allergic activities of fresh and aged black garlic extracts. *Int J Food Sci Technol*. 2012;47(6):1176-1182. doi:10.1111/j.1365-2621.2012.02957.x

55. Hwang S-L, Shih P-H, Yen G-C. Neuroprotective Effects of Citrus Flavonoids. *J Agric Food Chem*. 2012;60(4):877-885. doi:10.1021/jf204452y

56. Nakatani K, Atsumi M, Arakawa T, et al. Inhibitions of histamine release and prostaglandin E2 synthesis by mangosteen, a Thai medicinal plant. *Biol Pharm Bull*. 2002;25(9):1137-1141. http://www.ncbi.nlm.nih.gov/pubmed/12230104. Accessed September 12, 2018.

57. Chae H-S, Oh S-R, Lee H-K, Joo SH, Chin Y-W. Mangosteen xanthones, α-and γ-mangostins, inhibit allergic mediators in bone marrow-derived mast cell. *Food Chem*. 2012;134(1):397-400. doi:10.1016/J.FOODCHEM.2012.02.075

58. Chatuevedi N, Yadav S, Shukla K. *Diversified Therapeutic Potential of Avena Sativa: An Exhaustive Review*. Vol 1.; 2011. www.pelagiaresearchlibrary.com. Accessed September 17, 2018.

59. Aggarwal B, Yost D. *Healing Spices: How to Use 50 Everyday and Exotic Spices to Boost Health and Beat Disease*. Sterling Publishing; 2011.

60. Cardile V, Frasca G, Rizza L, Rapisarda P, Bonina F. Antiinflammatory effects of a red orange extract in human keratinocytes treated with interferon-gamma and histamine. *Phyther Res*. 2010;24(3):414-418. doi:10.1002/ptr.2973

61. Al-Khazraji SM. Studying the Analgesic, Anti-inflammatory and Antipyretic Properties of The Aqueous Extract of Petroselinum crispum in Experimental Animal Models. *IOSR Journal of Pharmacy*. 2015;5(9):17-23. www.iosrphr.org. Accessed September 17, 2018.

62. Liu H, Chen Y, Hu T, et al. The influence of light-emitting diodes on the phenolic compounds and antioxidant activities in pea sprouts. *J Funct Foods*. 2016;25:459-465. doi:10.1016/J.JFF.2016.06.028

63. Kim GJ, Choi HG, Kim JH, Kim SH, Kim JA, Lee SH. Anti-allergic inflammatory effects of cyanogenic and phenolic glycosides from the seed of Prunus persica. *Nat Prod Commun*. 2013;8(12):1739-1740. http://www.ncbi.nlm.nih.gov/pubmed/24555287. Accessed September 17, 2018.

64. Shin T-Y, Park S-B, Yoo J-S, et al. Anti-allergic inflammatory activity of the fruit of Prunus persica: Role of calcium and NF-κB. *Food Chem Toxicol*. 2010;48(10):2797-2802. doi:10.1016/j.fct.2010.07.009

65. Miguel MG, Neves MA, Antunes MD. Pomegranate (Punica granatum L.): A medicinal plant with myriad biological properties - A short review. *J Med Plants Res*. 2010;4(25):2836-2847. https://academicjournals.org/journal/JMPR/article-abstract/46EEE0023212. Accessed September 17, 2018.

66. Barwal S, Sunil A, Dhasade V, Patil M, Pal S, Subhash C. Antihistaminic effect of various extracts of Punica granatum Linn. flower buds. *J Young Pharm*. 2009;1(4):322. doi:10.4103/0975-1483.59321

67. Lee C-J, Chen L-G, Liang W-L, Wang C-C. Anti-inflammatory effects of Punica granatum Linne invitro and in vivo. *Food Chem*. 2010;118(2):315-322. doi:10.1016/J.FOODCHEM.2009.04.123

68. Meira M, Pereira Da Silva E, David JM, David JP. Review of the genus Ipomoea: traditional uses, chemistry and biological activities. *Rev Bras Farmacogn Brazilian J Pharmacogn*. 2012;22(3):682-713. doi:10.1590/S0102

69. Sadeghi H, Mostafazadeh M, Sadeghi H, et al. Anti-inflammatory properties of aerial parts of Nasturtium officinale. *Pharm Biol*. 2014;52(2):169-174. doi:10.3109/13880209.2013.821138

70. Karpagam T, Varalakshmi B, Suguna Bai J, Gomathi S. Effect of different doses of Cucurbita pepo linn extract as an anti-Inflammatory and analgesic nutraceautical agent on inflamed rats. *Int J Pharm Res Dev*. 2011;3:184-192. https://www.researchgate.net/publication/281304533. Accessed September 17, 2018.

71. Wang R, Wu G, Du L, et al. Semi-bionic extraction of compound turmeric protects against dextran sulfate sodium-induced acute enteritis in rats. *J Ethnopharmacol*. 2016;190:288-300. doi:10.1016/j.jep.2016.05.054

72. Yong YK, Zakaria ZA, Kadir AA, Somchit MN, Ee Cheng Lian G, Ahmad Z. Chemical constituents and antihistamine activity of Bixa orellana leaf extract. *BMC Complement Altern Med*. 2013;13:32. doi:10.1186/1472-6882-13-32

73. Lee W, Kim TH, Ku S-K, et al. Barrier protective effects of withaferin A in HMGB1-induced inflammatory responses in both cellular and animal models. *Toxicol Appl Pharmacol*. 2012;262(1):91-98. doi:10.1016/j.taap.2012.04.025

74. Chevallier A. *Encyclopedia of Herbal Medicine: 500 Herbs and Remedies for Common Ailments. 3rd Edition*. Dorling Kindersley Publishing; 2016.

75. Dharmananda S. Reducing inflammation with diet and supplements: the story of eicosanoid inhibition. Institute for Traditional Medicine (Portland, Oregon). http://www.itmonline.org/arts/lox.htm. Accessed June 23, 2017.

76. Gholamnezhad Z, Keyhanmanesh R, Boskabady MH. Anti-inflammatory, antioxidant, and immunomodulatory aspects of Nigella sativa for its preventive and bronchodilatory effects on obstructive respiratory diseases: A review of basic and clinical evidence. *J Funct Foods*. 2015;17:910-927. doi:10.1016/J.JFF.2015.06.032

77. Tembhurne S, Feroz S, More B, Sakarkar D. A review on therapeutic potential of Nigella sativa (kalonji) seeds. *J Med Plants Res*. 2014;8(3):167-177. doi:10.5897/JMPR10.737

78. Low Dog T, Johnson R, Foster S, Kiefer D, Weil A. *National Geographic Guide to Medicinal Herbs: The World's Most Effective Healing Plants*. National Geographic; 2012.

79. Sachan AK, Das DR, Kumar M. Carum carvi-An important medicinal plant. *J Chem Pharm Res*. 2016;8(3):529-533. www.jocpr.com. Accessed September 17, 2018.

80. Hussein A, Lobna M, Mohammed A, Mohamed G. Biochemical Effects of Chamomile Oil on Inflammatory Biomarkers in Gastroenteritis. *Int J Drug Dev Res*. 2009;9(2). http://www.ijddr.in/drug-development/biochemical-effects-of-chamomile-oil-on-inflammatory-biomarkers-ingastroenteritis.php?aid=19225. Accessed September 17, 2018.

81. Bhat SP, Rizvi W, Kumar A. Coriandrum Sativum on Pain and Inflammation. *International journal of Research in Pharmacy and Chemistry*. 2014;4(4):939-945.

82. Park HJ, Park JS, Hayek MG, Reinhart GA, Chew BP. Dietary fish oil and flaxseed oil suppress inflammation and immunity in cats. *Vet Immunol Immunopathol*. 2011;141(3-4):301-306. doi:10.1016/J.VETIMM.2011.02.024

83. Zaidi SF, Kim J-H, Tomoe Y, Usmanghani K, Kadowaki M. Effect of Pakistani medicinal plants on IgE/antigen- and ionophore-induced mucosal mast cells degranulation. *Pak J Pharm Sci*. 2014;27(4 Suppl):1041-1048. http://www.ncbi.nlm.nih.gov/pubmed/25016264. Accessed September 17, 2018.

84. Ravindran PN, Pillai GS, Balachandran I, Divakaran M. Galangal. *Handb Herbs Spices*. January 2012:303-318. doi:10.1533/9780857095688.303

85. Kiuchi F, Iwakami S, Shibuya M, Hanaoka F, Sankawa U. Inhibition of prostaglandin and leukotriene biosynthesis by gingerols and diarylheptanoids. *Chem Pharm Bull (Tokyo)*. 1992;40(2):387-391. http://www.ncbi.nlm.nih.gov/pubmed/1606634. Accessed September 17, 2018.

86. Pursell J. *The Herbal Apothecary: 100 Medicinal Herbs and How to Use Them*. Timber Press; 2015.

87. Singh S, Taneja M, Majumdar DK. Biological activities of Ocimum sanctum L. fixed oil--an overview. *Indian J Exp Biol*. 2007;45(5):403-412. http://www.ncbi.nlm.nih.gov/pubmed/17569280. Accessed September 17, 2018.

88. Choudhary GP. Mast cell stabilizing activity of Ocimum sanctum leaves. *Int J Pharma Bio Sci*. 2010;1(2). https://www.cabdirect.org/cabdirect/abstract/20113372323. Accessed September 17, 2018.

89. Rahman S, Islam R, Kamruzzaman M, Alum K, Mastofa Jamal AH. Ocimum sanctum L.: A Review of Phytochemical and Pharmacological Profile. *Am J Drug Discov Dev*. 2011:1-15. doi:1O.3923/ajdd.2011

90. Asha'ari ZA, Ahmad MZ, Wan Din WSJ, Che Hussin CM, Leman I. Ingestion of honey improves the symptoms of allergic rhinitis: evidence from a randomized placebo-controlled trial in the East Coast of Peninsular Malaysia. *Ann Saudi Med*. 2013;33(5):469-475. doi:10.5144/0256-4947.2013.469

91. Birdane YO, Büyükokurog -lu ME, Birdane FM, Cemek M, Yavuz H, Emin Büyükokurog -lu M. *Anti-Inflammatory and Antinociceptive Effects of Melissa Officinalis L. in Rodents.* Vol 158.; 2007. https://pdfs.semanticscholar.org/5878/238e3799fa869d5fa8add813b46e3da796ca.pdf. Accessed September 17, 2018.

92. Cheel J, Theoduloz C, Rodríguez J, Schmeda-Hirschmann G. Free Radical Scavengers and Antioxidants from Lemongrass (Cymbopogon citratus (DC.) Stapf.). *J Agric Food Chem.* 2005;53(7):2511-2517. doi:10.1021/jf0479766

93. Shin Y-W, Bae E-A, Lee B, et al. In Vitro and In Vivo Antiallergic Effects of Glycyrrhiza glabra and Its Components. *Planta Med.* 2007;73(3):257-261. doi:10.1055/s-2007-967126

94. Mukherjee D, Biswas A, Bhadra S, et al. Exploring the potential of Nelumbo nucifera rhizome on membrane stabilization, mast cell protection, nitric oxide synthesis, and expression of costimulatory molecules. *Immunopharmacol Immunotoxicol.* 2010;32(3):466-472. doi:10.3109/08923970903514830

95. Sharma BR, Gautam LNS, Adhikari D, Karki R. A Comprehensive Review on Chemical Profiling of Nelumbo Nucifera : Potential for Drug Development. *Phyther Res.* 2017;31(1):3-26. doi:10.1002/ptr.5732

96. Lecomte J. General pharmacologic properties of silybine and silymarine in the rat. *Arch Int Pharmacodyn Ther.* 1975;214(1):165-176. http://www.ncbi.nlm.nih.gov/pubmed/50765. Accessed September 17, 2018.

97. Thakur S, Verma A. Antihistaminic Effect of Moringa Oleifera Seed Extract. *Int J Pharm Res Allied Sci.* 2013;2(1):56-59. www.ijpras.com. Accessed September 17, 2018.

98. Atawodi SE, Atawodi JC. Azadirachta indica (neem): a plant of multiple biological and pharmacological activities. *Phytochem Rev.* 2009;8(3):601-620. doi:10.1007/s11101-009-9144-6

99. Sonika G, Manubala R, Deepak J. Comparative Studies on Anti-Inflammatory Activity of Coriandrum Sativum, Datura Stramonium and Azadirachta Indica. *Asian J Exp Biol Sci.* 2010;1(1):151-154.

100. Chandak R, Devdhe S, Changediya V. Evaluation of anti-histaminic activity of aqueous extract of ripe olives of olea-europea. *J Pharm Res.* 2009;2. http://jprsolutions.info/files/final-file-5691ddee522e91.46302541.pdf. Accessed September 17, 2018.

101. Persia FA, Mariani ML, Fogal TH, Penissi AB. Hydroxytyrosol and oleuropein of olive oil inhibit mast cell degranulation induced by immune and non-immune pathways. *Phytomedicine.* 2014;21(11):1400-1405. doi:10.1016/j.phymed.2014.05.010

102. Silva F V., Guimarães AG, Silva ERS, et al. Anti-Inflammatory and Anti-Ulcer Activities of Carvacrol, a Monoterpene Present in the Essential Oil of Oregano. *J Med Food.* 2012;15(11):984-991. doi:10.1089/jmf.2012.0102

103. Baser KHC. Chapter Four: The Turkish Origanum species. In: Kintzios SE, ed. *Oregano: The Genera Origanum and Lippia.* CRC Press; 2003:123-140. doi:10.1201/B12591-11

104. Grigoleit H-G, Grigoleit P. Pharmacology and preclinical pharmacokinetics of peppermint oil. *Phytomedicine.* 2005;12(8):612-616. doi:10.1016/j.phymed.2004.10.007

105. Inoue T, Sugimoto Y, Masuda H, Kamei C. Effects of peppermint (Mentha piperita L.) extracts on experimental allergic rhinitis in rats. *Biol Pharm Bull.* 2001;24(1):92-95. http://www.ncbi.nlm.nih.gov/pubmed/11201253. Accessed September 17, 2018.

106. Sharma SC, Sharma S, Gulati OP. Pycnogenol® inhibits the release of histamine from mast cells. *Phyther Res.* 2003;17(1):66-69. doi:10.1002/ptr.1240

107. Boskabady MH, Ghasemzadeh Rahbardar M, Nemati H, Esmaeilzadeh M. Inhibitory effect of Crocus sativus (saffron) on histamine (H1) receptors of guinea pig tracheal chains. *Pharmazie.* 2010;65(4):300-305. http://www.ncbi.nlm.nih.gov/pubmed/20432629. Accessed September 17, 2018.

108. Kang OH, Chae H-S, Choi J-H, et al. Effects of the Schisandra Fructus Water Extract on Cytokine Release from a Human Mast Cell Line. *J Med Food.* 2006;9(4):480-486. doi:10.1089/jmf.2006.9.480

109. Wilson L. Review of adaptogenic mechanisms: Eleuthrococcus senticosus, Panax ginseng, Rhodiola rosea, Schisandra chinensis and Withania somnifera. *Aust J Med Herbal.* 2007;19(3):126-138. https://search.informit.com.au/documentSummary;dn=406522201744304;res=IELHEA. Accessed September 16, 2018.

110. Kim HM, Lee EH, Cho HH, Moon YH. Inhibitory effect of mast cell-mediated immediate-type allergic reactions in rats by spirulina. *Biochem Pharmacol.* 1998;55(7):1071-1076. http://www.ncbi.nlm.nih.gov/pubmed/9605430. Accessed September 17, 2018.

111. Yang HN, Lee EH, Kim HM. Spirulina platensis inhibits anaphylactic reaction. *Life Sci.* 1997;61(13):1237-1244. http://www.ncbi.nlm.nih.gov/pubmed/9324065. Accessed January 26, 2019.

112. Eidi A, Oryan S, Zaringhalam J, Rad M. Antinociceptive and anti-inflammatory effects of the aerial parts of *Artemisia dracunculus* in mice. *Pharm Biol.* 2016;54(3):549-554. doi:10.3109/13880209.2015.1056312

113. Maham M, Moslemzadeh H, Jalilzadeh-Amin G. Antinociceptive effect of the essential oil of tarragon (Artemisia dracunculus). *Pharm Biol.* 2014;52(2):208-212. doi:10.3109/13880209.2013.824007

114. Russell N, Jennings S, Jennings B, et al. The Mastocytosis Society Survey on Mast Cell Disorders: Part 2- Patient Clinical Experiences and Beyond. *J allergy Clin Immunol Pract.* 2018;0(0). doi:10.1016/j.jaip.2018.07.032

115. Folkerts J, Stadhouders R, Redegeld FA, et al. Effect of Dietary Fiber and Metabolites on Mast Cell Activation and Mast Cell-Associated Diseases. *Front Immunol.* 2018;9:1067. doi:10.3389/fimmu.2018.01067

116. Snow R. "Mast Cell Activation Syndrome: ID, Explanation and Treatment" presented at the 27th Annual American Herbalists Guild Symposium, September 29 – October 2, 2016, Seven Springs, PA. Accessed February 19, 2018.
117. Turner H. Phone interview conducted on 7-13-18.
118. McIntosh K, Reed DE, Schneider T, et al. FODMAPs alter symptoms and the metabolome of patients with IBS: a randomised controlled trial. *Gut.* 2017;66(7):1241-1251. doi:10.1136/gutjnl-2015-311339

References Chapter 12: Holistic Healing

1. Sánchez-Borges M, Cardona V, Worm M, et al. In-flight allergic emergencies. *World Allergy Organ J.* 2017;10(1):15. doi:10.1186/s40413-017-0148-1
2. Chatterjea D, Martinov T. Mast cells: versatile gatekeepers of pain. *Mol Immunol.* 2015;63(1):38-44. doi:10.1016/j.molimm.2014.03.001
3. Noto H, Goto A, Tsujimoto T, Noda M. Low-carbohydrate diets and all-cause mortality: a systematic review and meta-analysis of observational studies. *PLoS One.* 2013;8(1):e55030. doi:10.1371/journal.pone.0055030
4. Kosinski C, Jornayvaz F, Kosinski C, Jornayvaz FR. Effects of Ketogenic Diets on Cardiovascular Risk Factors: Evidence from Animal and Human Studies. *Nutrients.* 2017;9(5):517. doi:10.3390/nu9050517
5. Harvey CJ, Schofield GM, Williden M, McQuillan JA. The Effect of Medium Chain Triglycerides on Time to Nutritional Ketosis and Symptoms of Keto-Induction in Healthy Adults: A Randomised Controlled Clinical Trial. *J Nutr Metab.* 2018;2018:1-9. doi:10.1155/2018/2630565
6. Zhang H, Tsao R. Dietary polyphenols, oxidative stress and antioxidant and anti-inflammatory effects. *Curr Opin Food Sci.* 2016;8:33-42. doi:10.1016/J.COFS.2016.02.002
7. Pizzorno J. *The Toxin Solution: How Hidden Poisons in the Air, Water, Food and Products We Use Are Destroying Our Health.* Harper Collins; 2017.
8. White GE, Wells GD. Cold-water immersion and other forms of cryotherapy: physiological changes potentially affecting recovery from high-intensity exercise. *Extrem Physiol Med.* 2013;2(1):26. doi:10.1186/2046-7648-2-26
9. Bleakley CM, Davison GW. What is the biochemical and physiological rationale for using cold-water immersion in sports recovery? A systematic review. *Br J Sports Med.* 2010;44(3):179-187. doi:10.1136/bjsm.2009.065565
10. Martel C, Belanger A, Luo X, Trescases-Thorin N, Thorin E. Intermittent Fasting with a High Fat Diet Reveals the Contribution of Mitochondrial Free Radicals to the Endothelium-Dependent Relaxation of Mouse Aorta. *FASEB J.* 2015;29(1):642-645. https://www.fasebj.org/doi/abs/10.1096/fasebj.29.1_supplement.642.5. Accessed September 19, 2018.
11. Pinarbasi A, Aksungar FB, Arslan DO, et al. SUN-P001: Metabolic and Mitochondrial Changes in an Intermittent Fasting Model in Humans. *Clin Nutr.* 2017;36:S53. doi:10.1016/S0261-5614(17)30624-6
12. Wegman MP, Guo MH, Bennion DM, et al. Practicality of Intermittent Fasting in Humans and its Effect on Oxidative Stress and Genes Related to Aging and Metabolism. *Rejuvenation Res.* 2015;18(2):162-172. doi:10.1089/rej.2014.1624
13. Choi IY, Piccio L, Childress P, et al. A Diet Mimicking Fasting Promotes Regeneration and Reduces Autoimmunity and Multiple Sclerosis Symptoms. *Cell Rep.* 2016;15(10):2136-2146. doi:10.1016/j.celrep.2016.05.009
14. Kulinski JM, Metcalfe DD, Young ML, et al. Elevation in histamine and tryptase following exercise in patients with mastocytosis. *J allergy Clin Immunol Pract.* 2018;0(0). doi:10.1016/j.jaip.2018.07.008
15. Afrin L. In-person interview conducted in St. Cloud, Minnesota on 9-16-17.
16. Peterson MR, Coop CA. Long-term omalizumab use in the treatment of exercise-induced anaphylaxis. *Allergy Rhinol.* 2017;8(3):170-172. doi:10.2500/ar.2017.8.0204
17. Eggleston PA, Kagey-Sobotka A, Proud D, Adkinson NF, Lichtenstein LM. Disassociation of the Release of Histamine and Arachidonic Acid Metabolites from Osmotically Activated Basophils and Human Lung Mast Cells. *Am Rev Respir Dis.* 1990;141(4_pt_1):960-964. doi:10.1164/ajrccm/141.4_Pt_1.960
18. Thong BY-H. Prevention of Anaphylaxis Based on Risk Factors and Cofactors. *Curr Treat Options Allergy.* 2016;3(3):212-223. doi:10.1007/s40521-016-0095-z
19. Feldweg AM. Food-Dependent, Exercise-Induced Anaphylaxis: Diagnosis and Management in the Outpatient Setting. *J Allergy Clin Immunol Pract.* 2017;5(2):283-288. doi:10.1016/j.jaip.2016.11.022
20. Kobernick AK, Jerath MR. Exercise-Induced Anaphylaxis Successfully Treated with Hydroxychloroquine. *J Allergy Clin Immunol.* 2016;137(2):AB49. doi:10.1016/j.jaci.2015.12.163
21. Barg W, Medrala W, Wolanczyk-Medrala A. Exercise-induced anaphylaxis: an update on diagnosis and treatment. *Curr Allergy Asthma Rep.* 2011;11(1):45-51. doi:10.1007/s11882-010-0150-y
22. Geller M. Diagnostic and Therapeutic Approach in Patients with Exercise-Induced Anaphylaxis. *Curr Treat Options Allergy.* 2016;3(2):181-188. doi:10.1007/s40521-016-0083-3
23. Shimizu T, Tokuda Y. Exercise-induced anaphylaxis. *BMJ Case Rep.* 2012;2012. doi:10.1136/bcr.01.2012.5671

24. Oropeza AR, Bindslev-Jensen C, Broesby-Olsen S, et al. Patterns of anaphylaxis after diagnostic workup: A follow-up study of 226 patients with suspected anaphylaxis. *Allergy*. 2017;72(12):1944-1952. doi:10.1111/all.13207

25. Mostmans Y, Blykers M, Mols P, Gutermuth J, Grosber M, Naeije N. Anaphylaxis in an urban Belgian emergency department: epidemiology and aetiology. *Acta Clin Belg*. 2016;71(2):99-106. doi:10.1179/2295333715Y.0000000060

26. Seneviratne SL, Maitland A, Afrin L. Mast cell disorders in Ehlers–Danlos syndrome. *Am J Med Genet Part C Semin Med Genet*. 2017;175(1):226-236. doi:10.1002/ajmg.c.31555

27. Horowitz R. *How Can I Get Better? An Action Plan for Treating Resistant Lyme and Chronic Disease*. New York, NY: St. Martin's Griffin; 2017.

28. Hamilton M. Phone interview conducted on 6-22-18.

29. American Heart Association. American Heart Association Recommendations for Physical Activity in Adults. https://www.heart.org/en/healthy-living/fitness/fitness-basics/aha-recs-for-physical-activity-in-adults#.WpHn8ainHIU. Accessed September 19, 2018.

30. Abera Tessema T. Significance of yoga in modern life. *Int J Yoga, Physiother Phys Educ*. 2017;2(5):123-125. http://www.sivanandadlshq.org/. Accessed September 19, 2018.

31. Vempati R, Bijlani RL, Deepak KK. The efficacy of a comprehensive lifestyle modification programme based on yoga in the management of bronchial asthma: a randomized controlled trial. *BMC Pulm Med*. 2009;9:37. doi:10.1186/1471-2466-9-37

32. Ifeoma OJ, Uchenna CU, Chukwuemeka EO. Effects of Yoga in Health and Aging: A Knowledge-Based Descriptive Study of Health Educators in Universities of Nigeria. *Am J Educ Res*. 2017;5(4):443-452. doi:10.12691/education-5-4-14

33. Tripathi S, Sharma P, Singh A, Sharma A. Ayurveda and Yoga Therapy for Allergy and Asthma. In: Vedanthan P, Nelson H, Agashe S, Mahesh P, eds. *Textbook of Allergy for the Clinician*. CRC Press; 2014:421. https://books.google.com/books?hl=en&lr=&id=X3vSBQAAQBAJ&oi=fnd&pg=PA421&ots=MP0hPZYeF7&sig=0at-ObPqHVan6DLOOnYe3ZWjypU#v=onepage&q&f=false. Accessed September 19, 2018.

34. Uno Y. Irritable bowel syndrome-how a low-FODMAP diet or yoga might help. *Aliment Pharmacol Ther*. 2018;47(3):444-445. doi:10.1111/apt.14433

35. Alikiani Z, Toloee ME, Jafari AK. The effects of Pilates exercise and caraway supplementation on the levels of prostaglandin E2 and perception dysmenorrhea in adolescent girls non-athlete. *Asian Exerc Sport Sci J*. 2017;1(1):11-16. http://journal.aesasport.com/index.php/aesa/article/view/11. Accessed September 19, 2018.

36. Ramos JS, Dalleck LC, Tjonna AE, Beetham KS, Coombes JS. The Impact of High-Intensity Interval Training Versus Moderate-Intensity Continuous Training on Vascular Function: a Systematic Review and Meta-Analysis. *Sport Med*. 2015;45(5):679-692. doi:10.1007/s40279-015-0321-z

37. Milanović Z, Sporiš G, Weston M. Effectiveness of High-Intensity Interval Training (HIT) and Continuous Endurance Training for VO2max Improvements: A Systematic Review and Meta-Analysis of Controlled Trials. *Sport Med*. 2015;45(10):1469-1481. doi:10.1007/s40279-015-0365-0

38. Pearson SJ, Hussain SR. A Review on the Mechanisms of Blood-Flow Restriction Resistance Training-Induced Muscle Hypertrophy. *Sport Med*. 2015;45(2):187-200. doi:10.1007/s40279-014-0264-9

39. Alyousif ZA. *The Effects of High Intensity Interval Training (HIIT) on Asthmatic Adult Males*.; 2014. http://utdr.utoledo.edu/theses-dissertations/1751. Accessed September 19, 2018.

40. Romero SA, McCord JL, Ely MR, et al. Mast cell degranulation and de novo histamine formation contribute to sustained postexercise vasodilation in humans. *J Appl Physiol*. 2017;122(3):603-610. doi:10.1152/japplphysiol.00633.2016

41. Schott C, Fozard J. Chapter 8: Hypotension and Shock. In: Murugan R, Darby J, eds. *Rapid Response System: A Practical Guide*. Oxford University Press; 2018:80. https://books.google.com/books?hl=en&lr=&id=DLNSDwAAQBAJ&oi=fnd&pg=PA75&dq=histamine+and+hypotension&ots=wTMCxIcDua&sig=B56FOm-887sYuhQPMwVqnzLQRwE#v=onepage&q&f=false. Accessed September 18, 2018.

42. Luttrell MJ, Halliwill JR. The Intriguing Role of Histamine in Exercise Responses. *Exerc Sport Sci Rev*. 2017;45(1):16-23. doi:10.1249/JES.0000000000000093

43. Buck TM, Romero SA, Ely MR, Sieck DC, Abdala PM, Halliwill JR. Neurovascular control following small muscle-mass exercise in humans. *Physiol Rep*. 2015;3(2):e12289. doi:10.14814/phy2.12289

44. Phungphong S, Kijtawornrat A, Wattanapermpool J, Bupha-Intr T. Regular exercise modulates cardiac mast cell activation in ovariectomized rats. *J Physiol Sci*. 2016;66(2):165-173. doi:10.1007/s12576-015-0409-0

45. Emhoff C-AW, Barrett-O'Keefe Z, Padgett RC, Hawn JA, Halliwill JR. Histamine-receptor blockade reduces blood flow but not muscle glucose uptake during postexercise recovery in humans. *Exp Physiol*. 2011;96(7):664-673. doi:10.1113/expphysiol.2010.056150

46. Ely MR, Romero SA, Sieck DC, Mangum JE, Luttrell MJ, Halliwill JR. A single dose of histamine-receptor antagonists before downhill running alters markers of muscle damage and delayed-onset muscle soreness. *J Appl Physiol*. 2017;122(3):631-641. doi:10.1152/japplphysiol.00518.2016

526

47. Halliwill JR, Buck TM, Lacewell AN, Romero SA. Postexercise hypotension and sustained postexercise vasodilatation: what happens after we exercise? *Exp Physiol*. 2013;98(1):7-18. doi:10.1113/expphysiol.2011.058065

48. Mccord JL, Pellinger TK, Lynn BM, Halliwill JR. Potential Benefit from an H1-Receptor Antagonist on Postexercise Syncope in the Heat. *Med Sci Sport Exerc*. 2008;40(11):1953-1961. doi:10.1249/MSS.0b013e31817f1970

49. Pal GK, Velkumary S, Madanmohan. Effect of short-term practice of breathing exercises on autonomic functions in normal human volunteers. *Indian J Med Res*. 2004;120(2):115-121. http://www.ncbi.nlm.nih.gov/pubmed/15347862. Accessed September 19, 2018.

50. Jerath R, Crawford MW, Barnes VA, Harden K. Self-Regulation of Breathing as a Primary Treatment for Anxiety. *Appl Psychophysiol Biofeedback*. 2015;40(2):107-115. doi:10.1007/s10484-015-9279-8

51. Goldstein LA, Mehling WE, Metzler TJ, et al. Veterans Group Exercise: A randomized pilot trial of an Integrative Exercise program for veterans with posttraumatic stress. *J Affect Disord*. 2018;227:345-352. doi:10.1016/j.jad.2017.11.002

52. Rehmeyer J. *Through the Shadowlands: A Science Writer's Odyssey into an Illness Science Doesn't Understand*. Rodale; 2017.

53. Smith T. Craniobiotic Technique. http://www.craniobiotic.com. Accessed September 19, 2018.

54. NMT Seminars. Introduction to Neuromodulation Technique. https://www.nmt.md/p/introduction-to-nmt. Accessed October 6, 2018.

55. Meglathery S. Chapter 7: Validating the Patient. In: Driscoll D, De A, Doherty C, Ferreira JP, Meglathery S PJ, ed. *The Driscoll Theory Newly Revised: The Cause of POTS in Ehlers-Danlos Syndrome and How to Reverse the Process*. Warnick Publishing; 2015.

56. Abrams D, His Holiness the Dalai Lama, Archbishop Desmond Tutu. *The Book of Joy: Lasting Happiness in a Changing World*. Avery Publishing; 2016.

57. Gauthier T, Meyer RML, Grefe D, Gold JI. An On-the-Job Mindfulness-based Intervention For Pediatric ICU Nurses: A Pilot. *J Pediatr Nurs*. 2015;30(2):402-409. doi:10.1016/j.pedn.2014.10.005

58. Alevizos M, Karagkouni A, Panagiotidou S, Vasiadi M, Theoharides TC. Stress triggers coronary mast cells leading to cardiac events. *Ann Allergy Asthma Immunol*. 2014;112(4):309-316. doi:10.1016/j.anai.2013.09.017

59. Goyal M, Singh S, Sibinga EMS, et al. Meditation programs for psychological stress and well-being: a systematic review and meta-analysis. *JAMA Intern Med*. 2014;174(3):357-368. doi:10.1001/jamainternmed.2013.13018

60. Faurot K (Kim) R, Gaylord S, Palsson OS, Garland EL, Mann JD, Whitehead WE. 715 Mindfulness Meditation Has Long-Term Therapeutic Benefits in Women With Irritable Bowel Syndrome (IBS): Follow-Up Results From a Randomized Controlled Trial. *Gastroenterology*. 2014;146(5):S-124. doi:10.1016/S0016-5085(14)60447-9

61. Househam AM, Peterson CT, Mills PJ, Chopra D. The Effects of Stress and Meditation on the Immune System, Human Microbiota, and Epigenetics. *Adv Mind Body Med*. 31(4):10-25. http://www.ncbi.nlm.nih.gov/pubmed/29306937. Accessed September 19, 2018.

62. Oschman JL, Chevalier G, Ober AC. Chapter 38: Biophysics of Earthing (Grounding) the Human Body. In: Rosch P, ed. *Bioelectromagnetic and Subtle Energy Medicine, 2nd Edition*. 2014:427-456.

63. Sung H-C, Lee W-L, Li H-M, et al. Familiar Music Listening with Binaural Beats for Older People with Depressive Symptoms in Retirement Homes. *Neuropsychiatry (London)*. 2017;7(4):347-353. doi:10.4172/Neuropsychiatry.1000221

64. Colzato LS, Barone H, Sellaro R, Hommel B. More attentional focusing through binaural beats: evidence from the global-local task. *Psychol Res*. 2017;81(1):271-277. doi:10.1007/s00426-015-0727-0

65. Isik BK, Esen A, Büyükerkmen B, Kilinç A, Menziletoglu D. Effectiveness of binaural beats in reducing preoperative dental anxiety. *Br J Oral Maxillofac Surg*. 2017;55(6):571-574. doi:10.1016/j.bjoms.2017.02.014

66. Wilkins L. The Research on Prayer and Healing: Past, Present and Future Challenges. *Baylor BEARdocs*. May 2015. https://baylor-ir.tdl.org/baylor-ir/handle/2104/9453. Accessed September 19, 2018.

67. Hiari T. A Thinking Patient: Twilah Hiari's Reflections on Diagnosis, Disability and Culture. www.athinkingpatient.com. Accessed September 19, 2018.

68. Super T's Mast Cell Foundation. https://supermastcell.org/. Accessed September 19, 2018.

69. Weinstock LB, Brook JB, Myers TL, Goodman B. Successful treatment of postural orthostatic tachycardia and mast cell activation syndromes using naltrexone, immunoglobulin and antibiotic treatment. *BMJ Case Rep*. 2018;2018. doi:10.1136/bcr-2017-221405

70. Bonamichi-Santos R, Yoshimi-Kanamori K, Giavina-Bianchi P, Aun MV. Association of Postural Tachycardia Syndrome and Ehlers-Danlos Syndrome with Mast Cell Activation Disorders. *Immunol Allergy Clin North Am*. 2018;38(3):497-504. doi:10.1016/j.iac.2018.04.004

71. Hamilton MJ. Nonclonal Mast Cell Activation Syndrome: A Growing Body of Evidence. *Immunol Allergy Clin North Am*. 2018;38(3):469-481. doi:10.1016/j.iac.2018.04.002

72. Russell N, Jennings S, Jennings B, et al. The Mastocytosis Society Survey on Mast Cell Disorders: Part 2- Patient Clinical Experiences and Beyond. *J allergy Clin Immunol Pract*. 2018. doi:10.1016/j.jaip.2018.07.032

73. González-de-Olano D, Domínguez-Ortega J, Sánchez-García S. Mast Cell Activation Syndromes and Environmental Exposures. *Curr Treat Options Allergy*. 2018;5(1):41-51. doi:10.1007/s40521-018-0151-y

74. Rastogi V, Singh D, Mazza JJ, Parajuli D, Yale SH. Flushing Disorders Associated with Gastrointestinal Symptoms: Part 1, Neuroendocrine Tumors, Mast Cell Disorders and Hyperbasophila. *Clin Med Res*. 2018;16(1-2):16-28. doi:10.3121/cmr.2017.1379a

75. Roizen G, Peruffo C, Maitland AL. Mast Cell Activation Disorders In The Setting Of Idiopathic CD4 Lymphopenia. *J Allergy Clin Immunol*. 2018;141(2):AB23. doi:10.1016/J.JACI.2017.12.072

76. Carter MC, Desai A, Komarow HD, et al. A distinct biomolecular profile identifies monoclonal mast cell disorders in patients with idiopathic anaphylaxis. doi:10.1016/j.jaci.2017.05.036

77. Daens S, Grossin D, Hermanns-Lê T, Peeters D, Manicourt D. Severe Mast Cell Activation Syndrome in a 15-year-old patient with hypermobile Ehlers-Danlos syndrome. *Rev Med Liege*. 2018;73(2):61-64. http://www.ncbi.nlm.nih.gov/pubmed/29517867. Accessed September 19, 2018.

78. Kumaraswami S, Farkas G. Management of a Parturient with Mast Cell Activation Syndrome: An Anesthesiologist's Experience. *Case Rep Anesthesiol*. 2018;2018:1-5. doi:10.1155/2018/8920921

79. Broesby-Olsen S, Carter M, Kjaer HF, et al. Pediatric Expression of Mast Cell Activation Disorders. *Immunol Allergy Clin North Am*. 2018;38(3):365-377. doi:10.1016/J.IAC.2018.04.009

80. Blanco D, Ruiz Sancho V, Barranco R, Fernández C, Bobolea I. Hipersensibilidad a antiinflamatorios no esteroideos, alergia a alimentos y síndrome de activación mastocitaria: relevancia del estudio alergológico completo y breve revisión del tema, a propósito de 2 casos. *Med Fam Semer*. September 2018. doi:10.1016/j.semerg.2018.04.006

81. Doherty TA, White AA. Postural orthostatic tachycardia syndrome and the potential role of mast cell activation. *Auton Neurosci*. May 2018. doi:10.1016/J.AUTNEU.2018.05.001

82. Chen M, Kim A, Zuraw B, Doherty TA, Christiansen S. Mast cell disorders. *Ann Allergy, Asthma Immunol*. 2018;121(1):128-130. doi:10.1016/j.anai.2018.03.027

83. Kesterson K, Nahmias Z, Brestoff JR, Bodet ND, Kau A, Kim BS. Generalized pruritus relieved by NSAIDs in the setting of mast cell activation syndrome. *J Allergy Clin Immunol Pract*. March 2018. doi:10.1016/j.jaip.2018.03.002

84. Bay JL, Sedarsky KE, Petersen MM. A case of neuropathic pain in monoclonal mast cell activation syndrome. *Ann Allergy, Asthma Immunol*. 2018;120(5):543-544. doi:10.1016/j.anai.2018.02.019

85. Ravi A, Meeusen J, Divekar R, Donato L, Hartz MF, Butterfield JH. Pediatric Mast Cell Activation Syndrome. *J Allergy Clin Immunol*. 2018;141(2):AB275. doi:10.1016/j.jaci.2017.12.876

86. Weiler CR, Alhurani RE, Butterfield JH, Divekar R. Systemic Mastocytosis (SM) and Mast Cell Activation Syndrome (MCAS); How Do They Differ? *J Allergy Clin Immunol*. 2018;141(2):AB275. doi:10.1016/j.jaci.2017.12.875

87. Casassa EA, Mailhol C, Tournier E, et al. Mast cell activation syndrome: High frequency of skin manifestations and anaphylactic shock. *Allergol Int*. 2018;0(0). doi:10.1016/j.alit.2018.07.003

88. Molderings GJ, Knüchel-Clarke R, Hertfelder H-J, Kuhl C. Mast Cell Activation Syndrome Mimicking Breast Cancer: Case Report With Pathophysiologic Considerations. *Clin Breast Cancer*. 2018;18(3):e271-e276. doi:10.1016/j.clbc.2017.12.004

89. Haenisch B, Molderings G. White matter abnormalities are also repeatedly present in patients with systemic mast cell activation syndrome. *Transl Psychiatry*. 2018;8(1):95. doi:10.1038/s41398-018-0143-5

90. Rechenauer T, Raithel M, Götze T, et al. Idiopathic Mast Cell Activation Syndrome With Associated Salicylate Intolerance. *Front Pediatr*. 2018;6:73. doi:10.3389/fped.2018.00073

91. Arndt KK, Viswanathan RK, Mathur SK. Clinical Characteristics of Patients in Allergy Clinic with Presumed Diagnosis of Mast Cell Activation Syndrome (MCAS). *J Allergy Clin Immunol*. 2018;141(2):AB50. doi:10.1016/J.JACI.2017.12.162

92. Valent P, Akin C, Bonadonna P, et al. Mast cell activation syndrome: Importance of consensus criteria and call for research. *J Allergy Clin Immunol*. 2018;142(3):1008-1010. doi:10.1016/j.jaci.2018.06.004

93. Sincero J. *You Are a Badass®: How to Stop Doubting Your Greatness and Start Living an Awesome Life*. Running Press; 2013.